This book is dedicated to Helen and to Fiona,
without whose indulgence and understanding
tolerance it could not have been completed.

CONTENTS

FOREWORD

The third edition of *Pathology for Surgeons in Training* indicates that the unusual format of this book has found a real niche in the ever expanding surgical literature available to young surgeons. That it is specifically directed to this group of doctors is important because they are faced with a wide range of pressures in their professional lives and yet have to find the time and the stimulus to acquire knowledge rapidly. This format with its focus specifically on the knowledge required for surgical examinations set by the Royal Colleges, provides a most useful learning and reference foundation. The previous editions of this book enjoyed considerable success and there is no doubt the new and revised addition which has been brought thoroughly up to date but has maintained the original style, will be equally well received.

Pathology is the foundation stone of surgical knowledge for clinical application. All subjects are extensively cross-referenced but also include where appropriate historical notes and suggestions for further reading which are most useful. The student is provided with the base knowledge and the opportunity to extend this as interest or necessity dictates. The very fact that the volume does not need to be read from cover to cover but acts much more as an anthology of Pathology only adds to its usefulness. The text is clear, well laid out and the knowledge contained is accurate.

I commend *Pathology for Surgeons in Training* not only to young surgeons but to established teachers, trainers and examiners as a certain way to ensure that they also keep their knowledge base up to date. Passing examinations is a means to an end but this revision text should not be considered simply as an examination crammer. It serves a much wider, more useful and longer lasting function.

Professor J G Temple
President, Royal College
of Surgeons of Edinburgh

PREFACE

Candidates preparing for the examinations for the diplomas of MRCS or AFRCS often feel a need for a compact guide allowing quick and highly selective revision of Pathology. The present volume is intended to meet this requirement. The subjects chosen include not only classical **Surgical Pathology** but a substantial component of **Microbiology**, **Haematology, Immunology, Clinical Chemistry** and **Blood Transfusion** as well as brief notes on such issues as **Audit, Computers, Imaging** and **Telepathology**.

This is not a textbook nor should it be read from cover-to-cover. The book has been prepared as an **A to Z guide** to the knowledge demanded by College examiners. It is planned so that postgraduate students can approach their chosen topics easily. To meet these aims, the contents, based on the syllabuses issued by the four surgical Colleges of Great Britain and Eire, are assembled for rapid, selective reference.

There is extensive **Cross-referencing** so that a candidate, wishing to revise Ischaemia, for example, is advised also to read Anoxia, Gangrene and Necrosis while an examinee, seeking rapid help with Cancer of the Colon, is referred to Carcinogenesis, Cancer Genetics and Tumours. For the same reasons, there is a comprehensive **Index**, arranged so that the major topics are clearly distinguished from those that have been given only incidental mention.

A difficulty that all recent surgical texts face is how to deal with the advances taking place in **Molecular Biology, Immunology** and **Genetics** and other subjects dominated by highly specialised techniques, a problem compounded by the jargon used by experts in these subjects. Here, we have compromised. All surgeons in training require to know that a susceptibility to colon and breast cancer, retinoblastoma and Wilms' tumour, chronic myelocytic leukaemia and xeroderma pigmentosa, may be inherited. They may be interested in the frequency of the heritable defects, the mode of inheritance and the chromosomal abnormalities that underlie some cancers. They cannot be expected to know the exact location and designation of the mutant gene loci associated with these tumours or even the number and location of any chromosomal defect.

The text includes **56 Tables**. Further summary Tables of normal haematological and chemical values are appended. There are **58 explanatory Diagrams** selected to illuminate points of importance and difficulty. The relevance of **History** to contemporary surgical practice may be denied but the authors believe that short comments on the founding fathers of Surgery and related subjects, add interest and assist candidates to place examination topics in context. Brief biographies of pioneers whose names are quoted in the text are therefore retained. No modern work can fail to take proper account of the impact made by the **Internet**. Consequently, a short note is included indicating how additional information can be obtained from **Web sites**.

D. L. Gardner
D. E. F. Tweedle
January 2002

ACKNOWLEDGEMENTS

We owe a particular debt to Mr P. K. Datta FRCSEd, Consultant Surgeon, Caithness General Hospital, whose long experience as an Examiner for the Royal College of Surgeons of Edinburgh has proved invaluable in designing this Edition, and to Dr. Stephanie J. Dancer FRCPath, Department of Laboratory Medicine, Vale of Leven District General Hospital, whose advice and guidance in this, as in the previous Edition, has enabled us to deal with the complex problems of Clinical Microbiology.

Our colleagues, Professor T.J. Anderson FRCPath., Western General Hospital, Edinburgh (Breast cancer); Mr A. Bleetman FRCSEd., Birmingham Heartlands Hospital (Accident and Emergency Surgery); Dr Jan Cullingworth, Ph.D. University of Edinburgh (Carcinogenesis); Mr. I D Gardner FRCS., Derbyshire Royal Infirmary (Surgery); Dr T Hewson PhD, University of Edinburgh (Immunology); Dr S. J. Howell MRCP, Christie Hospital, Manchester (Cancer studies); Dr. A. S. Krajewski FRCPath, Northampton General Hospital (Immunology); Dr A. M. Lessells, FRCPath, Western General Hospital, Edinburgh (Biopsy diagnosis); Dr D. F. Martin FRCP, University Hospital of South Manchester (Imaging); Mr. R. K. Tandon FRCSEd, Royal Wolverhampton Hospital (Orthopaedics); Professor W. A. Wallace, FRCSEd., Department of Orthopaedic Surgery, University of Nottingham (Internet), have given unstintingly of their time and energy in ensuring the accuracy of the text.

We acknowledge the expert advice of the Departments of Haematology and of Clinical Biochemistry (Dr S. W. Walker) of the Royal Infirmary, Edinburgh, and the guidance of the staff of the Scottish Blood Transfusion Service. We express our thanks to Mr I. Lennox, MMAA, formerly of the Department of Medical Illustration of the University of Edinburgh, who prepared the drawings with his customary skill and understanding, and to Mrs S. Jones M A of the Royal College of Surgeons of Edinburgh whose critical help with the manuscript has proved indispensable.

HOW TO USE THIS BOOK

THIS IS AN A TO Z REVISION TEXT FOR EXAMINATION CANDIDATES

IT IS FOR SIMPLE, QUICK REFERENCE, NOT FOR SYSTEMATIC READING

Using the **A to Z headings** and the **Index**, select the topic you want to revise, e.g. **Embolism**

READ IT

Then follow the guides to related topics. They are shown at right of column margins in the form:

Now read Coagulation (p. 95), Thrombus (p. 320)

READ THEM

Persuade your friends to ask you questions from the book.

Check the **Tables** e.g. for evaluation of coagulation factors prior to surgery.

Check the **Appendix.**

Read the snapshot **Biographies** when a name is given in the text. Learning about the history of a topic helps you to remember it.

When you have exhausted what this book tells you about a topic, look at the **Further Reading** list. It will guide you to larger references on the subject.

Search the **Web sites** recommended by your Internet tutor.

A

ABSCESS

An abscess is a localised collection of pus. Diseases dominated by abscess formation are suppurative.

Causes

There is a wide range of causes. They include physical and chemical injury, irritation and infection. The necrotic tissue of malignant tumours may resemble an abscess. Infection may be direct, indirect or blood-borne. Foreign bodies provoke abscess formation and stitch abscesses appear within the tracks of sutures. Abscesses form in infected surgical wounds and at sites of injuries that penetrate skin or other lining epithelia.

Infective agents

Every variety of extracellular, infective micro-organism may cause abscess. Cutaneous abscesses are usually due to *Staphylococcus aureus*. Intra-abdominal abscesses are initiated by gastro-intestinal commensals such as *Klebsiella pneumoniae*, *Escherichia coli*, Enterobacter spp., Bacterioides spp., Proteus spp., Clostridia spp., *Streptococcus intermedius* group and *Enterococcus faecalis*. Aerobic micro-organisms thrive at abscess margins but anaerobes such as *Actinomyces israelii* and micro-aerophilic organisms proliferate centrally. 'Cold' abscesses are caused by *Mycobacterium tuberculosis*: necrotic material accumulates without signs of acute inflammation. Abscesses attributable to protozoa, metazoa (worms) and fungi are described on pp. 282, 356 and 135, respectively.

Now read Bacteria (p. 30)

Structure

Abscesses form when persistent inflammation results in the accumulation of cell and tissue debris. An inflammatory exudate includes many dead and some living polymorphs but, occasionally, macrophages predominate. The causative micro-organisms, parasites or foreign bodies can often be recognised within the pus. Some may survive inside or outside phagocytic cells (p. 225, 270) in spite of antibiotic treatment.

The contents of an abscess may be fluid, semi-fluid, caseous or granular. The appearances are much influenced by the nature of the causal organism. Tuberculous pus, for example, appears like cream cheese and is caseous. Amoebic pus resembles orange–brown anchovy sauce. Staphylococcal pus is yellow, thick and viscous. Haemolytic streptococcal pus is thin, watery and blood-stained while the pus in *Pseudomonas aeruginosa* infections is green. Pus resulting from anaerobic infection is thin and often foul-smelling.

Pyogenic abscesses are common in the skin, subcutaneous tissues, mouth, peritoneal cavity and anorectal tissues. Perinephric, pelvic and subphrenic abscesses are also frequent. Those that derive from blood-borne infection are most frequent in the brain (p. 63), liver (p. 210), lung (p. 217) and bone (p. 54). Less commonly, abscesses develop in the pancreas and fallopian tubes.

Behaviour

Abscesses swell as the large molecules liberated by tissue destruction attract water by osmosis. Extension of the lesion, continued irritation and the persistence of infection contribute to the disorganisation and death of increasing numbers of cells. Their proteins are denatured. Overlying tissue dies. Abscesses 'point' and rupture through epithelial surfaces. Without this escape or effective surgical treatment, they resolve slowly. Granulation tissue forms a surrounding, pyogenic membrane. Finally, fibrosis leads to encapsulation and even to dystrophic calcification.

ACQUIRED IMMUNODEFICIENCY SYNDROME (AIDS)

AIDS (Acquired ImmunoDeficiency Syndrome) is a generalised disorder of immunity. It is caused by a human immunodeficiency virus (HIV).

The syndrome of AIDS is a growing, worldwide, health problem. The greatest number of cases is encountered in Africa. Here, more than 25% of some populations is infected. In South Africa, where there are 4×10^6 cases, the incidence of new cases is ~1600/day.

Causes

The HIV are retroviruses that infect the lymphocytes, macrophages and monocytes of body fluids. In North America, Europe and sub-Saharan and Central Africa the agent is HIV-1. In West Africa, a second strain, HIV-2, is found. Helper T lymphocytes (p. 173) are destroyed. The loss of these T-cells accounts for most features of the syndrome. Macrophages and monocytes remain virus reservoirs and HIV binds to the cells of the intestinal tract and central nervous system.

Now read Retroviruses (p. 350)

Transmission

The human immunodeficiency viruses are transmitted by venereal contact or parenterally, before or after birth. In Western countries, the infection is common among homosexual adults and intravenous drug abusers; in Africa, Latin America and the Caribbean, heterosexual adults and infants are implicated; in Asia, India, Eastern Europe and the Pacific rim, heterosexual and homosexual adults and drug abusers are the common targets.

- **Venereal infection**. This mode of transmission is principally by anal intercourse among homosexual and bisexual adults; the virus is conveyed in seminal lymphocytes. Heterosexual infection is becoming more frequent in Europe as are other sexually related diseases.
- **Parenteral infection**. This mode of transmission is commonplace in addicts who inject drugs intravenously. It may also afflict haemophiliacs given factor VIII from contaminated, pooled plasma. Prevention is complicated. Antibody tests occasionally yield false-negative results because of delay in antibody formation, so-called 'seroconversion'. Occupational exposure rarely leads to infection in doctors, dentists and other health workers (p. 159).
- **Transplacental infection**. Intra-uterine infection of the fetus may occur.
- **Neonatal infection**. Blood, amniotic fluid and breast milk convey the virus. Maternal IgM antibodies cross the placenta so that serological tests in the neonate are ambiguous.

Immunological changes

Cell-mediated

Failure of cell-mediated immunity caused by the destruction of T-helper (Th) lymphocytes is the key to understanding AIDS.

Now read Immunity (p. 171), Lymphocytes (p. 206)

HI virus envelopes bind to lymphocyte surface receptors, allowing virus particles to enter the cells (Figs 1 and 56). Within the lymphocytes, a viral enzyme, reverse transcriptase, writes ('transcribes') viral RNA onto lymphocyte DNA, conveying information about the structure of the virus to the host. The altered host DNA is integrated into the lymphocyte genome. However, HIV may remain in infected lymphocytes, unintegrated and dormant. When these cells are activated, often by coincidental infections such as cytomegalovirus (CMV), hepatitis B virus (HBV), Epstein–Barr virus (EBV) or a herpes virus, HIV replicates and kills them.

As AIDS progresses, there is a therefore a fall in the number of CD4 lymphocytes. As a result, T-cells no longer proliferate in response to other bacterial and viral antigens and cell-mediated immune reactions are progressively impaired. Diminished natural killer (NK) cell activity (p. 231) is also observed.

Antibody-mediated

In response to HIV, all infected persons form anti-HIV antibodies (p. 19). The antibodies may appear within days of exposure to the virus but the response can be delayed for as long as 6 months. Antibodies are against the HIV envelope glycoprotein that provokes polyclonal B-cell activity. Detecting anti-HIV

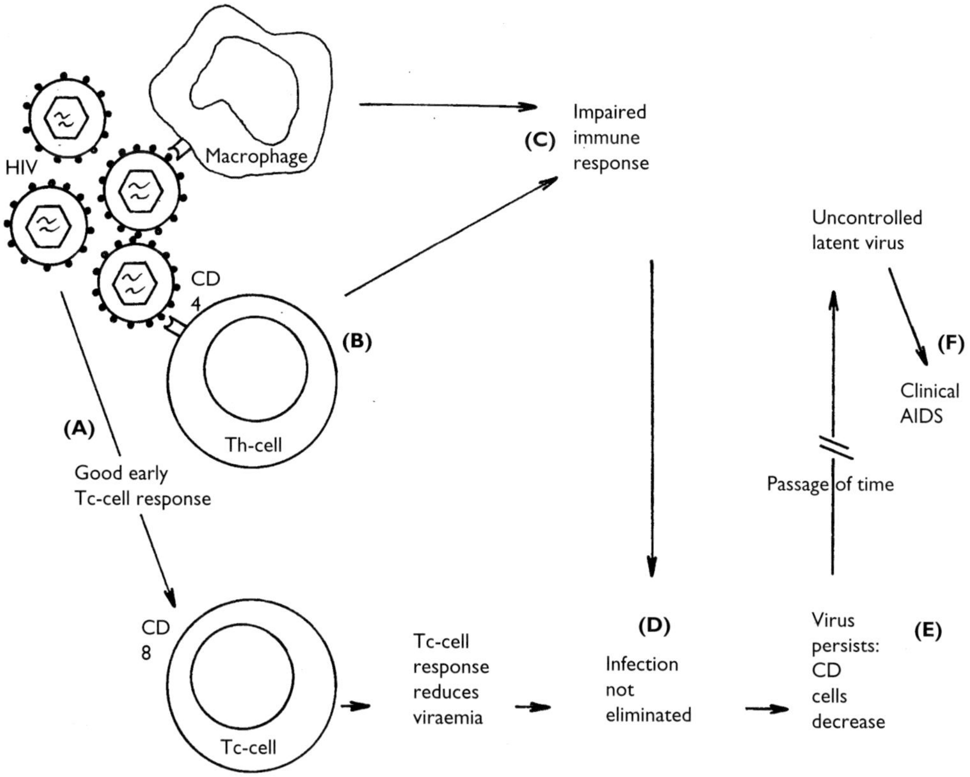

Figure 1 Pathogenesis of Acquired Immunodeficiency Syndrome (AIDS).
(A) CD8 T cytotoxic/cytolytic lymphocytes (Tc-cells) respond early and positively to HIV infection. Antivirus antibodies are also formed and viraemia lessens. (B) However, there is simultaneous destruction of T helper (CD4) lymphocytes (Th-cells) and virus gains entry to them causing (C) a failure of the cell-mediated immune response and (D) progressive inability to eliminate HIV. Virus persists (E) and patient remains permanently infectious. Eventually, impaired immunity provides opportunity for onset (F) of life-threatening opportunistic viral, bacterial or protozoal infections.

antibodies clinically allows infection to be confirmed but does not prove conclusively that the full syndrome will develop. Later, with the onset and increased severity of disease, antibody levels fall.

Structure

After a latent period that may be very long, secondary, opportunistic infection or cancer often progress rapidly, leading to death.

Opportunistic infection

Impaired immunity encourages opportunistic infection by viral, bacterial, protozoal and parasitic agents. Many of these organisms are not normally pathogenic. The most frequent are cytomegalovirus, *Mycobacterium tuberculosis*, and *Pneumocystis carinii*. herpes simplex and herpes zoster infections are also frequent. AIDS may encourage molluscum contagiosum and anogenital condylomata.

Many central nervous system and lung disorders are due to opportunistic infection. They include streptococcal, staphylococcal and Haemophilus infections. Oral candidiasis and hairy cell leukoplakia occur, the latter attributable to Epstein–Barr virus. Oesophageal ulceration due to Candida, cytomegalovirus and Herpes virus accompany diarrhoea, malabsorption, anorectal ulceration and proctitis.

Tumours

AIDS is often complicated by cancer. Kaposi's sarcoma (p. 49) is the most common malignant tumour. Squamous carcinoma of the mouth and cloacogenic anorectal carcinoma are unusually frequent and oesophageal carcinoma *in-situ* is encountered. The frequency of extranodal, B-cell non-Hodgkin's lymphoma (p. 223) is raised. Multiple myeloma may develop and brain cancer is increasingly common.

Now read Kaposi's sarcoma (p. 49)

Regional disease

Persistent generalised lymphadenopathy is the result of massive viral replication. The lymph nodes may be the site of bacillary angiomatosis (p. 222). Brain atrophy is associated with late, advancing immunosuppression. If intravenous drug abuse is continued, embolic infection and endocarditis often occur. When hepatitis B or syphilis co-exist, their effects are potentiated by HIV. Liver granulomas are due to mycobacteria.

Behaviour and prognosis

The clinical signs of infection at first resemble glandular fever. There is then a latent period that may be as long as 10 years. Prognosis in AIDS is related to the number of viral particles in the circulating plasma. Transmission is rare from persons with levels of less than 1500 viral copies of HIV-1/mL serum. Many antiviral drugs (Table 6) are available. They may be given alone or in double or triple combination. They slow the progression of HIV and AIDS but there is not yet any single drug that can effect a cure.

Now read Antiviral agents (p. 23)

Intensive HIV retroviral therapy has led to a decline in the morbidity of AIDS and the frequency of perinatal infection has been reduced. That immunity can be acquired has been suggested by recent studies of prostitutes in an African population. Vaccines are therefore under trial but none offers certain protection. There are separate treatments for the common bacterial, viral, fungal and parasitic infections that complicate AIDS. In the absence of treatment, death is the inevitable outcome. Male circumcision offers some protection.

HIV AND SURGERY

Virus is present in all body fluids. Surgeons and nurses are exposed whenever they operate on seropositive cases, and patients are at risk when examined or cared for by seropositive surgeons or health workers. Blood and blood products that have not been screened for virus must be avoided.

Patients as a threat to hospital staff

Great care is needed in the management of patients who have been exposed to HIV, whether seropositive or not. There is no entirely reliable drug for the treatment of staff who have been exposed. However, the overall risk to surgeons of acquiring needle-stick and other sharp instrument injury is relatively small, occurring in ~0.4% of operations. Saliva is of low infectivity.

Now read Needle stick injury (p. 362)

All HIV-positive patients are assumed to be infectious. Theatre procedures must be scrupulous. One theatre is selected for high-risk cases. Anaesthesia is induced in theatre. The anaesthetist wears protective clothing. All body fluids may contain virus so glasses, goggles and masks are worn. Impenetrable gowns and drapes are used. The risk of glove penetration during surgery (p. 142) varies according to the type and length of operation but may be as high as 30%. 'Double-gloving' (p. 143) is advisable. Occasionally, the use of steel-mail gloves is recommended. Instruments are passed only in containers, but disposable instruments may be adopted. Staples and diathermy are preferred to sutures. The increasing use of closed drainage systems has lessened the risk.

After an operation, gowns, shoes and gloves are discarded in reverse order and all instruments placed in a bag for return to the central sterilising unit. Endoscopic instruments are freed from virus by cleaning in detergent, followed by a minimum of 4 minutes exposure to 2% gluteraldehyde. For endoscopic retrograde cholangiopancreatography (ERCP) and colonoscopy, 10 minutes exposure to gluteraldehyde between **all** cases, is recommended. However, the elimination of coincidental hepatitis B virus and Cryptosporidium requires at least 30 minutes treatment and *Mycobacterium tuberculosis* 60 minutes. In cases of injury from high risk donors, individuals are expected to complete a 6 week course of prophylactic chemotherapy.

Now read Disinfection (p. 118), Sterilisation (p. 304)

Surgeons as a threat to patients

There is a small risk that surgical and dental patients may acquire HIV from hospital staff. The probability of transmitting HIV by needle-stick injury is ~0.14%. A doctor or nurse discovered to be HIV-positive is required by English law to report to the hospital manager and to colleagues and is banned from undertaking further invasive procedures.

ACTINOMYCOSIS

Actinomycosis is a bacterial disease caused by a variety of Gram-positive anaerobic or micro-aerophilic rods from the genus Actinomyces.

Causes

The species implicated in the majority of human infections is *Actinomyces israelii*. Many actinomycotic infections are, however, polymicrobial. Organisms such as Actinobacilli, Bacteroides spp., Staphylococcus spp. and Streptococcus spp. can be isolated in varying combinations, depending upon the site of infection.

Structure

Actinomycosis begins with a disruption of the mucosal barrier. Oral and cervico-facial infections develop after dental procedures or trauma. Pulmonary lesions follow aspiration (p. 217). Abdominal disease succeeds the surgical treatment of appendicitis or the ingestion of foreign bodies such as fishbones. Pelvic actinomycosis is associated with neglected intra-uterine contraceptive devices.

The lesions of actinomycosis are deep-seated, indolent and destructive. An acute inflammatory phase is soon superseded by a chronic reaction. Single or multiple indurated swellings develop and eventually suppurate centrally to yield abscesses that are often followed by sinus formation. *Actinomyces israelii* proliferates in the centre of the abscess. Fibrotic walls surround the lesions and sinus tracts close and re-form spontaneously. The rupture of a liver abscess through the diaphragm into the pleural cavity is one mechanism of spread.

Behaviour and prognosis

The diagnosis of actinomycosis rests upon the identification of sulphur granules in pus: crushed on a microscope slide, these aggregates of micro-organisms stain to show characteristic Gram-positive branching bacilli. Their isolation from a site other than the tonsils implies a pathological state. Surgical incision and drainage is still advocated despite the advent of efficacious antimicrobial therapy. Long-term intravenous treatment with penicillin followed by oral antibiotics (p. 17) cures extensive disease.

Nocardiosis

Nocardiosis has many features in common with actinomycosis. The infection is caused by the aerobic organism, *Nocardia asteroides*.

ADRENAL GLANDS

Each of the paired adrenal (suprarenal) glands comprises a cortex and a medulla. Although contiguous, these components function as separate organs.

Biopsy diagnosis of adrenal disease

Many adrenal diseases can be diagnosed by high resolution CT and MRI, and by isotopic scanning. Nodules as small as 5.0 mm in diameter can be detected. Fine needle aspiration under radiological guidance can sometimes be performed. The identity of functioning tumours is confirmed by adrenal vein catheterisation when blood and urine are collected for analysis.

ADRENAL CORTEX

The adrenal cortex has three zones, each secreting a distinct population of steroid hormones (corticosteroids). An outer **zona glomerulosa** synthesises mineralocorticoids, an intermediate **zona fasiculata** secretes glucocorticoids and an inner **zona reticularis** liberates weak adrenal androgens. The cortex is also a source of oestrogens. The synthesis of corticosteroids from adrenal or plasma cholesterol begins in the mitochondria of the cortical cells.

Now read Endocrine system (p. 126)

Cortisol

The most important corticosteroid in man is cortisol (hydrocortisone). This hormone comprises half of the total steroid production by the adrenal cortex. Cortisol stimulates gluconeogenesis from glycogen and from protein, raising the blood glucose concentration. It also promotes the renal retention of sodium and the loss of potassium but much less effectively than aldosterone. Cortisol modulates the correction of fluid imbalance in dehydration and the intracellular over-hydration of adrenocortical insufficiency. It facilitates the vasoconstrictive effects of catecholamines on arterioles, leading to an increase in systemic blood pressure. Erythropoiesis with leucocytosis and eosinophilia are stimulated. Lymphoid tissue atrophies. Antibody production falls and allergic responses are diminished. There is a reduction in the severity of inflammatory reactions and in the speed and adequacy of wound healing. In shock (p. 290), cortisol can stabilise lysosomal membranes if it is given before any further damaging stimulus.

The secretion of cortisol is modulated by adrenocorticotrophic hormone (ACTH - corticotrophin), a 39-amino acid polypeptide released from the corticotrophic cells of the anterior pituitary gland. In turn, these pituitary cells are regulated by a corticotrophin-releasing hormone (CRH) that passes to the anterior pituitary gland from the hypothalamus.

Aldosterone

Aldosterone increases renal tubular Na^+ re-absorption and K^+ and H^+ excretion. Comparable effects are recognised in the ileum and colon and the loss of Na^+ in sweat and saliva is diminished.

Aldosterone secretion is regulated by the **renin-angiotensin system** (p. 201). In response to lowered renal arteriolar blood pressure, juxtaglomerular cells liberate the enzyme renin which converts the prohormone protein angiotensinogen to angiotensin I. Angiotensin-converting enzyme (ACE) abbreviates this decapeptide to active angiotensin II. This molecule is an octapeptide acting directly upon the cells of the zona glomerulosa. It stimulates aldosterone secretion the release of which is influenced by potassium and by sodium.

Androgens

The principal androgen secreted by the adrenal cortex is dehydro-epi-androsterone (DHEA) but smaller amounts of androstenedione and testosterone are also liberated.

Adrenal cortical hyperfunction

Three syndromes of excess adrenal cortical activity (hyperadrenocorticalism) correspond to the three main classes of corticosteroid: Cushing's syndrome (excess glucocorticoid), Conn's syndrome (excess mineralocorticoid), and the adrenogenital syndromes (excess androgen).

Cushing's syndrome

Cushing's syndrome is encountered more often in women than men. Moon face, virilisation and the abnormal deposition of fat in sites such as the back of the neck attract attention and the individual may be described as resembling a 'lemon on a stick'. There is a proximal myopathy with muscle atrophy, abdominal striae and osteoporosis. Hypertension is characteristic. Abnormal collagen metabolism and maturation result in defective wound healing. The lowered glucose tolerance simulates diabetes mellitus.

The causes of excess glucocorticoid secretion are:

- Cushing's disease (p. 273).
- A functioning tumour of the adrenal cortex (p. 247). There is depressed ACTH secretion and atrophy of the remaining, normal adrenal tissue.
- The secretion of corticotrophin-releasing factor (CRF) from an ectopic source such as small cell bronchogenic carcinoma, islet cell tumour of the pancreas or thymic carcinoid tumour. Adrenal cortical hyperplasia may be extreme.

Changes closely similar to Cushing's syndrome are caused by therapeutic corticosteroid treatment when the bodily changes are said to be 'cushingoid'

Hyperaldosteronism

Excess aldosterone enhances sodium retention and potassium excretion. There is systemic hypertension but usually no dependent oedema. The muscles become weak and there may be flaccid paralysis. Hyperaldosteronism may be primary or secondary.

Conn's syndrome is **primary** hyperaldosteronism. It is usually caused by an adenoma of the adrenal cortex. However, the syndrome may be due to unilateral or bilateral adrenal cortical hyperplasia or, rarely, to primary adrenal cortical carcinoma.

Inappropriate secretion of excess aldosterone may

be **secondary** to cardiac failure or hepatic cirrhosis. The secretion of aldosterone is increased following injury or operation. The magnitude and duration of this increase are proportional to the severity of the accident or procedure; they are exaggerated if there are postoperative complications, particularly local or systemic sepsis. Secondary hyperaldosteronism may also be a consequence of increased secretion of renin from a kidney affected by renal artery stenosis or from a renin-secreting renal tumour. It is a component of Cushing's syndrome.

Adrenogenital syndrome

This rare disorder is attributable to a functioning tumour of cortical cells. It may also be due to an inherited disorder of steroid synthesis, the most frequent of which is 21-hydroxylase deficiency. Virilisation is one result.

Adrenal cortical hypofunction

Glucocorticoid hypofunction (hypo-adrenocorticalism) may be acute or chronic.

Acute

This uncommon disorder is exemplified by the haemorrhagic adrenal cortical necrosis of the Waterhouse–Friderichsen syndrome, a complication of meningococcal bacteraemia. It is also an occasional feature of other septicaemic or bacteriaemic states in which endotoxic shock is contributory. A closely similar condition of haemorrhagic adrenal infarction may follow episodes of hypotension during major abdominal surgery. Clinical signs include the acute onset of vomiting with resultant dehydration, hyponatraemia, hyperkalaemia, hypoglycaemia and hypotension.

Chronic (Addison's disease)

Chronic insufficiency is usually attributable to autoimmune adrenalitis (p. 28) but may be due to metastatic carcinoma. Tuberculosis is another cause.

Tumours

The adrenal cortex is a frequent site for metastases from carcinoma of the bronchus, breast, stomach, kidney and other sources.

Primary adrenal cortical tumours are uncommon. They may be functional or non-functional. Large, non-functional tumours are usually malignant as are those secreting androgens.

Benign

Adenoma

Adenomas are formed of clear or of compact cells, resembling those of the zona fasciculata and zona reticularis, respectively. Those that are functional secrete cortisol, aldosterone or sex steroids.

Malignant

Carcinoma

Carcinoma is distinguished from adenoma with difficulty. Indeed, the malignant behaviour of the neoplastic cells may not be suspected until metastases have been recognised.

ADRENAL MEDULLA

The secretions of the adrenal medulla exercise a less critical influence on surgical homeostasis than those of the cortex but they occupy central roles in responses to stress (p. 313) and sepsis (p. 178).

Tumours

Metastases from common primary sites, such as the bronchus, are frequent. Primary tumours are very uncommon.

Benign

Phaeochromocytoma

This is a rare tumour of the chromaffin cells of the adrenal medulla or of the extra-adrenal chromaffin cells of the organ of Zuckerkändl. The tumour may be bilateral and is occasionally part of a multiple endocrine neoplasia 2 (MEN 2) syndrome. Phaeochromocytomas are usually but not always benign. The neoplastic cells secrete the catecholamines, adrenaline and noradrenaline, as well as inappropriate hormones that include ACTH and vaso-intestinal polypeptide (VIP). The tumour is usually associated with hypertension and hyperglycaemia. Diagnosis is confirmed by the detection of high levels of vanillyl mandelic acid (VMA) in urinary samples collected over 24 hours. VMA is a metabolite of the catecholamines.

Now read Multiple endocrine neoplasia (p. 126)

Myelolipoma
Myelolipoma is a name for the uncommon finding of an island of haemopoietic and adipose tissue within the adrenal medulla.

Ganglioneuroma and neurofibroma
These are occasional benign tumours of the adrenal medulla and of the organ of Zuckerkändl.

Malignant

Neuroblastoma
This malignant tumour accounts for ~15% of cancer deaths in children. Although neuroblastoma may originate in any part of the sympathetic nervous system, the majority are intra-abdominal. Half of these tumours derive from the adrenal medulla. There may be a selective distribution of metastases so that those from a left adrenal tumour pass to the lung, those from a right-sided tumour to the liver. Chromosomal and genetic analyses (p. 91) assist prognosis.

AGEING

Ageing is the process of growing old. It is the aggregate of the degenerative changes in cells, tissues and organs that decides the life span. Age changes are both intrinsic and extrinsic. Together, they result in a decreased capacity to respond to environmental stress. They therefore exercise a significant influence on the results of surgery.

Intrinsic changes

There is a failure to replace effete cells in numbers sufficient to maintain normal tissue function and a time-dependent, irreversible deterioration in cell structure. Cells have a finite life span. Although clones of cells that appear 'immortal' can be selected in the laboratory, this is not the natural condition. Normally, cultured cells are restricted by a 'Hayflick limit' to a sequence of 48 divisions, after which death occurs. One explanation is that there is a continual accumulation of genetic errors on the basis of somatic mutation: the errors that occur invariably in DNA replication (p. 140) are not wholly repaired. A further view invokes programmed ageing, apoptosis (p. 89).

In **progeria**, premature ageing, there are many fewer cell divisions than normal before cell death.

Extrinsic changes

Another explanation for the changes of ageing is the gradual aggregation of free radical damage, the 'cumulative error' hypothesis. Such injury is caused, for example, by ionising radiation or by failed antioxidant defence mechanisms. Free radicals (p. 133) can lead to mitochondrial and nuclear DNA damage. Cells affected in this way cannot repair DNA. They form insoluble material like lipofuscin in heart muscle and secrete inadequate amounts of endocrine and paracrine molecules. A second, extrinsic cause may be the modification of tissue proteins by the accumulation of products such as those of glycosylation that cross-link and inactivate adjacent proteins.

AGEING AND SURGERY

Surgery is greatly influenced by problems created by the processes of ageing and by the altered responses of senescent tissues to disease. The aged are susceptible to cancer and atheroma. Morbidity and mortality are increased by comparison with younger individuals. Amyloid (p. 9) accumulates and osteoporosis is commonplace.

In operative surgery, the most common difficulties are nutritional and metabolic. Old persons are prone to protein malnutrition and often suffer from deficiencies of vitamins A, B and D. They are frequently anaemic. In the face of large changes in blood pressure and tissue perfusion, myocardial ischaemia may culminate in infarction.

Postoperatively, deep vein thrombosis and embolism are constant threats. Skeletal muscle atrophy prejudices survival. Immobility encourages thrombosis. It also diminishes respiratory movements and facilitates bronchopneumonia. Senescent tissues may be incapable of mounting normal defence reactions against infection. Respiratory capacity is limited. There is an impairment of renal function and inadequate urinary concentration. Cerebral function is often altered and episodes of hypotension may precipitate cerebral infarction.

AMOEBIASIS

Amoebiasis is a colonic infection caused by the intestinal protozoon, *Entamoeba histolytica*.

Cause

The disease follows faecal contamination of food or water but flies can convey amoebic cysts to foodstuffs. There is also a well-recognised risk of transmission between homosexual males: amoebiasis is a cause of diarrhoea in patients with AIDS. After ingestion, the vegetative amoebae that evolve may live for long periods in the gut without invading this tissue. Dysentery results when invasion begins. Infection may spread to the liver by the portal vein and ultimately to the lung and brain. Amoebic liver abscess is a common sequel; it is much more frequent in males than females. Abscess is usually single.

In diagnosis, free *E. histolytica* are sought in specimens of fresh, warm stool. However, they are often not detectable. To allow identification of the organism, secretions or biopsy specimens are stained by the periodic-acid/Schiff (PAS) method. Serological confirmation of diagnosis is sought by applying an enzyme-linked immunosorbent assay (ELISA) to the sample but indirect haemagglutination and polymerase chain reactions (p. 139) can also be used. The diagnosis of liver abscess is assisted by ultrasonic and CT scans, ultrasonically guided needle aspiration and serum haemagglutination tests.

Structure

Characteristic transverse ulcers with overhanging edges form in the wall of the colon (Fig. 53d, p. 334). They may be confused with those of Crohn's disease or ulcerative colitis. However, biopsy reveals unicellular amoebae with four small, darkly staining nuclei. Amoebic abscesses, such as those that frequently develop in the liver, contain orange–red pus resembling 'anchovy sauce'. Unlike other hepatic abscesses (p. 210), those of amoebiasis do not possess a well-developed pyogenic membrane although they are bounded by a thin wall of granulation tissue. Abscess formation may also occur in the lung and brain.

Now read Abscess (p. 1)

Behaviour and prognosis

Amoebic abscesses may rupture into the pleural, pericardial or peritoneal cavities. Unusual or rare complications of amoebiasis include toxic dilatation of the colon; perforation; and the formation of an amoeboma the appearances of which can be mistaken for those of cancer.

OTHER AMOEBAE

Acanthamoeba spp. can cause disseminated infection in immunocompromised individuals, for example after renal transplantation. Free-living amoebae such as *Naegleria fowleri* have been found in freshwater baths and tanks. This organism is capable of causing meningitis and can harbour *Legionella pneumophila* (p. 216).

AMYLOID

Amyloids are insoluble glycoproteins that cause organ failure when laid down in excess. The disorder caused by this process is amyloidosis (β-fibrillosis).

The amyloids are chemically distinct but have identical physical properties. Each molecule consists of an individual protein molecule and a smaller antigenic P-substance that is common to all the amyloids. The amyloids are divided into categories according to the chemical structure of the individual proteins.

All amyloids have a molecular arrangement described as a folded, beta-pleated sheet. This means that the dyes used in staining amyloid are incorporated in a similar laminar fashion between the sheets of the protein, giving a doubly refractile appearance when viewed with plane-polarised light. Congo red is one of the stains most commonly employed to identify amyloid: the red-stained material is seen in polarised light to be apple green, not red.

AMYLOIDOSIS

Excessive deposition of amyloids in tissues is amyloidosis (Table 1). When a cause for amyloidosis can be demonstrated, the condition is **secondary**. When no demonstrable cause can be found, the term idiopathic or **primary** amyloidosis is used. In Western countries, the commonest cause of secondary amyloidosis is rheumatoid arthritis but the disorder is also encountered in other chronic inflammatory conditions, bronchiectasis and chronic osteomyelitis. In less privileged countries, the chronic inflammatory causes of amyloidosis include tuberculosis and leprosy.

Biopsy diagnosis

In systemic amyloidosis, needle biopsy of the rectal mucosa or the kidney establishes the diagnosis.

Table 1 Types of amyloid of significance in surgery

Type of amyloid	Characteristics
Amyloid A (AA)	Deposited in blood vessel walls in chronic inflammatory diseases such as rheumatoid arthritis (p. 191) and Crohn's disease (p. 165)
Amyloid L (AL)	Laid down during the development of some immunocytic diseases and in plasma cell myeloma (p. 237). The material is an aggregate of Ig light chains or fragments of them
Amyloid β_2-microglobulin ($A\beta_2M$)	Accumulates in selected sites such as bone and carpal tunnel connective tissue after long-term renal dialysis using membranes of low permeability. In sporadic cerebral amyloid angiopathy the amyloid is β_4 peptide. It is found around blood vessels and in nearby giant cells
Amyloid calcitonin (ACAL) and amyloid intestinal vaso-active polypeptide (AVAPP)	Molecules that accumulate locally at sites of functioning endocrine tumours (p. 126, 247)

Autopsy diagnosis

With time, the spleen, kidneys, liver and other viscera become enlarged and pale. Iodine gives affected tissues a mahogany brown colour that resists decolorisation with sulphuric acid.

ANAEMIA

Anaemia is a reduction below normal (Appendix Table) in the concentration of haemoglobin in the circulating blood. However, account must be taken of the age, sex and race of an individual before measurements such as haemoglobin concentration become meaningful.

In anaemia, there is a diminution in the number of circulating red blood cells; in the concentration of haemoglobin in each cell; or in both. When the red blood cells retain their normal size, the anaemia is **normocytic**. An increase in red cell size is **macrocytosis**, a decrease **microcytosis**. When the haemoglobin concentration within the cell is raised, the term **hyperchromasia** is used. The converse condition is **hypochromasia**.

There are three main classes of anaemia: dyserythropoietic, haemolytic and haemorrhagic.

DYSERYTHROPOIETIC (DYSHAEMOPOIETIC) ANAEMIA

Dyserythropoiesis indicates a defect in the formation of haemoglobin.

Iron deficiency anaemia, usually microcytic and hypochromic, is commonplace in countries where parasitic disease and malnutrition are rife. It affects 30% of the world's population. However, there is a lower prevalence among those cooking in iron utensils. Iron deficiency anaemia is still surprisingly frequent in the UK and is often recognised in patients admitted for surgery. It is attributable to insidious blood loss and the escape of 10–20 mL/day soon results in a negative iron balance and the depletion of iron stores. Iron deficiency anaemia is characteristic of the Plummer–Vinson syndrome (p. 257, 375).

Now read Iron (p. 271)

Megaloblastic anaemia is a particular form of dyshaemopoiesis. It is common in vegans in whom it may lead to blindness. There is a defect both in the numbers and in the maturation of red blood cells due to a deficiency of cyanocobalamin (vitamin B_{12}, p. 352). Megaloblasts are large, haemoglobinised, red blood cells that retain an immature nucleus. There is an imbalance between nuclear and cytoplasmic maturation. In diseases of the **proximal** part of the small intestine, such as multiple diverticulosis, a blind loop syndrome with a change in gut flora leads both to iron deficiency and to megaloblastosis. Megaloblastic anaemia is also common after resection of the **distal** part of the small intestine. There is defective vitamin B_{12} absorption.

HAEMOLYTIC ANAEMIA

In haemolytic anaemia, there is excessive red blood cell destruction (p. 301). There are genetic and acquired causes. Hereditary spherocytosis is an example of the former, malaria of the latter. Micro-angiopathic haemolytic anaemia is described on p. 100.

Auto-immune haemolytic anaemia

In auto-immune haemolytic anaemia, anti-red blood cell auto-antibodies are formed.

Antibody binding is usually optimal at 37°C. The anaemia is of a 'warm antibody type'. Occasionally, antibody binds to the red cells best at low temperature; the anaemia is then of a 'cold antibody type'. Auto-immune haemolytic anaemia may complicate systemic lupus erythematosus (p. 29) or lymphoma (p. 223) and can be provoked by mycoplasmal pneumonia and by viral infections. In a further category, anaemia becomes severe in cold weather.

Iso-immune haemolytic anaemia

Iso-immune haemolytic anaemia is exemplified by haemolytic disease of the newborn (p. 46).

The red blood cells of a fetus may bear antigens, such as those of the Rhesus blood groups (p. 46), distinct from those of the mother. Some fetal red blood cells invariably cross the placental barrier, entering the maternal circulation. If anti-fetal red blood cell antibodies are then formed by the mother, they may pass back across the placenta. Entering the fetal circulation, they bind to fetal red blood cells and lead to haemolysis.

HAEMORRHAGIC ANAEMIA

Haemorrhagic anaemia is caused by acute or chronic blood loss for example in menorrhagia or in the presence of haemorrhoids (p. 12).

Now read Blood loss (p. 42)

OTHER FORMS OF ANAEMIA

Particular forms of anaemia accompany liver disease (macrocytic), renal failure and rheumatoid arthritis (hypochromic, normocytic), and pregnancy (hypochromic, normocytic or macrocytic).

Leuco-erythroblastic anaemia

In this condition, immature red and white blood cells and their precursors appear in the circulating blood. The cause is usually the presence of extensive metastatic tumour deposits in the bone marrow.

ANAL CANAL

The anal canal (Fig. 2a) is the distal end of the intestine. Most of the upper third of the anal canal is lined by large bowel mucosa. The middle third, the transitional zone, is lined mainly by transitional epithelium. The lower part is lined solely by squamous epithelium but unlike the skin of the peri-anal region, is devoid of hair follicles, sweat glands and sebaceous glands. These histological distinctions, originating embryologically, ensure that there are significant differences in the pathological responses of the various parts.

Biopsy diagnosis of anal disease

Anal disease outwith the canal may be apparent *naked eye* or at proctoscopy. Fungal infections can be diagnosed by the microscopy of cell scrapings. Anal warts are excised under local anaesthesia, but samples of suspected tumours are obtained under general anaesthesia.

DEVELOPMENTAL AND CONGENITAL DISORDERS

- If there is defective development of the anal canal above the levator ani muscle, there is no anal sphincter. In males the rectum usually opens into the urethra, in females into the posterior vagina. The lack of a sphincter results in incontinence.
- When there is anomalous development of the mid-part of the anal canal, there is an imperforate anal membrane, the rupture of which may lead to fibrous stenosis.
- Defects of the lower part of the anal canal, below the levator ani muscle, result in the opening of the anal canal onto the surface of the vulva or perineum, effectively constituting an ectopic anus. An opening below the levator ani muscle maintains continence.

Fissure

Anal fissure is a vertical, slit-like ulcer in the epithelium of the lower part of the canal. The majority of fissures occurs posteriorly, in a position designated 6 o'clock. In time, a so-called sentinel skin tag develops at the outer end of the fissure. The anal papilla at the inner end may hypertrophy, with the development of a fibrous polyp. Most fissures have no obvious cause although patients are usually constipated. Fissures are more common in parous than in nulliparous women and may be sited anteriorly ('12 o'clock'). Fissures are particularly common in Crohn's disease, less frequent in ulcerative colitis.

Haemorrhoids

Haemorrhoids are the dilated vascular spaces of the mucosa and skin of the anal canal. The spaces develop from naturally-occurring fusiform and saccular dilatations of the arteriovenous plexus that lies beneath the anal epithelium. The plexuses form cushions that aid continence. Haemorrhoids are a consequence of prolapse of these cushions due to episodic, increased pressure within the anal canal. They are more common in individuals who consume a typical low-fibre Western diet, particularly in those who are constipated and strain at stool.

- **Internal haemorrhoids** arise in the upper two thirds of the anus and are lined by columnar epithelium with an *intestinal* sensory innervation.
- **External haemorrhoids** are a late manifestation of internal haemorrhoids but can arise *de novo*. They are lined by modified squamous epithelium with a *cutaneous* innervation and are often exquisitely painful, particularly if haemorrhage produces a peri-anal haematoma. Thrombosis then occurs. In the absence of surgical intervention, the superficial component shrivels to become a painless skin tag.

INFECTION AND INFLAMMATION

Abscess

Anorectal abscesses are very common. They are classified anatomically (Fig. 2b) as peri-anal, ischiorectal, submucosal, intersphincteric or pelvirectal.

Peri-anal abscesses and other septic phenomena are common in patients suffering from AIDS. Anorectal sepsis is also frequent in patients with Crohn's disease. However, there is usually no demonstrable cause and it is assumed that abscess develops from a focus of infection in an anal gland, between the internal and external sphincters. Some anorectal abscesses originate from *Staphylococcus aureus* infection of a sebaceous gland.

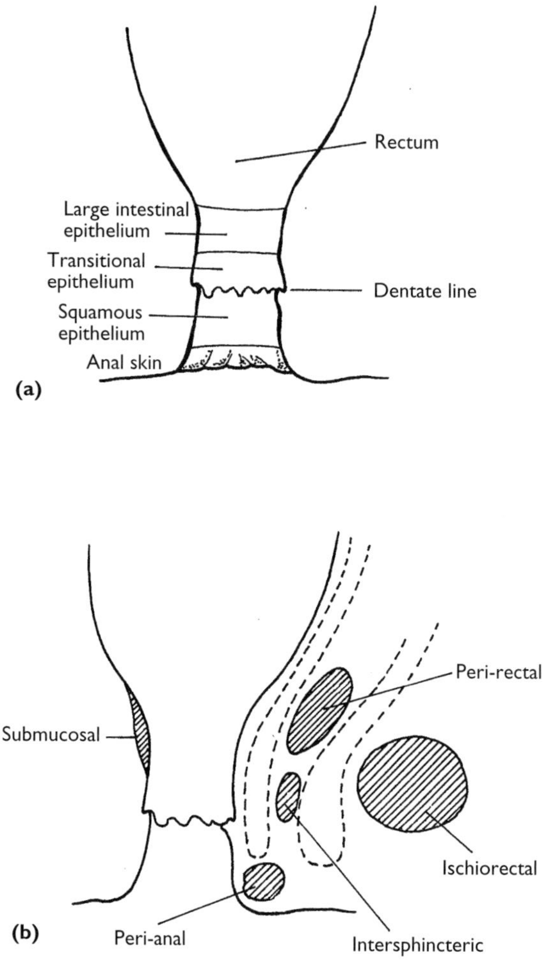

Figure 2 Anal canal.
(a) Anatomy of the anal canal. (b) Location of peri-anal and peri-rectal abscesses.

Bacteria isolated from anorectal abscesses include *Escherichia coli*, *Bacteroides fragilis*, *Enterococcus faecalis* and/or streptococci of groups A, C, G and, occasionally, B. The *Streptococcus intermedius* group may be implicated. The infection tends to extend downwards between the sphincters into the peri-anal region. Fistula formation (p. 132) may occur.

Fistula

The majority of fistulas *in ano* are not associated with gastro-intestinal disease but are a consequence of anorectal abscesses. However, they are a common feature of Crohn's disease and actinomycosis. Biopsy may reveal the granulomas typical of these conditions. Most fistulas are **simple**, with direct communication between the epithelium of the anus and the epithelium of the peri-anal skin. **Complex** fistulas pass through several components of the internal and external anal sphincters.

Granuloma and cloacogenic polyp

The tissues of the anal margin are susceptible to Crohn's disease. Granulomas in this location can be found in patients with no evidence of small or large intestinal disease.

Cloacogenic polyp is recognised in elderly persons as a ~15 mm diameter, polypoidal, inflammatory swelling. There is prolapse of the transitional zone mucosa. Microscopically, the polyp has a tubulovillous structure interspersed with islands of squamous epithelium that shows no evidence of dysplasia and has no malignant potential.

TUMOURS

Tumours of the anal margin are distinguished from those occurring within the anal canal.

Anal margin

Bowen's disease

Bowen's disease is a form of intra-epithelial neoplasia. It appears as diffuse red plaques of the perineal skin. The lesion has irregular edges. Ulceration is found in 6% of cases and the recognition of this condition suggests the presence of underlying, invasive carcinoma.

Condylomata acuminata

Anal warts are caused by human papilloma viruses (HPV) 6, 11, 16 and 18. The majority is transmitted sexually. In one individual, as many as several hundred warts may be recognised. They may also exist in the anal canal.

Paget's disease

Apocrine glands are frequent in the anal region and Paget's change suggests the presence of intraduct carcinoma of these glands. Eczematous skin changes accompany the characteristic presence of intra-epithelial Paget's cells in the deeper parts of the squamous epithelium. Paget's disease of the anal margin has been recognised in patients with carcinoma of the breast or rectum.

Now read Paget's disease of the breast (p. 68)

Squamous carcinoma

Squamous carcinoma of the anal margin closely resembles this form of tumour at other epithelial sites (p. 303). It is more common in the old than the young, and is more frequent in males than females. The structure is that of a well-differentiated, keratinising carcinoma. Ulcer formation is usual but the cancer may sometimes be nodular. Lymphatic spread to the regional inguinal lymph nodes is likely but, in spite of this tendency, there is a 5-year survival rate of ~80%.

Anal canal

Intra-epithelial neoplasia

Intra-epithelial neoplasia (AIN) is graded AIN I to AIN III and is associated with anal condylomata and with HIV-positivity. It is encountered in women with human papilloma virus (HPV) infection and cervical intra-epithelial neoplasia (CIN). In men it occurs frequently in homosexuals who engage in anal sexual practices. Microscopy reveals a dysplastic epithelium. AIN III may progress to invasive carcinoma, a phenomenon particularly associated with infection by HPV 16 (p. 80, 351).

Carcinoma

Carcinoma of the anal canal is very uncommon. In the UK, there are ~300 cases annually.

Causes
This is a disease of elderly women and of homosexual men. It is a progression from AIN.

Structure
The tumour occurs in the modified squamous epithelium of the lower anus or in the transitional zone in the upper anus, above the dentate line (Fig. 2). The majority of tumours are exfoliative squamous carcinomas but some are undifferentiated, small cell lesions. A few tumours resemble basal cell carcinoma

of the skin, from which they are distinguished histologically.

Behaviour and prognosis

The dentate line is a barrier to distal spread but proximal extension takes place, to pelvic and inguinal lymph nodes. Prognosis is related to the depth of the tumour, its size and the presence or absence of lymph node involvement. Spread through the wall of the anal canal with lymph node metastases is associated with recurrence in at least 50% of cases although the 5-year survival may be as high as 70%.

Malignant melanoma

Malignant melanoma (p. 227) of the anal canal is much less frequent than squamous carcinoma and accounts for only 1% of all malignant melanomas. The lesion arises in the transitional zone of the canal and forms a polypoidal mass. The tumour may not be pigmented but the cells contain melanosomes and express S100 protein. Lymph nodes are often involved by the time of diagnosis. Metastasis takes place to the liver and lungs. The prognosis is poor.

ANEURYSM

An aneurysm is a localised dilatation of the wall of the heart or of a blood vessel of any variety or size and with a lumen that communicates directly with that of a cardiac chamber or blood vessel.

TRUE ANEURYSMS

True aneurysms have a continuous wall and are classified structurally and functionally.

- **Morphologically** (anatomically) aneurysms may be saccular, fusiform, berry, dissecting, communicating or cirsoid.
- **Functionally** (causally), aneurysms may be congenital, atherosclerotic, traumatic, arteriovenous, ischaemic, mycotic (infective) or syphilitic.

Classification

There are many varieties (Fig. 3). In alphabetical order they are:

- **Arteriovenous**. Arteriovenous (AV) aneurysms may be congenital or acquired. Congenital AV aneurysms are recognised in lung and other tissues. Aorto-vena caval fistula may culminate in cardiac failure. Many acquired AV aneurysms are the result of injuries such as stab wounds that penetrate adjacent vessels simultaneously. The femoral artery and vein are particularly susceptible and arteriovenous aneurysm may form at this site after a knife has penetrated both blood vessels simultaneously.
- **Atherosclerotic**. Atherosclerotic aneurysms are the most common of all such lesions. The abdominal aorta below the origin of the renal arteries is the usual site but these aneurysms may arise from the wall of the popliteal artery or other vessels. The majority of atheromatous abdominal aneurysms are fusiform whereas most popliteal aneurysms are saccular.
- **Cirsoid**. A cirsoid aneurysm is the dilatation of a group of blood vessels resulting from a congenital malformation. There is arteriovenous shunting of blood.
- **Congenital**. Congenital saccular (berry) aneurysms are often found at the bifurcations of the intracerebral arteries. They are more frequent in women than men and can be recognised in more than 1% of adults. On average, they are ~5–10 mm in diameter. The source of the aneurysm is a defect in the internal elastic lamina. Rupture is most common at ~50 years of age and accounts for many cases of subarachnoid haemorrhage (p. 65).
- **Dissecting**. Now termed aortic dissection, this potentially fatal catastrophe originates as a tear in the intima of the aorta. Blood escapes into the defect, propagates in the media along the length of the vessel, and frequently ruptures externally. In type A dissection, the ascending aorta is affected; in type B, it is not.
- **Ischaemic**. After myocardial infarction, a left ventricular aneurysm may be found in regions of cardiac muscle necrosis. It forms a protruding, localised mass. Less often, the mural aneurysm develops in the muscular wall of the interventricular septum and is intracardiac.
- **Mycotic**. *Staphylococcus aureus* and *Salmonella typhi* are examples of bacteria with an affinity for arterial tissue where they cause destructive lesions with aneurysm formation. In Chagas' disease, small mycotic aneurysms characteristically form near the

apex of the left ventricle, a site at which *Trypanosoma cruzi* (p. 282) destroy cardiac muscle cells.

- **Syphilitic**. When early treatment has not been undertaken, the wall of the proximal part of the thoracic aorta is prone to the destructive effects of *Treponema pallidum* (p. 314). Saccular aneurysm of the aortic arch may result.
- **Traumatic**. Injury to an artery at the site of a surgical operation may cause aneurysm formation. Popliteal artery aneurysm, for example, is a rare complication of knee arthroplasty. Stab or missile injuries may lead to a similar result. Some traumatic aneurysms are arteriovenous.

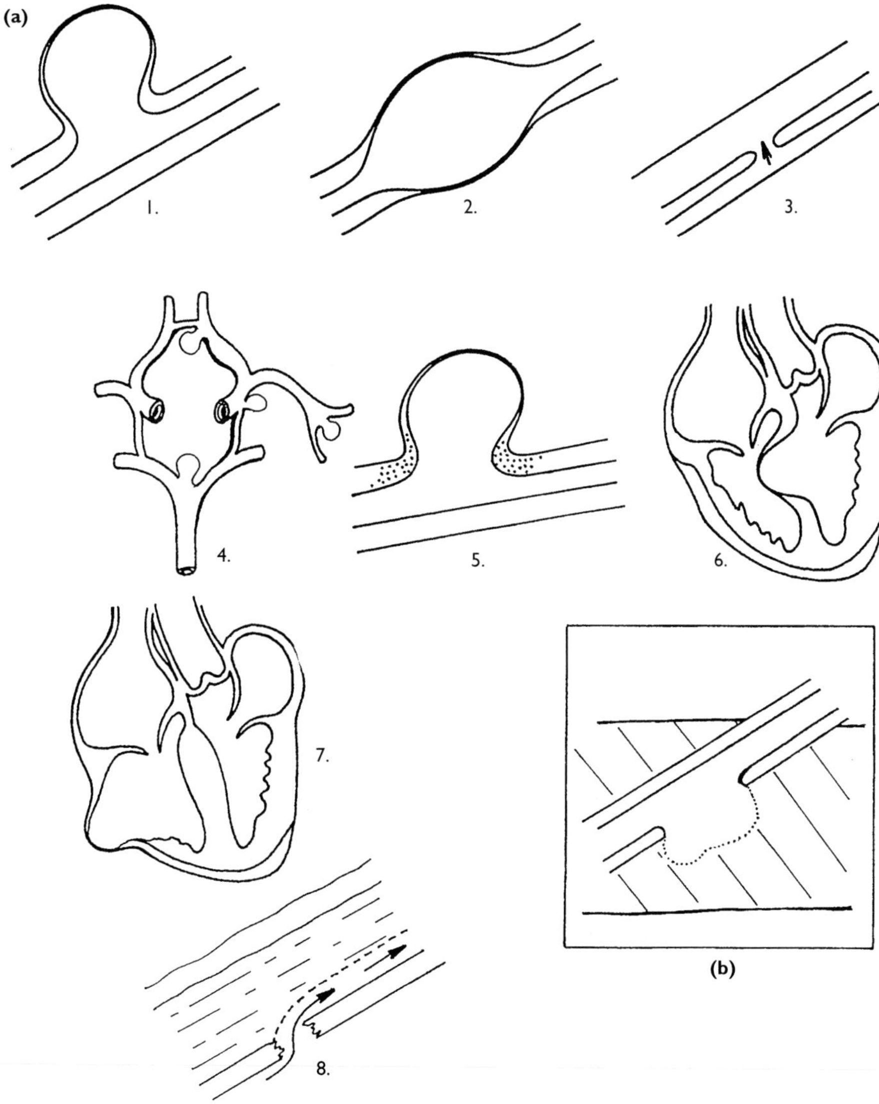

Figure 3 Aneurysms.
(a) True aneurysms. Aneurysm wall is formed by blood vessel(s). 1. Saccular. Note thin wall of dilated vascular segment; 2. Fusiform; 3. Arteriovenous, a form of fistula; 4. Congenital, berry aneurysms at bifurcation of arteries of circle of Willis; 5. Mycotic, the inflammatory reaction destroying arterial tissue at aneurysm margins; 6. Cardiac septal, of a form complicating septal infarction; 7. Cardiac lateral, at a site implicated by Chagas' disease; 8. Dissecting: blood tracks between intima and media or within media.
(b) False aneurysms. Aneurysm wall is formed by surrounding tissue.

FALSE ANEURYSMS

False aneurysms are blood-filled spaces in continuity with the circulation but with part of, or the entire wall, composed of non-vascular tissue. At least part of the wall is deficient. They form, for example, within the pancreas where they can be mistaken for pseudocysts.

COMPLICATIONS OF ANEURYSM

The principal complications of arterial aneurysm are thrombosis, rupture and mechanical disturbance of surrounding tissues. Aneurysm may be complicated by bacterial infection, for example in individuals with hepatic cirrhosis.

Thrombosis

Thrombosis within an arterial aneurysm extends insidiously. Emboli may break away from any surface where recent thrombus is exposed to the circulation.

Rupture

Aneurysmal rupture results in local bleeding and the disruption of nearby tissues. The posterior extension and rupture of an abdominal aortic aneurysm leads to bleeding into the retroperitoneal tissues. Anteriorly, bleeding takes place into the para-aortic tissues, tracking around the internal iliac arteries. Occasionally, a duodenal fistula may be created, with massive bleeding into the intestinal tract. Whether renal function is threatened depends on the site of the aneurysm which is often below the origin of the renal arteries. When subarachnoid haemorrhage complicates congenital aneurysm of the arteries of the circle of Willis, some blood inevitably escapes into adjacent cerebral tissue.

Mechanical effects

Aneurysms tend to enlarge. Mechanical and hydrodynamic effects result. The pulsatile walls of enlarging abdominal aortic aneurysms erode vertebral bodies posteriorly. The intervertebral discs are spared. The radiographic profile of the vertebrae appears 'scalloped'. In a similar fashion, saccular aneurysm of the arch of the aorta may erode sternal and rib bone anteriorly.

ANGIOGENESIS

Angiogenic factors are molecules that promote the growth of blood vessel endothelium. They catalyse the vascularisation of embryonic tissues and make possible the provision of a vascular supply for tissue and organ growth. In disease, angiogenic factors enable capillary buds to extend into the extracellular matrix of avascular tissues such as hyaline articular cartilage or cornea. They also assist the growth of blood vessels into healing infarcts. Angiogenesis is a characteristic of many chronic inflammatory diseases. In rheumatoid arthritis, for example, inflammation and the ingrowth of new, capillary buds, lead to the replacement of marginal cartilage by a rim of vascular granulation tissue. Angiogenesis plays a crucial part in neoplastic growth.

Angiogenesis in cancer

Angiogenesis is a host response in cancer (p. 76, 242). Explants of neoplastic tissue can survive if the mass is no more than 1 mm in diameter. Beyond this size, the establishment of a vascular network is critical to tumour cell growth. Conversely, a reduction in blood supply to a tumour that has already exceeded the critical size of 1.0 mm^3 may result in necrosis.

The provision of a tumour blood supply is stimulated by angiogenic factors derived either from neoplastic cells themselves e.g. vascular endothelial growth factor (VEGF), bFGF and thymidine phosphorylase, or from macrophages e.g. transforming growth factor alpha (TGFα). Malignant angiogenesis is regulated by a balance between angiogenic and anti-angiogenic molecules. Many anti-angiogenic compounds, such as VEGF receptor-inhibitor, inhibit the proliferation of new vessels but do not cause tumour regression. Others such as endostatin stop tumour growth which resumes, however, when treatment ceases. A further category including protamine blocks angiogenesis and can lead to tumour regression.

Now read Blood vessels (p. 48)

ANOXIA/HYPOXIA

Anoxia is the absence of oxygen from the whole or part of the environment. Hypoxia is a relative oxygen lack.

Tissues and organs range in degree of sensitivity to anoxia, from highly sensitive (central nervous system (p. 60), cardiac muscle, renal tubules) to relatively insensitive (skin, fascia, tendons, ligaments, aponeuroses – Table 2). Central nervous system neurones respire aerobically and tolerate anoxia for only 2–4 minutes before permanent injury or death are caused. Tissues such as articular cartilage that respire by anaerobic glycolysis can withstand long periods of hypoxia or anoxia.

All surgical and endoscopic procedures requiring intravenous sedation or inhalational anaesthesia are performed with constant monitoring of peripheral oxygenation by pulse oximetry.

Table 2 Relative oxygen consumption of some body tissues at 37° C

Organ	Oxygen consumption mL/min/kg
Heart	94
Kidney	61
Liver	44
Brain	33
Skeletal muscle	2–3
Articular cartilage	Very small

ANTIBIOTICS

Antibiotics are substances that inhibit the growth of micro-organisms. They are widely used in surgery (Table 3) and surgical prophylaxis and may be administered before, during or after an operation.

Anti-biosis means 'against life': antibiotics are cell poisons and exert injurious effects on human cells as well as on those of micro-organisms. In any infection, bacteria are initially fewer in number than the cells of the host but divide more frequently. As a result, antibiotics are generally more damaging to micro-organisms than to patients. Antibiotics can kill (bactericidal) or inhibit (bacteriostatic) the growth of micro-organisms, *in vivo* or *in vitro*.

Many antibiotics that were originally obtained from living organisms can now be synthesised. Others are manufactured by recombinant gene technology. Among the new antibiotics are members of known antibiotic families e.g. fluoroquinolone derivatives such as moxifloxacin; drugs produced by the anaerobic Actinomycetes spp. such as the streptogramins; and compounds manufactured by screening the inhibitors of defined bacterial targets.

Table 3 Mode of action of some antimicrobial drugs employed in surgery

Actions and class of antibiotic	Examples
Impair the synthesis of the structural glycopeptides of the bacterial wall	Beta-lactams penicillin, ampicillin, flucloxacillin, co-amoxyclavulanate, cephalosporins, imipenem Glycopeptides vancomycin
Affect the function of bacterial cytoplasmic membranes	Polymyxin, amphotericin B
Interfere with nucleic acid synthesis	Quinolones nalidixic acid, ciprofloxacin, metronidazole
Interfere with protein synthesis at the ribosomal level	Aminoglycosides gentamicin Macrolides erythromycin

Antibiotic therapy

Each hospital faces its own problems. In day-to-day surgery, a short, printed guide to first line antimicrobial prescribing should be available. The advice of a bacteriologist, based on the results of cultures, is desirable before deciding upon an antibiotic of choice.

- Cultures should therefore always be taken.
- Selection of antibiotic should be on the basis of the narrowest possible spectrum of antibacterial activity.

Fortunately, strains of organisms such as staphylococci that are resistant to penicillin may retain susceptibility to other agents, for example flucloxacillin, erythromycin, rifampicin, gentamicin, and vancomycin. Gram-negative organisms, especially coliforms, may display multiresistance to most, if not all, of the beta-lactam antibiotics, aminoglycosides and quinolones. Dual antibiotic therapy must sometimes be employed to treat infections caused by these organisms.

NATURAL ANTIBIOTICS

Natural, peptide antibiotics contribute to the innate resistance to invading pathogens of insects, plants and mammals. They have broad antimicrobial activity. Defensin is one member of this group; others include cecropins and magainins. The defensin family shows broad activity against Gram-positive and Gram-negative bacteria, fungi, mycobacteria and enveloped viruses. Natural antibiotics can be isolated from neutrophil polymorphs, macrophages, small intestinal epithelial cells and skin.

Now read Microbial defence (p. 231), Natural immunity (p. 171)

Lysozyme

Lysozyme (p. 371) is an enzyme with antibacterial properties. It is present in tears, nasal and bronchial secretions. Lysozyme has the properties of an antibiotic. Lysozyme and penicillin act by disrupting the same chemical components of bacterial cell walls.

ANTIBIOTIC RESISTANCE

Drug resistance extends to all known micro-organisms and affects pathogens as diverse as the *Mycobacterium bovis* associated with HIV-1 immunosuppression, and the malaria parasite. Many strains of common pathogenic bacteria such as *Staphylococcus aureus* now display multiple resistance to antibiotics and pose a challenge to safe surgery. Threatened by an antibiotic, bacteria mutate quickly: they have very short multiplication times (p. 32).

Now read Bacteria (p. 30)

One factor leading to resistance is the widespread commercial use of antibiotics to promote growth in animals. Ideally, antimicrobials used in this way should not be the same as those employed in man. The recent administration of avoparcin to animals may have been in part responsible for the emergence of vancomycin-resistant organisms in man.

Mechanisms of resistance

Resistance to an antibiotic is acquired by one of two mechanisms:

- **Selection**. Sensitive strains are largely eliminated. However, some resistant organisms persist. The proportion of resistant organisms increases until they predominate. In the case of penicillin, resistance is due to the presence in the resistant bacteria of the enzyme penicillinase.
- **Mutation**. Sensitive strains acquire resistance by mutation (p. 142). The genetic shift may be by transduction (e.g. penicillin resistance); by the acquisition of a plasmid containing a new genetic programme (e.g. gentamicin resistance); or by chromosomal change (e.g. streptomycin resistance).

An increasing proportion of bacteria is now resistant to more than one antibiotic. The frequency of resistance varies according to the extent to which an antibiotic is selected in a particular hospital. The proportion of antibiotic-resistant strains tends to rise if the use of a single antibiotic persists locally, particularly if the drug has a broad spectrum of action. It is desirable to minimise this threat by using an antibiotic for as short a period as possible.

Methicillin and vancomycin

There are particular problems with methicillin-resistant *Staphylococcus aureus* (MRSA), a global, nosocomial pathogen. The organism has become a serious threat to safe surgical practice. In England and Wales, the number of hospitals affected by epidemics of the organism rose from 40/month in 1993 to over 110 in 1996.

Until recently, the answer to MRSA has been the use of vancomycin. However, vancomycin-resistant *Staphylococcus aureus* (VRSA) now offers a new threat and other vancomycin-resistant micro-organisms such as the enterococci are an increasing challenge. The identification in a surgical patient of vancomycin-resistant MRSA *Staphylococcus aureus* demands isolation and immediate communication with the Hospital Infection Control Team. There are few therapeutic options. They include the use of the oxazolidinones and the parenteral streptogramin, quinupristin–dalfopristin.

Now read Hospital acquired infection (p. 159)

ANTIGENS AND ANTIBODIES

ANTIGENS

Antigens are natural or synthetic, organic molecules that can be recognised specifically when they have access to the immune surveillance system of an individual. They are often complex and are usually protein but may be polysaccharide, nucleic acid or lipid. Antigen molecules are of an almost infinitely varied nature. They may be parts of pathogenic micro-organisms; allergens; the cells of transplanted organs; or components of the tissues of an individual him/herself.

Now read Immunity (p. 171)

One part of an antigenic molecule, the **antigenic determinant,** reacts with cells or antibodies in the immune response and dictates its specificity. Another part, the carrier, determines the degree of response. The simplest part of an antigen molecule that can combine with a T-cell receptor (p. 173) or with antibody is an **epitope**. **Haptens** are small molecules or metal ions, not themselves antigenic, that can elicit antibody formation when attached to a large carrier molecule. Penicillin is one example.

The route by which an antigen reaches immunoreactive tissues influences the cellular events leading to immunisation (p. 175). Whether the antigen enters by intradermal, intravenous, respiratory or other pathway modifies the recipient's response, just as do the amount and concentration of antigen. Administered orally, many antigens are destroyed or changed by digestion so that antigenic reactivity is lost or specificity altered. Nevertheless, some protein antigens can be absorbed unchanged from the intestine, to be found in the circulation. Poorly understood mechanisms prevent these antigens from eliciting an immune response except in cases of food or milk allergy in **atopic** persons.

Antigens are more likely to provoke an immune response if they are retained locally, an effect that can be brought about artificially by substances such as killed mycobacteria in oil, which are therefore called **adjuvants**.

ANTIBODIES

Antibodies (Abs) are immunoglobulins (Igs) formed when B lymphocytes encounter antigen (Ag) (p. 172). They are glycoproteins. Antibodies circulate in the bloodstream and are present in the plasma, reaching most extracellular tissue spaces but not the cerebrospinal fluid. The variety of Ags to be recognised in the course of daily life is very large. Immunoglobulin structure reflects this requirement. The **Ag binding sites** of individual Igs are extremely varied. The **non-Ag-binding sites** of the same molecules are less diverse.

Structure of Igs

Each Ig molecule is formed of two 'heavy' and two 'light' amino acid chains (Fig. 4). The names of these chains indicate their relative molecular masses. The chains are assembled into whole Ab molecules after the process of translation (p. 140). The four chains in a molecule are linked together. Each chain has a variable (V) region or 'domain' and a constant (C) region. In turn, each domain comprises a series of units that are sequences of ~110 amino acids. Within each domain, a 'loop' of amino acids is formed by a double bond. Light chains have one V_L and one C_L unit whereas the much larger heavy chains have one V_L and three or four C_L units.

Antibodies are proteins and their structure at all levels of diversity is determined genetically. Each chain is coded by distinct genes. The genes for kappa light chains lie on chromosome 2, those for lambda chains on chromosome 22. All types of heavy chain are coded by genes that are located on chromosome 14.

Properties of Igs

- **Antibody-binding functions**. The sequence of amino acids of the V_L and V_H parts of the Fab region of the Ig molecule are highly variable. Together, these domains form an Ag-binding site unique to each Ab. The identity of this binding site determines the idiotype. It contains the antigen-binding sites characteristic of each Ig molecule and of the clone of B-cells from which it has been secreted (p. 172).
- **Biological functions** (Table 4). By contrast, the constant (Fc) regions of each molecule of one class share the same primary structure. This part of the molecule takes part in the many biological i.e. non-immunological, functions of these molecules such as binding to complement (p. 232).

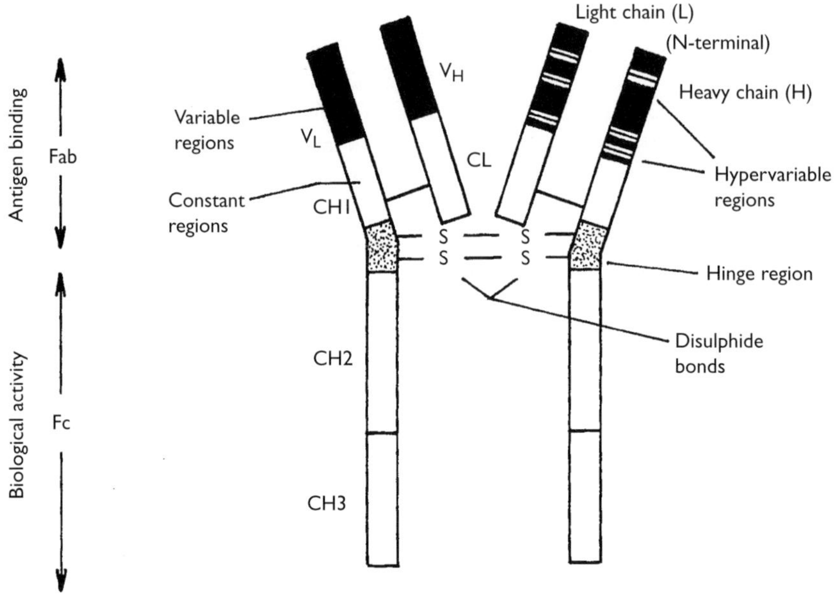

Figure 4 Antibody: immunoglobulin G.
Antibodies (immunoglobulins) are glycoproteins. Basic structure is of four polypeptides: two light (L) chains and two heavy (H) chains. (at left margin) Chains can be separated ('cleaved') to give two Fab fragments that comprise parts of molecule that bind to antigen, and Fc fragment that serves other functions such as combining with complement and binding to macrophages. (centre) Precise Ag binding site of IgG molecule is N-terminal quarter of H-chain together with N-terminal half of L-chain. There are five kinds of H-chain. They specify class of immunoglobulin (IgG, IgM, IgA, IgD, IgE). There are two kinds of L-chain (κ and λ). The five four-chain units of the very large IgM molecule, found mainly in the blood, are held together by a J-chain.

Immunoglobulin classes

On the basis of the type of heavy chain, Igs exist in five classes: G, M, A, D and E (Table 5.) The corresponding heavy chains are γ, μ, α, δ and ε.

- **Immunoglobulin G** (IgG) is the most abundant of the Igs. It combats micro-organisms and toxins extracellularly. IgG is the predominant Ab in the secondary response that follows a primary challenge by Ag (p. 172). IgGs bind macrophages and neutrophil receptors.
- **Immunoglobulin M** (IgM) is the first Ab to appear in a primary immune response (p. 172). IgM molecules are the initial form of Ab manufactured by the newborn child. They circulate as pentameters. The five subunits, each resembling the unit structure of IgG, are joined by a 15 kDa J chain.
- **Immunoglobulin A** (IgA) predominates in secretions such as the saliva, gastro-intestinal secretions, and milk. Two IgA units (monomers) are joined by a J chain and bound to a secretory glycoprotein.
- **Immunoglobulin D** (IgD) is a receptor for Ag on B-cell surfaces.
- **Immunoglobulin E** (IgE) prepares mast cells and basophil leucocytes in type I hypersensitivity reactions (p. 161).

Classification of Igs

Three forms of structural diversity classify Igs:

- **Isotypic**. The five classes described (above) define the **isotypes**. Each Ab isotype has a heavy chain Fc region with individual structural and biological properties distinct from Ab specificity.

Table 4 Biological properties of the immunoglobulins (Igs).

Properties	IgG	IgA	IgM	IgD	IgE
Complement fixation by					
classical pathway	++	±	– –	– –	
alternative pathway	–				
Crosses placenta	+	–	–	–	–
Fixes to homologous mast cells	–	–	–	–	+
Binds to macrophages, polymorphs	+	±	–	–	–

Table 5 Immunoglobulin (Ig) classes.

Ig class	IgG	IgA	IgM	IgD	IgE
Molecular mass of immunoglobulin (kDa)	150	170–420	900	180	190
Heavy chains each of ~440 amino acids	Gamma (γ)	Alpha α)	Mu (μ)	Delta (δ)	Epsilon (ε)
Molecular mass of heavy chains (kDa)	50–55	62	65	70	75
Light chains each of ~220 amino acids	κ or λ	κ or λ	κ or λ	κ or λ	κ or λ
Molecular mass of light chains (kDa)	~23	~23	~23	~23	~23
Serum concentration (mg/mL)	6–16	1.4–4.0	0.4–2.0	0.02–0.4	17–450 ng/mL
% total serum Ig	80	13	6	0–1.0	0.002

A single person is able to make the five different classes (isotypes) of Abs (Table 4) and to switch between these classes (**isotype switching**) at different phases of an immune response. Thus, in reacting to tetanus toxoid, the isotype of the first Ab produced is IgM whereas later in the immune response the isotype becomes IgG. Isotype switching causes a substitution of the non-Ag binding parts of Ig but a retention of the Ag binding site and therefore of Ab specificity.

- **Allotypic**. Immunoglobulins of an identical isotype are not the same in different members of a single species. There are slightly different amino acid sequences. These individual variations are attributable to different Ag determinants in C_L and C_{H2}. There is genetic diversity determined by allelic genes. The varied determinants are allotypic.
- **Idiotypic**. The key to Ab diversity lies in the continual mutations that occur among the genes coding for the amino acid chains that form the hypervariable (V) region of an antibody molecule. These regions are specific to one clone of plasma cells and enable an almost infinite range of Ags to be recognised.

ANTIGEN/ANTIBODY MEASUREMENT

Many techniques of measurement use radio-active isotopes as labels that can be measured with precision; these methods are the basis of radio-immunoassay.

Alternative, non-radio-active assays employ enzyme-conjugated reagents in a similar way to the avidin-biotin technique (p. 158).

Antigen measurement

Antigen is added to the material to be tested. Anti-immunoglobulin labelled with a radio-active isotope is then used to measure the quantity of Ag–Ab binding. The technique is very sensitive. Very small amounts of Ag can be assayed. Among them are polypeptide hormones, tumour markers, hepatitis B surface antigen and other proteins, as well as smaller molecules including digoxin, morphine-like compounds, steroids and the prostaglandins.

Antibody measurement

Antigen in known amount is stuck on beads of polymer or in plastic wells and incubated with the solution to be tested. An anti-Ig labelled with a radio-active isotope such as ^{125} iodine, ^{3} hydrogen, or ^{14} carbon is added. The amount of labelled Ab bound to this Ag–Ab complex is determined by counts of emitted gamma-rays or beta particles.

ANTINEOPLASTIC DRUGS

Antineoplastic, chemotherapeutic drugs are employed in the treatment of cancer.

The management of many forms of tumour is now in the hands of teams of surgical, medical, oncological and laboratory specialists. The best use of surgery may be before or after regimes of chemotherapy. In terms of the degree of their response to currently available chemotherapy, tumours may be classified:

- First, as being curable (testicular carcinoma, Wilms' tumour, Hodgkin's and non-Hodgkin's lymphoma and acute leukaemia).
- Second, as yielding a large and significant response (small cell carcinoma of lung; carcinomas of breast, bladder, anus, uterine cervix and ovary).
- Third, as yielding only minor, insignificant changes (non-small cell carcinomas of lung; carcinoma of colon, liver (hepatocellular), kidney, pancreas and prostate, as well as malignant melanoma, astrocytoma and Kaposi's sarcoma).

CLASSES OF CHEMOTHERAPEUTIC DRUGS

Antineoplastic, chemotherapeutic drugs are classified according to their chemical structure or by their biological properties.

- One class is active against dividing and non-dividing cells.
- A second class such as methotrexate and vincristine is effective in only one phase of the cycle of cell division (p. 84). They are **phase specific** and must be given repeatedly to be effective.
- A further class is active against cells in all phases of the cell cycle. They are said to be **phase non-specific** and tend to be effective only against slowly growing tumours.

Anticancer compounds are also classified according to the relationship between their mechanisms of action and the tumours against which they are most potent. Thus, antipurines are employed against acute leukaemia and breast cancer, oestrogens against prostatic cancer and steroids against lymphoma.

- **Antimetabolites.** These drugs are structural analogues of the nucleosides of DNA or of precursors or cofactors essential for the synthesis of the nucleic acids. Methotrexate, for example, is a structural analogue of folic acid (p. 352). It competes with this molecule, preventing nuclear maturation. Other antimetabolites include the pyrimidine-analogue compounds 5-fluorouracil, cytarabine, fludarabine and 6-mercaptopurine. Although 5-fluorouracil can be infused into the hepatic artery for the treatment of hepatic metastases, the other pyrimidine analogues find a place mainly in the treatment of the leukaemias.
- **Alkylating agents.** In these widely used anti-tumour compounds, alkyl groups are substituted for some of the hydrogen atoms, preventing DNA replication and RNA transcription. Melphalan and cyclophosphamide are examples. Irradiation with X-rays or gamma-rays has similar effects and these chemotherapeutic drugs are therefore said to be **radiomimetic**. Other alkylating agents include the nitroso-ureas and platinum-containing compounds such as cisplatin. The former are particularly effective against tumours of the central nervous system because of lipid solubility and good penetration. The latter are active against lung, ovarian, testicular, bladder, and head and neck tumours.
- **Antibiotics.** Many potent antibiotics, such as the anthracycline daunorubicin and its analogue

doxorubicin (adriamycin), inhibit the synthesis of DNA and/or RNA. They have a wide spectrum of activity and are myelosuppressive. However, doxorubicin, in particular, is also effective in the treatment of carcinomas of the lung, breast, stomach, bladder, prostate and thyroid.

- **Plant alkaloids.** These substances block the function of the protein of the microtubules essential for the mitotic division of cells (p. 86). Vincristine is such an agent.
- **Other anticancer drugs**. Further compounds include nitroso-ureas such as carmustine, and enzymes such as l-asparaginase.
- **Hormone receptor blockers**. Advances in endocrinology have led to increased understanding of hormone binding and activation. Tamoxifen is an agent that blocks oestrogen receptors. The use of this drug, which has been advocated for the prophylaxis of breast cancer (p. 67), carries a very slightly enhanced risk of the development of uterine endometrial carcinoma (p. 341).

COMBINATION CHEMOTHERAPY

Advantage is now often taken of the different modes of action of individual chemotherapeutic agents to devise combined regimes in which several different compounds are given together or in sequence.

DRUG RESISTANCE

Resistance to **single** chemotherapeutic drugs is the result of a number of different mechanisms, some indirect. For example, chemotherapy with drugs affecting a tumour-cell enzyme can induce the production of different forms of the enzyme that are less sensitive to the drug. Alternatively, as in the case of methotrexate, there may be increased synthesis of a tumour-cell enzyme upon which the chemotherapeutic drug exerts its anticancer effects.

Resistance to a **range** of cytotoxic drugs may be due to the expression by neoplastic cells, including those of colorectal, renal and pancreatic carcinomas, of a multiple drug resistance gene, *mdr-1*. This gene encodes P-glycoprotein, a membrane molecule. The protein provides an export system for anticancer drugs, which therefore attain only low intracellular concentrations.

ANTISEPSIS/ASEPSIS

Antisepsis is the prevention of the growth and multiplication of the micro-organisms that cause sepsis. Asepsis is the exclusion of these organisms from the tissues. The terms antisepsis and asepsis should be clearly distinguished.

ANTISEPSIS

Antiseptics (pp. 178, 373) are mild disinfectants, devoid of significant irritative and sensitising properties and therefore suitable for application to the skin. The disinfectants are described on p. 118.

Now read Disinfection (p. 118), Hospital acquired infection (p. 159), Sterilisation p. 304

ASEPSIS

Asepsis exists when live, pathogenic micro-organisms are excluded from the environment. In practice, the methods of antisepsis and asepsis are employed together. Before surgery, bacterial colonisation of the skin is reduced by bathing. Within the operating theatre all instruments, dressings and appliances used in surgery are sterilised, usually by heating them in an autoclave. The patient's skin, at and near an operating site, is prepared by shaving or depilation and washed with antiseptic.

The techniques of antisepsis and asepsis are effective against most vegetative forms of bacteria but spores, such as those of *Clostridium difficile*, and the transmissible agent of Creutzfeldt–Jakob dementia, are frequently unaffected. Even when operations are performed in specially designed theatres in which the site of operation is exposed only to filtered air, there remains a small incidence of wound infection caused by organisms that escape these exacting preventative measures.

ANTIVIRAL AGENTS

Antiviral agents may be natural or pharmacological. They act against viruses to destroy or inactivate them. The most important of the natural antiviral agents is the family of interferons.

Interferons

The interferons (IFN) are a family of small proteins formed by cells infected by virus.

Interferons are best formed in cells infected by viruses that do not cause cell death quickly. Liberated into the extracellular fluids, interferons bind to receptors on nearby, uninfected cells. Genes are activated within these cells, leading to the synthesis of enzymes that both degrade viral and host mRNA, blocking viral protein synthesis. Interferons have further, important properties. They include the inhibition of cell division; the increase of antigen expression; boosting the action of NK-cells; and amplification of the ability of some neoplastic cells to activate complement via the alternative pathway.

There are three interferon families:

- IFNα. Leucocytes manufacture IFNα. There are at least 14 proteins in this category.
- IFNβ. Fibroblasts and other cells make IFNβ.
- IFNγ. IFNγ is produced like a cytokine (p. 114) after sensitised T-cells have bound specific antigen.

Interferons are potent therapeutic agents. The presence of as few as 10–12 molecules is sufficient to enable a cell to resist viral infection. Interferons manufactured by recombinant gene technology are under trial for active protection against infection with herpes virus and HBV; they offer hope as agents in the therapy of breast, bone marrow and skin cancer although these prospective uses are complicated by the hazards of bone-marrow cell depression.

Antiviral drugs

An increasing number of effective antiviral agents has been discovered (Table 6). However, the emergence of strains resistant to antiviral agents is a growing problem. In retroviral infections such as AIDS (p. 2), the plasma viral load, like the numbers of Th CD4 lymphocytes in the circulating blood, is of prognostic significance. The aim of treatment is to suppress viral replication. One measure of success is a decrease in the number of virus copies in the plasma to below 5000/mL. Two or three drugs can be used in combination. The combination of two nucleosides together with a potent protease inhibitor is one example.

- **Antiviral agents in transplantation**. Ganciclovir started 10 days before operation and continued for 98 days post-operatively, is effective in preventing CMV infection in liver transplant patients.

Table 6 Examples of antiviral agents of use in surgery

Antiviral agent	Example
Those that block viral RNA or DNA synthesis	Zidovudine (AZT): useful for the control of asymptomatic HIV infection and for the treatment of AIDS and AIDS-related disorders Acyclovir: effective in the treatment of Herpes virus infections
Those that prevent viral penetration and uncoating	Amantidine: inhibits influenza virus A but not virus B
Those that inhibit viral protein synthesis	Interferons: effective in chronic hepatitis B and C infections

- **Anti-retroviral agents**. Zidovudine is a nucleoside analogue. Nevarapine is a new antiretroviral drug used in treating HIV. Lamivudine is another.
- **Protease inhibitors**. Ritonavir, a potent orally bio-available inhibitor of HIV-1 aspartyl protease, lowers the risk of complications after HIV infection and prolongs survival. Saquinavir, nelfinavir, abacavir and idinavir are similar compounds.

ARTERIES

The extent of the arterial circulation exerts a profound influence on the pathogenesis, anatomical location and severity of disease. For example, the degree of infarction of viscera such as the large intestine is determined by the territorial distribution of the intestinal arteries and the adequacy of the anastomoses between them. When a femoral artery is occluded, arterial circulation through the profunda femoris is often sufficient to maintain a circulation to the limb. In bone, osteomyelitis (p. 53) originates at the metaphyses in the end-arteries within which blood-borne staphylococci lodge.

The differential distribution of blood flow can be shown by injecting a microbubble contrast agent. The contrast agent contains galactose microparticles which dissolve in water to release bubbles small enough to pass through capillaries but large enough not to pass cell membranes. The surface tension of the bubbles, and thus their longevity, is reduced by the addition of palmitic acid, a lipid.

Arterial disease is an unavoidable feature of life in Western societies; it is much less frequent in African populations where malnutrition is endemic. Many arterial diseases are confined to individual races. Thus, Moyamoya disease, a spontaneous occlusion of the Circle of Willis, is encountered only in the Japanese.

Now read Blood vessels (p. 48)

Particular arteries are prone to individual diseases. The aorta is the site for saccular and dissecting aneurysm, the mouths of the renal arteries targets for intimal fibromuscular hyperplasia. The popliteal artery is susceptible to saccular aneurysm or, less commonly, to dissecting aneurysm, entrapment and thrombosis while the musculo-elastic arteries of the lower limb are common sites for medial sclerosis and atheroma.

Biopsy diagnosis of arterial disease

Arterial biopsy is only occasionally necessary. Thus, in giant-cell arteritis, a portion of the temporal artery is removed to allow histological confirmation of the diagnosis. Magnetic resonance imaging (MRI) and computed tomography can be used to 'look up' the aorta and its branches. This technique, **virtual angioscopy**, is employed to assess intracranial aneurysm (p.65).

DEVELOPMENTAL AND CONGENITAL DISORDERS

Severe malformations (p. 226) of arteries are incompatible with intra-uterine development and survival. One example is persistence of a vitelline artery. The vessel takes the place of the umbilical artery in the placental circulation. Blood is shunted from the caudal end of the embryo so that one lower limb does not form. The stillborn infant suffers from sirenomelia and appears to be a 'mermaid'.

Among the heritable abnormalities of arteries compatible with adult life are the defects in the elastic lamina of the vessels of the circle of Willis that lead to berry aneurysm (p. 65) and the arterial disorders of the Ehlers–Danlos syndrome (p. 190).

INFECTION AND INFLAMMATION

Thrombo-angiitis obliterans (Buerger's disease)

In thrombo-angiitis, a disorder of men, not women, parts of arteries and of the accompanying veins are foci for low-grade inflammation. Entire neurovascular bundles may be implicated, one explanation for the pain which is a hallmark of the disease. Arterial thrombosis is likely and the consequent ischaemia may culminate in gangrene. The legs are affected much more often than the arms. The cause of the disorder, to which cigarette-smokers are prone, remains uncertain. An association with the MHC antigens HLA-A9 and B5 (p. 330) suggests the influence of racial and genetic susceptibility.

Now read Veins (p. 344)

Arteritis

Inflammation of arterial walls may be caused by bacterial and fungal infection, infected emboli, trauma and by the injection of infected material such as the substances used by drug abusers. Bacteria that settle in arterial walls include *Staphylococcus aureus*, Salmonella spp. and *Pseudomonas aeruginosa*. The consequences of bacterial and fungal arteritis include mycotic aneurysm (p. 14).

Arteries are also susceptible to the damaging effects of small immune complexes (p. 161) which lodge in the vessel wall and incite inflammation, with focal, segmental vascular destruction. This form of vasculitis is characteristic of systemic auto-immune connective tissue diseases such as rheumatoid arthritis and polyarteritis nodosa.

ARTERIALISATION

The word arterialisation is used in two ways.

- In a first sense, a vein is said to be arterialised when it is placed in functional continuity with an artery. One example is the use of part of a saphenous vein to construct a coronary artery bypass. A similar approach employs a vein to receive arterial blood directly in procedures designed to relieve distal limb ischaemia: the vein forms new smooth muscle, becomes thicker and stronger but remains susceptible to arterial disease, particularly atheroma.

- In a second sense, venous blood is said to be arterialised when it is exposed to oxygen in the lungs.

ARTERIOSCLEROSIS

Arteriosclerosis means a 'hardening of the arteries'. The word is used very freely to indicate all forms of degenerative arterial disease and it therefore includes atheroma, atherosclerosis and Mönkeberg's medial sclerosis. Arteriolosclerosis is an analogous term for diseases of arterioles such as those affected in systemic hypertension.

ATHEROMA

The word atheroma means 'porridge'. Atheroma is the progressive accumulation of lipid-rich plaques in the arterial intima. Medium-size and large musculoelastic, systemic arteries are particularly at risk but the endocardium, the intima of veins that transport blood at arterial pressures and the lining of lung arteries in cases of pulmonary hypertension, are also affected.

Causes

Factors predisposing to atherogenesis are genetic and acquired. Age, sex, diet, sedentary occupations, endocrine disorders such as diabetes mellitus and myxoedema, hypertension and cigarette smoking are among the known causes.

- **Race**. Atheroma is prevalent in well-nourished, Western societies. It is infrequent in African populations existing on low calorie diets containing little animal fat.
- **Heredity**. The smooth-muscle cells of an atheromatous plaque are monoclonal (p. 83). A neoplastic-like transformation of vascular smooth-muscle cells may be a factor in the genesis of the arterial lesion.
- **Age and sex**. Although atheroma is first encountered clinically in young and middle-aged men, the vascular changes originate in childhood. The frequency of severe disease is much higher in men than women until the age of 45–50 when, after the menopause, the frequency of atheromatous lesions complicated by thrombosis or aneurysm is as high in adult females as it is in males. Atheroma is less severe among athletes than among those who do not practice regular, vigorous exercise.
- **Hydrodynamics**. Atheroma is commonplace at sites of turbulent blood flow such as the most proximal parts of the coronary arteries and in regions of high blood pressure and rapid flow. Turbulent blood flow and mechanical injury to the endothelium precipitate endothelial disturbance.
- **Coagulation mechanisms**. Endothelial injury may be caused by free oxygen radicals (p. 133). It provokes platelet adherence. Atheroma is not initiated if blood platelets are absent. Platelets adhere to the connective tissue collagen exposed by endothelial cell loss and are activated; they liberate platelet-derived growth factor (PDGF) that acts upon medial smooth-muscle cells.
- **Lipids**. The accumulation of lipid (p. 207) in the intima is central to atherogenesis. Populations with high living standards, a high intake of fat containing saturated fatty acids and high plasma levels of low-density lipoproteins (LDL) have an incidence of atheroma much greater than identical ethnic groups living in conditions of malnutrition. Lipid accumulates in the arterial intima at sites of smooth-muscle multiplication but these cells themselves may synthesise lipid or avidly phagocytose lipid micelles. By contrast, high-density lipoproteins (HDL) are protective; they collect cholesterol from peripheral sites, a process known as **reverse cholesterol transport** and deliver it to the liver and sterol-metabolising organs. HDL deficiency, which may be heritable, may therefore promote atherogenesis.

Structure

Arterial smooth muscle cells migrate into the intima and multiply. The cells synthesise new collagen and proteoglycan. There is low-grade inflammation. The intima increases in thickness and extent. Subsequently, secondary thrombus forms and this material, covered by a neo-endothelium, becomes a yellow atheromatous plaque. When thrombi form on the surface of the plaque, or other changes such as intramural haemorrhage occur, the lesion is described as 'complicated'. The limited, simple, plaques of early life become hard and thickened owing to the formation of new collagen. The term **atherosclerosis** is then used to describe the ageing lesion in which deposits of calcium occur.

The anatomical lesions of atheroma and atherosclerosis are located mainly at the sites of origin of the cerebral, coronary, intestinal, renal and limb arteries.

Partial occlusion by the plaque itself, superadded thrombosis, regional ischaemia and infarction or gangrene are the most common pathological results. Aneurysms develop. They may be saccular, fusiform or dissecting (p. 14). The common consequences of atheroma are stroke, myocardial infarction, intestinal infarction, renal ischaemia, secondary hypertension and lower-limb gangrene.

Behaviour and prognosis

When atheroma affects smaller, muscular arteries, such as those of the brain, the presence of the plaques may be sufficient to impede blood flow significantly. However, many of the circulatory changes caused by atheroma are due to superadded thrombosis, aneurysm, dissection or embolisation.

Because of the high frequency of atheroma in Western society, the disorder has become of great surgical importance. The more slowly developing results of atheroma, such as angina pectoris and aneurysm, can be treated by surgical techniques such as angioplasty, vascular grafting or the implantation of substitute plastic vessels.

Much effort has been directed to identifying ways of preventing atheroma. The possibility of using local gene therapy to alter the behaviour of the cells of atheromatous plaques has heightened hopes of effective treatment.

MECHANICAL INJURY AND TRAUMA

Arteries are resistant to minor trauma and their walls are very resilient. They tolerate tensile, compressive and shear stress and are torn with difficulty. However, severe physical injury, for example by high-velocity projectiles such as rifle bullets, is immediately destructive and penetrating injuries lead to profuse haemorrhage.

Arteries are susceptible to accidental or deliberate incision. Occupational injuries of this kind, encountered in butchers, shoe makers and lathe workers, may culminate in aneurysm. Similar injuries are frequent in assaults. Mechanical penetration by needle puncture is quickly followed by healing but larger stab wounds, such as those incurred during arterial catheterisation or caused by knives, may result in the delayed development of false aneurysms (p. 16).

Arteries are not immediately damaged by ionising radiation but 'endarteritis' (endarterial fibromuscular hyperplasia) often develops after irradiation (p. 186) and interferes with tissue healing if further surgery is required. Arterial walls resist most chemical injuries; however, strong acids applied externally or local injections of steroidal anaesthetic agents can cause sufficient disturbance to lead to local thrombosis. Arteries also resist external neoplastic cell infiltration as long as blood flow is active. When thrombosis occurs and the movement of blood ceases, cancer cells readily penetrate arterial walls.

Thrombosis and embolism

Many of the disorders outlined above lead to arterial thrombosis, a common complication of diabetes mellitus. Arterial embolism is a frequent result of endocardial thrombosis complicating myocardial infarction. When there is patency of the cardiac septa, thrombus originating in the venous system may lead to 'paradoxical' arterial embolism (p. 124).

Now read Thrombus (p. 320)

ASBESTOS – ASBESTOSIS

Asbestos is a carcinogen. There is an increased probability of bronchial carcinoma, a synergistic and carcinogenic relationship with cigarette smoking, and the likelihood of mesothelioma of the pleura (p. 274). The risks of neoplasia are dose-related so that only those workers with prolonged, heavy exposure are liable to develop either cancer.

Asbestos was an important commercial product. The various forms of asbestos are minerals; they are fibrous, hydrated silicates. There are two principal forms of the mineral: serpentine asbestos like chrysotile (curly, flexible fibres), and amphibole asbestos (straight, stiff, brittle fibres). Although both forms are actively fibrogenic, in terms of mesothelioma the less prevalent amphiboles are much more pathogenic than the more common serpentines. The flexible serpentines are impacted in the upper respiratory tract and removed by ciliary action. The stiff amphiboles align themselves in the air stream, reach the alveoli, penetrate epithelial cells and lodge in the interstitial tissues.

Asbestos proved to be an excellent insulating material and was used to lag boilers and pipes, to make brake linings and for fire-proofing. During the manufacture of asbestos-containing materials, a fine, fibrogenic dust was created and inhaled. Prolonged inhalation culminated in **asbestosis**, a diffuse pneumoconiosis scheduled for compensation as an industrial disease and often complicated by the development of tuberculosis.

Now read Mesothelioma (p. 274)

ATROPHY

Atrophy is a decrease in the size of one or more cells of a tissue or of a part or organ.

The umbilical tissues atrophy following birth and embryonic rudiments such as those of the branchial clefts wholly or partly atrophy at this time. Muscle and bone atrophy accompanies disuse. Pressure, ischaemia, nerve injury or mechanical obstruction may each contribute to atrophy under particular circumstances.

The atrophy of nerves is a special case. Following proximal injury, Wallerian degeneration interrupts the structure of axons peripheral to the site of disruption (p. 248). In another example, the kidney and liver are frequently the site of simultaneous atrophy and aplasia. When a small kidney is recognised in the presence of a normal-sized ureter, the reduction in size of the kidney may be assumed to be atrophic, not aplastic: renal aplasia would be accompanied by a correspondingly small ureter. The atrophy of heart muscle cells in old age is 'brown' atrophy: a lipofuscin pigment accumulates inside the cells and a diminishing quantity of contractile protein leads to the reduced size of the cell.

Sudeck's atrophy

Sudeck's atrophy, also known as 'reflex sympathetic dystrophy', is an acute disorder of bone and of the overlying soft tissues, usually of the hand or foot, at the site of an injury. There are two stages: first, a hot-phase, with a disorder of the circulation provoked by sympathetic nervous system hypertonus; second, a cold phase, with consequent, trophic changes in the tissues. There is osteoporosis. Vitamin C may be preventative.

Now read Hypertrophy (p. 144)

AUDIT

In clinical terms, audit is the monitoring and measuring at regular intervals of the results of different surgical treatments undertaken in different institutions. In financial terms, it describes an examination and verification of accounts.

Clinical audit centres on the continuing collection and appropriate analysis of data to enable improvements to be made in practice. The greatest difficulty is to ensure that such assessments are made on comparable populations of patients. Some surgical specialties such as cardiac surgery lend themselves easily to meaningful assessment. Pre-operative assessment is standardised. There are well recognised outcomes and only a limited number of operations is performed. In other specialties such as gastro-intestinal surgery, outcomes are more difficult to judge due to the great variety of diseases encountered and the many different operations undertaken. The process of audit should be interdisciplinary, confidential, democratic, and involve all members of a clinical team. Each meeting should be chaired by a consultant on a rotational basis and minutes should be kept, distributed and agreed.

Now read Trauma (p. 332)

AUTO-IMMUNE DISEASE

Auto-immune reactivity

Auto-immunity is a description for an immunological or hypersensitivity reaction directed against antigens of the 'self'. There is a breakdown of tolerance.

Now read Tolerance (p. 175)

B- and T-cell suppressor activity diminishes with age. The increased tendency for auto-immune diseases in the old may be a result of this change. Either humoral or cell-mediated reactions occur against self-antigens and the disturbance caused in this way may be sufficiently severe to lead to tissue injury. As well as the failure to recognise self-antigens with the initiation of a correspondingly inappropriate immune response, there may be a similar failure in the aged to recognise foreign antigens. This defect may help to explain the increased incidence of malignant disease.

Among the disorders that may be initiated and the causative antibodies are:

- **Chronic active hepatitis** (anti-smooth muscle).
- **Primary biliary cirrhosis** (anti-mitochondrial).
- **Diabetes mellitus** (anti-cell surface insulin receptors).
- **Rheumatoid arthritis** (soluble, circulating, anti-immunoglobulins – rheumatoid 'factors').
- **Systemic lupus erythematosus** (anti-dsDNA).
- **Rheumatic fever** (anti-heart muscle surface molecules).
- **Pernicious anaemia** (anti-soluble, non-circulating intrinsic factor).
- **Goodpasture's syndrome** (anti-lung and anti-kidney basement membranes).

AUTOPSY

Autopsy is the procedure of determining the site, nature and extent of disease by personal inspection and examination of a body after death, i.e. *post-mortem*. It is the only certain means of deciding the reasons for death and ultimate outcome of surgical procedures. A search for factors that may have contributed unexpectedly to death and the inspection of operation sites in patients who have died is therefore integral to good surgical practice.

Under British law, signed consent must be obtained from the 'next of kin' before an autopsy may be performed. An autopsy conducted without the consent of a relative, or without instruction by the appropriate official may constitute a criminal offence. 'Next of kin' may authorise an autopsy provided that enquiries have shown that the deceased had not expressed an objection. However, no organs may be retained for examination or for teaching, unless written consent has been granted. Consent for an autopsy should not be sought if a death has already been reported to the Procurator Fiscal in Scotland or to the Coroner elsewhere in Great Britain as a body becomes their 'property' until it is released. The body is examined and disposed of according to their instructions. If, after an autopsy, there is reason to suspect that death was unnatural or accidental, the legal officers must be informed. In Scotland, the Procurator Fiscal then decides on the appropriate course of action. In the remainder of Great Britain, an inquest is called by HM Coroner.

Without statutory obligation, it is customary for deaths from accident, suicide or homicide to be notified. Throughout Britain, all deaths are reportable that occur after anaesthesia, particularly if the patient has not regained consciousness and when death may have resulted by mishap. In England, deaths occurring within 24 hours of admission to hospital are reported as are all uncertifiable deaths throughout Great Britain. In cases reported to the Fiscal or Coroner, tissue or organs needed for transplantation cannot be removed without their consent.

B

BACTERIA

Bacteria are very small, free-living, unicellular organisms.

- **Cocci** are spherical. Streptococci grow in chains. Staphylococci multiply in clusters. Meningococci, gonococci and pneumococci form pairs.
- **Bacilli** are rod-shaped cells.
- **Vibrios** are short, curved rods.

Many bacteria found in man depend upon the life of the native tissues. Some are commensal and survive in symbiosis. Other bacteria of surgical significance are parasitic. The advantages of symbiosis are often mutual and may be crucial to survival. For example, bacteria thrive in the distal part of the small intestine and synthesise nutritional substances such as vitamin K that are essential to the host.

Cell structure

- **Plasma membrane**. The living material of a bacterium is circumscribed by a thin plasma membrane (Fig. 5). There are no mitochondria and metabolic processes that may be aerobic or anaerobic take place largely within the membrane.
- **Cell wall.** The plasma membrane is covered by a peptidoglycan cell wall (Fig. 6).
- **Capsule**. Occasionally, there is an additional protective polypeptide or polysaccharide capsule.
- **Genetic material**. There is no nucleus but only a coil of dsDNA together with minute, circular plasmids that also contain DNA.

Motility

- **Flagellae**. Some bacteria are motile. Movement is made possible by helical, filamentous flagella composed of strongly antigenic proteins, flagellins.

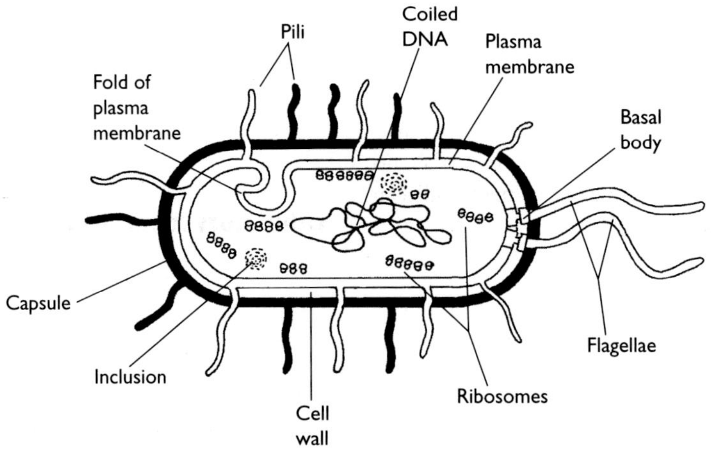

Figure 5 Bacterial cell.
Surface of bacterium is formed by complex cell wall beyond which may be capsule, pili and flagellae. Cell wall surrounds the plasma membrane. Many bacterial cell functions are undertaken by systems that are part of this membrane. Cytoplasm contains numerous ribosomes. Genetic information is carried by circular coil of dsDNA loosely termed a chromosome; it differs in structure from mammalian chromosomes. There is no nuclear membrane. Some DNA is also present outside the bacterial 'chromosome'; it is in the form of small, circular plasmids.

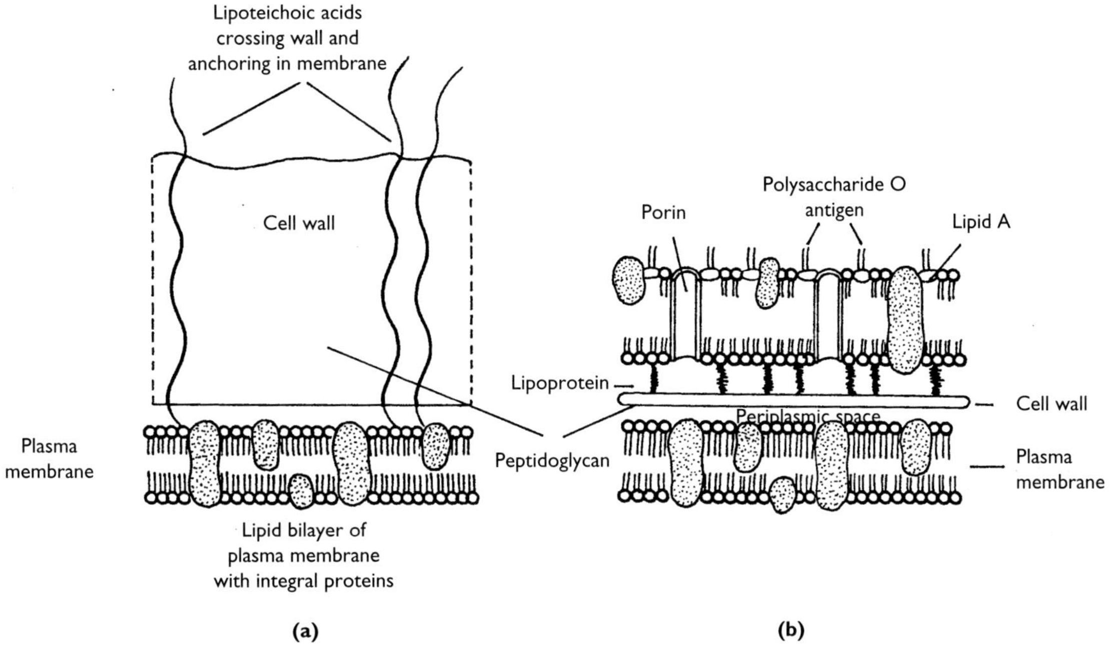

Figure 6 Bacterial cell wall.
Cell wall structure determines whether bacteria are Gram-positive or Gram-negative. Much of bacterial cell wall is peptidoglycan.
(a) Gram-positive bacteria. Peptidoglycan forms a thick layer outside the plasma membrane.
(b) Gram-negative bacteria. Peptidoglycan layer is thin and anchored to lipoprotein in peptidoglycan layer. Lipopolysaccharides of membrane are a form of pathogen conserved molecular pattern. They are synthesised only by bacteria, not by host, and are recognised by receptors of the innate immune system. In some bacteria, of which *Streptococcus pneumoniae* (the pneumococcus) is an example, there is a further outer layer of high molecular weight polysaccharide that protects bacterial cell against phagocytosis, thereby ensuring virulence and pathogenicity.

- **Pili**. Pili enable organisms to attach to the surface of a host epithelial cell by means of molecules termed adhesins. *Escherichia coli* attach to uro-epithelium but gonococci have pili that play no part in movement. The presence of many pili can deter phagocytosis.

Spores

Some bacteria package themselves into spores and enter a resting phase. *Clostridium tetani* (p. 94) is one example: the organisms have a drumstick-shaped structure with a round, projecting, terminal spore. They can survive long periods in adverse environmental conditions and can be carried in dust and soil. Spores are particularly resistant to heat, drying, ultraviolet light, ionising radiation and disinfectants. Germination takes place when the environment becomes less hostile. Organisms such as *Bacillus anthracis* (anthrax) and *Clostridium perfringens* (gas gangrene – p. 137) do not form spores in living tissues.

Laboratory identification of bacteria

To identify an organism from a particular patient or outbreak of infection requires a combination of many or all of the methods used in a medical microbiology laboratory. They include microscopy, culture and biochemical tests. Other procedures may be necessary, especially if a suspect organism cannot be cultivated or a rapid diagnosis is demanded. These additional methods include:

- **Bacterial components**. Searching for characteristic parts of the bacteria such as cell wall components or extracellular toxins. One example is the direct toxin test for *Clostridium difficile*.

- **Antibody formation**. Demonstrating a high or rising titre of antibodies against a causative organism such as *Salmonella typhi*.
- **Gene sequences**. Identifying specific gene sequences in clinical material or from isolated organisms such as *Mycobacterium tuberculosis*.

Some micro-organisms can be recognised by light microscopy without any prior preparation of a sample. Thus, ova, cysts and parasites may be identified in a stool. Bacteria, however, cannot be imaged in this way and must be stained with a combination of dyes to aid identification.

Gram's stain

Gram's stain (p. 17) is particularly useful for this purpose. It enables the provisional identification of bacteria in smears or sediments of pus, cerebrospinal fluid, blood, synovial fluid, pleural and other exudates. The method is also of value for detecting bacteria in tissue sections and wound swabs and after the successful cultivation of micro-organisms in the laboratory.

The mechanism of the stain relates to bacterial structure (Figs 5 and 6). It allows bacteria to be divided into two classes, Gram-positive and Gram-negative:

- In **Gram-positive** bacteria, the cell wall is thick and contains other large molecules.
- In **Gram-negative** bacteria, the cell wall is thin but covered by an outer membrane of lipoprotein and lipopolysaccharide.

A third category of organism, the Mycobacteria, and Nocardia such as *Nocardia asteroides,* contain a wax that stains poorly with Gram's method. These bacteria are acid-fast (p. 237) and require a different staining procedure, the Ziehl–Neelsen reaction.

On the basis of the Gram stain, sufficient evidence can be obtained to permit appropriate antibiotic treatment to be chosen. Three examples are:

- The recognition of Gram-positive cocci such as *Streptococcus pneumoniae* in a case of post-operative pneumonia.
- The detection of Gram-negative bacilli such as *Escherichia coli* or other coliforms in a patient with urinary infection.
- The finding of the Gram-positive sulphur granules of *Actinomyces israelii* in an abdominal abscess.

Bacterial growth and culture

In searching for the cause of a bacterial infection, priority is often given to growth of the responsible micro-organism by culture. It is therefore useful to understand how bacterial growth takes place.

Bacterial growth

Bacteria divide by simple binary fission: a cross-wall extends inwards and splits the cell into two equal parts. Before division occurs, the cells increase in size. There are large differences in the frequency of bacterial bisection. The rate of bacterial cell division depends on the genus as well as on the conditions of growth. Thus, the schism of coliforms such as *Escherichia coli* can occur every 15–20 minutes and continues until the available energy sources are exhausted. By contrast, *Mycobacterium tuberculosis*, the tubercle bacillus, divides only once every 12–24 hours.

An initial **lag phase** of bacterial growth (Fig. 7) is succeeded by a **logarithmic phase**. The rate of multiplication then remains stationary before declining and ultimately ceasing. After 2–5 hours, sufficient growth has often occurred to permit preliminary identification by physicochemical techniques such as chromatography. After 18–20 hours, enough bacteria have formed to cause a tube of broth in an incubator at 37°C to become turbid, a rough indication of the time taken for significant wound infection to be established clinically.

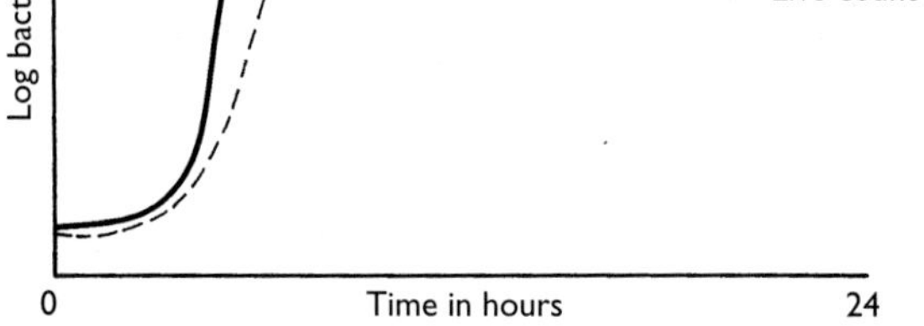

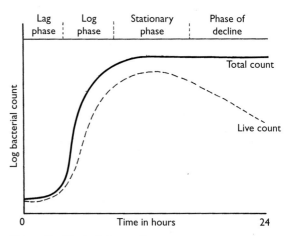

Figure 7 Bacterial growth.
Bacteria inoculated into growth medium multiply very rapidly by binary fission. Figure shows an initial short lag phase before division begins; then a period (the log phase) of accelerated growth in which bacterial cell numbers increase exponentially; and finally a stationary phase, followed by growth cessation. Curves compare total numbers of bacteria with numbers that are viable and can cause disease.

Bacterial recovery

Although culture may not always be essential for diagnosis, it is necessary if tests of antibiotic susceptibility (sensitivity) (p. 17) are to be performed.

Swabs or other samples obtained from the patients, wounds, staff or fomites are introduced into an appropriate growth medium. The nutritional requirements of the suspect bacteria – sources of energy, salts, amino acids and cofactors – must be present, as well as substances preferred by individual organisms (Table 7).

Growth media are prepared so that they support the multiplication of as wide a range of bacteria as possible. Such media are easily and cheaply produced from hydrolysed horse serum protein to which are added warm, liquid agar; meat extract; yeast; and sodium chloride. Sometimes the whole medium is made synthetically. Media are poured into sterile plastic Petri dishes or tubes where the gel solidifies. Bacteria grow on the surface of the gel initially as pinhead-size colonies.

Many pathogenic bacteria grow poorly on simple substrates; they prefer blood agar, a medium that allows the assessment of types of haemolysis (p. 145). Culture media are adjusted to suit the requirements of fastidious micro-organisms.

- **Salmonellae**. Indicators added to the growth media are employed to demonstrate changes in pH. This is of importance in the diagnosis of salmonellosis and enteric fever (p. 127) since intestinal pathogens do not ferment lactose. Bile salts are also added. In their presence, these pathogens thrive but many bacteria do not.

Table 7 Conditions regulating bacterial growth

Environmental requirement	**Comment**
Oxygen	Occasionally, additional carbon dioxide is required, as with Campylobacter and Haemophilus spp.
Temperature	Optimum temperature for growth is 37°C for most human pathogens (but 30°C for MRSA – p. 18, 304)
Water	Drying impairs growth and may lead to spore formation
pH	Many organisms grow best at a neutral or slightly alkaline pH
Light	Ultraviolet light, including daylight, is inhibitory

- **Mycobacteria**. Certain slowly growing organisms, such as *Mycobacterium tuberculosis* (p. 237), grow best on complex media including coagulated egg and glycerol.
- **Anaerobic bacteria**. Other bacteria, such as *Clostridium perfringens* (p. 93) and *C. difficile* (p. 103) are anaerobic and only grow in atmospheres from which oxygen has been excluded. The common anaerobic streptococci and Bacteroides are sought under these conditions. An anaerobic environment may also assist the identification of aerobes such as *Streptococcus pyogenes* (p. 312). One device used to culture anaerobes is the Gaspak system.

Laboratory tests

Laboratory tests may confirm bacterial identity absolutely or be sufficient only to suggest strongly the presence of a particular organism. Procedures used most frequently include:

- **Oxidase**. The reagent contains a chemical that turns purple on exposure to an oxidase-producing organism. The test is used to differentiate a Pseudomonas-type bacterium (oxidase-positive) from a coliform (oxidase-negative).
- **Catalase**. If an organism is catalase-positive, it produces bubbles of oxygen when brought into contact with hydrogen peroxide. Staphylococci are catalase-positive; streptococci are catalase-negative.
- **Coagulase**. Coagulase-positive organisms cause plasma to clot. The test distinguishes *Staphylococcus aureus* from other staphylococci. In this way, virulence and a threat to surgery are high-lighted.
- **Lancefield grouping of streptococci**. Beta-haemolytic streptococci such as *Streptococcus pyogenes* (p. 312) can be assigned to a Lancefield group. A latex particle test identifies clumping when particles and organisms are mixed.
- **Biochemical tests for Enterobacteriaeciae**. These biochemical systems assist the identification of Gram-negative bacteria. A colour change denotes a positive result. The reactive strips bear numbers and the organism is identified from a reference manual.
- **Latex agglutination tests**. Organisms recovered from an agar plate or samples taken directly from a patient are added to latex particles conjugated with antibodies to a particular organism. One example is the recognition of *Streptococcus pneumoniae* from blood, sputum or urine.

Bacteriuria

Bacteriuria is the presence of bacteria in the urine.

Specimens of urine obtained from normal, healthy females are often contaminated. Urinary infection is 14 times more common in women than men. 'Significant bacteriuria' is said to be present when a correctly collected midstream specimen contains more than 10^5 organisms or colony forming units (CFU)/mL. When abnormal numbers of leucocytes, together with bacteria, are recognised by the microscopy of a wet film, antibiotic susceptibility tests are set up. The results of these tests and of culture are available within 24 hours.

The identification of Mycobacteria in urine samples requires special procedures.

BACTERIAL TYPING

The investigation of outbreaks of hospital infection caused by apparently similar micro-organisms demands molecular typing. If the precise identity of organisms recovered from separate samples is not proven, it may transpire that the similarity of the bacteria is coincidental both in time and space.

Typing greatly assists the exact identification of the source of an outbreak of infection. It helps to decide whether a patient, a member of staff, equipment or an environmental agent such as the air supply is responsible. Traditionally, typing methods have relied upon the characterisation of **phenotypic** properties such as biotype, serotype, phage type, antibiotic susceptibility or even the appearance of the isolated bacteria on culture media. Although these methods are cheap and easy to perform, they lack discrimination. The techniques of **genotyping** used in molecular biology have therefore been developed and applied increasingly in medical microbiology. These methods include:

- **Plasmid analysis**.
- **Total genomic DNA digestion and display**, e.g. Southern blotting, ribotyping, pulsed field gel electrophoresis.
- **Polymerase chain reaction** (PCR)-based methods.

Now read Polymerase chain reaction (p. 139)

BACTERAEMIA AND SEPTICAEMIA

Bacteraemia

Bacteraemia is the presence of bacteria in the bloodstream.

Small numbers of bacteria are present periodically in the blood of normal persons. Transient bacteraemia may occur after brushing the teeth and bacteraemia is recognised following procedures such as sigmoidoscopy. The organisms are quickly destroyed in normal subjects but may initiate the infection of abnormal cardiac valves, prostheses or canulae. They represent a hazard to immunosuppressed individuals. Patients with cardiac valvular disease are therefore given antibiotics during the period of any surgical operation, including endoscopy, and during dental extractions and manipulations.

Septicaemia

Septicaemia is the multiplication of bacteria in the blood. It is associated with a failure of bactericidal mechanisms to destroy organisms released into the circulation.

Blood culture

Blood culture is used to detect bacteria present in the circulation.

Patients should have received no antibiotics for at least 48 hours prior to blood sampling. At least six attempts to recover bacteria should be made before the method is abandoned. When a patient has already been treated with antibiotics, their effects can be blocked by adding inhibitory agents to the culture media. For example, para-aminobenzoic acid (PABA) competes with the tetracyclines, while penicillinase destroys penicillin.

The number of circulating organisms is often small. Relatively large volumes of blood are therefore used to inoculate a variety of culture media. The natural bactericidal or bacteriostatic actions of the blood are minimised by the culture medium and can be further reduced by adding substances to inhibit antibacterial action. Initial tests for bacteraemia are now often made by an automated radiometric culture technique. Multiple samples are grown overnight to seek early evidence of infection.

Ten millilitres of blood is taken by venepuncture after treating the skin with an antiseptic. The blood, withdrawn by pre-sterilised plastic syringe, is introduced into culture bottles the tops of which must be sterile. The media currently used support the growth of most pathogenic bacteria. The addition of a bile salt, sodium taurocholate, assists the recovery of *Salmonella typhi* and *S. paratyphi*. Bacteroides and

Clostridia spp. are of particular importance in surgical bacteriology. Cultures are set up in an anaerobic jar to enable their identification.

BACTERIOPHAGE

Bacteriophages (phages) are viruses that multiply in bacteria.

Now read Virus (p. 347)

Virulent phages cause the host bacterium to lyse. Large bacteriophages resemble syringes in shape and function; the head contains double-stranded DNA. There is a hollow tail with a base plate where the virus attaches to the bacterial cell wall. Phage DNA is transferred to the bacterium through the tail by the process of transduction. The DNA is integrated into the genome of the bacterial cell that manufactures new phage protein and nucleic acid. Eventually, the parasitised bacterial cell is disrupted by lysis.

Advantage can be taken of the phage typing of bacteria to trace sources of surgical infection.

BACTEROIDES

Bacteroides is an important Gram-negative, non-sporing genus of anaerobic bacilli. The main pathogen is *Bacteroides fragilis.* Bacteroides spp. are prolific commensals of the lower intestinal tract of man. Bacteroides are also frequently present in the mouth and oropharynx and may exist in the lower genito-urinary tract in the female.

Bacteroides spp. are not invasive but often cause localised diseases such as acute appendicitis, acute cholecystitis, abscesses associated with diverticulitis and acute salpingitis. Metabolic disorders such as diabetes mellitus and immunosuppression impair host resistance. Bacteroides can cause infection after abortion or childbirth and can provoke bacterial vaginosis. At sites of local tissue injury, as in surgical procedures on the large intestine, Bacteroides may induce local infection. Less often, they gain access to the bloodstream and metastatic infection may ensue. The brain is one target. Post-operative bacteraemic shock (p. 291) is another result. Bacteroides are relatively resistant to the penicillins but respond to metronidazole and to the lincomycins (p. 17).

BILE

Bile, the exocrine secretion of liver cells, is an aqueous solution of bile acids, bile pigments, and inorganic ions in which cholesterol and phospholipids are suspended in micellar form. Abnormalities in the proportions of these constituents contribute to the development of biliary calculi. Bile is a vehicle for the excretion of toxic substances of high molecular weight.

BILE ACIDS

Cholic acid and chenodeoxycholic acid are conjugated with taurine (from meat) and glycine (from vegetables) to form water-soluble detergents, the bile acids. They are essential for the emulsification of triacylglycerides in the small gut and assist in their enzymatic hydrolysis. There is an enterohepatic circulation and the sum of the bile acids in the bile ducts, intestines and blood constitutes a **metabolic pool**.

The many causes of obstruction to the outflow of bile include calculi; tumours; and fibrosis of the biliary tract or pancreas. Obstruction culminates in jaundice (p. 189), steatorrhoea and the excretion of bile acids in the urine. The synthesis of bile acids is reduced in the presence of hepatocellular disease, a condition that may also promote steatorrhoea. A reduction in the pool of bile acids may follow disease or resection of the distal ileum, the main site for the reabsorption of these substances in the enterohepatic circulation. The incidence of biliary calculi in these patients is much increased.

A proportion of the bile acids is deconjugated in the bowel by bacterial action. In patients with abnormally large bacterial populations, for example in incomplete intestinal obstruction or with a blind intestinal loop, the concentration of the bile acid metabolites may be very high, a defect that may contribute to the development of large-bowel cancer. The reflux of bile acids into the stomach and oesophagus is one cause of gastritis and oesophagitis and may contribute to the development of gastric carcinoma (p. 309).

BILE PIGMENTS

Bile pigments are derivatives of haem, the oxygen-carrying porphyrin of the haemoglobin molecule. The main pigment is bilirubin.

Bilirubin

- **Unconjugated bilirubin**. Each day, ageing red blood cells are broken down in large numbers in the mononuclear macrophages of the reticulo-endothelial system, particularly in the sinusoidal cells of the red pulp of the spleen. Eighty per cent of circulating bilirubin comes from this source. Haem is freed from the red cells and converted to bilirubin, a water-insoluble, iron-free molecule that becomes soluble when bound to plasma albumin. Normally more than 90% of measurable serum bilirubin is in this state, the form in which it is carried to the liver for conjugation within hepatocytes. Even in excess, unconjugated bilirubin cannot be excreted by the renal glomeruli nor secreted by renal tubules.
- **Conjugated bilirubin**. Within liver cells, released from albumen, bilirubin is conjugated with glucuronic acid enabling it to be excreted in the bile. The water-soluble glucuronides formed in this way can be excreted by the kidney. The excess is easily recognised in the urine.
- **Urobilin**. In the small gut, bilirubin glucuronide is converted by bacterial action to a mixture of colourless compounds described as faecal urobilinogen ('stercobilinogen'). Oxidation converts these colourless substances to an orange–red faecal urobilin. The majority of the faecal urobilinogen is absorbed from the gut and, like the bile acids, recirculated in the bloodstream. A small fraction is excreted in the stool, producing its characteristic colour. The fraction of the re-absorbed, circulating urobilinogen excreted as urinary urobilinogen is normally too small to be detected by the usual chemical tests.

Now read Jaundice (p. 189), Liver (p. 208)

BILIARY TRACT

The bile duct system and the gall bladder are a single functional entity.

Biopsy diagnosis of biliary disease

Exfoliative cytology of bile is specific but insensitive, providing a diagnosis in only one third of cases. A negative result has little value. Cytological examination of specimens obtained by brushing at endoscopic retrograde cholangiography or by fine needle aspiration has greater sensitivity and specificity but less than from cholangiographic appearances alone.

DEVELOPMENTAL AND CONGENITAL DISORDERS

The biliary tree is a frequent site for congenital anomalies. The commonest defect of the gall bladder is a so-called Phrygian cap in the fundus, proximal to a constriction of the body. Agenesis, atresia, hypoplasia and duplication of the gall bladder are uncommon but, in their presence, there is a greater than normal risk of the formation of biliary calculi and of the development of malignant bile duct tumours.

Biliary atresia

Biliary atresia is a congenital obliteration of the bile ducts by fibrous tissue It occurs in 1 birth in every 14000. The incidence is the same in both sexes. The liver displays the feature of cholestatic jaundice but the frequent presence of giant cells, identified at biopsy, makes a distinction from neonatal hepatitis difficult. The cause is unknown. Jaundice is not usually evident at birth but develops soon afterwards. Biliary atresia has been attributed to viral infection. However, foetal cystic dilatation of intrahepatic bile ducts has been identified *in utero* or in neonates and the condition is often associated with other congenital anomalies, suggesting a genetic cause. The condition may be classified according to the extent of the ductal involvement:

- **Type I**. Atresia is confined to the bile duct.
- **Type II**. Atresia is confined to the common hepatic and bile ducts.
- **Type III**. Atresia involves the right and left hepatic and the common hepatic and common bile ducts.

Choledochal cysts

Choledochal cysts and diverticula are dilatations of the extra-hepatic bile ducts. Various classifications have been proposed according to the site, number and size of the cysts. They are commoner in the distal, lower part of the bile duct than in the proximal part and occur more frequently in females than males, more often in orientals than occidentals. Often asymptomatic, choledochal cysts may give rise to pain and jaundice. These complaints are particularly likely if the cyst is complicated by choledocholithiasis, cholangitis, pancreatitis or malignant change, all conditions more common in individuals without cysts.

Choledochocoele

A choledochocoele, one type of choledochal cyst, is a localised dilatation of the distal common bile duct within the wall of the second part of the duodenum. It may cause biliary obstruction.

Caroli's disease

Caroli's disease, a further type of choledochal cyst, is an uncommon, apparently congenital condition in which there are multiple dilatations of intra- and extra-hepatic bile ducts. The intra-hepatic ducts are extensively involved. Occasionally, however, the disorder is confined to the ducts draining a single hepatic lobe. The condition, sometimes asymptomatic, must be distinguished from sclerosing cholangitis (p. 38). Cholangitis, septicaemia and cholangiocarcinoma are possible complications.

METABOLIC DISORDERS

Calculi

Forty per cent of females and 20% of males form biliary calculi (gallstones). The incidence increases with age. Three varieties of calculi are encountered: cholesterol; mixed; and pigmented. Eighty per cent are mixed or cholesterol; no more than 20% are pigment calculi.

Mixed calculi

The majority of biliary calculi in Western patients are 'mixed'. The calculi are light brown and of variegated shape and size. They are heterogeneous, containing predominantly cholesterol but also bile pigment and calcium salts. The centre of the calculus is likely to comprise cholesterol or bile pigment with successive layers of other substances deposited upon them. The large number and relatively rapid growth of mixed calculi within a fibrotic gall bladder wall leads to mutual compression. The stones become multifaceted.

Mixed calculi were thought to arise on the basis of a minute nidus of bacteria, insoluble crystals, or particulate or cellular debris but this view is no longer supported. However, Salmonella spp. can occasionally be isolated from gallstones.

Cholesterol calculi

Pale yellow, crystalline cholesterol stones are uncommon. They are large, ovoid, smooth-surfaced, and often single ('solitaire'). Some cholesterol calculi form in patients who excrete excess biliary cholesterol but the majority are due to a decrease in the bile salt pool. Cholesterol calculi are particularly likely to form in patients with hepatocellular disorders or following disease or resection of the terminal ileum (p. 164). They arise in women taking contraceptive pills and during the last trimester of pregnancy: there is hormonally-induced stasis in the biliary tree.

Pigment calculi

Pigment calculi, composed of calcium bilirubinate, are multiple, small, black, friable and irregular in shape. They are more common among Africans and Asians than in Europeans. Pigment calculi are formed by the excretion of excess bile pigment and are frequent in patients with congenital haemolytic anaemia (p. 11). By contrast with cholesterol stones, they contain less than 1% cholesterol.

Effects of biliary calculus

A calculus impacted in the common bile duct is liable to cause obstructive jaundice. A calculus lodged in Hartmann's pouch obstructs the outflow of mucin. The glandular secretions accumulate and produce a **mucocoele**. If infection supervenes, it gives rise to **empyema** (p. 126) of the gall bladder. The origin of the infecting organisms is sometimes obscure. Although the micro-organisms found in patients with cholangitis are usually enteric, there is little to confirm that the infection is ascending in nature. Rarely, a calculus may ulcerate through the wall of the gall bladder into the duodenum and thence into the ileum where intestinal obstruction may result, the condition of **gallstone ileus.** Gall bladders containing calculi frequently become the site for cholecystitis. It is not certain that carcinoma of the gall bladder is more common in patients with biliary calculi than in the general population, but chronic inflammation predisposes to the development of cancer.

Cholesterosis

In this frequently asymptomatic condition, found in ~10% of otherwise normal individuals at autopsy, the mucosa of the gall bladder contains histiocytes laden with lipid. The lipid appears as yellow flecks within the pale red mucosa, giving a strawberry-like appearance. Excessive absorption of cholesterol from supersaturated bile may be the underlying mechanism. Co-existent calculi are uncommon.

INFECTION AND INFLAMMATION

Cholecystitis

Acute

In the majority of patients, acute cholecystitis is a bacterial infection associated with the presence of one or more calculi. The causative organisms are usually *Escherichia coli,* Klebsiella spp., *Streptococcus faecalis,* Bacteroides spp. or *Clostridium perfringens.* The gall bladder wall is hyperaemic and the external surface is covered by a fibrinous exudate. If a gallstone impacts in Hartmann's pouch or in the cystic duct, empyema of the gall bladder may develop with subsequent gangrene, perforation and peritonitis.

Chronic

Chronic cholecystitis may be provoked by chemical mechanisms as well as by bacterial infection. The wall of the gall bladder, shrunken and atrophic, contains much fibrous tissue; it may be distorted by the development of Rokitansky–Aschoff sinuses, herniations of the epithelium through the now fibrotic muscle coat. When pronounced, these changes are termed **cholecystitis glandularis proliferans**. Histologically, this change must be distinguished from neoplasia. Episodes of acute inflammation due to intermittent impaction of stones in Hartmann's pouch are common. Occasionally, obstruction of the cystic duct provokes the secretion of mucin and the gall bladder becomes a **mucocoele**. Dystrophic calcification (p. 73) culminates in the appearance termed 'porcelain gall bladder'.

Acalculous cholecystitis

Acalculous cholecystitis is uncommon and may be acute or chronic. It is seen most frequently in patients in intensive care units and in those suffering from burns and severe, prolonged sepsis. The condition is associated with dehydration, intravenous feeding, multiple blood transfusions and assisted ventilation. Bile stasis and ischaemia may be responsible.

Cholangitis

Cholangitis is provoked by the presence of a calculus in the bile duct. Infection is a consequence of obstruction and stasis. The usual cause is the migration of a gallstone from the gall bladder into the common bile duct via the cystic duct. Intermittent obstruction of the biliary tree results, with jaundice and cholangitis. Bacteraemia and septicaemia may ensue. Cholangitis is rarely the result of ascending infection. Following endoscopic sphincterotomy or choledochojejunostomy, the free reflux of the duodenal contents into the bile duct can be easily demonstrated radiographically. Cholangitis is uncommon in such individuals.

Primary sclerosing cholangitis

Primary sclerosing cholangitis is an uncommon disease of unknown aetiology that may have an immunological basis. It is more common in males, particularly in patients suffering from ulcerative colitis or Crohn's disease (p. 165). In the majority of patients, the condition affects both the intra- and extra-hepatic bile ducts with numerous strictures and dilatations. In about 20% of cases, the changes are confined to the extra-hepatic ducts. There is gross, concentric, periductal fibrosis. Hepatic failure, varices and cholangiocarcinoma are frequent complications. The untreated disease may pursue an indolent course although progressive deterioration of a patient's condition is usually followed by death within 10 years of onset. Patients with severe, advancing sclerosing cholangitis can be treated successfully by liver transplantation.

MECHANICAL INJURY AND TRAUMA

The biliary tree is implicated in liver injury resulting from road-traffic and aeroplane accidents; stab wounds (p. 357); and explosions.

TUMOURS

Benign

Benign tumours of the gall bladder and bile ducts are rare. However, the biliary tract may be involved in familial adenomatous polyposis (p. 105). The adenomas display the customary predilection for malignant change. Adenomyomatosis describes changes seen in chronic cholecystitis with the development of Rokitansky–Aschoff sinuses.

Malignant

Cholangiocarcinoma

Cholangiocarcinoma may develop at any site within the biliary tree (Fig. 8). The cancer is most frequent at the junction of the right and left hepatic ducts when it is designated a **Klatskin tumour**.

Causes

Carcinoma of the **gall bladder** is four times more frequent in females than males. In most countries it is uncommon before the age of 50 years. The significance of the association of carcinoma with cholelithiasis is debatable although microscopic foci of malignant change can be found in up to 1% of gall bladders removed for calculus. High concentrations of the elements cadmium, lead and chromium have been reported in the bile of patients with gall bladder carcinoma. Like carcinoma of the stomach, colon, uterus and cervix, there is an increased incidence in individuals of blood group A.

In Europe, cholangiocarcinoma of the **bile ducts** is infrequent but the tumour is relatively common in patients suffering from sclerosing cholangitis, Caroli's disease or choledochal cysts. In the UK, the incidence is ~1:40 000 ($25/10^6$) population per annum. There is little difference between the prevalence in men and women. The frequency is high in South America, Israel and South-East Asia where the disease is related to infestation by the liver flukes *Clonorchis sinensis*, *Opisthorchis viverrini* and *Opisthorchis felineus* (p. 356).

Structure

The tumour arises within the liver or in the extra-hepatic bile ducts and their branches (Fig. 8).

- **Intra-hepatic** cholangiocarcinoma is a single, ill-defined, irregularly shaped, firm, white mass with stellate processes extending into the liver substance. Occasionally, additional, satellite nodules proliferate nearby.
- **Extra-hepatic** cholangiocarcinoma arises as a small nodule spreading locally to encase the hepatic artery and portal vein. Some tumours are polypoid.

Histologically, irregular ductules lined by well-formed cuboidal or columnar cells lie within much fibrous tissue. The macroscopic, scirrhous character of the tumour and the fibrous microscopic reaction make differentiation from primary sclerosing cholangitis difficult. There are no pathognomonic immunohistochemical tests. When tumours of the lower end of the bile duct are considered, a distinction between bile duct carcinoma and carcinoma arising in the duodenum, the ampulla of Vater or the pancreas may be difficult. In this location, almost all tumours are adenocarcinomas. They are usually mucin-secreting.

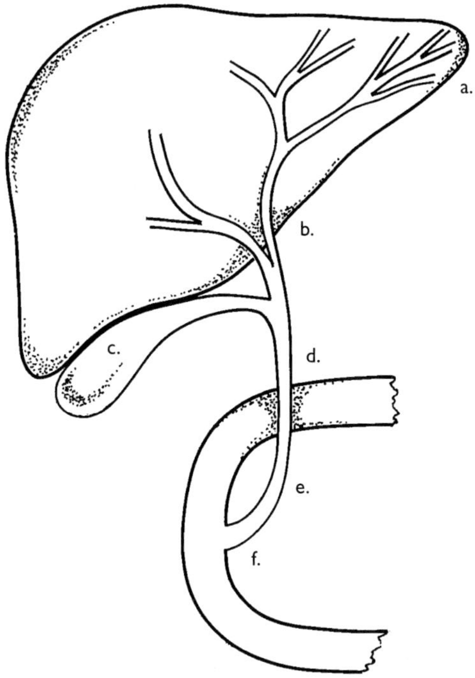

Figure 8 Location of carcinomas of biliary tree. There are six principal sites: (a) intra-hepatic (peripheral); (b) hilar; (c) gall bladder; (d) upper bile duct (supraduodenal); (e) lower bile duct (retroduodenal or retroperitoneal); (f) ampullary.

Behaviour and prognosis

- **Intra-hepatic**. The prognosis in those with carcinoma of the gall bladder is poor. Direct invasion of the gall bladder bed occurs early when the 5-year survival is only 1%. Overall, it is less than 5%.
- **Extra-hepatic**. After surgical resection of carcinoma of the extra-hepatic bile ducts, the mean survival period is 12 to 18 months with an occasional patient surviving 5 years. After resection of carcinoma of the distal bile duct, the 5-year survival is ~25%.

BIOPSY

Biopsy is the removal of tissues or cells from a living patient, and their examination for diagnosis and prognosis. Biopsy is often employed for other reasons, for example, to assess endocrine status, or to judge the progress of a disease in response to treatment. In practice, it is imperative to record the precise location from which a specimen is obtained and desirable to draw a diagram of this site.

SMALL BIOPSIES

Superficial specimens sufficient for diagnosis can be obtained by scraping or shaving a skin surface or by passing a spatula, brush or swab across a mucosal surface. Techniques of this kind are used in the diagnosis of diseases such as leukoplakia (p. 207), and in oral, pharyngeal, bronchial and gastric diagnosis. However, they do not yield enough tissue for the assessment of the depth and extent of a tumour. Small lesions sited more deeply are also sampled by a variety of forms of needle or trocar. Lesions of limited extent are frequently explored during endoscopy or conventional surgical operation.

Needle biopsy

Specimens for diagnosis can often be obtained by percutaneous needle puncture from deeper structures, such as those within the thoracic or abdominal cavities. The needles are guided by ultrasonography, by CT or MRI (p. 169). If the material is sufficiently soft, adequate samples can be obtained by fine-needle aspiration. With denser tissues, a device such as a Trucut needle is necessary to remove a core specimen. The needle incorporates a circumferential guillotine. Needle biopsy is employed on a very large scale for the study of tissues ranging from breast and thyroid to synovium. The dissemination of tumour cells along needle tracts is an uncommon hazard but may be encountered in the biopsy of tumours such as hepatocellular carcinoma, mesothelioma and some sarcomas.

Now read Bone biopsy (p. 50)

Fibre-optic endoscopy and biopsy

Endoscopy is the examination of the interior of the body by means of an instrument that incorporates an optical viewing system and a source of light. Instruments for endoscopy may be rigid or flexible. Flexible endoscopes contain parallel bundles of very fine glass fibres along which light can pass without distortion. Images are displayed on monitors and can be digitised and recorded on video tape or disk.

The genito-urinary, the respiratory and the gastro-intestinal tracts can be examined from either end. Laparoscopy enables the coelomic cavities to be inspected. The heart and the larger arteries are accessible via a brachial or femoral artery. In addition to widespread use in visual diagnosis, endoscopes contain channels through which small pieces of tissue or fluid can be collected for biochemical, cytological or histological examination.

Now read Imaging (p. 169)

Sentinel lymph node biopsy

The search for a sentinel lymph node is becoming accepted practice in the initial investigation of an increasing proportion of tumours, in particular malignant melanoma (p. 227) and those of the breast. Its use in the assessment of colorectal, vulvar, thyroid, skin (non-melanoma), head and neck, and uterine tumours is under consideration.

A blue dye or a radionuclide is injected into the affected region. Labelled nodes are identified by a search conducted by non-invasive gamma counter or intra-operatively. The former method enables sentinel nodes to be identified before an incision is made and gives guidance during dissection. The highest success rates come when the two approaches are combined. Suspect nodes are excised and examined histologically. Not only does a scan pinpoint a sentinel node: it also allows subsequent confirmation that all nodes, with their tumour cell deposits, have been removed.

LARGER BIOPSIES

Larger biopsies are obtained by incision or excision.

- **Incisional biopsy**. In this procedure, no attempt is made to remove a lesion wholly. Since the choice of a biopsy site is subjective, it is always possible that foci of particular importance such as the growing edge or point of maximum invasion of a malignant tumour will escape notice. Simple enucleation of a circumscribed lesion is influenced by this possibility.
- **Excisional biopsy.** In the case of suspected tumours, excision minimises the risks of implanting cancer cells at the operation site and diminishes the hazards of disseminating micro-organisms. Excisional biopsy guarantees the preparation of microscopic sections that represent a disease process fully. Nevertheless, excisional biopsy of a tumour that has extended locally or excision of a single lymph node, compromise fields of dissection for lymphadenectomy. Under these circumstances, fine needle aspiration biopsy may be preferable.

Conveyance

In general, the surgeon requires a responsible report on a biopsy at the earliest possible moment. Therefore specimens, properly identified, should be delivered promptly to the laboratory. Health and Safety regulations demand that samples are conveyed safely. Unfixed material, including slides from suspect lymphomas and fresh tissue for some forms of immunostaining, are transported in sealed containers. In many cases, however, the interpretation of a biopsy section may be impossible without fixation. These fixed samples are immersed in strong jars containing a fluid that prevents drying and autolysis (putrefaction). The samples should never be allowed to adhere to the walls of the container.

Fixation

Fixatives prevent autolysis and putrefaction and harden tissues. A fixative is usually a fluid; occasionally it is a gas. The volume of fixative in a container to be carried to a laboratory should be not less than ten times the volume of the specimen. The fixative used most commonly for light microscopy is neutral, buffered 4% formalin, a 10% solution of the 40% formaldehyde supplied commercially. Cell preparations and smears, spread on slides, are fixed by an alcohol spray immediately. Small fragments of skin are placed in Bouin's fluid. For electron microscopy (EM), expert guidance is often required but buffered gluteraldehyde at 4°C is generally used for fixation.

Processing, microtomy and staining

The techniques used for the processing, sectioning and staining of biopsy specimens do not differ from those employed in Histology.

Now read Histology (p. 157)

FROZEN SECTION

Frozen sections enable a surgeon to perform the most relevant operation in particular circumstances. They are not made merely to provide a rapid diagnosis and are seldom final. The advantage of freezing is that it offers an alternative to the hardening that results from fixation. If possible, the pathologist should be given advance warning when the procedure is required. Frozen sections are employed:

- **Diagnosis**. To provide a diagnosis when unexpected appearances are seen at operation.
- **Staging**. To confirm tumour staging by the recognition of the presence or absence of lymph node or tumour metastases.
- **Adequacy**. To establish the adequacy of excision of a tumour by defining a resection margin.
- **Identification**. To confirm the removal of a tissue such as parathyroid gland when its identity is in doubt.

Frozen sections prepared are of poorer quality than those obtained by fixation and paraffin embedding. There are some conditions, therefore, such as malignant melanoma and papillary carcinoma of the thyroid, that cannot be diagnosed by frozen section. As a result of the varied quality and limited size of the material to be examined, there is a small false-negative rate; the false-positive rate should be extremely low.

BIOPSY REPORTS

Reports are dictated by histopathologists, keyed in, printed, checked and finally authorised by the consultant in charge. In some hospitals, reports can be dispatched via a telephone – or cable network. The reports are generated on the recipient's printer. In many hospitals reports are still conveyed by hand or sent by surface mail.

Retrospective access to biopsy reports is regulated strictly by a heirarchy of a confidential 'need-to-know' character, necessitated by the adoption of a laboratory and hospital computer network.

BLEEDING – HAEMORRHAGE

Bleeding is likely to follow injury to the heart, arteries, capillaries, veins and all vascular tissues. It ceases when vascular contraction and plugging of the lesion by platelets are followed by the formation of a thrombus.

Now read Coagulation (p. 95), Haemostasis (p. 146)

BLEEDING TIME

The bleeding time measures the duration of haemorrhage from a small skin wound made with a needle or stylet. It varies from 1 to 9 minutes. An excessive bleeding time is usually due to a combination of failure of vascular contraction and either thrombocytopenia or thrombocytopathia.

Abnormalities of platelet function and of coagulation are described on pp. 99 and 100, respectively.

EXCESSIVE BLEEDING

Small haemorrhages into the skin, epithelium or peritoneum are **petechiae**. Larger areas of flat haemorrhages are **ecchymoses**. If bleeding produces a swelling, the lesion is a **haematoma**.

Purpura

Purpura (Lat: purple) describes either petechiae or ecchymoses.

- **Non-thrombocytopenic purpura** may be due to disease of small vessels or to hereditary or acquired defects of platelet function.

  Purpura is a feature of meningococcal septicaemia, typhus and other rickettsial diseases, and some childhood viral diseases. Capillaries are damaged by microbial toxins although thrombocytopenia and disseminated intravascular coagulation (DIC) may contribute to the injury.
- **Thrombocytopenic purpura** is described on p. 99. There is a deficiency in the number of blood platelets.
- **Henoch–Schönlein purpura** is a disorder of young people that follows infection, usually streptococcal. It is an immune complex disease (p. 161) and complexes can be demonstrated in affected tissues. In addition to the skin lesions, there is bleeding into the gut wall, producing abdominal colic and even intussusception. Acute glomerulonephritis occurs and death may follow.

Telangiectasia

Telangiectasia is a persistent disorder in which there are multiple, dilated blood vessels. In clinical practice, telangiectasia is distinguishable from purpura: the vascular lesions disappear when pressure is applied to the skin with a glass slide. Bleeding into the gastro-intestinal tract is often due to telangiectasia. **Hereditary haemorrhagic telangiectasia** is inherited as an autosomal dominant trait.

BLOOD LOSS

Blood loss may be slow and clinically imperceptible, at an obvious rate, or disastrously rapid.

A continual, **slow** blood loss, often from capillaries or small veins, leads to hypochromic, microcytic, iron-deficiency anaemia (p. 10).

The very **rapid** loss of blood, from arteries, large veins or ruptured viscera, results in haemorrhagic shock.

Now read Shock (p. 290)

If acute haemorrhage is not fatal, vasoconstriction of peripheral and visceral arterioles maintains arterial blood pressure. The circulating blood volume is reduced but there is no immediate alteration in the packed cell volume. In the absence of intravenous or intra-arterial transfusion, the circulating blood volume is then gradually restored by the passage of interstitial tissue water into the bloodstream. This diffusion of water results both from an increased capillary osmotic pressure and from a lowered arteriolar filtration pressure. There is a consequential fall in the red blood cell and haemoglobin concentrations, and in the packed cell volume. Ultimately, accelerated haemopoiesis, recognised by the presence of reticulocytes in the circulation, restores the normal red blood cell mass and haemoglobin concentration.

Small wounds of very vascular tissues, such as the scalp or liver, may be responsible for disproportionately severe bleeding and a substantial blood loss. Surgeons often underestimate the amount of blood lost during operation. The volume of blood collected in aspiration ('suction') apparatus should be measured. Swabs should be weighed and an allowance made for the drying of blood by evaporation. In severe injuries, it is convenient to estimate a loss of 500 mL of blood from each superficial wound as large as an open human hand or from each deep wound the size of a closed human fist.

Table 8 Volume of blood lost at sites of common fractures

Site of fracture	Blood loss (L)
Humerus	0.5–1.0
Radius + ulna	0.5
Femur	0.5–1.5
Tibia + fibula	0.5–1.0
Pelvis	1.0–3.0

Haemorrhage may be **concealed**. For example, bone is very vascular and, at the site of simple fracture, much blood may be lost both from the injured bone and from nearby, lacerated muscle (Table 8). Other causes of concealed haemorrhage include: injuries to abdominal viscera with the intra- or retroperitoneal accumulation of blood; concealed accidental haemorrhage; and *abruptio placentae*. The rapid loss of blood into the gastro-intestinal tract is generally revealed as haematemesis or melaena. In haemoptysis, blood loss is rarely massive.

Bone marrow after blood loss

In adult patients with anaemia due to chronic blood loss, yellow marrow in sites such as the shaft of the femur turns red as it once again begins to produce red blood cells. After a single, large, acute haemorrhage there is no immediate increase in the quantity of the red bone marrow. However, a qualitative change is soon detected, with an increase in the relative number of red blood cell precursors. An increase in the relative proportion of basophilic erythroblasts heralds the onset of new red blood cell formation. Reticulocytes are released into the peripheral blood, the process of **reticulocytosis**.

Now read Anaemia p. 10)

BLOOD-BORNE INFECTION

It is characteristic of the initial phase of microbial disease that the majority of infecting viruses and rickettsia, but few bacteria and fungi, enter the blood. The majority of bacteria are killed by the innate, microbial defence mechanisms (p. 231). Later, many bacteria proliferate in the blood and other tissues, releasing toxins that cause severe disease.

The presence of micro-organisms in the blood is intermittent and may be clinically silent. The spread of micro-organisms takes place within the systemic, pulmonary or portal circulations initially but retrograde emboli and paradoxical routes are possible. Micro-organisms may also be carried free in the plasma, in erythrocytes, leucocytes or platelets, or in a combination of these compartments (Table 9).

Catheter-related bloodstream infection (CRBSI)

Intravascular catheters are widely used in abdominal and cardiothoracic surgery as well as in the treatment of trauma, in transplantation and in cancer therapy. Within as little as 24 hours after catheterisation, viable micro-organisms are present inside a biofilm that adheres to the surfaces of almost all catheters. The organisms are those present on the skin. They comprise staphylococci; diphtheroids; streptococci, including enterococci; candida; but rarely Gram-negative bacteria (p. 32).

The organisms gain access to the bloodstream from the site of insertion, or from the hub of a catheter. In the latter case, they come from the hands of surgical personnel, a hazard that is increasingly likely when indwelling catheters require repeated disconnection and manipulation. The films in which bacteria lodge are formed of host proteins. They include fibronectin and fibrinogen and are resistant to the defencive actions of macrophages and antibodies. The risk of disseminated infection is related to the number of bacteria on the catheter surfaces.

Table 9 Examples of micro-organisms carried in the blood in human disease

Organism	Free in plasma	Within CD4 lymphocytes	Within mononuclear phagocytes	Within polymorphs	Within red blood cells
Virus	Poliovirus Yellow fever virus	HIV	EB virus Measles virus HIV		Colorado tick fever virus
Bacteria	*Streptococcus pneumoniae* *Bacillus anthracis*			Pyogenic bacteria	*Bartonella bacilliformis*
Protozoa	*Trypanosoma cruzi*		*Leishmania donovani* *Toxoplasma gondii*		*Plasmodium falciparum*

Diagnosis is made when the number of bacterial colonies in samples taken through the catheter is at least five times greater than the number obtained after contemporaneous, conventional peripheral blood sampling.

SYSTEMIC BACTERIAL DISEASE

In systemic bacterial disease, bacteria enter the blood, the state of bacteraemia (p. 34). Foci of metastatic infection form when there is a localising factor, such as a congenitally bicuspid aortic valve or when resistance is impaired. Endocarditis may follow streptococcal bacteraemia after dental manoeuvres and osteomyelitis may succeed transient *Staphylococcus aureus* bacteraemia. Widespread foci of blood-borne infection are regular features of some bacterial diseases. Typhoid (*Salmonella typhi*) and anthrax (*Bacillus anthracis*) are examples.

Now read Bacteraemia (p. 34)

SYSTEMIC VIRAL DISEASE

In systemic viral disease, the organisms reach the blood quickly after crossing an epithelial surface. **Primary viraemia** results. Thus, in measles, viruses multiply briefly at an infected site such as a bronchiole. They pass through lymphatics and lymphoid tissue to the blood. Distant organs such as the brain are invaded. The blood is re-seeded and a massive **secondary viraemia** develops, with the infection of a further series of target organs. A rash or exanthem develops.

Now read Virus (p. 347)

The frequency of viraemia in systemic viral disease explains why blood, plasma and blood products are important sources of common viruses, such as those of hepatitis (p. 152), and why blood transfusion can be hazardous.

BLOOD TRANSFUSION

Even under the best conditions of surgical practice, the transfusion of blood and blood products is not without risk. In the United States of America it is necessary to obtain formal consent. Such consent is not required in the UK but may become necessary in the future.

Blood can be transfused **directly**, from one individual to another, or **indirectly** when the blood given is fresh or stored. In modern practice, direct transfusion is unusual.

AUTOLOGOUS TRANSFUSION

Concern about the transmission of AIDS, hepatitis and Creutzfeld–Jacob disease (CJD) has led to an increase in autologous transfusion. Blood for transfusion may be taken from a patient before operation (pre-operative autologous donation – PAD) or collected during an operative procedure (intra-operative salvage – IS). The autologous blood is restored to the individual during or after surgery. This process conserves available stocks of blood and minimises the risks of transfusion. However, it is only practicable when the patient has no active, infective or malignant process. For PAD the individual must be young and healthy with no significant pre-operative anaemia and no cardiovascular disorder. Autotransfusion is employed increasingly after severe trauma complicated by haemothorax.

HETEROLOGOUS TRANSFUSION

In the great majority of cases in the UK the source of blood for transfusion is another individual or group of individuals. Allogeneic (p. 329) transfusion depends upon identifying the red cell antigens of the donor and ensuring compatibility between these cells and the plasma antibodies of the recipient. Incompatible blood transfusion is hazardous and potentially fatal.

COLLECTION AND STORAGE OF BLOOD FOR TRANSFUSION

Whole blood is collected and stored in a pack. Blood, separated from plasma, is also kept as a suspension of red blood cells or as red blood cells in an additive solution. Initially, whole blood is taken into a nutrient, anticoagulant solution consisting of citrate, phosphate and dextrose. Centrifugation separates the plasma which is used to prepare platelet suspensions and a variety of products ranging from Factor VIII and hepatitis B immunoglobulin to albumen and fibrinogen. In the UK, the white blood cells are also removed to minimise the risk of transmitting CJD (p. 351): the blood is said to be 'leucocyte-depleted'.

The optimum temperature for storing blood is 2–6°C; at this temperature, bacterial proliferation is greatly slowed but not entirely prevented. The blood is stored in a refrigerator used for this purpose only.

After removal from the refrigerator prior to a transfusion, blood is allowed to warm slowly. Occasionally, it is heated actively in a properly maintained and validated blood warmer. If blood has not been used within a period of 30 minutes after a pack has been opened, it must not be used unless the transfusion can be completed within 5 hours after it has been taken from the refrigerator. After 30 minutes, the blood must not be returned to the refrigerator for later transfusion.

Under special circumstances, whole blood can be stored for periods of up to 3 months if it is mixed with glycerol as a cryoprotectant, rapidly frozen, and held at −90°C, a technique that requires costly equipment.

With storage, red blood cells accumulate water and tend to haemolyse. The oxygen-carrying capacity of the remaining cells diminishes and they lose glucose. Potassium escapes into the extracellular fluid in which the cells are stored and the pH rises. After 35 days, all stored blood must be discarded. In European practice, such is the demand for blood or red blood cells that they are rarely kept for more than 28 days.

In the UK, it is a legal obligation for all details of a transfusion to be recorded in a patient's clinical notes.

BLOOD SUBSTITUTES

Perfluorocarbon emulsions and haemoglobin solutions have been developed that can transport about half as much oxygen as whole blood. They are being tested as blood substitutes, for transfusion.

BLOOD GROUPS

The surfaces of human red blood cells bear many heritable antigens the specificity of which is regulated by a series of allelic genes. The presence of these antigens has enabled 22 blood groups to be designated. An individual is said to be of a particular group when his or her red cells bear the appropriate antigen. The groups of major clinical significance are ABO and Rh. The remaining groups only occasionally elicit adverse reactions following transfusion and are of greater significance for genetic and other red cell studies.

When blood is transfused into a recipient whose red-cell antigens are different from those of the donor, there is **incompatibility** (p. 329). Adverse reactions follow and antibody formation is provoked. Serious reactions are likely when a second transfusion is attempted.

Now read Antigens and Antibodies (p. 19)

ABO blood groups

Human red blood cells inherit either A or B antigenic substances, both or neither. Therefore, four ABO blood groups are designated (Table 10) depending on whether antigens A and B exist together (group AB), separately (groups A or B) or not at all (group O). The situation is complicated by the fact that the plasma of each individual already contains natural, complementary antibodies. The serum of persons who are of group A contains antibodies (called agglutinins) against the red-cell antigens (called agglutinogens) of group B and *vice versa*. When the red cells bear both A and B antigens, the group is AB and no serum agglutinin is present. When the group is O, haemagglutinins against both A and B agglutinogens are identified; adverse reactions are therefore probable on the first occasion of an incorrectly matched blood transfusion (see below).

Because the ABO antigens and antibodies were shared within a single species, man, they were described as **iso-antigens** and **iso-antibodies**, respectively. The prefix 'iso' signified equal. However, care is necessary in the use of this terminology because, in immunology, the prefix 'iso-' has come to mean identity of genetic constitution of individuals (p. 21).

The haemagglutinins are, for the most part, IgM antibodies (p. 20). After birth, they form naturally in response to normal exposure to the bacterial polysaccharide antigens of the gut that resemble the A and B antigens. The individual reacts immunologically only to polysaccharides absent from his/her own red blood cells, so that a person who has inherited only group A red-cell antigen forms only anti-B haemagglutinins and *vice versa*.

Rhesus blood groups

The word Rhesus is the generic name for the monkey, *Macaca mulatta*. For evolutionary reasons not yet fully understood, the Rhesus (Rh) antigen is present on the surface of the red blood cells of the majority of humans. In the UK, 85% of individuals are said to be Rh-positive. However, there are large racial differences in frequency and in south-east Europe, in the Middle East and in China, only 55% of the populations are Rh-positive.

The Rh antigen is coded by three pairs (alleles) of closely related genes, Cc, Dd and Ee, so that each individual locus is CDe, cDe, CDE, and so on. The most frequent of the dominant genes is D; most Rh-positive individuals in the UK are D rather than C or E. If a Rh-negative patient is transfused with Rh-positive blood, anti-Rh antibodies may be formed. Repeated transfusion provokes increasingly high antibody titres and may result in accelerated transfusion reactions with haemolysis and the other undesirable effects characteristic of incompatible blood transfusion.

An analogous situation arises when a Rh-negative mother bears an Rh-positive child. Fetal red blood cells escape across the placental barrier and stimulate antibody formation by the maternal immune system. Anti-Rh, IgG (but not IgM) antibodies then pass back into the fetal circulation. Binding to fetal red blood cells, IgG antibodies fix complement and causes haemolysis. The resulting **haemolytic disease of the newborn** may be mild and associated only with transient postnatal jaundice. However, high serum concentrations of bile pigment tend to accumulate in the basal ganglia and can culminate in the severe neurological syndrome of kernicterus.

BLOOD GROUP INCOMPATIBILITY

Blood for transfusion is said to be incompatible with that of a recipient when it includes red-cell antigens that can react with natural (e.g. ABO) or acquired (e.g. Rh) antibodies present in the recipient's serum, or when it contains high titres of antibodies able to combine with the recipient's red blood cell antigens.

Table 10 The ABO blood groups. The frequency in a population varies with race

Group	Genotype	Red-cell antigens (agglutinogens)	Serum antibodies (agglutinins)	Population frequency (UK) (%)
AB	AB	A + B	None	3
A	AA or AO	A	Anti-B	42
B	BB or BO	B	Anti-A	9
O	OO	None	Anti-A and anti-B	46

Normally, blood for transfusion should be of the same ABO group as that of the recipient.

Transfusion is usually permissible only when the ABO and Rh groups of both donor and recipient have been established and after a compatibility test (cross-matching) has been performed in the laboratory. This second test is necessary since, very occasionally, transfusion reactions may result from severe incompatibility to one of the rarer blood group systems, the identification of which is not part of routine blood grouping.

Rh-negative blood of group O, so-called **universal donor** blood, may be transfused in emergency situations only if it has been shown to contain low titres of anti-A and anti-B iso-agglutinins.

COMPLICATIONS OF TRANSFUSION

Blood transfusion may be complicated by hydrodynamic, thrombotic, haemorrhagic, infective and immunological phenomena. Electrolyte disturbances, particularly hyperkalaemia, are not infrequent. Cool blood may induce signs of hypothermia, particularly during operations in anaesthetised patients whose thermoregulatory mechanisms are disturbed. If large volumes are to be transfused, they should be given through a 'heating coil' immersed in water held several degrees above body temperature. Blood packs, however, should not be warmed directly.

Hydrodynamic

Blood is supplied in plastic bags and air embolism during transfusion is very rare. Formerly, air embolism could be induced if air was injected into bottles to increase the rate of blood flow. Micro-aggregates of red and white blood cells and platelets form in stored blood. They are removed by filters of small pore size inserted into the transfusion set. Intravenous infusion of large volumes of any fluid may precipitate heart failure and oedema. This is particularly likely to occur following the infusion of blood and other oncotic fluids that do not leave the circulation quickly.

Thrombotic and haemorrhagic

Inflammation of the vessel wall can be caused mechanically by a needle or catheter. Thrombosis commonly follows but thrombo-embolism is very rare. The amount of anticoagulant in stored blood is insufficient to produce hypocalcaemia and coagulopathy even after large transfusions. If there is bleeding following transfusion, a haemolytic reaction to the transfusion of incompatible blood should be suspected. Lysis of incompatible cells releases thromboplastic substances and disseminated intravascular coagulation (DIC) may develop (Fig. 21).

Infective

At ambient temperatures, blood is an excellent medium for culturing bacteria.

Bacterial

Although there has been much emphasis upon the transmission of viral infection, morbidity in the UK from bacterial contamination is more common than the transmission of HIV. The bacteria most likely to be transmitted are coagulase-negative *Staphylococcus aureus* and Gram-negative bacilli such as Pseudomonas spp.

Viral

In the UK, blood for transfusion is screened for HIV1 and 2 and for hepatitis B and C. As a result, and because of the need for leucodepletion (see Prions below) the cost of each unit of blood has risen sharply.

- **HIV types 1** and **2**. In the UK HIV (p. 350) is transmitted in only one case in every 2 million transfusions. In the USA, the frequency is four times higher. In sub-Saharan Africa, the risk of transmitting these viruses is many times greater still.
- **Hepatitis B**. The risk of transmitting hepatitis B (p. 152) is much increased by the infusion of pooled plasma but this is not a hazard that should occur in a well-run Transfusion Service.
- **Hepatitis C**. The risk of transmitting hepatitis C (p. 155) is now greater than that of transmitting hepatitis B. Eighty per cent of patients infected with hepatitis C become chronic carriers and in the UK one of every 15 000 donors carries the virus. The incidence of carriers in other parts of the world may be as high as 20%. In the UK prospective donors are now subject to stringent interview and serological testing for anti-HVC antibodies, a procedure begun in 1991. In the absence of this practice, many haemophiliacs throughout the world have been infected with HBC; it has become the most common cause of their death.

- **CMV and other viruses**. Cytomegalovirus, EB virus, human T-cell lymphotropic virus types I and II, HAV and HGV (Table 29) are among others that may be conveyed by blood transfusion.
- **Prions**. There is debate concerning the risk of transmitting the infective agents of CJD and of new-variant CJD (p. 351) by transfusion. The World Health Organisation has concluded that there is no evidence that CJD has ever been transmitted by blood or by blood products. There remains a theoretical risk that the disorder can be conveyed by white blood cells.
- **Parvovirus**. This is a transfusion-transmissable ssDNA virus found in blood and blood products. It poses a particular risk to patients with haemophilia who are dependent on receiving Factor VIII (p. 97) concentrate. Little is known of the pathogenicity of the TT virus (TTV), another transfusion transmissible ssDNA agent.

Now read Virus (p. 347)

Parasitic

Common parasitic diseases such as malaria are transmissible by blood transfusion.

Immunological

Allergic reactions such as urticaria and fever occur after 1% of blood transfusions. The reactions are due to antigens in the donor blood, other than blood group agglutinogens, to which the recipient is hypersensitive or to antibodies from donors who are hypersensitive to antigens in the recipient's blood. Anaphylaxis is rare.

Haemolytic reactions

Haemolytic reactions are due to the transfusion of incompatible blood. This mistake is almost always caused by a clerical error in the laboratory or ward. It is the commonest incident reported to the Serious Hazards of Transfusion (SHOT) Committee in the UK. If a haemolytic reaction is recognised early and the transfusion stopped, the only consequence may be the development of haemolytic jaundice. If the reaction is severe, haemoglobinaemia, haemoglobinuria and renal tubular necrosis are likely. Death may occur.

BLOOD VESSELS

Now read Arteries (p. 24), Veins (p. 344)

ENDOTHELIUM

Capillary endothelial cells play key roles in angiogenesis (p. 16). Arterial and arteriolar endothelial cells regulate atherogenesis. Venous and venular endothelial cells modulate inflammation and repair, haemostasis, thrombosis and tumour spread (p. 246).

Endothelial cells

Endothelial cells form numerous biologically active molecules. One of the most important, endothelium-derived relaxing factor (EDRF), is nitric oxide (p. 134). Among others are: coagulation and anti-coagulation factors; molecules promoting and inhibiting fibrinolysis; potent vasoconstrictors such as endothelin; and the endothelial cell adhesion molecules that determine polymorph margination.

Endothelialisation

Endothelial cells extend over and cover internal vascular surfaces after the normal cell lining has been lost. They rapidly line the inner surfaces of synthetic vascular grafts.

DEVELOPMENTAL AND CONGENITAL DISORDERS

Malformations of arteries are outlined on p. 25.

Dysplasia

In renal dysplasia (p. 85), for example, there may be reduplication of the vessels, stenosis of the mouth of a renal artery, and constriction of an artery passing to an ectopic, pelvic kidney.

TUMOURS

The diagnosis of tumours suspected to arise from vascular endothelial cells can now be assisted by the demonstration of markers, molecules such as factor VIII-related antigen, vWF (p. 101), CD 31 and CD 34.

Benign

Many congenital lesions thought to be vascular tumours are found to be hamartomas (p. 146).

Haemangioma

In heritable disorders such as the Osler–Weber–Rendu syndrome, angiomas are multiple and occur at sites as varied as the skin, mucosae, liver and spleen.

- **Capillary haemangiomas** are localised, but not encapsulated, deep-red meshworks of capillary-size vessels that contain red blood cells. They are one form of cutaneous 'birthmark' but are also found as solitary lesions in the viscera.
- **Cavernous haemangiomas** are seen as clearly defined, uniformly red–purple masses in the skin, lips and tongue and within the liver and other organs. They are formed of large, sinus-like, blood vascular channels.

Glomus tumour

Glomus tumour is an exquisitely tender, small, blue–purple island within the skin of the fingers or toes. The tumour centres upon a convoluted arteriole. There is an endothelial cell-lined vascular component, the channels of which are separated by a connective tissue and smooth-muscular stroma; and a population of cuboidal, myoid cells. Many myelinated and non-myelinated nerve fibres are present.

Glomus jugulare tumour

Glomus jugulare tumour originates in the glomus tissue in the wall of the jugular vein. It extends within the middle ear or cranium and is recognised as a highly vascular, aural polyp.

Chemodectoma

Chemodectoma describes a non-functioning, glomus-like tumour that arises in vascular organs, such as the carotid body, that have a specialised chemoreceptor function. Unlike chromaffinoma (p. 7), a population of 'chief' cells lying within a connective tissue stroma does not give a chromaffin reaction.

Malignant

Haemangio-endothelioma

Haemangio-endotheliomas are rare, slow-growing, vascular tumours of endothelial origin that occupy an intermediate position between benign haemangioma and angiosarcoma. Some are of a solid, cellular character. They are recognised in the viscera, where they are close to, or arise from, a large vein or artery.

One example is **spindle cell haemangio-endothelioma**, a tumour found in the skin or subcutaneous tissues of young men, mainly involving the distal extremities. It may recur locally but does not metastasise.

Angiosarcoma

The development of angiosarcoma is a rare complication of radiotherapy for breast carcinoma. Several other causes of angiosarcoma have been identified including occupational exposure to vinyl chloride, and AIDS. Although some of these rare tumours are recognised in the skin, others arise in the liver. Angiosarcoma of the head and neck, and especially of the scalp, is encountered in the skin of elderly persons. The malignancy of angiosarcoma contrasts with a high degree of histological differentiation.

Kaposi's sarcoma

Fully-developed Kaposi's sarcoma is a particular form of biphasic angiosarcoma. There are four variants (Table 11).

Causes

More than 100 years ago, Kaposi (p. 372) described the occasional, sporadic occurrence of small, purple nodules on the skin of elderly Eastern Europeans. A closely similar condition is endemic in Uganda, while African children are susceptible to an aggressive form of the disease that affects lymph nodes rather than the skin. Now, Kaposi's sarcoma has attracted attention because of its recognition in homosexual and bisexual males, but not drug abusers, with AIDS. The initiating agent in these immunocompromised individuals is believed to be human herpes virus 8 (HHV 8) (p. 351). The tumour may be promoted by factors released from normal cells that lead to angiogenesis.

Structure

There is a focal proliferation of small blood vascular channels from which red blood cells escape, and a fibrosarcoma-like proliferation of spindle cells. The lesions are multiple, small skin patches which arise on the head and neck, limbs, trunk and hard palate; and

Table 11 Variant forms of Kaposi's sarcoma

Variant	Risk group	Median survival
Classic (Kaposi, 1872)	Elderly East European or Mediterranean men	Decades or years
Endemic	African children or adults	Years or months
Immunosuppression or transplant-associated	Organ transplant recipients	Years or months
Epidemic or AIDS-associated	HIV infected persons, especially homosexual or bisexual men	Months or weeks

visceral lesions that appear in the alimentary tract, liver and lymph nodes.

Now read AIDS (p. 2)

Behaviour

By contrast with the sarcomas recognised in Uganda a century ago, the AIDS associated tumour is aggressive and affects not only the skin but the mouth, gut and lymph nodes. The lung is implicated and inexorable progression leads to death.

Haemangiopericytoma

Haemangiopericytomas are spindle cell tumours that arise in the subcutaneous tissue of the limbs or in the connective tissues of the retroperitoneum. The component cells lie outside the endothelium. Continued growth and metastasis are probable.

BONE

An understanding of the mechanisms and time sequence of bone formation, growth and maturation is necessary in order to comprehend the nature of most bone diseases.

Biopsy

Bone biopsy demands special techniques. In the search for metastatic tumour deposits or other bone disease, a serrated ~30 mm rotary cutting trephine is used, operated manually or by motor. The target for biopsy is selected after ultrasonic, CT or MRI scans have indicated the likely sites of lesions. The samples are **decalcified**, cut by heavy-duty microtome, and stained with haematoxylin and eosin (p. 158). Bone for the diagnosis of metabolic disease is taken from the iliac crest posterior to the anterior, superior iliac spine. The ~8 × 20 mm core is examined **undecalcified**. Stains are used that demonstrate osteoid seams.

Osteoid can be labelled and bone growth assessed by preliminary, oral doses of the fluorescent antibiotic tetracycline which binds to osteoid but, inconveniently, also to dentine. Young teeth retain their fluorescence permanently, to the embarrassment of 'disco' goers.

Biochemistry

Biochemical markers applicable to the diagnosis of metabolic bone disease include serum calcium, phosphate, alkaline phosphatase (bone formation), and urinary hydroxyproline (bone resorption).

Now read Biopsy (p. 40)

DEVELOPMENTAL AND CONGENITAL DISORDERS

Bone is subject to an extremely wide range of local and systemic, developmental disorders. Many are asymptomatic. The defects range from abnormally shaped skulls to supernumerary fingers and toes. Cervical rib is occasionally responsible for a thoracic outlet syndrome in which vascular and nerve compression result in limb ischaemia and pain. Osteogenesis imperfecta and chondrodystrophia fetalis are examples of generalised disease.

Osteogenesis imperfecta

Osteogenesis imperfecta (OI), the brittle bone syndrome, is a group of rare, inherited defects of the type

1 collagen molecule. Type 1 OI is an autosomal dominant characteristic but other types are inherited as autosomal recessive abnormalities. The defect results in diminished bone and dentine formation. Multiple fractures of the fragile bone; thin, blue sclerae; and cardiac valve abnormalities are characteristic. Imaging techniques may reveal skeletal fractures *in utero*.

Chondrodystrophia fetalis (achondroplasia)

Achondroplasia, the so-called 'circus dwarf anomaly', is an inherited defect of bones that grow by endochondral ossification. It is inherited as an autosomal dominant characteristic. When one parent is affected, the disorder is therefore expressd in 50% of the children. The mutant gene on somatic chromosome 4 codes for FGFR3, a protein that regulates the action of fibroblast growth factor (FGF) on cartilage. The long bones and those of the spine are conspicuously abnormal so that the individual, who may be male or female, is of short stature. The cranium is unaffected and the brain and intelligence are normal. Typically, the columns of chondrocytes at the growing ends of the long bones are short and irregular. Individuals with the disorder enjoy lives of normal duration and often find employment in theatres, circuses or the cinema.

GROWTH AND ENDOCRINE DISORDERS

Bone is prone to every form of nutritional and metabolic disturbance and readily shows the adverse influences of insufficient or excessive use. At sites of injury or irritation, new bone forms exostoses. Osteophytes, a comparable variety of exophytic bone growth, extend at the edges of joints affected by osteoarthritis, at the margins of ageing vertebrae, and in 'bunions'.

Atrophy

Bone quickly atrophies under conditions of decreased use or persistent or intermittent pressure. Atrophy is an important complication of bed rest but surprisingly small amounts of daily exercise are prophylactic.

Cyst

Simple bone cysts increase slowly in size at their sites of origin at the growing ends of long bones. The proximal end of the humerus is prone to this disorder.

Fibrous dysplasia

Fibrous dysplasia is one of the many localised bone diseases that simulate a neoplastic process. Islands of immature, 'woven' bone form in single or multiple sites. The lesions are expansile but circumscribed. The ribs, jaw, femur and tibia are often affected. Growth of the lesions ceases after puberty but pathological fracture is a common complication.

Myositis ossificans

Myositis ossificans is described on p. 238.

Paget's disease of bone

Paget's disease of bone (p. 374), osteitis deformans, is a frequent **local** disorder, affecting single or multiple islands of cranial, vertebral, pelvic, tibial or femoral bone in elderly persons. Rarely, the disorder is **generalised**. The aetiology is obscure. Paramyxovirus infection, autoimmunity and disordered endocrine regulation of bone growth have been implicated.

Excess osteoblastic new bone formation accompanies vigorous osteoclastic bone re-absorption leading to a mosaic pattern. The affected bone, heavy, dense and of low mechanical strength, becomes highly vascular, enabling easy recognition by isotopic scans. The local increase in blood flow may become so large that high-output cardiac failure develops. Paget's disease is an identified cause of osteosarcoma in the elderly.

There is a beneficial response to therapeutic calcitonin and to biphosphonates.

Osteitis fibrosa cystica (von Recklinghausen's disease)

In hyperparathyroidism (p. 267), parathyroid hormone (PTH) is secreted in excess. The source of PTH is usually either parathyroid adenoma or hyperplasia. Osteoclastic bone resorption is catalysed. The process is initiated by osteoblasts that retract from bone margins and secrete collagenase, exposing bone to vigorous phagocytosis. Osteoclasts burrow into the mineralised material, creating resorption lacunae. There is simultaneous but less active, new bone formation. Bone architecture is destroyed locally. Misshapen trabeculae appear. Marrow spaces fill with fibroblasts. The affected tissue is highly vascular. Haemosiderin escapes and the result, in untreated cases, is the presence of increasingly large islands of soft, brown tissue that becomes acellular, gelatinous and cystic and easily recognised by conventional radiography or CT scanning

METABOLIC DISORDERS

Osteomalacia/rickets

The normal growth, mineralisation and morphology of bone depend on the availability of adequate amounts of calcium and vitamin D.

Osteomalacia results from the inadequate mineralisation of bone matrix (osteoid), formed normally and in normal amounts (Fig. 9). The serum concentrations of calcium and phosphate are low but serum alkaline phosphatase activity is elevated. Before the growth of bone ceases and while endochondral ossification continues, the effects of inadequate mineralisation are more complex and the disease is called **rickets**.

The causes of osteomalacia/rickets are:

- Inadequate dietary vitamin D and calcium.
- Defective absorption of vitamin D.
- Defective utilisation of vitamin D.

Osteomalacia affects 4% of the elderly people of Western Europe and is an intractable problem in countries where social and religious practices prevent exposure to sunlight, the agency that promotes the synthesis of a vitamin D in the skin. Vitamin D deficiency (p. 351) is common among all elderly and housebound people. However, subclinical deficiency is also frequent in populations of surgical patients. It is a risk factor for bone loss and fracture. In the old, and in infants, dietary deficiencies can be corrected easily. Osteomalacia is diagnosed

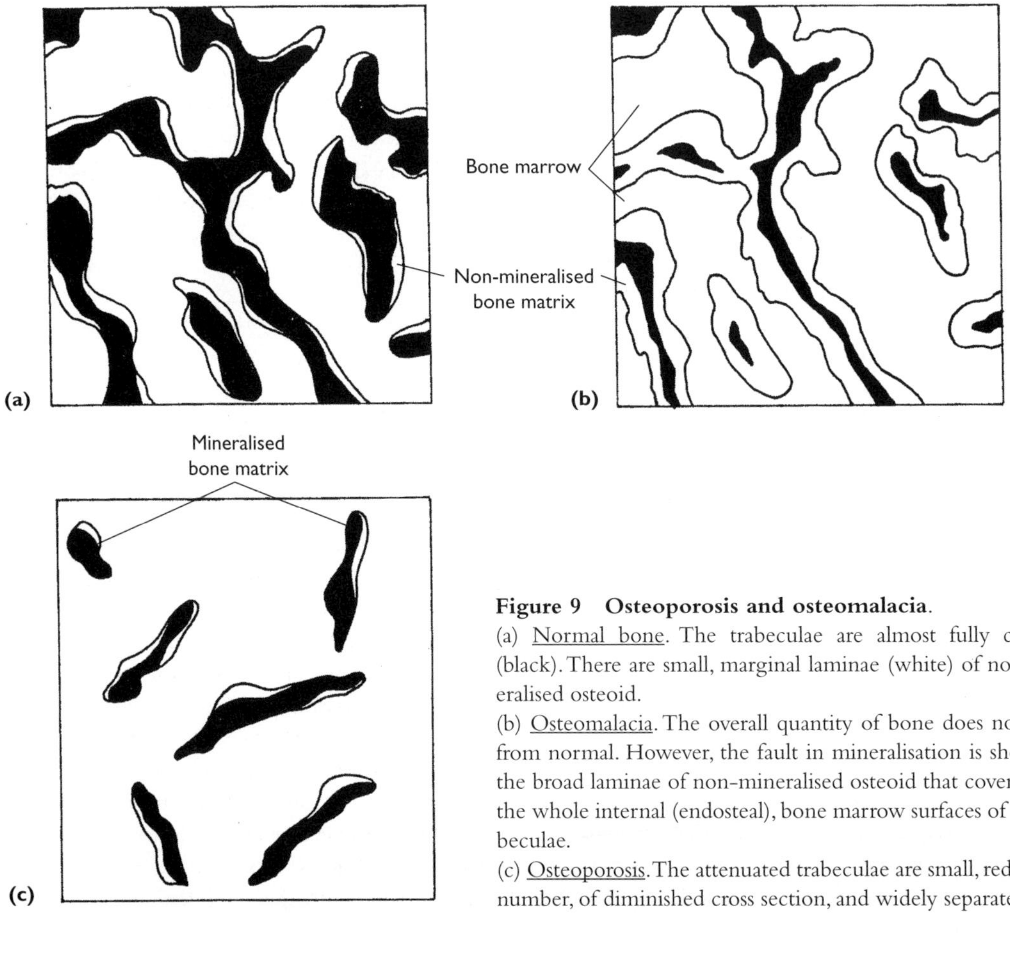

Figure 9 Osteoporosis and osteomalacia.
(a) Normal bone. The trabeculae are almost fully calcified (black). There are small, marginal laminae (white) of non-mineralised osteoid.
(b) Osteomalacia. The overall quantity of bone does not differ from normal. However, the fault in mineralisation is shown by the broad laminae of non-mineralised osteoid that cover almost the whole internal (endosteal), bone marrow surfaces of the trabeculae.
(c) Osteoporosis. The attenuated trabeculae are small, reduced in number, of diminished cross section, and widely separated.

sensitively by biopsy of the iliac crest (p. 50). The seams of non-mineralised bone can be measured and the response to treatment followed closely.

Osteomalacic bone is weak; pathological fracture readily occurs. Zones of incomplete pseudofracture, Looser's zones, are characteristic. They are detectable in the bone cortex, by X-ray. In vertebral bone, the appearance of 'rugger-jersey' spine is diagnostic. A particular form of osteomalacia occurs after prolonged renal dialysis with soft water containing aluminium. Osteomalacia is one of several forms of renal bone disease.

Now read Calcium (p. 74), Vitamin D (p. 351)

Osteoporosis

Osteoporosis is a local or systemic skeletal disease characterised by a low bone mass and micro-architectural deterioration, with a consequent increase in bone fragility (Fig. 9). The bone mineral density, best monitored at the lumbar spine, is at least 2.5 SD below that of the mean peak value in young adults. Unlike osteomalacia, the bone formed in osteoporosis is fully mineralised. Nevertheless, osteoporotic bone is mechanically weak. Pathological fracture is therefore commonplace. The femoral neck and the vertebrae are particularly vulnerable.

Throughout life, bone is continually lost and replaced. The balance of this daily turnover becomes negative in the most common forms of osteoporosis. Imperceptibly, bone loss comes to exceed bone formation. Since there is neither any fault in calcium metabolism nor abnormally raised bone destruction, serum concentrations of calcium, phosphate and alkaline phosphatase are normal and there is no increase in the excretion of calcium. However, the urine may contain an excess of collagen metabolites.

Osteoporosis is commonplace in the elderly of both sexes (senile osteoporosis) but is more severe in women than men. It is particularly likely in immobilised patients and is a hazard for those who seldom exercise. Astronauts travelling in 'space' were shown to be at risk because of weightlessness. Inadequate nutrition is a contributory factor. Osteoporosis occurs frequently in women after the menopause (postmenopausal osteoporosis). The disorder is provoked (systemically) by drugs such as corticosteroids and (locally) by inflammatory disorders such as rheumatoid arthritis. Osteoporosis also results from endocrine diseases such as hyperthyroidism and Cushing's syndrome. Protein malnutrition and heritable diseases such as osteogenesis imperfecta are other causes.

Tumours, such as metastatic carcinoma, leukaemia or myeloma, lead to a form of osteoporosis by destroying bone directly. The result is hypercalcaemia and an increased urinary excretion of calcium and hydroxyproline.

In diagnosis, conventional X-rays offer little assistance: the earliest recognisable change equates with a loss of ~25% of bone mass. However, changes of the order of 1% are demonstrable by dual photon absorptiometry. Quantitative CT and ultrasonography are also of value. Iliac-crest biopsy remains the most sensitive method of diagnosis. The degree of bone change can be measured microscopically.

INFECTION AND INFLAMMATION

Osteomyelitis

Osteitis is bone inflammation whereas osteomyelitis is inflammation of the medullary cavity of bone. However, the term osteomyelitis is generally taken to mean any form of bone infection.

The cause of osteomyelitis in the young is usually bacterial and the most frequent agent is *Staphylococcus aureus*. Haemophilus is another cause in children. Characteristically, the organisms gain access to the bloodstream from a small and undetected skin lesion such as a boil. Bacteria lodge in the end-arteries of metaphyses, particularly those of the femur or tibia. An abscess forms.

Now read Staphylococcus (p. 303)

Osteomyelitis is also a complication of trauma. Infection with *Pseudomonas aeruginosa* may follow compound fracture in road-traffic accidents or after intravenous drug abuse. Among other bacteria associated with osteomyelitis are Streptococcus spp. and Salmonella spp. especially *Salmonella typhi* in patients with sickle-cell disease. Fungal, parasitic and viral forms of osteomyelitis are occasionally recognised so that *Histoplasma capsulatum* var. *duboisii*, for example, frequently induces bone disease in poor, subtropical and tropical countries.

- The inert, dead bone is a **sequestrum**.
- The envelope of periosteal new bone surrounding the site of infection is an **involucrum**.

In the absence of antibiotic treatment, tissue destruction extends. Small, additional, intra-osseous abscesses form, accompanied by bone necrosis. As a longstanding, chronic abscess increases in size, a track may form, communicating with the skin and allowing the escape of pus through an opening or **cloaca**. Infection rarely spreads through the epiphysis to the nearby joint. Among the complications of persistent and inadequately treated disease is amyloidosis (p. 9).

Vertebral osteomyelitis

Blood-borne infection occasionally leads to the localised destruction of bone adjoining a vertebral end-plate. *Staphylococcus aureus* is the most frequent cause but *Escherichia coli*, Haemophilus and Salmonella are occasionally agents.

Brodie's abscess

The metaphyses of long bones such as the tibia may be sites for subacute or chronic localised osteomyelitis. An abscess forms. The contents may be sterile and the lesion is circumscribed by a radio-opaque lamina of reactive new bone.

Tuberculous osteitis

Mycobacterium tuberculosis evokes a particular form of osteomyelitis of bone near infected joints. Tuberculosis of bone is frequently termed osteitis rather than osteomyelitis and is sometimes given special designations such as Pott's disease (p. 375), tuberculous vertebral osteitis.

Tuberculous osteitis is a result of blood-borne infection with *Myco. tuberculosis* (p. 237). It is a worldwide form of chronic destructive bone disease. In populations not protected by BCG vaccination (p. 333), tuberculous osteitis is frequent in young persons but in Western countries it is more often recognised in the elderly. The incidence of tuberculous osteitis is increasing in large cities where AIDS and poverty combine to constitute a susceptible population. Immigrants are particularly at risk. Mycobacteria, conveyed to bone from pulmonary, lymph node or renal sources via the bloodstream, lodge near the epiphyses. The vertebrae are especially vulnerable but no bone formed by endochondral ossification is spared and the elbow, wrist, hip and knee joints are often implicated.

An acute inflammatory response is followed by granuloma formation with caseous necrosis and bone death but without reactive new bone formation. Vertebral bodies are progressively destroyed; they collapse, leading to angulation of the spine (gibus) and scoliosis or kyphoscoliosis. The sheath of a psoas muscle may be penetrated, allowing a 'cold' abscess (p. 1) to present below the inguinal ligament. In the absence of treatment, tuberculous vertebral osteitis extends to the spinal membranes. Tuberculous meningitis is one result; spinal cord compression, culminating in paraplegia, is another.

Now read Tuberculosis (p. 332)

MECHANICAL INJURY AND TRAUMA

Fracture

Fracture is the breaking of a hard material or tissue. The term is applied to both bone and cartilage.

In the majority of fractures (Fig. 10), there is a loss of continuity of cortical bone caused by **tensile** or by **shear stress**. In other cases, for example in the vertebrae, mechanical force reduces the volume of bone and the fractures are the result of **compressive stress**. Fracture may be a natural response by normal tissue to excessive direct or indirect force. Alternatively, fracture may occur in abnormal tissue that is unable to withstand physiological stresses. It is **pathological**. According to their anatomical form, fractures are classified as transverse, oblique or spiral. When there are many small fragments of bone, the fracture is **comminuted**. When bone fragments penetrate the skin or an epithelial surface, the fracture is **compound**.

In ageing populations, falls cause a large proportion of fractures. Among those aged over 60 years in the UK, the age-adjusted incidence in males rose from $4840/10^6$ persons in 1970 to $8400/10^6$ in 1995. In females, the corresponding figures were $11670/10^6$ and $19110/10^6$ persons. In younger populations, road traffic accidents are the predominant cause.

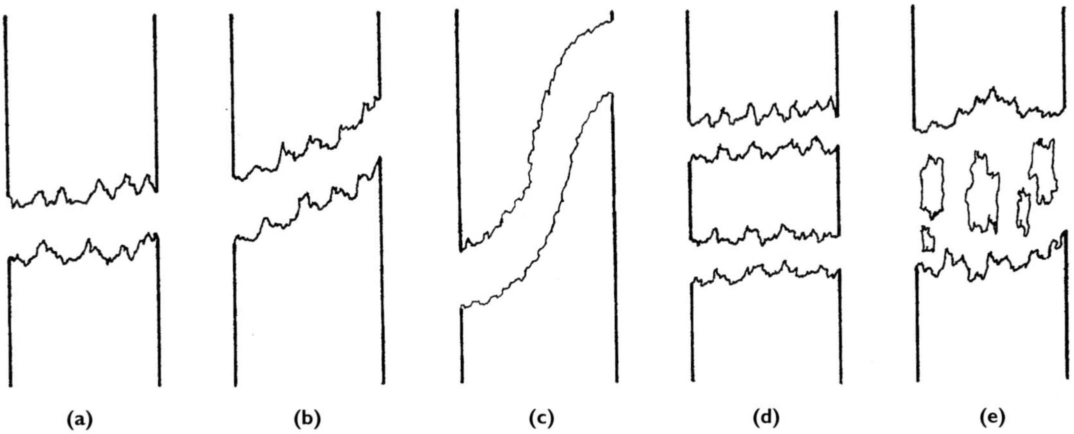

Figure 10 Bone fracture classification.
Anatomical form and appearances of fracture reflect nature and direction of compressive, tensile or shear forces that caused injury. Forces may be direct (impact) but are often exerted obliquely or during rotation. Categories are: (a) transverse; (b) oblique; (c) spiral; (d) segmental; (e) comminuted.

Fracture healing (Fig. 11)

Although the rate of healing of fractures is enhanced by immobilisation, very slight movement is of benefit.

Haematoma

Immediately after fracture, blood escapes in large amounts from injured periosteal, endosteal and marrow blood vessels and from those of nearby soft tissue. Blood coagulates in extravascular planes, forming a haematoma between and around the fractured bone ends. The extent of the haematoma is affected by the degree to which the bone ends are displaced. Fragments of ischaemic bone are scattered at the fracture site. Inflammation is excited by the local tissue injury. Polymorphs and then macrophages accumulate and engulf and destroy cell and tissue debris.

Granulation tissue

Within a few hours of fracture, repair begins. Capillary endothelial buds and dividing fibroblasts extend from adjacent viable tissue into the haematoma. The increased vascularity results in local osteoporosis of nearby bone. Type I bone collagen is laid down, together with a randomly arranged, non-collagenous matrix rich in proteoglycan. The response is the formation of granulation tissue that fills the space between the bone ends after 2–7 days.

Provisional callus

Within 1–2 days of injury, osteoblasts of the surviving periosteal and endosteal surfaces are activated. Together with the fibroblasts of the granulation tissue, these osteoprogenitor cells synthesise a disorderly microskeleton of extracellular osteocollagen that, with the associated proteoglycan, is called **osteoid**. Alkaline phosphatase formed by these cells catalyses the deposition of bone mineral in this extracellular matrix. The mineralised osteoid is described as **woven bone**. This material gradually fills the space between the fractured bones, extending to form a spindle-shaped mass external to the bone contours. It is the **provisional callus**. During the 5–15 days after injury, it has a splint-like, supportive function. Particularly beneath the periosteum, islands of cartilaginous matrix are seen. They are more extensive where there is relative ischaemia and larger when immobilisation is incomplete and healing delayed.

Definitive callus

Within 14–21 days, phagocytic osteoclasts start to remove the woven bone of the provisional callus and degradation of this mineralised tissue begins. The cells do not digest cartilage. Resorption of callus is accompanied by a vigorous, further process of orderly, lamellar bone synthesis. It forms a **definitive callus**. Arrays of activated osteoblasts synthesise osteocollagen and proteoglycan, and catalyse mineralisation by means of their alkaline phosphatase.

Remodelling

Influenced by the stresses of weight-bearing and movement, and by piezo-electrical forces, the excess external (subperiosteal) and internal (medullary) callus is now gradually and insidiously remodelled, restoring the shape and architecture of the bone to meet the stresses of normal movement and load-bearing.

Fractures of normal bones in **childhood** heal completely although the growth of a long bone after fracture can be excessive. Fractures involving epiphyseal plates threaten bone growth and may cause deformity; their significance is predicted by the Salter–Harris classification. In the very young, CT and MR scans and X-rays made years later may reveal no residual signs of fracture. By contrast, anatomical restoration of fracture sites **in the adult** is never entirely perfect and the location of a healed fracture can be identified as a permanent zone of subperiosteal roughening.

Delayed union (healing)

The healing of uncomplicated fractures may be delayed by:

- Excessive movement.
- Infection.
- Deficient blood supply.
- Systemic disease.
- Malnutrition.
- Old age.

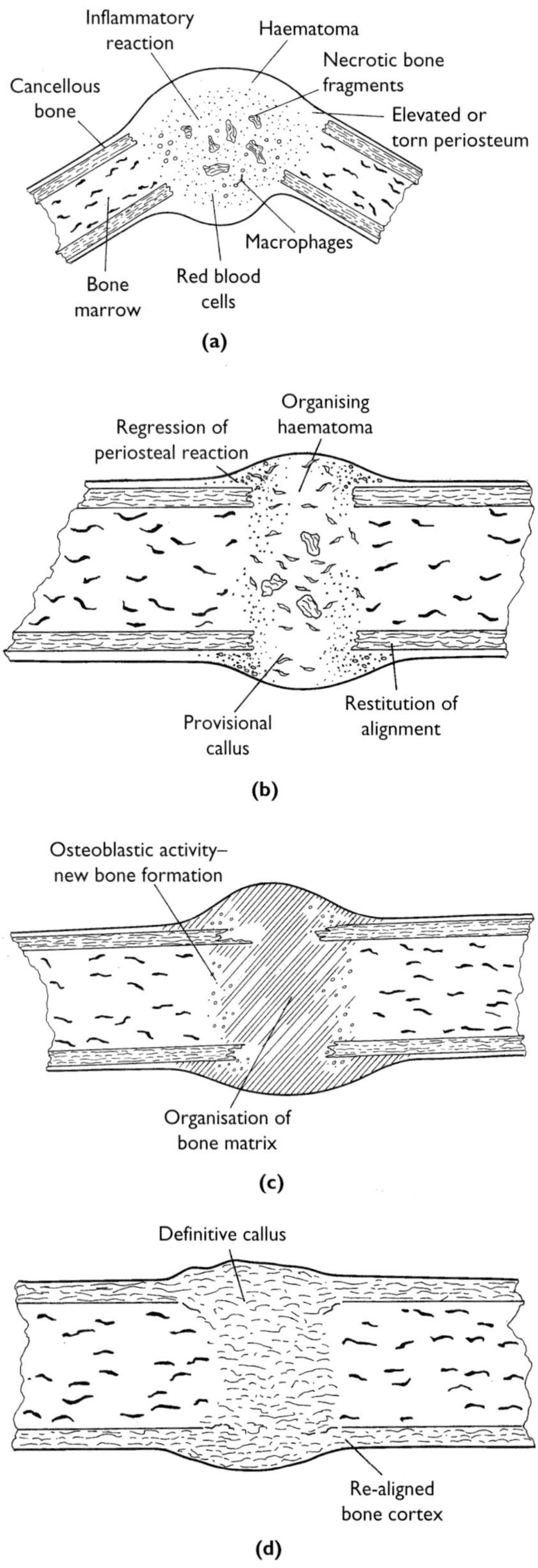

Figure 11 Bone fracture healing.

(a) Haematoma and necrosis. Immediate effects of uncomplicated fracture include displacement of bone ends; extensive local bleeding; necrosis of bone fragments; and onset of local inflammation.

(b) Provisional callus. Macrophages engulf dead tissue. Capillaries grow out from live bone ends; collagenous, fibrous tissue forms; and osteoid is laid down as temporary ('provisional') callus.

(c) Bone formation. Periosteal and trabecular bone osteoblasts catalyse osteoid deposition, new bone formation and mineralisation.

(d) Remodelling. Definitive callus undergoes slow process of remodelling taking place over many months. Childhood fractured bone resumes normal shape; adult fractured bone retains evidence of displacement and periosteal reaction.

Delayed healing is characteristic of compound fractures.

Movement

Shearing movements disturb granulation tissue and exacerbate inflammation. Distraction may also delay union, whereas impaction accelerates healing.

Infection

Bacterial infection prolongs and exaggerates the inflammatory response at fracture sites. Pus may accumulate. Abscesses form and osteomyelitis leads to ischaemic necrosis.

Ischaemia

Fractures can injure the arterial blood supply to bone and joint tissue irretrievably. Bone necrosis is an early consequence. More often, ischaemia is partial, and the growth of granulation tissue and the formation of osteoid simply impaired. Delayed healing is more likely where arterial supplies are precarious, as in fractures of the neck of the femur or of the scaphoid, or where blood vessels are abnormal, as in the aged.

Systemic disease

Renal failure with uraemia, diabetes mellitus and malnutrition are examples of systemic disorders in which fracture healing is often prejudiced.

Non-union (absence of healing)

Any sufficiently severe or prolonged, local or systemic factor predisposing to delayed healing may result in a failure of the union of a fracture. An example is the interposition of the tendon of the tibialis posterior between the bone fragments in fracture of the medial malleolus. Again, soft tissue may lie between the opposed parts of a fractured bone. Union is then impossible.

Occasionally, a pseudarthrosis (p. 283) may form at the site of non-union.

Fibrous union

Fibrous union is, in effect, repair as it is seen in soft, non-mineralised connective tissue. Fibrous union therefore represents defective mineralisation and may result from any of the numerous local or systemic causes of this process.

Pathological fracture

Pathological fractures are produced by the application of normal forces to diseased bones.

The causes are heritable and acquired. Pathological fracture may be a complication of any generalised disease in which there is reduced bone strength; it may also result from local bone disorders. A common explanation is metastatic carcinoma. Comparable fractures may be due to simple cysts or primary bone tumours. Examples of disorders in which decreased strength accompanies **reduced bone density** include osteoporosis, osteomalacia, osteitis fibrosa cystica and osteogenesis imperfecta. Examples of diseases in which decreased strength is associated with **increased bone density** include Paget's disease of bone and osteosclerosis. Abnormally dense bone is often weak.

Pathological fractures can heal readily, provided the cause is effectively treated. However, in those cases where fracture is due to the presence of primary or secondary neoplastic tissue, healing is inevitably delayed or prevented.

Spontaneous fracture

Spontaneous fractures are caused in normal bone by the sudden application of relatively small, unexpected forces. A normal lower limb bone can break readily when a single step down a stair is taken in darkness; there is no protective, reflex contraction of the skeletal muscles acting about the nearby joints.

Stress or **fatigue fractures** are caused by the repetitive application to normal bone of small forces, each episode alone being insufficient to produce a fracture. Fatigue fractures of the tarsal and metatarsal bones are common among joggers and soldiers ('march fracture'), and among ballet dancers. Avulsion of the spinous process of the seventh cervical vertebra ('clay-shovellers' disease') and lateral epicondylitis ('tennis elbow') are other examples.

TUMOURS

Tumours of bone are metastatic or primary (Tables 12 and 13). The former are very much more frequent than the latter.

Table 12 The most frequent primary benign bone tumours

Tumour	Site of origin	Pathological features	Radiological features	Behaviour
Osteochondroma	Metaphysis of long bones	Extending cortical island of bone covered by cartilage	Orderly exophytic bone processes	Excision is curative Metaphyseal aclasis is multiple form
Osteoid osteoma	Long bones, spine	Osteoblastic focus. Margin of bone sclerosis	Radiolucent centre Isotopic scan	Pain, alleviated by aspirin. Curettage is curative
Osteoblastoma	Long bones Posterior arch of vertebrae	Osteoblast-rich tissue	Circumscribed lytic or calcified island	May recur after curettage
Giant cell tumour	Epiphysis of long bone	Dark brown; zones of necrosis; multinucleate, giant cells; spindle cells	Radiolucent, solitary	Unpredictable. Although majority benign, may recur
Chondromyxoid fibroma	Metaphysis of tibia, metatarsals	Islands of myxoid tissue. May resemble chondrosarcoma	Defined lytic lesion	May recur after curettage
Chondroblastoma	Epiphysis of long bones e.g. femur, humerus	Chondroblast islands, chondroid matrix	Lytic lesion, sclerotic margin	May recur after curettage

Table 13 The most common primary malignant bone tumours

Malignant tumour	Site of origin	Pathological features	Radiological features	Behaviour
Osteosarcoma Parosteal osteosarcoma is a distinct category with better prognosis	Long bones, particularly near knee	Sarcoma cells always form osteoid or bone	Bone destruction with lysis or sclerosis and periosteal extension	5-year survival improving with controlled chemotherapy
Chondrosarcoma	Pelvis, ribs, femur, humerus	Large cartilage masses with focal calcification	Expanding bone lesion with thickening of cortex	Radical surgery can cure usual low-grade tumours
Ewing's sarcoma	Diaphysis or metaphysis of long bones, pelvis, ribs, scapula	Round cell tumour with special staining characteristics	Destructive and lytic lesion	A tumour of children, adolescents. Chemotherapy improves 5-year survival
Fibrosarcoma	Metaphysis of long bones	Cell structure determines grading	Bone lysis and destruction of cortex	Prognosis relates to grade. Lung metastases in high-grade tumours
Malignant fibrous histiocytoma	Metaphysis of long bones	Microscopic appearances distinct from fibrosarcoma	Aggressive tumour with bone lysis and destruction	May arise on basis of Paget's disease, bone infarction, irradiation
Chordoma	Sacrococcygeal region or skull base, from notochordal remnants	Large, destructive gelatinous masses	Variegated zones of bone lysis and focal calcification	Inexorable, slow local growth but seldom metastasise

Metastatic

The most common primary sources of cancer metastatic to bone, are the bronchus, breast, prostate, kidney and thyroid, in descending order of frequency. Thyroid metastases are usually derived from follicular carcinomas. Carcinomas of the pancreas, colon, stomach and ovary are other, less frequent sources.

The majority of metastases are **osteolytic**. Metastatic cells release parathormone-related protein (PTH-rP). Osteoclasts are stimulated and bone is resorbed. Transforming growth factor beta (TGF-β) and peptides like insulin-like growth factor-1 (IGF 1) are also released. They cause further bone destruction and stimulate proliferation of tumour cells. The zones of rarefaction that result are readily detected by radiography or by CT scans.

A much smaller proportion of metastases is **osteosclerotic**. Whether secondary deposits are bone-destroying or bone-forming is not directly related to their microscopic structure or grade. The most common and most important example of osteosclerotic metastasis is carcinoma of the prostate.

Primary

With few exceptions, primary benign and primary malignant bone tumours are diseases of young persons. The exceptions are multiple myeloma and most cases of chondrosarcoma.

Benign

Osteochondroma (p. 83), osteoid osteoma, osteoblastoma, giant cell tumour, chondromyxoid fibroma and chondroblastoma are the most frequent, although none is common (Table 12).

Osteoid osteoma

Osteoid osteoma is a tumour of the shaft of the long bones of young males. The lesion evokes nocturnal pain that is characteristically relieved by salicylates. The tumour is recognised by CT, MR or radio-isotope imaging. It grows slowly as an island of cells that form immature, woven bone in a minute island or 'nidus' that evokes surrounding radio-opaque osteosclerosis. Treatment by curettage is curative but incomplete removal can permit recurrence.

Malignant

The incidence of primary bone tumours for England and Wales is ~0.007/1000 persons. In Scotland about 40 new cases are recognised annually. Osteosarcoma, chondrosarcoma, Ewing's sarcoma, fibrosarcoma and malignant fibrous histiocytoma are the most frequent primary tumours (Table 13). Osteosarcoma in older persons is a complication of Paget's disease of bone. Chordoma is rare.

Osteosarcoma

Osteosarcoma is the most common primary malignant bone tumour of younger individuals.

Causes In the young, genetic mutations are suspected. In older individuals, half the cases recognised are in those with Paget's disease. Exposure to ionising radiation as a consequence of atomic plant accidents or following atomic explosions is a rare cause.

Structure Arising in the cavity of the metaphyses of long bones, the neoplasm penetrates and destroys the bone cortex, extending beneath, and raising the periosteum. At this site, new bone formation is provoked. A radio-opaque, 'sun-ray' striation is characteristic but the classical description of a Codman's triangle of reactive new bone in the angle between the normal and the elevated periosteum is not pathognomonic.

Further growth involves the epiphyseal plate so that the epiphysis and sometimes the adjoining synovial tissues are implicated. The numerous osteoblastic cells of which the tumour is formed are relatively large, with plump, deeply basophilic nuclei and relatively little cytoplasm. Mitotic figures are seen and may be abnormal. The microscopical recognition of osteoid or calcified bone matrix is of help in diagnosis since it provides evidence of the direction of tumour cell differentiation.

Behaviour and prognosis As with malignant fibrous histiocytoma and other primary, malignant bone tumours, suspicion of osteosarcoma demands immediate referral to a regional centre specialising in the treatment of bone cancer. Evidence of metastasis is frequently obtained at the time of first examination. Initial biopsy may be necessary but chemotherapy or radiotherapy, together with methods such as arterial embolisation, may be used before major surgery is attempted.

Resected specimens are subject to meticulous histological examination. Prognosis is closely related to the extent of the tumour; to the presence or absence of signs of distant metastasis; to evidence of the character and degree of differentiation of the neoplasm; and to signs of its response to therapy. The cells of osteosarcoma lie close to thin-walled marrow blood vessels and the tumour metastasises via the bloodstream to the lungs at a very early stage.

OSTEONECROSIS

Bone receives a large supply of oxygenated blood. Any agency that interrupts the supply to bone of oxygen or essential metabolites is likely to lead to bone death. The common causes of necrosis are injuries to bones supplied by single 'end-arteries'.

The most frequent site of osteonecrosis in childhood is the lateral femoral condyle (Perthes' disease). Death of the femoral head epiphysis in childhood may be due to effusion resulting from viral synovitis or trauma. Other sites of childhood osteonecrosis include the carpal lunate (Keinbock's disease), the navicular (Köhler's disease) and the second metatarsal (Freiburg's disease). Bone death is a complication of uncontrolled decompression in divers. Alcoholism and systemic lupus erythematosus are also predisposing diseases. However, there are many other cases in which no explanation for bone death is known.

Experimental evidence has shown that osteocyte injury occurs within 1–2 hours of the onset of ischaemia. In human osteonecrosis, light microscopic evidence of bone marrow cell death is recognisable within 2–3 days of loss of oxygen or arterial blood supply. Overt bone cell loss is not seen so soon.

Osteochondritis dissecans

In osteochondritis dissecans, a zone of knee subchondral femoral bone dies. The overlying cartilage, an avascular tissue, separates from the necrotic bone. The cartilage remains viable and constitutes a loose body within the joint within which it can provoke injury to the other articular bearing surfaces. Impaired joint movement with 'locking' is a consequence.

The aetiology of osteochondritis dissecans is uncertain. The condition occurs relatively often in athletic teenagers. The sites at which the condition may occur, and the subsequent course of the disease, suggest that ischaemia caused by trauma is important.

TRANSPLANTATION – BONE GRAFTING

The successful, historical use of dead bone in grafting rested on its lack of immunogenicity. The transplant acted as an inert microskeleton into which new, osteoprogenitor cells grew slowly.

Viable bone and cartilage grafts demand the same procedures of immunosuppression as other forms of transplant (p. 329).

BRAIN

Until recently, the regeneration or repair of brain and spinal cord cells was regarded as impossible. However, the transplantation of fetal dopamine-secreting cells (p. 7) has been shown to ease the symptoms of Parkinson's disease and implanted testicular Sertoli cells (p. 319) can stimulate CNS nerve cell re-growth.

Biopsy diagnosis of brain disease

Tissue is obtained by needle – or by open biopsy. In the diagnosis of tumours, smears of brain tissue are employed.

RESPONSE TO HYPOXIA OR ISCHAEMIA

Anoxia and ischaemia

The viability of central nervous system neurones depends upon a continual supply of oxygen and glucose. The cells are therefore highly sensitive to decreased cerebral arterial blood flow. Provided the blood pressure does not fall below 50–70 mmHg, an autoregulatory mechanism maintains an adequate blood supply. At lower pressures, the brain suffers from the effects of the diminished oxygenation.

The severity of the effects of cerebral ischaemia is much influenced by site and duration.

- **Site**. When cerebral ischaemia is focal and incomplete, neuronal injury is anatomically selective.

The boundary zones between adjacent vascular territories are vulnerable: they are furthest from incoming arterial blood. The effects of ischaemia are felt particularly by the neurones of the hippocampus, the deeper layers of parts of the parietal and occipital cortex, and the Purkinje cells of the cerebellum.

- **Duration**. The effects of sustained hypotension or prolonged cardiac arrest are much more severe than those of transient hypotension. If the injury is **transient**, changes in neuronal structure are recognised with difficulty. Indeed, alterations in the number and appearance of the astrocytes give a more reliable indication of the disorder than alterations in nerve cell structure. If ischaemia is **sustained**, cerebral infarction is likely.

Severe but transient falls in blood pressure causing focal, cerebral ischaemia, are frequent in elderly patients undergoing major surgical procedures involving general anaesthesia. Those with carotid, vertebral and cerebral artery atheroma are particularly susceptible. A preceding episode of myocardial infarction predisposes to this life-threatening occurrence, or myocardial infarction may take place during an operation. In younger patients, fainting during otherwise simple dental procedures, conducted in an upright, sitting position, is another cause of cerebral ischaemia or infarction.

The earliest tissue changes of cerebral ischaemia or anoxia are detectable biochemically and by electron microscopy. Within 2–3 minutes of the onset of ischaemia, neuronal mitochondria swell and the neurones appear vacuolated. No alteration in structure is detectable by light microscopy until a patient has survived for 12 hours or more. Neuronal death, loss of myelin and a polymorph infiltrate follow. Irreversible cell injury is indicated by loss of Nissl substance, cytoplasmic eosinophilia and nuclear pyknosis. Fine granules appear on the neuronal surface, nuclear shrinkage continues and cytoplasmic staining weakens before the dead cell is digested and removed by phagocytic microglia. Subsequently, macrophages replete with myelin are seen. The phagocytosis of necrotic neurones is **neuronophagia**, a process characteristic of some acute viral infections of the central nervous system. Infarcted cerebral tissue slowly softens. The eventual outcome, in survivors, is a cyst-like cavity containing a faint yellow, watery fluid.

ASTROCYTOSIS AND GLIOSIS

Astrocytes are the predominant glial cells. Microglia are macrophages. The other neuroglia are oligodendrocytes and the ependymal cells. There is an analogy between astrocytes and fibroblasts: both cells are supportive and reparative.

Astrocytosis

When neurones are lost, astrocytes multiply. The division of astrocytes is a response to hypoxia or hypoglycaemia. The presence of paired or clustered astrocytes is evidence of neuronal loss. Multinucleate, giant forms may be present and the cell body may swell. These fattened cells are called gemistocytic astrocytes (**gemistocytes**). Astrocytes are found near inflammatory, ischaemic or neoplastic lesions and in oedematous white matter. They also appear, in excess, in special circumstances such as the encephalopathy of chronic liver failure (p. 209).

Gliosis

Gliosis is the proliferation of the cytoplasmic fibrillary processes of astrocytes. Although gliosis is occasionally physiological, it generally represents a repair mechanism.

RESPONSE TO INTRACRANIAL DISEASE

The brain is a water-rich and highly vascular gel, surrounded by incompressible cerebrospinal fluid and contained within the rigid cranium. In adult life, this structure cannot increase in capacity. Any lesion occupying cranial space is liable to exert widespread hydrodynamic effects upon the brain, irrespective of the nature of the lesion or of the anatomical site. There is a threat to cerebral structure and function. The swelling of brain tissue itself contributes to the dangers of raised intracranial pressure. This swelling is due either to cerebral oedema or to increased cerebral blood flow. The results are important in cases of head injury where vasodilatation contributes critically to the swelling.

The presence of an expanding intracranial lesion therefore prejudices brain structure and function, directly and indirectly. Frequent space-occupying lesions include intracerebral haemorrhage; benign and malignant primary, and metastatic neoplasms;

subdural venous and extradural arterial haemorrhage; abscess; and arterial aneurysm. The hydrodynamic effects of such lesions can be compensated initially by small changes in the volume of intracranial blood and by a reduction in the volume of the cerebrospinal fluid (CSF). Particularly in the presence of quickly expanding lesions, however, compensation rapidly fails and a rise takes place in the CSF pressure.

The results of this failure are crucial to survival. The effects depend upon the location and size of the lesion (Fig. 12). They include flattening of the gyri, subfalcine herniation of the cingulate gyrus, uncal herniation and coning of the medulla. The transmission of pressure to the pons may produce bilateral pontine haemorrhages. Internal, non-communicating hydrocephalus can arise. Compression of medullary centres may threaten respiration, cardiac output, blood pressure and thermoregulation. Coma follows.

If a patient survives, but the rise in intracranial pressure is sustained, the inner table of the skull may display bone atrophy due to pressure from the cerebral gyri.

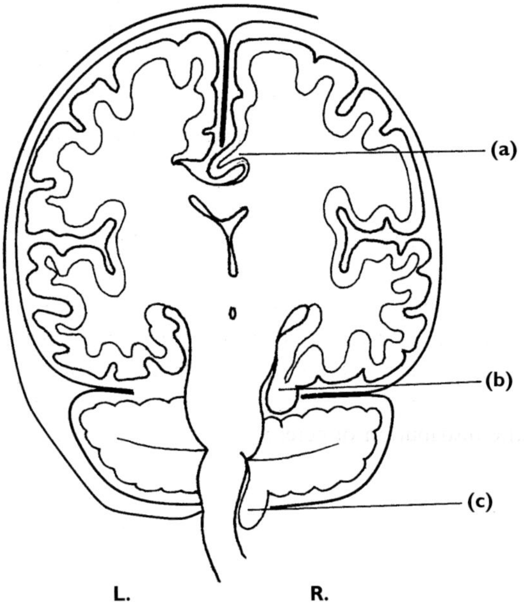

Figure 12 Effects of raised intracranial pressure. Increase in volume of right cerebral hemisphere, for example, due to slowly expanding tumour mass, displaces brain substance laterally and downwards. Results include (a) subfalcine herniation; (b) uncinate herniation; and (c) tonsillar herniation.

Hydrocephalus

Hydrocephalus is the abnormal or excessive accumulation of cerebrospinal fluid (CSF) within the cranium. The disorder leads to dilatation of the cerebral ventricles and raised intracranial pressure.

- In **obstructive** hydrocephalus, there is a block in the flow of CSF in the ventricular system or between the ventricular system and the spinal cord.
- In **communicating** hydrocephalus, there is obstruction to the absorption of CSF but no block.

One cause of hydrocephalus is bacterial meningitis; the inflammatory exudate obstructs the flow of the CSF from the third to the fourth ventricles, or from the fourth ventricle to the subdural spaces. In infancy, in which hydrocephalus may accompany spina bifida, brain atrophy and enlargement of the cranium are sequels.

Supratentorial expanding lesions

Space-occupying lesions situated above the tentorium cerebelli cause an increase in the volume of the affected cerebral hemisphere. The cerebral gyri flatten, the ipsilateral ventricle decreases in volume and there is a shift of midline structures, such as the falx cerebri, towards the contralateral side. In the face of a continuing increase in the size of a lesion, with rising CSF pressure, herniation of brain tissue is probable. Herniation takes place in two anatomical locations: under the margin of the falx cerebri (**subfalcine or supracallosal**) and through the opening of the tentorium (**tentorial**).

Infratentorial expanding lesions

Space-occupying lesions below the tentorium are liable to provoke a further displacement of brain tissue, leading to impaction of the cerebellar tonsils into the foramen magnum with compression of the medulla and the respiratory centre. Infratentorial lesions produce raised intracranial pressure more rapidly than do supratentorial lesions.

Medullary 'coning' (p. 61) may follow injudicious lumbar puncture in the presence of raised intracranial pressure.

DEVELOPMENTAL AND CONGENITAL DISORDERS

Neural tube defects

Spina bifida

Spina bifida describes defective fusion of the neural arches during embryonic development. The fault is associated with dietary folic acid deficiency and assumes several varieties.

Spina bifida cystica
In a small number of children, there are severe defects, the condition of **spina bifida cystica**. The majority of cases take the form of **meningomyelocoele**. There is a defect in the skin, vertebral arches and meninges, associated with cystic change in the spinal cord, syringomyelia, or other abnormality. The prospects for recovery are poor. In a minority of cases, the defect is a **meningocoele** in which the disorder is restricted to the skin, vertebral arches and meninges. The spinal cord is almost unaffected. Meningocoele can be corrected surgically, sometimes *in utero*.

Spina bifida occulta
One in every seven asymptomatic adults displays radiological absence of one or more vertebral arches. In some otherwise normal individuals, one or several lumbosacral spinous processes are absent.

INFECTION

The brain is prone to viral, bacterial, protozoal, helminthic and fungal infections. Inflammation of the brain is **encephalitis**, that of the meninges **meningitis**. Bacterial meningitis is most commonly caused by *Streptococcus pneumoniae*, *Neisseria meningitidis*, *Haemophilus influenzae* and by miscellaneous streptococci and staphylococci. It is particularly frequent in those with deficient splenic function (p. 302).

- **Direct infection**. Bacteria may be conveyed to the brain by penetrating injury in compound fracture of the skull, from the pituitary fossa, nasal sinuses or air passages. Micro-organisms may also pass to the meninges and brain from the sphenoid bone in chronic suppurative otitis media. Meningitis is likely to result.
- **Indirect infection**. Bacteria and viruses also reach the brain via the arterial bloodstream. Brain abscess is a complication of pyaemia and bronchiectasis. Encephalitis is one result of measles and other virus infections.

Brain abscess

Brain abscess is rare: it follows local or systemic disease and may be single or multiple. The incidence of brain abscess in the UK is now only 4 cases/10^6 persons/year. The main effects of abscess are those of a space-occupying lesion (p. 61).

Direct spread of infection from a paranasal sinus, from the middle ear or from the mastoid process are the commonest routes. The infecting organisms are usually *Streptococcus pneumoniae*, *Streptococcus pyogenes*, *Haemophilus influenzae*, *Pseudomonas aeruginosa* or *Bacteroides fragilis*. Blood-borne infection occurs in patients with bronchiectasis, bacterial endocarditis or congenital heart disease; it is infrequent in immunocompromised patients. Abscess following penetrating injury is the least common form and is due to infection by staphylococci, streptococci, coliforms or anaerobes.

Tuberculosis

In patients with pulmonary or other forms of tuberculosis, *Mycobacterium tuberculosis* is conveyed to the brain via the bloodstream. Vasculitis of the arteries of the base of the brain, meningitis and tuberculoma are the most frequent results.

Now read Tuberculosis (p. 332)

MECHANICAL INJURY AND TRAUMA

The brain is a hydrated gel held within the rigid cranium. A series of connective tissue septa divides the gel into compartments with firm or hard edges. The location of these boundaries strongly influences the distribution of cerebral injuries. Direct and indirect head trauma lead to primary or secondary brain damage respectively. Such injuries are a frequent cause of death. Young males are especially vulnerable. The causes include:

- Injuries that are the **direct** result of moving objects such as missiles.
- Injuries that are **indirect** and result from the physical effects of sudden acceleration or deceleration, as in car and aeroplane accidents.

The consequences are severe if there is angular movement with a sudden rotation of the skull. Missile injuries caused by objects such as high-velocity rifle bullets are especially damaging because of the great transfer of energy that takes place at impact (p. 358).

Head injury is frequently complicated by intracranial bleeding (p. 65)

Now read Wounds (p. 357)

Primary brain damage

Primary brain damage occurs at the site of impact of an object of small area such as a hammer, but is more widespread if the area of contact is large. The frontal poles, orbital gyri and temporal lobes suffer cerebral contusion. Due to the movement of the brain on impact, and the situation of the bony prominences of the skull and dural attachments, contusion of the brain is commonplace on the side opposite to the point of impact and constitutes a **contrecoup** injury. The brain is susceptible to shear strain and torsion so that, in addition to impact contusion, a widespread form of diffuse axonal injury occurs, affecting populations of neurones in sites such as the brain stem.

Secondary brain damage

This is usually the consequence of intracranial haemorrhage and haematoma. According to its location, a haematoma may be extradural, subdural or intracerebral (p. 65). The consequences of secondary damage can be minimised by ensuring adequate oxygenation and ventilation, by maintaining an adequate blood pressure and by the early evacuation of any haematoma.

TUMOURS

Metastatic

Nearly one-third of all intracerebral tumours is metastatic. The sites from which these tumours originate include the lung, breast, gastro-intestinal tract and kidney, in descending order of frequency. Malignant melanoma frequently metastasises to the meninges and cerebral tissues; they are commonly the sites of malignant lymphoma.

Now read Neoplasia/Tumours (p. 246)

Primary

The majority of primary brain tumours (Table 14) arise from the neuroglia. They are gliomas. In the UK, the annual incidence of primary brain tumour is ~130 /10^6 population.

Table 14 Classification and frequency of intracranial tumours

Nature of tumour	Frequency (% of total)
Glioma (total)	38
Astrocytoma grades III and IV (glioblastoma)	20
grades I and II	10
Ependymoma	6
Medulloblastoma	2
Meningioma	17
Pituitary adenoma	5
Schwannoma	5
Other primary tumours	9
Lymphoma	3
Metastases	23

Astrocytoma

Astrocytoma is the most frequent primary brain tumour (Table 14). It occurs in adults and in children. The tumour may be multifocal and both cerebral hemispheres may be implicated. It is a slowly growing lesion that merges imperceptibly with the surrounding cerebral tissue. The mass is of cystic structure. Sometimes, the tumour can be categorised by a single cell type, for example, fibrillary or protoplasmic astrocytes. Other neoplasms show cellular heterogeneity.

There are four grades. The prognosis is closely related to microscopic structure. Well-differentiated, grade 1 astrocytoma is formed of mature astrocytes surrounded by many neuroglial fibres. At the other end of the scale of differentiation, the rapidly growing grade 4 astrocytoma, designated **glioblastoma**, comprises a population of pleomorphic cells. The tumour has many small blood vessels that display endothelial hyperplasia.

Ependymoma

Ependymoma is an uncommon tumour of children that usually arises within the fourth ventricle. Individual tumour cells resemble epithelial cells. They are arranged around small blood vessels from which they are delineated by collagenous tissue. Tumour cells seed into the subarachnoid space.

Medulloblastoma

Medulloblastoma is a further tumour of childhood. It arises in the posterior fossa of the skull and appears as a friable mass that may extend into the fourth ventricle. Medulloblastoma grows quickly. The poorly differentiated cells extend throughout the subarachnoid space. There is a resemblance to some neuro-ectodermal tumours and the densely packed cells often form rosettes.

Meningioma

Meningiomas originate from the arachnoid granulations. They arise at any point along the lines of reflection of the dura mater that adjoin the intracranial venous sinuses and are therefore encountered in a parasagittal site or near the sphenoidal ridge. Meningioma may also arise from the dura mater of the spine, causing spinal cord compression. Microscopically, there is a characteristic whorled structure within which calcified psammoma bodies appear. The majority are benign although recurrence may occur several years after resection.

Ganglioblastoma

Ganglioblastoma is a highly malignant and anaplastic tumour of adults.

Cavernous angioma

This tumour-like vascular malformation, described on p. 49, occurs in ~0.5% of people. In ~50%, it is inherited as an autosomal dominant characteristic. Two loci have been identified, on chromosomes 3 and 7.

VASCULAR DISEASE

Now read Anoxia/hypoxia; (p. 16), Ischaemia (p. 187)

Intracranial haemorrhage

Intracranial haemorrhage may be traumatic (p. 63) or spontaneous. Spontaneous haemorrhage is a frequent cause of death. It is often a result of untreated systemic hypertension. Bleeding into the cerebral tissues takes place from micro-aneurysms and is most common in the territories supplied by the middle cerebral and posterior inferior cerebellar arteries. Less frequent causes are disorders of coagulation including leukaemia; angioma and hamartoma; haemorrhage into tumours such as glioblastoma multiform; and arteriovenous malformations.

Extradural haemorrhage and haematoma

Arteries that adjoin vulnerable parts of the skull are susceptible to the effects of manual blows and other injuries. The middle meningeal artery is one example; it lies beneath the thin temporal bone. Haemorrhage from a torn middle meningeal artery is a feature of trauma sustained during boxing. A lucid interval is followed some hours later by lapse into coma. The result of the arterial injury is bleeding beneath the bone of the skull, external to the dura mater. Cerebral compression is an early result.

Subdural haemorrhage and haematoma

The sagittal and other venous sinuses are prone to tears when the elderly suffer head injuries as a result of falls. Venous blood escapes slowly and accumulates beneath the dura, forming a haematoma. Signs of raised intracranial pressure develop slowly over a period of days or weeks.

Subarachnoid haemorrhage

The sudden onset of subarachnoid haemorrhage is more common in older females than in males. The mean age of onset is ~50 years. Some blood escapes into nearby cerebral tissue causing disruption. Bleeding is usually from a saccular aneurysm (Fig. 3) found at the bifurcation of one of the principal intracerebral arteries. The aneurysm results from a congenital defect in the elastic laminae of the vessel. Much less often, mycotic aneurysms rupture.

Now read Aneurysm (p. 14)

Intracranial venous thrombosis

Focal intracranial infection is liable to provoke thrombosis of nearby veins. In compound fracture with osteomyelitis, or in acute frontal sinusitis, thrombosis of the superior sagittal sinus is an occasional complication. Compound fracture through the ethmoid bone promotes bacterial infection from the nasal passages. In chronic suppurative otitis media with osteomyelitis of the mastoid bone, lateral sinus thrombosis may develop. Marantic thrombosis of cerebral veins occurs in malnourished and dehydrated children.

BREAST

The lobules of the female breast do not develop until puberty. They regress at the menopause. Throughout pre-menopausal life, the structure of the female breast is influenced by periodic alterations in the levels of circulating female sex hormones. These cyclical changes are always taken into account in the diagnosis of female breast disease in which the overriding demand is for the early recognition of cancer.

Biopsy diagnosis of breast disease

In primary diagnosis, samples of tissue are obtained by fine-needle aspiration, by core-cutting, Trucut-type needle or by excisional biopsy. Intra-operative identification of small lesions detected by mammography can be facilitated by pre-operative insertion of two or more localising needles, under radiological guidance. Biopsy in the management of breast cancer is discussed on p. 68.

GROWTH DISORDERS

Gynaecomastia

Gynaecomastia is excessive enlargement of the male breast. The most frequent causes include chronic liver disease and anti-androgen treatment for prostatic carcinoma. There are other rare causes. They include oestrogen secretion by a feminising tumour of the adrenal cortex; ectopic hormone secretion by bronchial carcinoma; occupational exposure to oestrogens; or the use of drugs such as digitalis and cimetidine. Gynaecomastia is also encountered transiently in adolescents and is a feature of chromosomal abnormalities such as Klinefelter's syndrome.

Fibrocystic change

Fibrocystic change affects the breast tissue of women between puberty and the menopause. It is present in 10% of all individuals, but is commoner in multipara and is unrelated to the onset of breast cancer. However, some of the microscopic appearances recall those of carcinoma *in-situ* and care is required in diagnosis.

Epithelial hyperplasia

The excessive multiplication (hyperplasia) of epithelial cells is a feature of many forms of breast disease. Two forms are described: 'usual' and 'atypical'. In the former, orderly nuclei of uniform structure are found in hyperplastic epithelium that may obliterate the duct lumen. In the latter, the appearances simulate those of cribriform carcinoma *in-situ*. A papillary pattern is recognisable.

Cyst formation

Breast cysts are commonplace. They are often multiple and result from local obstruction of ducts draining breast lobules. The thin-walled cysts appear blue but contain a fluid that may become yellow if there has been previous intracystic bleeding. Local dilatation of ducts draining breast lobules results from obstruction.

Adenosis and fibro-adenosis

The terms adenosis and fibro-adenosis indicate simply that the glandular acini of the breast have increased in size.

Sclerosing adenosis

Sclerosing adenosis is a proliferation of the lobular units drained by the breast ducts. It is a focal change often detected in normal breast tissue. A disorderly proliferation of the cells of a twin-layered glandular epithelium, without nuclear atypia, accompanies hyperplasia of the intralobular connective tissue stromal cells. Focal calcification gives rise to a fine-speckled appearance radiologically, mimicking the changes seen in carcinoma *in-situ*. There is no increased risk of malignancy.

Fibrosis

X-ray or CT scans of the adult female breast requently reveal small, radial 'scars'. The presence of a scar calls for examination of breast tissue by needle core biopsy. The scars represent a relative increase in the quantity of stromal fibrous tissue, part of the raised collagen content of breast tissue that occurs with advancing age. In accordance with the anatomy of the breast lobules, the collagen has a radial orientation.

Mammary duct ectasia

This is a symptomless disorder of multiparous females who have not undertaken breast feeding. Progressive dilatation of the larger mammary ducts provokes a nearby inflammatory reaction.

Focal lobular hyperplasia (fibro-adenoma)

In focal lobular hyperplasia, well-defined, small, mobile masses are formed. They are circumscribed foci of hyperplasia, not tumours. They often regress spontaneously. There is no increased risk of malignant change. The lobules comprise a loose intralobular connective tissue stroma within which are varying numbers of epithelial tubules. They are most commonly recognised between the ages of 15 and 25 years. The distinction between pericanalicular and intracanalicular forms has no significance.

INFECTION

Abscess

Famously associated with Joseph Lister's (p. 373) relief of Queen Victoria's axillary lesion, breast abscess occurs most often in the lactating gland. The most frequent causes are *Staphylococcus aureus* and *Streptococcus pyogenes*.

TUMOURS

Malignant

Carcinoma

Breast cancer is 100 times more frequent in the female than in the male. In Western societies, breast cancer is the leading cause of death among women aged 40–55 years, and the commonest cause of female cancer deaths overall. The mortality rate is 3.5% of all women. In England and Wales, there were 620 cases/10^6 persons in 1992. There are large racial differences and the incidence of breast cancer in Japan is only one-fifth of that in the USA.

Now read Carcinogenesis (p. 76), Neoplasia/Tumours (p. 242)

Causes

No single cause has been identified although viruses have been implicated. Many risk factors are known. The majority exert only a slight or moderate influence. They include a family history of breast cancer; early menarche; nulliparity; late age at first childbirth; late age at menopause; and exposure to ionising radiation.

A family history of bilateral breast cancer or of breast cancer at an unusually early age, while rare, represents a very high relative risk for the development of the disease. In half the observed cases with a family history of breast cancer, the neoplasm is associated with the inheritance of the *BRCA-1* or the *BRCA-2* genes (Table 18). Carriers of *BRCA-1* have ~50% chance of developing breast cancer by the age of 50 years, 85% by the age of 70 years. They also have a greatly increased risk of developing cancer of the ovary (p. 260). Cancers in women inheriting the *BRCA-1* germline are more commonly aneuploid, highly proliferative, high grade, oestrogen receptor-negative, than other, sporadic, hereditary breast cancers. But there is no difference in the recurrence rate or death rate. It is of interest that the prognosis is better in *BRCA-1* than in hereditary but non-*BRCA-1*-related cases. One reason may be that *BRCA-1* cancers do not express the *c-erbB-2* gene (Table 17) while many are medullary (p. 68).

Structure and origin

Mammographic screening enables impalpable lesions to be identified before invasion or metastasis have occurred. By this means, a reduction of deaths by 30% has been claimed in the UK.

The identity of the cell of origin of carcinoma of the breast influences prognosis. It was believed that all epithelial tumours originated from the cells of breast ducts or lobules, the majority from the former. However, many tumours previously regarded as ductal in origin are of doubtful origin and are classified as 'not otherwise specified' (NOS) or of 'no specific type' (NST).

A diagnosis can be made by fine needle aspiration cytology. Needle core biopsy yields sufficient tissue for paraffin section microscopy. The degree of differentiation of a tumour influences survival but to a lesser extent than tumour behaviour estimated by staging. Small tumours of low pathological grade and with no vascular invasion have a low probability of relapse. The precise identification of single cancer cells within the biopsy can be facilitated by immunohistochemical tests.

Duct carcinoma *in-situ* (DCIS) *In-situ* change accounts for ~17% of all new cases of breast cancer. It can be diagnosed by mammography in symptomless females and is often recognisable in normal breast tissue examined *post-mortem*. There is a proliferation of dysplastic epithelial cells within an intact duct basement membrane. The lesions assume a variety of patterns that are **solid**, **comedo**, **cribriform** or **micropapillary**. In comedo DCIS, there is central necrosis of the islands of cells that have filled the ducts. In the cribriform variety, many foci of necrosis are seen within islands of malignant cells.

Duct carcinoma Up to 75% of patients with a palpable malignant breast tumour have a ductal carcinoma. The majority is composed of cords and processes of infiltrating cancer cells within a dense, collagen-rich stroma that gives a tumour its property of 'cutting like an unripe pear'. The old designation 'scirrhous' (hard) has been abandoned. The arrangement, relative numbers and properties of the carcinoma cells, the extent of cell death and the presence or absence of mucin secretion allow detailed categories to be defined so that **medullary**, **mucoid**, **squamous** and **tubular** tumours are described. The medullary structure is prognostically favourable despite the high mitotic and nuclear grades of these cancers. 'Inflammatory' carcinoma is a term applied when lymphatics draining the breast are obstructed by neoplastic cells, causing oedema and hyperaemia.

Lobular carcinoma *in-situ* Lobular carcinoma *in-situ* (LCIS) precedes invasive cancer but less frequently than duct carcinoma *in-situ*.

Lobular carcinoma Invasive lobular carcinoma accounts for approximately 10% of breast cancers in the UK but is difficult to identify by mammography. The characteristic lesions are often bilateral and may be multifocal. In analogy with ductal carcinoma, **alveolar**, **solid**, **tubulo-lobular** and **pleomorphic** variants are described.

Paget's disease Paget's disease (p. 374) of the female breast is an unilateral, chronic, eczema-like lesion of the nipple and areola associated with intraduct carcinoma. Patients with Paget's disease represent less than 5% of all mammary carcinomas; they are relatively elderly. The tissue change that causes the eczematous reaction is the presence in the epidermis of large, pale, vacuolated, malignant (Paget) cells with hyperchromatic nuclei. Paget cells are frequently seen to be undergoing mitotic division. It is believed that they represent intra-epidermal spread from the underlying carcinoma. Histologically, Paget's disease of the breast is distinguished from carcinoma *in-situ* (p. 244) and from intra-epithelial malignant melanoma (p. 227).

Paget's disease of the anal margin is described on p. 13, Paget's disease of the penis on p. 268.

Behaviour and prognosis

The contribution of the histopathologist is an integral part of the management of breast cancer, which is best undertaken in centres where a group comprising surgeons, laboratory scientists, oncologists and radiotherapists meet often and regularly. The single most important factor in determining prognosis is staging according to the TNM system (p. 244). Prognosis depends upon the presence or absence of lymph node metastases, tumour size and histological grade, in that order. The prognosis is significantly worse with large tumour masses than with smaller and is related to the expression of tumour markers.

From the various procedures described on p. 244, the behaviour of the tumour and its probable response to treatment can be predicted and a judgement made on prognosis. Needle aspiration permits the identification of tumour markers. Oestrogen (ER)-positive tumours have a slightly better prognosis than ER-negative cases but their influence on prognosis is much less than TNM staging. The presence of progesterone receptors (PgR) is sought: they indicate an intact oestrogen-ER pathway. The expression and identity of genes (p. 77) may prove significant in classifying breast cancer and in predicting prognosis, but few studies have been completed to assess their prognostic value.

Significance of metastasis

The factors that regulate metastasis are multifactorial.

Now read Metastasis (p. 246)

The 10-year disease-free survival rate for patients without axillary lymph node involvement is 80%. The presence of tumour cells within regional lymph nodes significantly modifies both the choice of treatment and the prognosis. Lymphadenectomy is therefore an essential procedure. When doubt remained about involvement of the axillary lymph nodes by tumour, it was the practice to perform an 'axillary clearance' surgically. This time-consuming procedure often resulted in disfiguring blockage to regional lymphatic drainage, a swollen arm, and, occasionally, the development of angiosarcoma (p. 49).

It was then recognised that the identification of the lymph node closest to the tumour on the drainage path could yield invaluable evidence of metastatic spread. This node was a 'sentinel' (p. 40). Most sentinel nodes were axillary. However, 20% to 86% of lymphatic drainage from breast tissue is to the internal mammary nodes. It is therefore not surprising that ~8% of sentinel nodes are extra-axillary and that ~3% are exclusively non-axillary. The microscopical examination of sentinel nodes may be by frozen section but intra-operative imprint cytology is both convenient and more precise. The sensitivity of sentinel node biopsy is further increased when sections or imprints are taken from more than one level of the tissue sample and when immunohistochemical tests for cancer cells are made.

Mortality

Although the death rates from breast cancer in young and middle-aged women in the UK had been rising, it is now clear that between 1987 and 1997 there was a significant, relatively rapid and continuing decline in the overall mortality. In 1989, among women aged 20–69, $\sim 500/10^6$ died from breast cancer. In 1999, the corresponding figure was $\sim 380/10^6$. Radiotherapy itself can reduce breast cancer mortality but can increase mortality from other causes and early surgery alone is curative in more than 50% of cases. The observed recent decrease in mortality is, however, attributable not to a single form of treatment but to the prompt investigation of breast lumps, the use of mammographic screening, precise histopathological diagnosis, the expeditious use of surgery and treatment with hormones and cytotoxic compounds. Tamoxifen is credited with the greatest contribution to this dramatic advance. Chemotherapy has played a smaller part.

Prophylaxis

No certain way is known of preventing breast cancer. Bilateral prophylactic mastectomy can protect against the occurrence of breast cancer in women at very high risk such as those inheriting the *BRCA-1* gene. The expression of tumour genes that may contribute to the proliferative capacity and metastatic potential of a breast cancer may change during the menstrual cycle. This observation may explain the better response to surgery that is observed in patients from whom a tumour has been removed during the luteal phase of the cycle.

Now read TNM system (p. 244)

Rare tumours

All forms of sarcoma of the breast are uncommon or rare and **angiosarcoma** is no exception. A proportion of these tumours is well differentiated and may be mistaken for benign haemangioma, an impression confirmed microscopically. **Osteosarcoma** has been described. **Phyllodes tumour** ('cystosarcoma phyllodes' or giant fibro-adenoma) is a very uncommon lesion that develops in older women. A large, lobulated mass causes unilateral breast enlargement. The cut surface of the mass resembles that of a young cabbage. There is a cellular connective tissue stroma. Epithelial cells line elongated clefts. Only 10% of cases recur after excision and malignant change is rare.

BRONCHUS

In Western countries, the bronchi are often seriously damaged by chronic bronchitis. Patients with this disorder and the consequential emphysema are poor surgical risks. The bronchi are also the most common sites for primary cancer, just as the lung is a frequent target for carcinomatous metastases.

Biopsy diagnosis of bronchial disease

Diagnostic cytological examinations are made on sputum or on bronchoscopic aspirates. Procedures for bronchial biopsy are discussed on p. 214.

Now read Lung (p. 214)

TUMOURS

Benign

Adenoma

Adenoma is most common in those aged 40 years or less. It comprises less than 5% of the primary tumours of the bronchi and lungs.

Malignant

Carcinoma

Malignant tumours of the lung account for 12.8% of all cancer cases and for 17.8% of cancer deaths worldwide. The majority of these tumours originates in the bronchi or bronchioles.

In Europe, carcinoma of the bronchus is the most frequent cause of death from malignant disease in males and the second most frequent cause of death in females after breast cancer. In England and Wales, there were 730 cases/10^6 adults in 1992.

Causes

The single most important known cause is cigarette smoking. The age and sex incidence reflect cigarette-smoking patterns in an earlier generation. During the past 20 years, there has been a steady increase in smoking among young females, a decline among older men. The prevalence of bronchial cancer in present day society mirrors this trend. In the USA and in Scotland female deaths from bronchial cancer now exceed those from breast cancer. Passive cigarette smoking is associated with an increased risk but many other forms of air pollution are pathogenic. The incidence of bronchial cancer is high in urban areas. The inhalation of asbestos and other silicates, radon, chromium, nickel, cadmium and arsenic carries a greatly increased risk of the development of bronchial carcinoma.

Structure

The World Health Organization designates four histological types of bronchial carcinoma. However, from a surgical perspective and for planned treatment, there are two main categories of carcinoma: small cell and non-small cell. The latter class includes squamous cell carcinoma, adenocarcinoma and large cell carcinoma.

Small cell carcinoma

These tumours constitute ~20% of bronchial cancers. They are associated with cigarette smoking. They grow rapidly and are highly malignant. A number of variants are recognised, including undifferentiated small cell carcinoma, a category formerly called oat cell carcinoma. Small cell tumours are central in location: they arise from the larger bronchi and form expanding masses within the mediastinum where they invade lymph nodes. They can be identified by bronchoscopy but metastasise early. Uniform sheets of small cells are separated by only limited quantities of intercellular stroma. Small cell carcinomas synthesise and may secrete a variety of ectopic hormones suggesting that they originate from bronchial neuro-endocrine cells.

Non-small cell carcinoma

- **Squamous carcinoma** is the most frequent in Europe, accounting for ~40% of lung tumours. Its origin is particularly associated with cigarette smoking. The tumour is central in location: it arises from the proximal parts of the bronchial tree at sites of squamous metaplasia. It is endobronchial and may cavitate. Bronchial obstruction results in lung collapse, bronchopneumonia and haemoptysis. Metastasis is relatively late. Because of this proximal location, diagnosis by bronchoscopy and exfoliative cytology is relatively simple. However, early extension of the necrotic, cavitating mass to involve the structures of the mediastinum often renders surgical resection difficult.
- **Adenocarcinoma** is more common in women than in men, accounting for ~20% of bronchial carcinomas. There are several forms: broncho-alveolar or alveolar cell; acinar; papillary; and solid. They arise more frequently in small, peripheral bronchi or bronchioles than in the larger, central bronchi. For this reason, they are not accessible to bronchoscopy and the results of the diagnostic cytological examination of sputum are often negative. Microscopically, the tumour recalls the appearance of metastatic carcinoma from sites such as the large intestine, pancreas, gastric epithelium and ovary. Muco-epidermoid and cribriform variants of adenocarcinoma are recognised. The glandular acini of the tumours stain positively for carcino-embryonic antigen (CEA), helping to distinguish them from mesothelioma (p. 274) which may also have an acinar structure.
- **Large cell carcinomas** account for ~10% of lung

cancers. They arise in the lung periphery and cavitate, forming soft, necrotic masses. The tumour forms sheets of uniform, large cells that show little differentiation. However, electron microscopy suggests that they may be poorly differentiated variants of squamous carcinoma or adenocarcinoma.

Behaviour and prognosis

In general, the prognosis of bronchial carcinoma is related to the category of tumour and to staging. Staging assessment is by the TNM system but takes into account the state of the chest and mediastinum and the patient's performance status, that is, the result of pulmonary function studies together with the capacity of the patient to tolerate recommended forms of treatment.

Mortality The overall 5-year survival rate is less than 10%. For small cell tumours, chemotherapy is the backbone of treatment. Surgery is restricted to those with stage I or stage II disease, the type most likely to be operable although fewer than 1 in 7 is suitable for resection. Small cell carcinomas respond best to chemotherapy but their 5-year survival rate is no more than 5%.

The 5-year survival for stage I squamous carcinoma is ~40–67%. For stage II, the figure is 25–55%, for stage III (locally or regionally advance disease) treated by radiotherapy alone, the evidence suggests that the 5-year survival is ~5–10 % with a mean survival time of 10 months or less.

Metastasis Direct spread of bronchial carcinoma to mediastinal tissues often causes superior vena caval obstruction. A tumour located at a lung apex is liable to cause Pancoast's syndrome:

- Painful neuropathy of the arm, due to the spread of cancer cells into the brachial plexus.
- Horner's syndrome, the result of infiltration of the cervical sympathetic nerve plexus.
- Bone pain from metastases within the vertebral bodies and first rib.
- Perivascular infiltration around the subclavian artery and vein.

Lymphatic spread results in hilar and mediastinal lymphadenopathy. Blood-borne metastasis to the liver, contralateral lung, brain, bone and adrenals is very frequent. It is a particular feature of bronchial carcinoma that no body organ or tissue is spared, so that metastasis to a distal phalanx, a tarsal bone or to the base of a molar tooth may be the first sign of the disease.

Other bronchial tumours

Carcinoid

Carcinoid (p. 82) of the bronchus is a neuro-endocrine tumour. There is a capacity for local invasion but regional metastasis is recognised in only 25% of cases, distant metastasis in 5%. Carcinoids are therefore said ambiguously to be of 'low-grade malignancy'. Bronchial carcinoid tumours extend into the lumen of a bronchus but also beyond the bronchial wall. They assume a dumb-bell shape and the nearby mucosa remains intact, without ulceration, so that diagnostic cytological examination is negative. Like other neuro-endocrine tumours (p. 126), 50% of the cells are argyrophilic, but only 20% are argentaffin. In the small proportion (5%) that metastasise, the carcinoid syndrome (p. 82) may develop.

BURNS AND SCALDS

Burns are injuries caused by excessive dry heat. Closely similar injuries are caused by exposure to caustic chemicals. Burns are usually of external body surfaces, although hot gases may burn the trachea and bronchi. There is a direct relationship between the extent of injury and both the temperature to which the skin is exposed and the duration of the exposure. A hot water bottle at 45–55°C left in contact with a limb overnight can cause injuries comparable with a flash burn at 10 000°C for 0.001 second.

Scalds result from excessive moist heat.

Now read Heat excess (p. 151), Hypothermia (p. 162)

SEVERITY

Burns can be classified according to the depth of injury and the area of the body surface involved. They may be superficial, with destruction of part of the thickness of the skin, or deep, with whole-thickness skin loss. A convenient method for estimating the surface area involved in adults is the so-called 'rule-of-9s'. The anterior and posterior surfaces of the trunk, and that of each lower limb approximate to 18% of the body surface; each upper limb and the head represent 9%; and the perineum 1%. In children, these figures are modified since the head of the child comprises a larger percentage of the total body surface than that of the adult, the limbs a smaller proportion.

EFFECTS

The most important immediate effects of a severe burn are shock (p. 290) and fluid loss. The severity of these disturbances is in proportion to the area of the body that has been injured. Formulae have been devised for calculating the amount of fluid required to correct the fluid imbalance, based upon the area of skin involved.

In cutaneous burns, if the applied heat is sufficient, a central zone of coagulation or carbonisation is surrounded by zones of partial injury where cell function is disturbed but not lost. Inflammation develops at the circumference to this zone. However, red blood cells lyse within venules and thrombi occlude vessels at the margin of the burn. There is increased capillary permeability and protein leaks into the extravascular tissues, producing oedema.

HEALING

Following a superficial cutaneous burn, the surviving epithelial cells multiply rapidly in a process of re-epithelialisation. They derive from the residual basal cells. There is no scarring.

Deeper burns re-epithelialise slowly from the cells of undamaged hair follicles, sweat and sebaceous glands in a process that occupies ~14 days. There may be scarring.

No regeneration of skin can occur in full thickness burns. There are no residual epithelial elements and healing takes place not by regeneration but by fibrous repair (p. 131, 285). The granulation tissue formed in this way undergoes contraction but is subsequently covered by the centripetal ingrowth of cells from the adjacent epithelium. The scar tissue is often grossly disfiguring and keloid formation (p. 195) is likely. Contracture (p. 112) is a common complication.

In even more extensive, deep burns, bacterial infection is common, accounting for more than half of the subsequent deaths. The local actions of the immune response are impaired due to a deficient local vascular circulation and an impaired local concentration of immunoglobulins. Opportunistic Gram-negative organisms such as *Pseudomonas aeruginosa* and MRSA are prevalent. *Ps. aeruginosa* is responsible for 60% of deaths in outbreaks of infection in burn units. In survivors of deep burns, skin grafting is used to reduce early fluid loss and to aid healing. Autologous split-thickness skin grafting is employed but in the case of extensive injuries, donor sites are often inadequate. In the UK, it has been suggested that banks of cryopreserved skin for allografting should be established in National Blood Transfusion Centres. However, the transmission of HIV by donor skin has already been reported so that donors require careful selection and screening.

OUTCOME

In the UK, with a population of ~55 × 10^6 persons, there are 150 000 burn injuries every year accounting for 6% of patients attending Accident and Emergency (A&E) departments. Twelve thousand cases are admitted to hospital and ~600 of these individuals die. More than half of all patients are children.

In 1945 only 50% of those with 40% burns survived. Today, 50% of those with 80% burns survive. The probability of death from burns has greatly declined and is now no more than 4%. The success of modern treatment is attributable to the early excision of burn wounds; advances in critical care; the topical and systemic administration of antibiotics; and above all, to access to specialised, multidisciplinary centres. However, there remain three large risk factors:

- Age over 60 years.
- Burns of more than 40% of the body surface area.
- Inhalation injury.

When none of these three factors is present, the mortality is ~0.3%. With one factor, the mortality is ~3.0%; with two, it becomes ~33% and with three, more than 90%.

C

CACHEXIA

Cachexia describes the weakness, weight loss and wasting that occur in chronic physical and mental diseases. The condition is distinguished from malnutrition (p. 229) and is particularly evident in patients with cancer. The wasting of cachexia is attributable to diminished food intake combined with disturbed gastro-intestinal function; disuse atrophy; and an increased catabolism of tissues resulting from raised body temperature. The intermediary metabolism of tissues in neoplastic tissue may differ from normal but it has not been possible to isolate any single substance responsible for this difference.

CALCIFICATION

Calcification is the deposition of insoluble, inorganic calcium salts, in living tissues. Calcification is an essential part of bone formation and is closely dependent on normal concentrations of vitamin D, parathormone and calcitonin. Bone mineral comprises calcium phosphate and calcium carbonate, together with small amounts of sodium, magnesium, fluoride and other deposits. The calcium salts are present as a mixture of crystalline calcium hydroxyapatite and amorphous calcium phosphate. The hydroxyapatite crystals – delicate, needle-shaped and 100 nm long – accumulate in clusters in relation to bone collagen (osteocollagen). They are laid down under the influence of osteoblastic alkaline phosphatase.

As bone forms in zones of endochondral ossification, the matrix becomes provisionally mineralised by the deposition of crystalline calcium hydroxyapatite. Provisional calcification is only possible when vitamin D is available. Where mineralisation is proceeding during appositional bone growth, the mineral deposited is insoluble amorphous calcium phosphate. The formation of insoluble calcium hydroxyapatite crystals follows.

PATHOLOGICAL CALCIFICATION

Pathological calcification is a common consequence of local or systemic disease. It may be heterotopic, metastatic or dystrophic. The mineral is calcium hydroxyapatite but other insoluble calcium salts, particularly calcium pyrophosphate, are often deposited.

Heterotopic calcification

In heterotopic (ectopic) calcification, bone mineral is deposited at sites where it is not normally found.

Metastatic calcification

In metastatic calcification, the deposition of calcium takes place in tissues that are structurally and functionally **normal**. It is a sequel to excessively high plasma levels of this element. One cause is hyperparathyroidism, another excess vitamin D. The mineral is precipitated in parts such as arterial walls, gastric mucosa, lungs and the renal interstitium. Metastatic calcification is also encountered in multiple myeloma, sarcoidosis and carcinoma of the breast and may be caused by the excessive intake of vitamin D or calcium.

Dystrophic calcification

Dystrophic calcification, occurs in **abnormal** tissues. The circulating and extracellular fluid levels of calcium, phosphate, parathormone, vitamin D and calcitonin are normal. The process is commonplace in ageing tissues and is recognised, for example, in the radial and popliteal arteries, in Mönckeberg's medial sclerosis. Dystrophic calcification within the abdomen follows acute pancreatitis. It occurs in the walls of abscesses; foci of chronic, fibrocaseous tuberculosis; sites of parasitic infestation; cysts; and densely fibrotic scar tissue after surgical wound infection. Calcification is also frequent in complicated atherosclerosis (p. 26) and in the walls of aneurysms and cardiac valves, particularly the aortic. Some common malignant tumours such as gastric carcinoma undergo focal dystrophic calcification. Sand-like psammoma bodies may be formed as they are in meningiomas (p. 65). Radiographic and microscopic recognition of calcification in the form of calcium hydroxyapatite is a valuable diagnostic sign of carcinoma of the breast.

Calcinosis

Calcinosis is a form of dystrophic calcification. Calcifying tendinitis is an example. Systemic sclerosis is another. CREST syndrome describes systemic sclerosis with **C**alcinosis, **R**aynaud's phenomenon, o**E**sophageal hypomotility, **S**clerodactyly and **T**elangiectasia. Idiopathic calcinosis of the scrotum may represent the calcification of multiple epidermoid cysts. **Tumoral calcinosis** is a rare, familial form that occurs in young, negroid individuals and affects soft tissues anterior to the shoulder joint.

CALCIUM

Calcium (Ca) is essential for normal life. Extracellular concentrations of ionic calcium (Ca^{2+}) regulate transmembrane potentials and the contractility of muscle cells; low concentrations initiate myofibrillar relaxation. Calcium ions are necessary for the coagulation of blood (p. 95) and calcium salts are essential for the formation, growth and maintenance of bone.

The serum concentration of Ca is normally 2.30–2.65 mmol/L. Approximately 40–50% is physiologically active, free, **ionised** Ca^{2+}. A further 40–50% is **non-ionised** and bound to plasma protein, principally to albumin. The remaining 5–10% of Ca is in the form of complexes with organic acids. The differential distribution of serum Ca between the two main moieties is dependent upon plasma pH. Hypo-albuminaemia leads to a fall in **total** serum Ca without altering muscle contractility, nerve conduction or coagulation. Because total serum Ca is measured when a laboratory assay is requested, the concentration of plasma proteins should be considered when assessing the significance of the results.

In addition to the 70 mmol of calcium of extracellular and intracellular fluid, bone contains ~27 000 mmol mostly in the form of hydroxyapatite. Isotope studies suggest that only 125 mmol is freely exchangeable. Calcium balance is regulated by intestinal absorption, renal excretion and the avidity of storage in bone. These processes are controlled actively by parathormone, vitamin D and calcitonin and permissively by growth hormone, cortisol, the sex hormones and tri-iodothyronine (T3). Consequently, abnormal serum concentrations of Ca may result from a very wide variety of disorders.

HYPERCALCAEMIA

The most frequent causes of raised blood Ca concentrations are osteolytic metastases from cancers of the bronchus, breast and kidney. In bronchial carcinoma, there is an inappropriate secretion of parathormone-like polypeptides. Very high levels of Ca occur in primary hyperparathyroidism. Hypercalcaemia is also characteristic of multiple myeloma; sarcoidosis; Paget's disease of bone; prolonged immobilisation; the treatment of osteomalacia with excess vitamin D; hypervitaminosis D of infancy; hyperthyroidism; and hypo-adrenocorticalism.

Hypercalcaemia causes the release of excess gastrin so that peptic ulceration (pp. 121 and 308) is common, particularly in patients with hyperparathyroidism. Pancreatitis is also frequent; its cause is unknown but it is possible that Ca may induce the conversion of trypsinogen to trypsin within the pancreatic ducts.

In all forms of hypercalcaemia, metastatic calcification (p. 73) of the limb and coronary arteries is likely. The kidneys are affected and nephrocalcinosis may culminate in renal failure.

Now read Hyperparathyroidism (p. 267)

HYPOCALCAEMIA

The many causes of osteomalacia/rickets (p. 52) contribute to hypocalcaemia. Renal disease and hypoparathyroidism resulting from surgical or radiation injury to the parathyroid glands exert the same effect. Tetany (p. 319) is one sign.

Now read Osteomalacia/Rickets (p. 52)

Low serum concentrations of calcium accompany acute pancreatitis. They are due to intra-abdominal saponification of fat and to hypo-albuminaemia. Hypocalcaemia may also occur in chronic pancreatitis. It is attributable to increased faecal excretion associated with steatorrhoea. Rare causes of hypocalcaemia include renal tubular disease, the effects of diuretics such as frusemide; malignant hyperpyrexia; and leukaemia.

CALCULUS

A calculus (stone) is a concretion formed in an excretory duct or fluid-containing viscus. Lithiasis is the formation of calculi. Biliary (p. 37) and urinary (p. 338) calculi are commonplace. Salivary (p. 288), prostatic (p. 278) and pancreatic (p. 263) calculi are found less frequently.

In the past, niduses such as bacteria or debris resulting from inflammation were thought to be responsible for the origin of all calculi (p. 374). Now, the majority of these objects are thought to derive from the secretions of the ducts and organs in which they are found. Substances of low molecular weight, such as calcium salts, are held in solution by adsorption to macromolecules including glycoproteins and mucins. Calculi may therefore be formed either by an increase in the concentration of the crystalloid or a decrease in the concentration of the carrier molecules.

Primary calculi

Primary, metabolic calculi arise in the absence of local disease. They are formed solely of crystalloids such as cholesterol or cystine. Cholesterol, bilirubin, cystine and xanthine are inherently radiolucent but may contain small quantities of calcium or magnesium salts that render them opaque.

Secondary calculi

Secondary calculi consist largely of radio-opaque salts of calcium or magnesium. They form around foreign bodies such as sutures, desquamated cells, microorganisms or as deposits upon existing, primary calculi.

EFFECTS OF CALCULI

Calculi, particularly those of the biliary tract (p. 37), are frequently discovered incidentally during a radiological or autopsy study. However, many calculi that cause disease are symptomless. The presence of a calculus in a duct is suspected when signs develop of partial or complete obstruction to the outflow of secretions. Obstruction persists until the calculus is passed spontaneously or removed surgically. Obstruction due to calculi is commonly followed by infection within the duct. If obstruction is partial or intermittent, there may be proximal dilatation of the duct. If obstruction is complete, all glandular secretion ultimately ceases. Fibrosis of the obstructed organ often follows.

CARBOHYDRATES

Carbohydrates are macronutrients, a designation that describes the principal dietary components, carbohydrate, lipid and protein. Carbohydrates have the general formula $C_x(H_2O)_y$. However, the term is frequently applied to derivatives produced by oxidation or reduction such as sorbitol ($C_6H_{14}O_6$). The name 'sugar' is restricted to monosaccharides such as glucose and to disaccharides such as sucrose.

Now read Lipids (p. 207), Proteins (p. 281)

Carbohydrate is stored in the liver and skeletal muscle as glycogen. The quantity conserved amounts to ~400 g in a 70 kg man. In starvation, this reserve is exhausted rapidly. Glucose is then manufactured solely by the catabolism of amino acids in the process of **gluconeogenesis**. The brain and other glycolytic tissues require a minimum of 80 g/day of this sugar. The supply is essential even when ketosis and keto-adaptation (p. 231) are maximal as they are in established malnutrition. In this condition, the daily breakdown of at least 80 g of skeletal and visceral muscle protein is demanded.

CARCINOGENESIS and CANCER

Carcinogenesis describes the mechanisms that lead to the initiation, development and growth of a cancer, that is, a malignant neoplasm (p. 242). Carcinogens are agents that can cause neoplasms to form and grow. Some circumstances predispose to carcinogenesis; others are directly causative. The actions of all carcinogens are irreversible. Their effects persist throughout life. They are additive and are exerted over long time periods of time.

Now read Neoplasia (p. 242)

A **precancerous** state is one in which a potential for uncontrolled cell growth, invasion and metastasis has been initiated but in which no alterations in cell structure or function are apparent microscopically.

A cancer cell proliferates in a clonal manner (p. 83). In its relationships to nearby, normal cells, each daughter cell of this clone displays the same selective growth and survival advantages as the parent cell. The expansion of the clones continues until the population of clonal cells is sufficiently large to be recognisable as a **tumour** (p. 242).

The common agency responsible for all forms of cancer is disturbed regulation of cell division (p. 84) and survival. The propensity for deregulation is inherited or acquired. It is due to the mutation of genes, the protein products of which normally control cell division, cell survival and protein synthesis. In carcinogenesis, at least six mutations must accumulate before deregulation becomes effective.

- **Non-heritable cancer**. In the majority of cancers, there is no demonstrable, inherited predisposition.
- **Heritable cancer**. In the small proportion of cases in which there is an inherited predisposition, the mutations have usually been spontaneous. Occasionally, they represent the influence of a virus. In inherited, familial tumour predisposition, a dominant mutation is already present in one of the germ cell lines and is therefore inherited by every cell in the body. In the more common, heritable but non-familial cases, a recessive mutation is present in one of the germ cell lines. A further, second mutation is necessary before the emergence of a clone of cancer cells can take place. Both of these mutations must be at the same location on each of a pair of homologous chromosomes: the involved genes can therefore be designated alleles.

PREDISPOSITION TO CANCER

Race, locality, age, occupation, and social class are among the factors predisposing to cancer.

Race

There are wide differences in the geographical prevalence of cancers (Table 15). To describe these differences, a number of agreed definitions are used:

- **Incidence** is the number of persons with a defined form of tumour falling ill within one year. The probability of an individual in a particular group being diagnosed as having a particular cancer within one year is the incidence rate. For separate groups of a similar age this becomes the age-specific incidence rate. The figure can be adjusted for age when it becomes the age standardised incidence rate. Cumulative incidence rates are summed for each year of age.
- **Prevalence** is the number of cases of a tumour existing in a population at a given moment.

Locality

Cancers such as those of the liver and nasopharynx, infrequent or rare in the West, are commonplace in South-East Asia. Persons of a similar ethnic origin may display different frequencies of particular tumours according to where they live (Table 15). Within individual countries, there are further differences so that cancer of the lung is more common in northern parts

Table 15 Cumulative incidence rates (%) between 20 and 70 years for cancer of the female breast

Locality/race	Rates
United States	
White	10.6
Black	8.1
Japanese	8.2
United Kingdom	5.3
Japan	2.5
Africa	
Black	1.1

of the UK than in southern. Rarely, as in the case of mesothelioma of the pleura (p. 274), local differences are attributable to proximity to sources of carcinogens.

Age

Some tumours occur exclusively in children. Examples are retinoblastoma (p. 286), nephroblastoma (Wilms' tumour) (p. 200) and medulloblastoma (p. 65). Table 16 shows that, in adults, several common cancers are rare before the age of 40 years whereas others are distributed evenly across the age range. At the other end of the age spectrum, few breast cancers but relatively large numbers of colon cancers are found in those aged over 90 years.

Occupation

There have been many historical examples of industries in which cancer has been a hazard. These occupations include radiology, and the mining of shale oil, asbestos and uranium.

Social class

On the basis of the recognition of five social classes, there is a higher prevalence of gastric cancer, for example, in the lowest class, class V.

MECHANISMS OF CARCINOGENESIS

The key to carcinogenesis lies in the many changes (mutations) in the genes (oncogenes and tumour suppressor genes) coding for proteins that initiate or regulate cell growth, differentiation or death. To understand carcinogenesis it is therefore necessary to know how cells grow, divide and die.

Now read Control of cell division (p. 86)

The activation of oncogenes and the de-activation of tumour suppressor genes have four principal actions:

- Increased growth promotion.
- Decreased growth suppression.
- Decreased apoptosis.
- Decreased DNA repair.

In addition, the behaviour and outcome of a cancer is strongly influenced by any propensity for metastasis (p. 246) and by factors controlling angiogenesis (p. 16).

Activation of oncogenes

An oncogene is a gene that can transform a cell, that is, induce the production of a neoplasm.

Oncogene activation affords an important key to understanding carcinogenesis. Cellular oncogenes display a close similarity to the transforming oncogenes of retroviruses. Oncogenes originate by mutations in proto-oncogenes, gene sequences found in normal cells. Proto-oncogenes play an essential part in coding for proteins regulating cell growth and division. Activation of oncogenes, initiated by viral, physical or chemical agents, results from:

- Mutations in oncogene DNA.
- Chromosomal translocations that move oncogenes to new sites in the genome.
- Amplification of oncogenes.
- Abnormal transcriptional regulation (p. 140).

Table 16 Relative frequency of cancer in different age groups

Cancers of childhood	Adult cancers: <1% diagnosed before age 40 years		Adult cancers: 3–5% diagnosed before age 40 years	Adult cancer evenly distributed across the age spectrum
Rhabdomyoblastoma	Myeloma	Oesophagus	Breast	Uterus (cervix)
Medulloblastoma	Bronchus	Colon	Ovary	Thyroid
Nephroblastoma	Larynx	Rectum	Kidney	Sarcoma
Ependymoma	Stomach	Prostate	Mouth	Malignant melanoma
Acute leukaemia	Pancreas Endometrium	Bladder	Lip Pharynx	Non-Hodgkin's lymphoma

The proteins encoded by oncogenes resemble those coded by proto-oncogenes (Table 17). However, oncogenic products lack the regulatory functions exercised in normal cells by those of proto-oncogenes; their expression is independent of the external signals that modulate normal cell growth and differentiation. When activated, there is deregulation of the control of proliferation, resulting in cell transformation.

Table 17 Mode of action of oncogenes and the tumours that may result.

Mutation in genes encoding	Resultant neoplasm
Growth factors such as PDGF-β e.g. *sis*	Astrocytoma
Growth factor receptors such as EGF receptors e.g. *c-erb B-1*	Squamous carcinoma of bronchus
Secondary signalling proteins e.g. *ras*	Chronic myeloid leukaemia
Transcription factors e.g. *myc*, *N-myc*	Burkitt's lymphoma; small cell carcinoma of bronchus
Cyclins e.g. *L-myc*	Breast, oesophageal, skin carcinomas; lymphomas

Loss of tumour suppressor genes

Tumour suppressor genes prevent cancer growth. Mutations that lead to the inactivation of these genes encourage carcinogenesis. In some tumours, the deleted or altered gene codes for a protein that normally suppresses the synthesis of tumour growth factors in response to signals originating in another pair of genes. These tumour suppressor genes describe a DNA sequence that acts as a dominant suppressor of malignancy. Particular interest is centred on a tumour suppressor gene locus on chromosome 17 (*p53*) that encodes a protein designated p53. Point mutations at this locus are frequent features of a large variety of cancers in man. The p53 protein is thought to act as a 'guardian of the genome'. It co-ordinates the response to DNA damage by inducing either growth arrest, to allow DNA repair, or apoptosis (Table 18).

Another well-recognised example of this phenomenon is the inheritance of a defective copy of the *RB-1* gene, located within 13q14, establishing a familial risk of the development in children of retinoblastoma (p. 286). The presence of *RB-1* prevents retinoblastoma whereas its loss or inactivation predisposes to the growth of this cancer. Therefore, if the other, normal *RB-1* allele is lost by spontaneous mutation or through the action of environmental carcinogens, a malignant tumour develops.

Defective apoptosis

A family of genes regulates apoptosis (p. 89). *bcl-2*, for example, is anti-apoptotic. The protein products of this proto-oncogene permit cells to live for excessive periods. Thus *bcl-2* protects lymphocytes so that they survive in lymphoid and haemopoietic tissues. A mutation in *bcl-2* results in it becoming an oncogene. The development of follicular lymphoma (p. 223) is an example of the consequences of this mutation.

Defective DNA repair

During cell division, DNA does not always replicate accurately. DNA also suffers damage from ultraviolet light, exposure to chemicals and other factors. However, these defects rarely result in cancer. The reason is the existence of DNA repair mechanisms:

- **Nucleotide excision repair**. One such system repairs the cross-linking of nucleotides. It is defective in xeroderma pigmentosum (p. 362).
- **Mismatch repair**. A second system repairs the mismatches between individual bases but does not affect cell division directly. Thus, patients who develop hereditary, non-polyposis colon cancer (p. 106) inherit one or more mutated, mismatch repair genes. The mutations render colon epithelial cells susceptible to a second mutation, a second 'hit', leading to deregulation of cell division.
- **Telomere shortening**. A third system, catalysed by the enzyme telomerase reverse transcriptase, can reverse the process in human cancer by which telomeres (p. 91) do not shorten.

CHANGES IN CELL KARYOTYPES IN CANCER

Chromosomal abnormalities are frequent indications of the abnormalities of cell division characteristic of most cancers.

- **Quantitative changes**. Abnormal **numbers** of chromosomes (aneuploidy – p. 92) are found in the majority of malignant tumours and are a

Table 18 Mode of action of tumour suppressor genes and the tumours that may result from their defective action

Site of suppressor	Protein products	Gene	Action of gene	Neoplasms	
				Somatic	**Inherited**
Plasma membrane	Growth inhibitory factors	e.g. *BRCA-1*	Binds to cell surface and inhibits cell growth	Female breast cancer	Female breast cancer
Beneath plasma membrane	Cell adhesion molecules	e.g. *APC*	Cytoplasmic protein linked to E-cadherin on cell surface and involved in signal transduction	Carcinomas of stomach, pancreas, colon (p. 105)	Familial adenomatous polyposis coli
Cytoplasm	Signal transduction molecules	e.g. *NF2*	Regulates cell growth e.g. in Schwann cells; involved in cytoskeletal organisation	Neurilemoma, meningioma	Neurofibromatosis, acoustic neuroma, meningioma
Nucleus	Cell cycle regulation	e.g. *RB*	Initiates cell cycle arrest	Carcinomas of lung, breast, colon; retinoblastoma	Retinoblastoma, osteosarcoma.
	Cell cycle and apoptosis regulation	e.g. *p53*	Initiates growth arrest and apoptosis in response to variety of stimuli	Majority of cancers	Multiple carcinomas; rare genetic syndromes

distinguishing feature of precancerous states such as intra-epithelial neoplasia of the uterine cervix. The number of chromosomes is often in the ranges 40–50 or 60–90. Chromosomal numbers of 37 or 38 are frequent in carcinoma of the breast.

- **Qualitative changes**. There are simultaneous abnormalities of **form**. Bizarre chromosomal structures, some very large and long, are commonplace. They are markers for malignancy. Examples are given on p. 199.

Now read Chromosomes (p. 90), Genes (p. 138), Inheritance (p. 182)

ENVIRONMENTAL CAUSES OF CANCER

Many neoplasms arise as a result of environmental agencies. The principal known agents are ionising radiation, chemical substances and micro-organisms, particularly viruses. For environmental reasons not yet understood, Japanese women who have settled in America now have rates of breast cancer closer to those of native, white Americans than to those of native Japanese. The low rates of breast cancer in Asia are not simply due to differences in genetic susceptibility. Most chemical and physical cancer-producing agents are highly reactive and damage many sites other than those controlling neoplastic transformation.

Viral carcinogens

Both DNA and RNA viruses can cause tumours and are transmitted either horizontally, for example by contact, from individual to individual; or vertically, across the placenta.

DNA viruses

Oncogenic DNA viruses change the genetic structure of host cells permanently. DNA virus genome is integrated directly into the host chromosomes. However, the virus does not multiply and does not kill the host cells.

RNA viruses

To be oncogenic, an RNA virus must first reverse transcribe to complementary DNA by a unique enzyme system. The enzyme is **reverse transcriptase**. Its presence in a cell is highly indicative of the influence of retroviral RNA. RNA viruses that are oncogenic often multiply within transformed cells. Of the RNA tumour viruses, the Rous sarcoma virus has one gene (*src*) necessary for cell transformation but not for viral replication. The *src* oncogene codes for a single protein (src) with tyrosine kinase activity that may be responsible for some of the complex changes of cancer cell transformation. Normal cells have similar genes that have oncogenic potential; they are cellular proto-oncogenes (p. 77).

Viruses causing tumours

- **Epstein–Barr virus (EBV)**. EBV (p. 351) is associated with nasopharyngeal carcinoma (China, Malaysia, northern Africa, Alaskan Eskimos); Hodgkin's disease (USA); and a variety of neoplasms of the lymphoid tissues of which the most important is Burkitt's lymphoma in Uganda (p. 224). The geographic distribution is not accounted for by the fact that EB virus and the malarial parasite are both carried by mosquitoes, but because malaria disturbs the surveillance mechanism of the immune system. Transformed, malignant B-cells grow unhindered: T-helper cells (p. 173) are compromised.
- **Rous sarcoma virus**. Rous sarcoma virus (p. 375), the cause of a transmissible chicken sarcoma, was the first oncogenic virus discovered.
- **Mammary tumour viruses**. Mammary neoplastic viruses cause breast carcinomas in mice. In 1936, Bittner identified female mice with a high or a low incidence of mammary neoplasia. Mothers of a high-incidence strain conveyed cancer to suckling offspring of a low-incidence strain who were not at risk when suckled by mothers of a low-incidence strain. The virus was transmitted in the milk.
- **Human papilloma viruses**. Human papilloma viruses (HPV) are associated with and may cause skin, uterine cervical, anal and other tumours. Infections with HPV 1, 2 and 4 lead to common warts (p. 354). HPV 6, 11 and 30 are associated with condyloma acuminata (p. 294). HPV 6 and 11 have also been detected in laryngeal papilloma. The greatest interest lies, however, in the relationships between HPV and uterine cervical neoplasia. CIN 1 (p. 340) is accompanied by HPV 6 and 11; CIN 2 and 3 by HPV 16 and 18; and overt cervical cancer by HPV 16, 18 and 31.

Now read Uterus, cervix (p. 340)

Chemical carcinogens

The first evidence of the part that chemicals could play in carcinogenesis was Pott's (p. 375) description of scrotal cancer in those who had been chimney-sweeps as boys. Soot contains coal tar that is carcinogenic because of the presence in tar of hydrocarbons such as 3,4-benzpyrene. These hydrocarbons are found in the air of industrial towns, the exhaust gases of internal combustion engines, and in cigarette smoke. At least 11 classes of inorganic and organic chemicals are known to be carcinogenic. Many thousands of individual compounds have been incriminated (Table 19).

Hydrocarbons

Carcinogenic polycyclic hydrocarbons bear a generic resemblance to cholesterol and the steroid hormones. Paradoxically, these carcinogens are very similar to inert molecules. Whether an individual compound is an active carcinogen or an inactive compound is determined by small but critical changes in structure. Thus, 1:2,5:6-benzanthracene is a potent carcinogen while 1:2,3:4-dibenzanthracene is inactive. Carcinogenic activity is related to water solubility and an ability to react with DNA.

Aromatic amines

Carcinogenic aromatic amines attracted attention after the rise of the synthetic aniline dye industry. Aniline is not carcinogenic but derivatives of the associated compounds beta-naphthylamine and benzidine have this property. Naphthylamine induces

Table 19 Some important chemical carcinogens

Chemical carcinogen	Source	Target organ
Azo dyes e.g. dimethylaminoazobenzene ('butter yellow')	Artificial colouring agents	Liver
Aminofluorenes e.g. 2-acetylaminofluorene	Insecticides	Liver
Nitrosamines e.g. dimethylnitrosamine	Solvents	Urinary bladder
Alkylating agents, linking directly to DNA e.g. methylmethanesulphonate	Manufacture of polymers	Liver
Microbial toxins e.g. aflatoxin	Fungal contamination of peanuts	Liver
Inorganic compounds e.g. silicate	Asbestos	Lung

bladder cancer in species with glucuronidase. Beta-naphthylamine is converted to the carcinogen 1-hydroxy-2-aminonaphthalene in the liver, where it is safely conjugated with glucuronic acid. The deconjugation of this soluble product in the bladder permits local carcinogenesis that is therefore remote, tissue selective, and species specific.

In experimental studies, two stages in chemical carcinogenesis are demonstrable. A single, small amount of benzpyrene applied to the skin is without visible, external effect. The subsequent repeated application to the same site of an irritant but non-carcinogenic substance, such as croton oil, leads to neoplastic growth. The benzpyrene is said to **initiate** carcinogenesis; the croton oil **promotes** carcinogenesis. Initiation is irreversible, promotion is reversible. The croton oil acts as a co-carcinogen, but many agents are effective by themselves and are complete carcinogens.

Physical carcinogens

Ionising radiations exemplify the adverse, carcinogenic actions of physical carcinogens (Table 20). The particulate or wave-form radiations (p. 186) remove electrons from intracellular molecules, creating free radicals that can react with DNA. The mitotic phase of cell division is most susceptible to this injury. Consequently, cell populations in tissues such as the testis, bone marrow, small intestinal epithelium and lymph nodes, where cell divisions are numerous, are particularly vulnerable. By contrast, tissue such as brain, hyaline cartilage and cornea are tolerant of high doses of ionising radiation.

Squamous carcinoma of the hands of radiologists was recognised within a few years of the introduction of X-rays for diagnostic radiology (p. 185). Ionising radiations, particularly X-rays and gamma-rays, are potent cytotoxic agents; they are also effective carcinogens. Particulate radiation, in the form of neutrons and alpha-particles, exerts a similar effect. Beta-particles (electrons) are carcinogenic provided they gain access to cells after injection, inhalation or ingestion. Although solar, ultraviolet light (UVL) is less potent than ionising radiation as a carcinogen, it is of importance because exposure is often repetitive and prolonged. The influence of solar UVL is limited to exposed skin surfaces. At these sites, malignant melanoma, basal cell carcinoma and squamous carcinoma are readily induced, particularly in white people working in hot climates. These cancers are also frequent in regions where individuals are exposed for long periods to direct sunlight or to ultraviolet light penetrating cloud.

Now read Irradiation (p. 185)

Table 20 Some important physical carcinogens

Source of radiation	Consequences
Atomic bomb explosions	Leukaemia
Nuclear reactor accidents	Carcinoma of breast, lung and thyroid
Ingestion of uranium (miners)	Bronchial carcinoma
Ingestion of radon (watch dial-painters)	Osteosarcoma
Angiography with thorotrast (thorium dioxide)	Haemangiosarcoma Cholangiocarcinoma

CARCINOID

Carcinoids are functioning tumours of the cells of the diffuse endocrine system. They secrete several amines, particularly 5-hydroxytryptamine (5-HT).

In order of decreasing frequency, carcinoids arise from the enterochromaffin cells of the appendix, small intestine, rectum, colon, oesophagus and stomach. Identical but very uncommon tumours also occur in the bronchus, breast, thymus, liver, gall bladder, lung and ovary. The neoplasms are small, yellow and grow slowly. They invade the intestinal wall and may penetrate it. Microscopically, nests of cells of a uniform structure are closely related to a meshwork of small, thin-walled blood vessels.

Appendiceal carcinoids metastasise infrequently. They are encountered often by chance, when appendicectomy is undertaken in young adults.

Small intestinal carcinoids grow to a larger size, may be multiple and metastasise to the liver, lymph nodes, lungs and bone. Metastases of the liver, in particular, lead to the carcinoid syndrome.

CARCINOID SYNDROME

The carcinoid syndrome is a vasomotor disturbance with facial flushing and cyanosis, intestinal hypermotility, episodes of bronchoconstriction and right-sided cardiac disease. Malabsorption may result in a pellagra-like (p. 352) skin disorder. The syndrome arises in individuals in whom a carcinoid tumour, usually of the small intestine, has formed large hepatic metastases. The cells of carcinoids and their hepatic metastases secrete 5-HT, histamine, kallikrein and prostaglandins. They may also form ACTH, insulin, gastrin, calcitonin and other hormones.

The principal cause of the symptoms and signs of the carcinoid syndrome is 5-HT. This compound is readily degraded by healthy liver tissue. In the presence of large hepatic metastases, 5-HT is released into the inferior vena cava and promotes pulmonary valvular stenosis and endocardial fibrosis. 5-HT is then degraded in the pulmonary circulation to 5-hydroxyindole-acetic acid (5-HIAA) This metabolite is excreted in the urine where its presence provides diagnostic information. The other symptoms and signs of the carcinoid syndrome are attributable to bradykinin and the prostaglandins, compounds not metabolised in the lung. They therefore gain direct access to the systemic circulation.

CARTILAGE

The three forms of cartilage – hyaline, fibro- and elastic – are susceptible to different classes of disease. Cartilage is an avascular tissue and therefore cannot be a primary site of inflammation. It can, however, be injured or destroyed by inflammation arising in adjoining, vascular sites such as synovia.

DEVELOPMENTAL AND CONGENITAL DISORDERS

A very large number of developmental anomalies is known. Some are heritable. Achondroplasia (chondrodystrophia fetalis) is described on p. 51, metaphyseal aclasis (multiple ecchondromatosis) in Table 12 on p. 58. Multiple enchondromatosis appears in two forms: Maffucci's syndrome and Ollier's disease.

TRAUMA AND INJURY

The effects of trauma are exemplified by tears of the fibrocartilaginous meniscus of the knee joint. Effusion and disability result. Long-term, there is a predisposition to osteoarthritis, particularly if the meniscus is excised rather than repaired. The fibrocartilages of intervertebral discs are disrupted in severe spinal injuries with bone fracture.

TUMOURS

Benign

Enchondroma

Enchondroma is a single, symptomless tumour of the cylindrical bones of the hands or feet, although occasionally it is detected in long bones including the femur and humerus. The tumour is formed of islands of cartilage in which the matrix appears soft and blue–grey. Pain and swelling may follow local injury and pathological fracture is a complication.

Enchondroma of a long bone may simulate

chondrosarcoma but this malignant tumour does not arise in the small, tubular bones of the hand and foot. Several or many enchondromas are found in **multiple enchondromatosis**. Together with multiple soft tissue haemangiomas, they are also encountered in Maffucci's syndrome. In both of these rare conditions, there is a significant risk of malignant transformation.

Osteochondroma

In osteochondroma, a single, hard, irregular and enlarging mass is noticed arising, for example in a phalanx of a child or adolescent. The tumour is a developmental disorder at a metaphysis. There is formation of a bony outgrowth covered by a cap of cartilage. Enchondral ossification takes place in the neoplastic cartilage. Rarely, osteochondromas are multiple, a condition inherited as an autosomal dominant characteristic to which the term metaphyseal aclasis (**hereditary multiple ecchondromatosis**) is applied. A small number of these individuals develop low-grade chondrosarcoma, a change more likely when the initial lesion is sited in the axial skeleton.

Malignant

Chondrosarcoma

Chondrosarcoma is a malignant tumour of older adults.

Causes

There is predisposition to the development of the tumour in individuals with rare forms of heritable cartilage disorder such as metaphyseal aclasis. The common sites of origin are pelvis, shoulder, ribs and other parts of the axial skeleton. Swelling or discomfort draw attention to the tumour which may, however, reach a very large size before treatment is sought.

Structure

The radiolucent mass is punctuated by speckled calcification. Histologically, the cells of chondrosarcoma extend into and fill bone marrow spaces. The neoplastic cells are, however, devoid of the characteristic features of malignancy such as high nucleocytoplasmic ratios, nuclear pleomorphism and mitotic activity. The recognition of early, low-grade chondrosarcoma is particularly difficult.

Behaviour and prognosis

Chondrosarcoma is resistant to radiotherapy and chemotherapy. Radical surgery is therefore often indicated. The tumour tends to recur locally and may grow as an island of implanted cells at a site of biopsy. For these reasons, the surgical management of chondrosarcoma can only be properly undertaken in centres where excellent facilities for imaging co-exist with appropriate surgical expertise. Osteosarcoma or malignant fibrous histiocytoma may develop concomitantly with chondrosarcoma in a process still misleadingly called dedifferentiation.

CELL

Cells (Fig. 13) are the structural and functional units of all human tissues. The body is formed of ~10^{13} of these units. The number of cells/unit volume of tissue, the cell density, of different tissues varies from very high (intestinal epithelium, lymph nodes) to very low (fibrocartilage).

A **clone** is a collection of cells, organisms or nucleic acid sequences, all derived from the same ancestral cell. Unless mutation has taken place, each contains identical genetic information.

CELL STRUCTURE

- **Plasma membrane**. Every human cell (Fig. 13) is bounded by a plasma membrane. It is a lipid bilayer in which proteins are embedded.
- **Nucleus**. With the exception of mature red blood cells and platelets, each cell contains one or more nuclei in which is concentrated all the chromosomal DNA (p. 90). The nucleus, separated by a double membrane from the non-nuclear content of the cell – the cytoplasm or cytosol – includes a smaller nucleolus in which ribosomes are assembled.
- **Endoplasmic reticulum**. Continuous with the outer membrane of the nuclear envelope is the endoplasmic reticulum (ER). Rough ER bears the ribosomes engaged in protein synthesis (p. 140). Smooth ER lacks ribosomes and is closely concerned with lipid metabolism. The sacs of the Golgi apparatus process and package large molecules before they are either delivered to other organelles, or secreted.
- **Cytoplasm**. The cytoplasm contains a skeleton of protein filaments including the centrioles and microtubules.

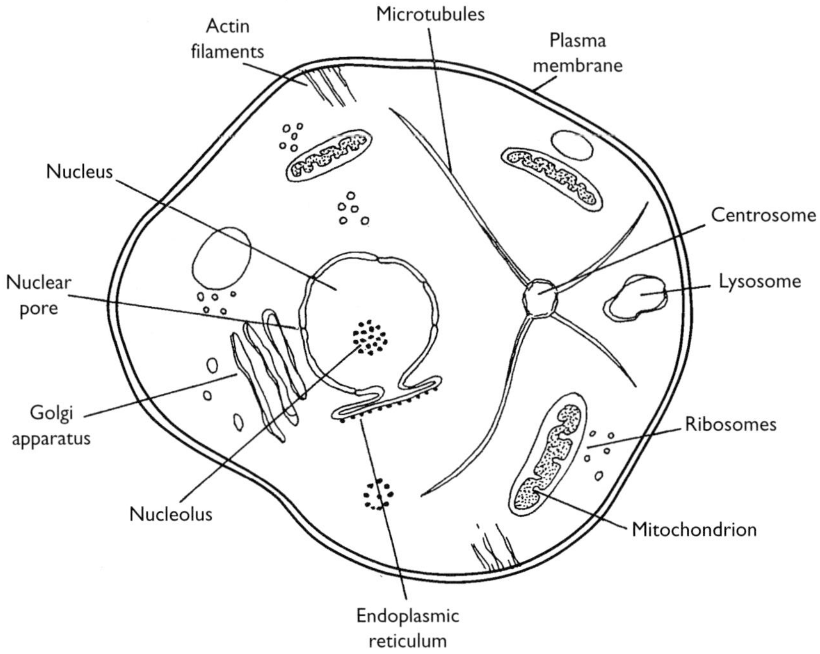

Figure 13 Cell structure.
Diagram depicts main features found in majority of human cells. There are wide differences in detailed structure between, for example, cardiac muscle cell rich in contractile filaments and plasma cell with much cytoplasmic RNA. Some cells, such as erythrocytes and platelets, have no nuclei.

- **Cytoplasmic filaments**. All cells contain fine, delicate cytoplasmic filaments identifiable by monoclonal antibodies. Occasionally, as in muscle, the number of filaments is very large. The filaments in muscle are thick (myosin) and thin (actin and tropomyosin B). Other filaments, intermediate in diameter between actin and myosin, are prekeratin tonofilaments, vimentin, desmin, neurofilaments and glial fibrillary protein. Intracytoplasmic filaments help to identify cancer cells, degenerative diseases and metabolic disorders. Actin and myosin filaments are found in striated-muscle neoplasms, tonofilaments in squamous carcinoma. Increased numbers of neurofilaments are present in ageing neurones and in nerve cells in Alzheimer's and other neurological diseases. Glial fibrillary protein is found in glial scars and some astrocytomas. Desmin filaments are prominent in heart muscle in some cardiomyopathies and after treatment with anabolic steroids. Vimentin filaments predominate in ageing and degenerate chondrocytes; in synovial cells in rheumatoid arthritis; and in synovial sarcoma.
- **Mitochondria**. Mitochondria are the powerhouses of the cells, using oxygen to make high-energy ATP. They contain a distinctive form of DNA.
- **Lysosomes**. Within the cytoplasm are scattered lysosomes (p. 225) and peroxisomes that generate and destroy hydrogen peroxide.

Now read Mitochondrial DNA (p. 141)

CELL GROWTH AND DIVISION

Normal growth

The continual multiplication of cells is necessary to replace the large number lost by desquamation (skin), exfoliation (gastro-intestinal), senescence, apoptosis and injury.

There is a cycle of cell division. In tissues such as those of the lining epithelia, cells divide frequently and continuously throughout life. At other sites, such as arteriolar smooth muscle, division is very infrequent. Skeletal muscle cells do not divide after maturation and red blood cells and platelets are anucleate. Neurones do not divide but regenerate by molecular replacement.

The cycle of cell division (Fig. 14) may be as brief as 8 hours (intestinal crypt cells) or as long as 100 days (heart muscle cells). In a single 24-hour cycle, 90% of the time is occupied by rest between divisions. There is a series of phases of division:

- **G0 phase**. A cell in the G0 phase has left the cell cycle and is senescent.
- **G1 phase**. The cycle of division begins with a phase of high synthetic activity. The cell enlarges, manufactures new proteins and prepares to copy the nuclear DNA.
- **Restriction point**. Near the end of G1 is a restriction point (checkpoint). A family of proteins called cyclins and cyclin-dependent kinases (CDKs) form elaborate complexes to allow a dividing cell to pass these points when there is no significant defective DNA and when the cell has enlarged sufficiently.

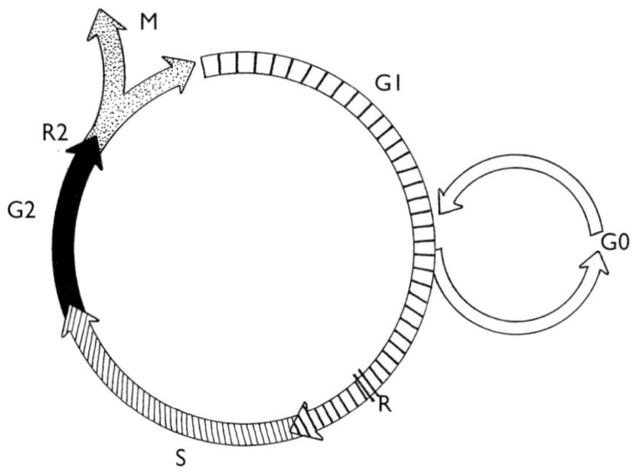

Figure 14 Cell division.

M: Somatic cell division takes place in process of mitosis. After mitosis, cell may divide again (as shown) or stop cycling temporarily or permanently.
G1: Cell enlarges, manufactures new proteins, and prepares to copy DNA.
R: Restriction point. Here, 'decisions' are made whether to divide or not.
G0: In a period of indefinite length, cell may rest.
S: Nuclear DNA now replicates in preparation for division. Complement of chromosomes is duplicated.
G2: Cell prepares to divide again.

- **S phase**. Nuclear DNA is then replicated. This is the time when each chromosome divides to form a pair of identical 'sister chromatids'.
- **G2 phase**. A further phase follows in which the enlarged cell, with its duplicated chromatids, prepares to divide.
- **Restriction point**. A second checkpoint follows. It is passed when sufficient DNA is replicated and when the cell has achieved a viable size.
- **M phase**. Now there is nuclear, then cytoplasmic division.

Abnormal growth

A number of terms designate different abnormalities of cell growth:

- **Aplasia** describes complete cessation of cell growth and multiplication.
- **Hypoplasia** is a reduction in the frequency of cell division relative to the rate normal for an individual tissue or organ.
- **Hyperplasia** is an increase in the number of cells in an organ or tissue.
- **Metaplasia** is the change of one type of differentiated tissue to another differentiated type. An example is the translation of the normal pseudostratified columnar ciliated epithelium of the bronchus into stratified squamous epithelium under the influence of chronic irritants or carcinogens such as those of cigarette smoke.
- **Dysplasia.** The term dysplasia is used in two distinct ways.

  In the first, dysplasia represents a loss of, or reduction in, the degree of differentiation of cell types. Dysplastic changes are frequently precancerous. Dysplastic glandular cells lose their nuclear polarity. The size of the nuclei increases so that the nucleocytoplasmic ratios rise, approaching those of embryonic or 'blast' cells. The chromosome number increases, deviating from the diploid number. The abnormally large number of chromosomes is reflected in the high nuclear chromatin content. Among these large, deeply staining nuclei, mitotic figures become numerous. The appearances of the tissue merge with those of carcinoma in-situ (p. 244). In stratified squamous epithelium, there is a loss of the capacity of the cells to form keratin and the emergence of cells resembling those of the young stratum germinativum.

  In the second, dysplasia describes an abnormality

of organ growth. Renal dysplasia is one example. A small, poorly formed kidney may contain cartilage and is accompanied by other abnormalities of the genito-urinary tract.

- **Anaplasia** is a loss of structural differentiation. It is a feature of poorly differentiated malignant tumours (p. 243).
- **Neoplasia** is described on p. 242.

Mitosis

Mitosis is the process by which the duplicated genetic material of the cell divides in half during somatic cell division. One member of each chromosomal pair passes to each daughter cell. Each daughter cell has a complete chromosomal set. Mitosis may lasts for as little as 1–2 hours.

Control of cell division

Cells divide when instructed to do so by their neighbours. The cells of a tissue therefore form a complex, interdependent association the size, shape and degree of differentiation of which are determined genetically. However, cell division is also influenced by signals coming from more remote sources. Some are endocrine but the most important are polypeptide growth factors.

Many molecules are involved in the events leading to cell division (Fig. 15). The majority are proteins or polypeptides. The necessary transfer of high energy phosphate is catalysed by phosphokinases.

- **Growth factors** (p. 144) bind to specific receptors at the cell surface.
- **Growth factor receptors**. Receptors are activated following this binding. They are 'transmembrane', part external to the cell, part within it. One part becomes phosphorylated, i.e., acquires phosphate, and sends signals to other proteins within the cytoplasm.
- **Secondary signalling proteins**. Secondary signalling is involved in transducing signals from the cell receptors (Fig. 15) to the nucleus. The signals are sent via proteins the most important of which are the *ras* family and the GTP-binding proteins, particularly the G proteins. Another secondary signaller, protein kinase C, is activated after calcium stores are mobilised.
- **Transcription factors**. Within the nucleus are genes such as *jun*, *myc* and *fos* that encode transcription factors. They are intimate regulators of DNA synthesis (p. 139) and cell division and can act in a positive or negative manner.
- **Cell cycle clock**. The initiation and frequency of cell division is regulated by a group of nuclear proteins, the cell cycle clock. These proteins integrate the many growth-regulating signals received by each cell. When the signals are stimulatory, the cell enters a cycle of division. When they are inhibitory, division ceases (Fig. 15).

The nuclear proteins that control the cycle of division are cyclins D, E, A and B. They act by combining with and activating a further group of enzymes called cyclin-dependent kinases (CDKs). To enable their action, a molecular 'switch' operates at restriction points (Fig. 15) in the cycle of division. When the switch is 'on', cyclin/CDK complexes bind high energy phosphate that comes from a common cell source, ATP, and transfer it to pRB, the protein coded by *RB1*, the retinoblastoma (p. 286) gene.

RB is the 'universal brake'. It acts to stop the cell cycle, an action it exerts by sequestrating transcription factors. When phosphorylated, the brake stops working, transcription factors are released, catalysing the production of proteins necessary for the progression of the cell through its cycle of division. *RB1* is absent from children with the inherited form of retinoblastoma (p. 286).

In normal cell division, the DNA of telomeres (p. 91) is progressively lost. Consequently, when the shortening of DNA strands reaches a critical length, cell division ceases. Normal cells do not express telomerase, an enzyme that stimulates telomeric DNA formation. In cancer, this is changed (p. 78).

Now read DNA (p. 139), Growth factors (p. 144)

Meiosis

Meiosis is reduction division, the process by which the germ cells divide to form gametes, the spermatozoa and ova, each of which has only 23 chromosomes. At fertilisation, half of the 46 chromosomes of the zygote derive from each parent cell.

Now read Carcinogenesis (p. 76), Neoplasia (p. 242)

CELL SURFACE RECEPTORS

Although steroid and thyroid hormones can cross the plasma membrane, most signalling molecules cannot.

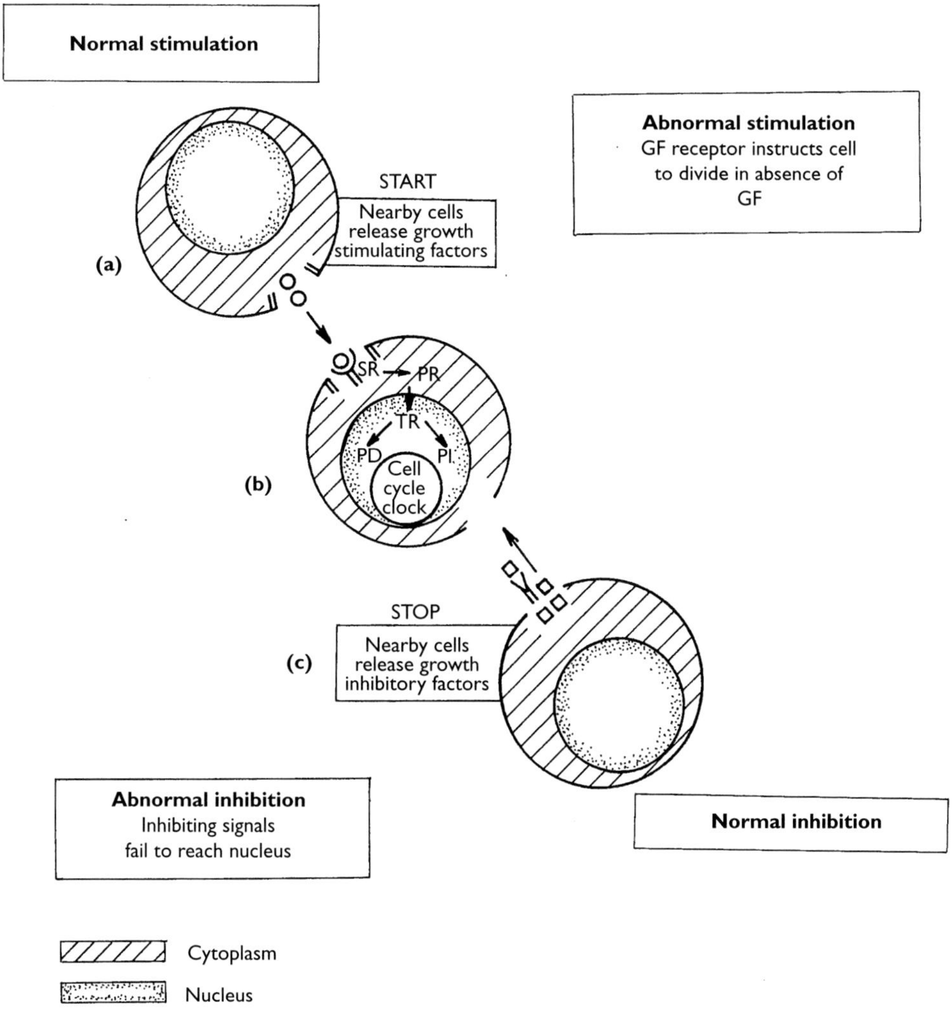

Figure 15 Cell growth and its regulation.
Understanding of regulation of cell growth is necessary to comprehend carcinogenesis.
(a) Start. Signalling pathways inside cell receive growth-stimulating signals from other cells in a tissue. External signals are initiated by secretion of growth factors. These proteins pass through intercellular spaces and bind to receptors on target cell surfaces. Receptors are transmembrane proteins traversing plasma membrane and projecting into cytoplasm.
(b) Transcription. When growth-promoting signals enter cell, chain of further, stimulating signals is initiated and reaches nucleus.
(c) Stop. Within nucleus, transcription factors respond and activate groups of genes that code for the proteins required to initiate, catalyse and conclude cycle of cell division.
PD: proteins triggering cell division, within nucleus; PI: proteins inhibiting cell division, within nucleus; PR: cytoplasmic relay proteins; SR: cell surface receptors; TR: transcription factors.

Their receptors must therefore span the plasma membrane, detecting the signal in the extra-cellular matrix and relaying it, in a different form, to the interior of the cell.

There are three classes of cell surface receptors: ion-channel-linked receptors; G-protein-linked receptors, the most important; and enzyme-linked receptors. G-protein-linked receptors (guanosine triphosphate-binding protein receptors) are polypeptides that extend seven times across the plasma membrane.

CELL JUNCTIONS

The cells of epithelia and solid viscera are attached to each other by specialised structures called junctions, of which desmosomes are one example. In addition, cells are bound to each other and/or to nearby extracellular matrix molecules by electrostatic forces and by families of cell adhesion molecules (CAMs).

ADHESION MOLECULES

These important molecules include **selectins** that bind leucocytes and platelets to endothelial surfaces; **integrins; cadherins**; and the molecules of the **immunoglobulin gene superfamily** (p. 20). Adhesion molecules not only play key roles in cellular processes: they are active in tissue repair, immune functions, the aggregation of platelets, and tumour invasion.

Integrins

Integrins are a family of cell surface, linked proteins. Some integrins anchor cells to molecules of the extracellular matrix (ECM) such as fibronectin, collagens, von Willebrand factor and vitronectin while acting as cues for migration, signal differentiation and growth. Others mediate cell-to-cell interactions.

Integrins are heterodimers, that is, they are formed of two different parts, α and β, each of which stretches (transmembrane) across the plasma membrane of a cell. More than 20 forms of integrin are recognised. The binding of integrins depends on the presence of Ca^{2+} or Mg^{2+} ions but is weak compared to the binding of hormones to their receptors. Inside the cell, integrins link, for example, to actin filaments (p. 84) in stress fibres. The signalling systems conveyed by integrins may be bidirectional, inside $\rightarrow$ out or outside $\rightarrow$ in.

A heritable defect in $\alpha_{IIb}\beta_3$ integrin I is a feature of thrombasthenia. A heritable fault in β_2 integrin results in **leucocyte adhesion deficiency**, a cause of repeated bacterial infections.

Cell–cell adhesion molecules (CAMs)

Two classes of protein enable the selective adhesion of cells within individual tissues and organs. The first class is Ca^{2+}-dependent, the second Ca^{2+}-independent. The cadherins exemplify the former, members of the immunoglobulin superfamily the latter.

- **Cadherins**. E-cadherin binds epithelial cells, N-cadherin nerve and muscle cells, and P-cadherin placental and epidermal cells.
- **Immunoglobulin superfamily**. These molecules play important roles in organ growth and development. N-CAM is one example. It is expressed by most nerve cells.

CELL MOVEMENT

Many individual cells are freely mobile. The movement of cells is exemplified by the behaviour of neutrophil polymorphs in bacterial infection. Within 30 minutes of the stimulus, increased numbers of circulating polymorphs adhere to vascular endothelium and begin to emigrate from the bloodstream towards the organisms. In cell culture, fibroblasts travel in an analogous manner across a glass surface. They extend a leading edge that attaches to the surface before pulling the rest of the cell forwards. Changes in cell shape, movement during cell division, the extension of epidermal squamous cells across a healing excised wound (p. 359) and the movement of young fibroblasts during the growth of granulation tissue, are the result of molecular changes in cytoplasmic microtubules, actin filaments and intermediate filaments.

Now read Chemotaxis (p. 179), Metastasis (p. 246)

CELL ORGANISATION

At an early stage of embryonic development, individual cells begin to assemble into units that become organs, such as the kidneys, or tissues, such as bone and cartilage. Organogenesis and the movement and fusion of various embryonic components are controlled by regulatory genes. In epithelia, cells rest upon defined but semipermeable basement membranes formed of types IV and VII collagen, and of proteoglycan and glycoproteins such as laminin. To establish malignant disease, it is necessary that cancer cells penetrate basement membranes. Proteinases make this possible. A comparable process is essential to the spread of bacteria such as *Mycobacterium tuberculosis* from lung and intestinal surfaces into these tissues. Basement membranes thicken with age and this process is an integral part of the renal and vascular disorders frequently present in diabetes mellitus (p. 117).

CELL DEATH

The death of cells may be the result of irreversible injury caused by hypoxia, ischaemia, nutritional deficiency, heat, cold, trauma, infection, immunological or other disturbance. As metabolism fails, a process of non-programmed **autolysis** begins. The death of single cells may be programmed and takes place by **apoptosis** (see below). Cell death cannot be demonstrated reliably by structural change alone but rests upon evidence of the loss of crucial functions, such as the failure of oxidative phosphorylation.

Now read Death (p. 116)

Cells that respire very vigorously by oxidative metabolic pathways are exquisitely sensitive to agents damaging or blocking these pathways. When metabolism ceases, the integrity of the plasma membrane and of the intracellular membranes quickly fails. Subsequently, the microscope demonstrates cytoplasmic eosinophilia and the lysis (**karyolysis**), fragmentation (**karorrhexis**) or compaction (**pyknosis**) of nuclei. Cells that respire less actively or are less dependent on oxidative phosphorylation show these changes after longer periods and some, such as the chondrocyte which respires anaerobically, may survive under adverse conditions for periods as long as a few days or even up to 2–3 weeks.

Autolysis

Autolysis is the destruction of cells by their own enzymes. It is self-digestion. When cells suffer irreversible injury due, for example, to hypoxia or to a metabolic poison, the active processes by which the cell and organelle walls maintain their special functions are disorganised. The mitochondria, cytoskeleton and plasma membranes suffer damage. There is a breakdown in sodium and potassium transport so that the cell accumulates water. Cytoplasmic vacuolation occurs, microfilaments disintegrate, lysosomal enzymes are activated and released into the cytoplasm and autolysis takes place. Aerobic respiration ceases, H^+ ions accumulate in the dying cells and intracellular pH falls. Hydrolytic, glycolytic and proteolytic enzymes leak from damaged lysosomes and digest the injured cells and the surrounding extracellular matrix. The resultant degraded membranous material is removed by phagocytosis (p. 270). Autolysis is accelerated by high body and ambient temperatures and slowed by a reduction in temperature.

Apoptosis

Apoptosis, formerly termed necrobiosis, is the programmed death of individual cells. It is an inherited characteristic of universal importance enabling the maturation of normal tissues in embryogenesis as well as the death of abnormal cells in cancer. It is regulated by growth factors.

Apoptotic cells shrink. The nuclear chromatin condenses and is broken down. The cell becomes a small, eosinophilic shell that breaks into pieces, apoptotic bodies. They are engulfed by phagocytes and changed to secondary lysosomes (p. 225). Apoptosis is an energy-dependent, physiological process. It maintains the balance between organ growth and atrophy, is a normal feature of organ development and ageing, and does not provoke inflammation. Apoptosis is also the means by which cells are removed quickly from target organs such as the breast and prostate when trophic hormones are withdrawn. It provides a mechanism for regulating the balance of cell numbers in the skin, gut and lymphoid organs.

Since apoptosis destroys immature lymphocytes that bind auto-antigens, defective apoptosis predisposes to auto-immune disease (p. 28), just as the blocking of apoptosis may delay immunodeficiency. Susceptibility to AIDS is decreased by promoting apoptosis; fewer CD4 lymphocytes are deleted than normal. Apoptosis is also an efficient way of removing cells undergoing malignant transformation as a result of a genetic defect. *C-myc* and the *p53* tumour suppressor gene (p. 78) may promote apoptosis. By contrast, abnormal apoptosis can facilitate cancer by the action of oncogenes that suppress apoptosis such as *bcl-2*.

Drugs may increase the susceptibility of cells to apoptosis, amplifying the effects of chemotherapy on cancer cells or decreasing their susceptibility in AIDS.

CHEMOTAXIS

Chemotaxis is the unidirectional movement of leucocytes towards chemical agents at sites of injury or inflammation.

Among the agents responsible for chemotaxis are the components of complement (p. 232), products of bacteria and polymorphs, lymphokines (p. 115) and substances formed in injured tissues. The components of complement that are chemotactic include C5 fragments, the C567 complex and a C3 fragment. They can be generated both by antigen–antibody interaction and, directly, by bacterial, plasma and tissue proteases. Movement takes place along a gradient of chemical concentration. Polymorphs move rapidly and can pass through endothelial cell junctions by amoeboid movement. They accumulate at injured sites within 30 minutes. Monocytes move much more slowly.

Now read Complement (p. 232), Leucocytes (p. 204), Phagocytosis (p. 270)

CHOLESTEROL

Cholesterol is a lipid. It is an organic hydrocarbon that is widespread in nature and is found in all normal diets and synthesised in all body tissues. Ninety-five per cent of all cholesterol is within cells; 5% is in the blood. The ring structure of cholesterol is common to many classes of biological compounds including steroid hormones, bile acids, vitamins and drugs like digoxin.

Cholesterol and cholesterol esters, all insoluble in water, are carried in the circulation as low-density lipoproteins (LDL), particles formed of cholesterol, other lipids and proteins. Cell-surface receptors allow LDL into cells. The absence of these receptors results in very high levels of LDL. Raised concentrations of LDL may be associated with a predisposition to atheroma (p. 26), cholelithiasis (p. 37) and their complications. Plasma concentrations of cholesterol and LDL are high in diabetes mellitus and in much less common hereditary conditions such as the hyperlipoproteinaemias. In familial hypercholesterolaemia, for example, there are mutations in the gene encoding the LDL receptor. Low concentrations of LDL, with an increase in the high-density lipoprotein (HDL) fraction, are protective against these disorders.

Now read Atheroma (p. 26), Diabetes mellitus (p. 117)

CHROMOSOMES

Chromosomes are the forms or packets in which the genetic material of the cell (DNA) is organised. Many genetic diseases are due to chromosomal abnormalities and severe defects are commonplace in tumour cells (p. 78).

Chromosomes are extremely long threads of DNA. They can only be visualised as discrete structures during metaphase. In the clinical diagnosis of suspected genetic disease, cultured lymphocytes are arrested at this point in the cycle of cell division (p. 84) by the cell poison, colchicine. Between divisions, the nuclear chromatin is coiled into a tangle of delicate strands that appear as punctate bodies inside the nuclear membrane. The proteins that accompany DNA coil round the long molecule, turning it into a highly condensed structure called **chromatin**.

Now read Cell division (p. 84)

Each chromosome has a bifid structure (Fig. 16). The two arms of a chromosome are sister **chromatids**. One arm is short (p), the other long (q). The arms are united at a centromere.

Autosomes and sex chromosomes

Forty six chromosomes (the **diploid** number) are present within each normal human somatic cell. The twenty three pairs constitute the **haploid** number; it is the number of chromosomes and chromatids remaining after meiotic (reduction) division (p. 86). A cell with a normal number of sets of chromosomes is **euploid**. The presence of intact pairs rather than single chromosomes demonstrates that two copies of every DNA genome are necessary for normal cell function. The 46 chromosomes comprise 44 non-sex **autosomes** and two **sex chromosomes**. In the nucleus of a female somatic cell, there are two X chromosomes. In the male somatic cell, there is one X and one Y chromosome. In the female cell, one of the X chromosomes is inactivated at a very early stage of

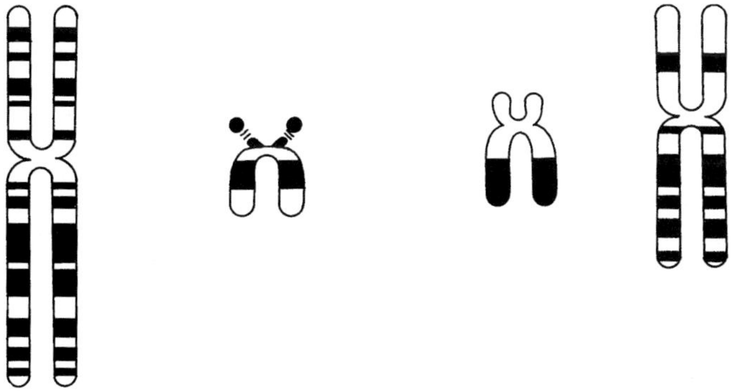

Figure 16 Chromosome structure.
Among somatic chromosomes, chromosome 2 is one of largest, chromosome 21 the smallest. The relatively large female X sex chromosome contains very much larger number of genes than the small male Y chromosome. Giemsa staining defines chromosome bands. Bands are negative (pale) or positive (dark). Numbering of bands increases from centromer (c) to telomere

fetal development. The other exerts a dominant, controlling influence as Lyon demonstrated. Each female cell, like each male cell, therefore has only one active X chromosome.

Cytogenetics – low resolution diagnosis

Spread on slides, chromosomes from cultured cells are arranged and numbered to give a **karyotype**. The normal karyotype is 46,XX for a female cell, 46,XY for a male. The autosomes are numbered from 1 to 22, beginning with the largest. Absence or additions of chromosomes are readily described. Using the Giemsa staining technique, every chromosome can be shown to have an individual **banding pattern** (Fig. 16). The bands are numbered according to an international system. Darkly-stained bands contain fewer than 20% of human genes. The intervening, light bands comprise the remainder and include most human genes. Disorders affecting these regions are associated with severe disease.

The structural unit of the chromosome is the **nucleosome**. Each nucleosome is made up of short (~200 base pairs) lengths of DNA associated with a protein, a histone. The structure is orderly, with the proteins acting as wedges. The nucleosomes, attached to each other by a shorter piece (~60 bp) of linker DNA, resemble a string of beads. These strings, in turn, are organised into coils or supercoils by other, non-histone proteins. From these units are formed the chromatids and, ultimately, the chromosomes.

Chromosomes contain three specialised DNA sequences essential for chromosome replication, separation and partition:

- A **replication origin**, where duplication of DNA starts.
- A **centromere**, that permits a single copy of each chromosome to be pulled into the daughter cell during cell division.
- A **telomere** located at each end of a chromosome.

Telomeres contain nucleotide sequences that enable the ends of the chromosomes to be copied. Without a telomere, some DNA could be lost each time a DNA molecule is replicated. The enzyme telomerase adds multiple copies of the telomere DNA sequence to the chromosome ends (p. 139). In this way, new strands of DNA are completed. Telomeres protect DNA from attacks by nucleases.

Molecular cytogenetics – high resolution diagnosis

The entire genetic structure of two chromosomes has been mapped and the mapping of others is nearing completion. The sequencing of chromosomes 21 and 22 (Fig. 16) was completed in 2000. Chromosome 21 is small; it carries 225 genes whereas chromosome 22 has 545. When a disease such as Down's syndrome (p. 92) has been traced to a chromosome, it is possible that the new understanding may enable the function of the gene(s) predisposing to the disease to be identified. Refinements in chromosmal analysis that have led to this new knowledge include:

- **Chromosmal painting** is used in cancer cell studies. A DNA probe hybridises to the whole length of one pair of chromosomes.
- **Fluorescence *in-situ* hybridisation** (FISH) enables a gene to be localised to a particular region of a chromosome. The duplication or deletion of parts of a chromosome can be identified.
- **Comparative genomic hybridisation** is valuable in defining tumour DNA.

CHROMOSOMAL ABNORMALITIES

Chromosomal abnormalities are very common. They are recognised in 8% of clinically apparent, normal pregnancies and in 50% of aborted fetuses. Many abnormalities cause large defects that can be seen when the karyotype is studied. Most are acquired early, during the formation of the gamete; in fertilisation; or during early mitotic cell division in the embryo. Although some acquired abnormalities can be shown to be the result of exposure to ionising radiation or to the action of chemicals, viruses or hormones, there is often no demonstrable cause. Occasionally, chromosomal abnormalities are inherited.

Alteration in numbers of chromosomes

- In **monosomy**, one chromosome is missing from each cell. Autosomal monosomy is rare but monosomy X is common among spontaneously aborted human embryos.
- In **trisomy**, there is one additional chromosome in each cell. One cause is *non-dysjunction*, a defective segregation of chromosomes.
- In **heteroploidy**, there is an abnormal number of complete haploid sets of chromosomes.
- In **aneuploidy**, there is an alteration in the total number of chromosomes in the somatic cell from the normal, euploid number other than a multiple of this number.
- In **polyploidy**, there is an extra set or sets of chromosomes. *Triploidy* (69 = 23 × 3 chromosomes) or *tetraploidy* (92 = 23 × 4 chromosomes) are lethal conditions. They are found in 15% of spontaneous abortions. There are exceptions: Purkinje cells are normally tetraploid and megakaryocytes are octaploid, having 184 chromosomes.

Alteration in shape or form of chromosomes

- In **deletion** there is the loss of part of a chromosome.
- In **translocation** there is the movement of part of one chromosome to another. Both deletion and translocation are encountered in the abnormal karyotypes seen in most malignant tumours.
- In **duplication**, there is an extra copy of a chromosomal segment.
- In **inversion**, there is a re-arrangement of material within a chromosome.

Congenital autosomal anomalies

Autosomal abnormalities are usually incompatible with life.

Now read Malformation (p. 226)

Down's syndrome

In Down's syndrome, a worldwide disorder affecting one in every 600 births ($1660/10^6$ individuals), a small additional chromosome 21 is present, leading to **trisomy 21**. The diploid number is increased to 47. The karyotype is 47,XY,+21. The cause of the abnormality is non-dysjunction. In nine cases out of 10, the additional chromosome is maternal. The defect may arise early during meiotic cell division; during the formation of the gametes; or later, after the zygotes have formed. In a few children with Down's syndrome, the defect is different: the long arms of chromosome 21 are translocated to another chromosome.

Many embryos with trisomy 21 undergo spontaneous abortion. Down's syndrome is more common among children of older mothers, not fathers. At age 40, the age-related risk in mothers is 1:110. The flat occiput, upward slanting palpebral fissures, flat nose, small mouth and short fingers are characteristic. There is defective cerebral development and mental retardation. Cardiac malformations occur in 40% of cases. Duodenal atresia is relatively common. Later, dementia, leukaemia and non-specific immunodeficiency are additional hazards. However, the life span is only slightly diminished.

Congenital sex chromosome anomalies

In live children, abnormalities of sex chromosomes are more common than autosomal anomalies. The relatively trivial effects of aneuploidy of the sex chromosomes are due, first, to the small size of the Y chromosome which carries little genetic information except the determination of sex and, second, to the partial suppression in most normal cells of one X chromosome. Examples include Klinefelter's, the XYY and Turner's syndromes.

Klinefelter's syndrome

With a karyotype of 47,XXY, this is present as an anomaly in 1 in 600 'males'. The presence of the Y chromosome determines that part of the male phenotype is expressed but there is testicular and seminiferous tubule atrophy and no germ cells. Gynaecomastia and slight learning difficulties are clinical signs.

Turner's syndrome

The syndrome occurs in 1 in 2000 newborn females but many die before birth. The karyotype (45,X) represents the loss of the second X chromosome. The disorder is expressed as small stature but normal intelligence in infertile women with hypoplastic ovaries and failure to menstruate. There may be aortic coarctation.

Chromosomal abnormalities and cancer

In cancers, chromosomal abnormalities are conspicuous and genetic mutations commonplace (p. 78). A predisposition to carcinogenesis is sometimes heritable.

Now read Carcinogenesis (p. 76), Inheritance (p. 182)

CIRCADIAN RHYTHM

Chronobiology is the study of body rhythms that vary in frequency from fractions of a second (firing of neurones) to years (population variations). These rhythms regulate the many functions that control homeostasis. The customary human Circadian rhythm is driven by a built-in body 'clock' located in the suprachiasmatic nucleus of the hypothalamus. The natural rhythm has a time interval of 24 hours although after prolonged periods in the dark, without a clock, it becomes 24.3 hours.

With sleep, there is an increase in the 'darkness' hormone, melatonin, in prolactin and in growth hormone; a drop in body core temperature; a reduction in urine volume; and maximum perceived fatigue. Mood is lowest in the early morning when both the blood pressure and cortisol secretion rise. Glucose tolerance decreases during the day and there is insulin resistance at night. Although gastric emptying and gastro-intestinal hormone secretion are largely regulated by the ingestion of food, their underlying activity is rhythmic. Immune mechanisms, neurotransmission and cell proliferation, display circadian changes.

The results of surgical operations are influenced by Circadian rhythms. In the same way, many drugs are handled differently at different times. Anti-cancer drugs may be employed at times when tumour cells are most susceptible to treatment, host cells most resistant. The 5-year survival of cases of ovarian cancer is improved when doxorubicin and cisplatin are administered in the morning, and the therapeutic efficiency of growth factors such as granulocyte-macrophage CSF and erythropoietin is improved when they are given at optimal circadian times.

CLOSTRIDIA

Clostridia are common anaerobic bacteria that can cause potentially fatal human diseases including tetanus and gas gangrene (p. 137).

Clostridia are large, Gram-positive, metabolically active, spore-bearing, saprophytic organisms. The spores germinate in warm, moist conditions when there is very little oxygen. The majority of clostridia grow in soil, water or decomposing plant and animal material. Some, notably *Clostridium perfringens* (*Cl. welchii*) and *Cl. sporogenes*, inhabit the human intestinal tract, invading the tissues and blood at death to cause putrefaction. A few, behaving as opportunistic pathogens, produce disease when vegetative forms develop and attack injured or devitalised tissue. These pathogens all liberate powerful exotoxins.

Clostridium perfringens and *Cl. septicum* are causes of gas gangrene. *Cl. tetani* causes tetanus and *Cl. botulinum* botulism. Their spores resist the actions of many commonly used antiseptics and disinfectants. *Cl. perfringens* forms four main exotoxins: alpha (α), beta (β), epsilon (ε) and theta (θ). Alpha-toxin is the principal cause of the toxaemia of gas gangrene. It is a heat-stable lecithinase and produces necrosis and haemolysis. Some strains of *Cl. perfringens* also form an enterotoxin that can lead to food poisoning. *Cl. difficile* is the cause of antibiotic-associated diarrhoea. In adults, the organism can survive antimicrobial treatment, multiply and produce potent toxins that may lead to severe and potentially fatal pseudomembranous colitis (p. 103). The cephalosporin group of antibiotics is particularly associated with this disorder.

Now read Gas gangrene (p. 137)

TETANUS

Tetanus is a sporadic neurological disorder in which increased skeletal muscle tone and spasms are caused by the bacterial exotoxin of *Clostridium tetani*, tetanospasmin. The disease results when devitalised tissue provides a micro-environment for the germination of the bacterial spores.

Causes

The spores of *Cl. tetani* soil are found in damp soils, particularly in agricultural countries where horses are employed. In Asian countries where it is customary to apply cow dung to the newborn umbilicus, fatal neonatal tetanus is common. Spores are also recognised in dust or dirty clothing and even in improperly sterilised surgical catgut. They are occasionally identified in air entering operating theatres. The presence of other forms of bacterial infection, particularly those caused by pyogenic cocci and *Cl. perfringens*, predispose to the growth of *Cl. tetani*.

Tetanus is a major cause of death in poor, agricultural populations living in hot climates and therefore remains the sixth most frequent of all bacterial diseases worldwide. It has been a disease of accident and war. In earlier times, before immunisation became widespread, every infantry battle was followed by great numbers of fatal cases. Tetanus began days or even weeks after fighting ceased, in wounded with muscle ischaemia or gangrene. Stab and puncture wounds, even though very small, may be potent causes. Fatal cases in Western populations can result from a single prick by a rose thorn or a splinter. Tetanus is still occasionally encountered in those injured in civilian accidents.

Toxin

Tetanus toxin (tetanospasmin) is a polypeptide neurotoxin. It is formed by the vegetative forms of *Cl. tetani*. It binds locally to motor neurone terminals, enters the axons, and is transported within the axon to the nerve cell bodies of the spinal cord and brain stem. The toxin migrates across the motor nerve synapses to the presynaptic terminals. Both the central and autonomic nervous systems are affected although, because of the blood–brain barrier, the toxin cannot enter the brain itself.

Tetanospasmin blocks the release of inhibitors of neurotransmission so that the resting, firing rate of the motor neurones increases. The consequential heightened numbers of stimuli leads to rigidity of the muscles supplied by the affected neurones. Recruitment of signals results in muscle spasms. In local tetanus, only muscles supplied by affected nerves react. In generalised tetanus, increased muscle tone and muscle spasms develop when tetanospasmin gains access to the bloodstream and spreads to other terminals.

Prevention

The most effective safeguard against tetanus is the proper surgical treatment of wounds although antibiotics help to prevent the growth of *Cl. tetani*. **Active immunisation** (p. 175) offers protection if immunity is maintained by booster injections of toxoid at less than 10-year intervals. In non-immunised patients with contaminated wounds, **passive immunisation** (p. 175) can be achieved by the intramuscular injection of human anti-tetanus immunoglobulin. This protein is prepared commercially from pooled plasma obtained from selected human donors. Anaphylaxis may still occur after injection but is much less frequent than formerly when anti-tetanus serum was harvested from horse serum, as it still is in some countries.

BOTULISM

Botulism is a rare form of food poisoning caused by the toxin of *Clostridium botulinum*. The toxin causes a paralysis that may be fatal.

Clostridium botulinum is a widely distributed saprophyte, present in soil and vegetable matter. Spores are formed that can resist the sterilising action of moist heat at 100°C for several hours. They germinate in foods such as meat and sausage that have been improperly canned or bottled and are found in imported honey. In infancy, *Cl. botulinum* is an occasional cause of neonatal gastro-enteritis. After germination, the organism forms one of the most potent of known toxins. The toxin acts on the parasympathetic nervous system. Taken by mouth, the toxin is absorbed from the gut and exerts its effects on cholinergic motor end-plates, causing paralysis of muscles including those of the diaphragm, pharynx, larynx and eye.

Botulinum toxin can be used to treat chronic anal fissure. Its use represents a form of chemical denervation.

COAGULATION

Coagulation of blood, blood clotting, is the principal factor in haemostasis. In the living circulation, the function of the coagulation system is the formation of a haemostatic plug, terminating bleeding. Coagulation is initiated by a complex sequence of molecular events, many enzymic, that combine to protect the body against the adverse effects of blood loss. The system is a cascade of interacting proteins and cofactors. The ultimate objective is the conversion of the soluble plasma protein fibrinogen into the insoluble substance fibrin, and thus the formation of a coagulum. The components of the system can be studied and measured in the laboratory, individually or in groups.

Coagulation does not normally take place within the circulation: the formation of a coagulum is prevented by the simultaneous, balanced and antagonistic mechanism of fibrinolysis (p. 130). The components of the blood interact with the walls of the blood vessels which manufacture and secrete fibrinolysins and other lytic agents.

If coagulation takes place *in vivo*, it is pathological and is designated **thrombosis** (p. 320). Tissue injury results.

Now read Haemostasis (p. 146)

COAGULATION MECHANISM

Coagulation is an interrelated sequence of reactions, catalysed by enzymes and modified by cofactors. The process is a cascade of amplified response that culminates in the formation of a coagulum or clot. There is an analogy with the amplified cascades of complement activation (p. 231) and with antibody formation in the immune response (p. 171).

Coagulation involves extrinsic and intrinsic pathways. The consequences of their activation are the conversion of prothrombin to thrombin by activated thromboplastin, and the polymerisation of fibrinogen to fibrin under the influence of the enzyme thrombin.

The coagulation mechanism implicates numerous proteins in a sequence of activation. Many of the proteins are enzymes. The primary and secondary, amino acid composition of the majority of these molecules is known, as are their genomes. International agreement designates a roman numeral for each component. Fibrinogen is factor I. The activated state of each enzyme is shown by adding a suffix to the numbered factor. Activated factor VII, for example, is termed factor VIIa. The nomenclature proceeds in a retrograde fashion corresponding to the sequence of reactions within the cascade. Some factors are named after the first individual in whom a particular inherited disorder of haemostasis was identified. The existence of a factor VI is now doubted.

In addition to the coagulation cascade, other platelet and lipid factors involved in coagulation have been identified and designated by Arabic numerals. Platelet factor 3 is the only one of importance: it is a phospholipoprotein and acts with plasma thromboplastin to convert prothrombin to thrombin.

- **Factor I**, fibrinogen, is a plasma protein produced by the liver. In health, 75% of fibrinogen is in the plasma, 25% in lymph. The conversion of fibrinogen to fibrin is brought about by the proteolytic enzyme, thrombin. The fibrin clot that forms is stabilised by factor XIII. After coagulation has occurred, the fluid that remains lacks fibrinogen. It is called **serum**. The concentration of fibrinogen in the blood increases after surgical operations, often doubling by the 10th postoperative day. After this time, the concentration falls rapidly to normal levels (Appendix Table), a sequence similar to that of the platelet count.

- **Factor II**, prothrombin, is an inactive glycoprotein found normally in the blood and manufactured by the liver. In coagulation, prothrombin is converted into an active form, thrombin, by activated thromboplastin in the presence of Ca^{2+}.
- **Factor III**, thromboplastin, is an ubiquitous lipoprotein present in cell membranes and 'exposed' after injury. The term 'thromboplastic activity' is often used to describe the properties of this molecule. The activity can be produced intrinsically, from the blood, or extrinsically, from the tissues.

The extrinsic system

Tissue thromboplastin, extrinsic prothrombin activator, is rapidly formed following local trauma in the presence of factors IV, V, VII and X (Fig. 17). The initiating event is the release of tissue factor, a protein present in fibroblasts and macrophages and liberated following tissue damage. After combining with phospholipids, it binds with factor VII. The complex initiates the proteolysis of factor X.

- **Factor IV**, ionic calcium (Ca^{2+}), helps to accelerate the conversion of fibrinogen to fibrin. Calcium ions are also essential for other reactions in coagulation. In practice, hypocalcaemia is never sufficiently severe to interfere with coagulation or thrombosis.
- **Factor V**, pro-accelerin, is a labile plasma protein destroyed by heat.
- **Factor VII**, pro-convertin, is a heat-stable factor present in serum.
- **Factor X**, Stuart–Prower factor, is a thermolabile protein present in serum.

The intrinsic system

Blood thromboplastin, intrinsic prothrombin activator, is formed by factors IV, V, VIII, IX, XI, XII and platelet factor 3 (Fig. 18).

Initially, there is activation of factor XII as a result of contact of blood with a foreign surface. The early stages of the sequence are slow. Once thrombin has been formed, the process is greatly accelerated.

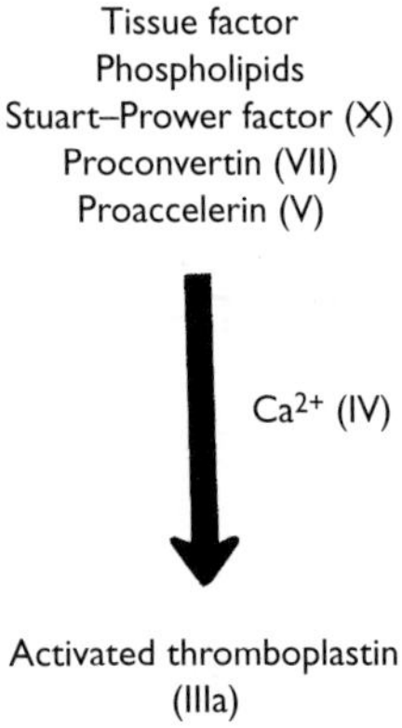

Figure 17 Blood coagulation: extrinsic system. Local tissue injury is responsible for the activation of a sequence of enzymes that finally catalyse tissue thromboplastin.

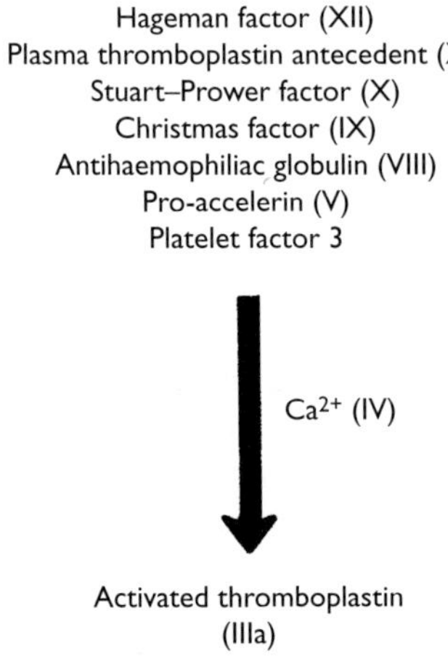

Figure 18 Blood coagulation: intrinsic system. Initiating event is activation of Hageman factor (factor XII) due to contact of blood with foreign surface. Contact initiates and amplifies cascade of molecular events that leads to activation of tissue thromboplastin.

- **Factor VIII**, is anti haemophiliac factor (p. 100). It is a large protein that regulates the activation of factor X by proteases generated in this pathway.
- **Factor IX** is a pro-enzyme, converted to an active protease by factor XIa or by the tissue factor-VIIa complex.
- **Factor XI** is a 160 kDa protein activated via the intrinsic pathway and converted to an active protease, XIa.
- **Factor XII** is Hageman factor. It is a protein that undergoes conversion to an active protease that catalyses the formation of kallikrein (p. 180) and the activation of factor XI (Fig. 18).
- **Factor XIII,** fibrin stabilising factor, is a transglutaminase that stabilises fibrin clots by forming cross-links between adjacent chains of fibrin.

Final common pathway

The last two stages of the coagulation cascade represent a final common pathway (Fig. 19)

The ultimate part of clot formation is the production of a network of fibrin resistant to digestion by plasmin. Peptide bonds form between fibrin polymers under the enzymic control of activated factor XIII (XIIIa).

Fibrinogen is modified by the release of fibrinopeptides A and B from the α- and β-chains of the parent protein. The modified molecule becomes a fibrin monomer. It polymerises as an insoluble polymeric gel. This polymer is stabilised by cross-linking of the individual chains, a process also brought about by factor XIIIa.

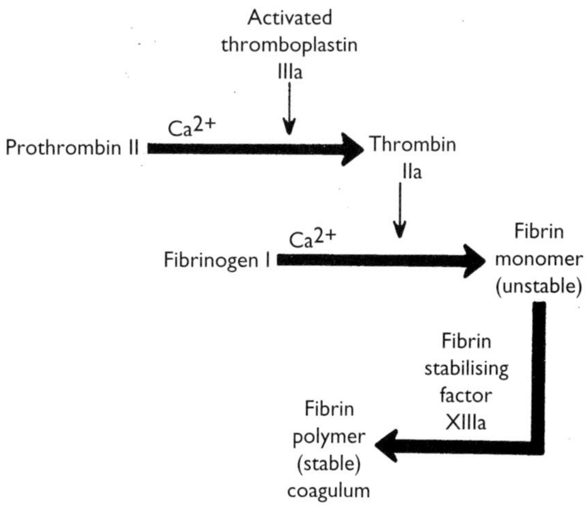

Figure 19 Blood coagulation: final common pathway. Activated thromboplastin from both intrinsic and extrinsic coagulation cascades initiates ultimate production of insoluble fibrin polymer to form coagulum (clot). Role of thromboplastin and of Ca^{+} in catalysing definitive conversion of thrombin to fibrinogen is indicated. This step precedes the polymerisation of fibrinogen to form insoluble fibrin.

CLOT LYSIS AND BLOOD VESSEL REPAIR

These important processes begin immediately after the formation of the haemostatic plug. The fibrinolytic system is activated by three agencies: Hageman factor (XII) fragments, urokinase and tissue plasminogen activator. Tissue plasminogen activator is the most important. It diffuses from the endothelial cells of nearby blood vessels, converting plasminogen, which is adsorbed from the fibrin clot, into the enzyme plasmin. Plasmin then degrades the fibrin clot into small fragments that are removed by the mononuclear macrophage system. Any plasmin entering the circulation is quickly inactivated. Patients who are deficient in plasmin inhibitor bleed because of unrestrained fibrinolysis.

Now read Fibrinolysis (p. 130)

REGULATION OF THE PLASMA COAGULATION SYSTEM

At a site of injury, the fluidity of the blood is influenced by the vigour of blood flow. Continued, rapid flow reduces the concentration of reactants in the coagulation pathways and the converse holds true. Regulation is also effected by the adsorption of coagulation factors to endothelial surfaces and by the presence of many inhibitors in the plasma. The most important inhibitors are anti-thrombin and the protein C/protein S system.

Anti-thrombin

This molecule forms complexes with all the serine protein coagulation factors except factor VII, neutralising thrombin in a process accelerated by heparin.

Protein C/protein S system

Protein C and protein S are synthesised in the liver under the control of vitamin K. Protein C inactivates plasma cofactors V and VIII and stimulates the release of tissue plasminogen. Protein S is a cofactor for protein C and enhances its activity.

Table 21 Assessing the coagulation system

Test	Significance
Bleeding time	The significance of the bleeding time is described on p. 42.
Capillary fragility (Hess's test)	A positive test is the occurrence of purpura below a tourniquet applied to the arm for 5 minutes at a pressure between diastolic and systolic blood pressure. There is a poor correlation with the platelet count and positive tests have been obtained in normal people. It is positive in scurvy (p. 353).
Platelet count	Thrombocytopenia exists when blood platelet counts fall below 100×10^9/L, thrombocythaemia when platelet counts rise above 500×10^9/L.
Platelet adhesion	Platelet counts are performed before and after exposure to foreign surfaces such as cellophane and glass.
Platelet aggregation	The amount of light transmitted through a suspension increases as the platelets aggregate.
Clot retraction	The clot from healthy blood begins to retract 30–60 minutes after a sample is taken. In the presence of thrombocytopenia, the clot is like a jelly and does not retract
Fibrinogen concentration	The plasma concentration of fibrinogen is normally 1.5–4 g/L.
Whole blood clotting time	In glass tubes, the clotting time is 5–15 minutes. In silicon-coated tubes it is 20–60 minutes. The normal clotting time demands an effective intrinsic system, adequate final common pathway and normal platelet function.
Thromboplastin generation test	This test assesses the individual factors involved in the intrinsic system. If plasma adsorbed onto aluminium hydroxide is incubated with serum, platelets and calcium, clotting occurs in 8–10 seconds. If clotting is delayed, the deficient factor can be ascertained by replacing either the patient's plasma, serum or platelets with normal plasma, serum or platelets, respectively.
Prothrombin time (PT)	The patient's plasma is incubated with calcium and a brain extract that provides extrinsic thromboplastic activity. The time taken for a clot to form is compared with a control plasma and expressed as a ratio. The test assesses the extrinsic system and the final common pathway.
Kaolin–cephalin clotting time (KCCT)	The patient's plasma is added to calcium and cephalin, a phospholipid, in a glass tube. The phospholipid makes the test independent of the platelet count. The glass provides a foreign surface for activation of factor XII. The time taken for a clot to form is compared with a normal control. The KCCT is a more sensitive method of assessing the intrinsic coagulation system, and the final common pathway, than the whole blood clotting time.

PROPAGATION OF THE CLOT

The plug of platelets and fibrin formed during haemostasis does not normally propagate beyond the site of injury because only a small amount of each coagulation enzyme is converted to its active form. Nevertheless, there are circumstances under which propagation may occur (p. 321).

COAGULOPATHIES

The term coagulopathy is given to a defect in the coagulation mechanism (p. 95). In most laboratories, it is possible to measure the concentration of the individual coagulation factors. If this facility is not available, it may be possible to deduce from simple tests which factor is deficient in the patient's plasma or serum. Some factors are sensitive or resistant to heat or freezing. Others can be adsorbed onto aluminium hydroxide.

ASSESSING THE COAGULATION SYSTEM

Tests used to assess the common pathway, the extrinsic system, the intrinsic system, or a combination of these mechanisms, are summarised in Table 21.

ASSESSMENT OF BLEEDING DISEASE BEFORE SURGERY

Bleeding diseases encountered in surgery can be assessed adequately by four tests:

- The platelet count.
- The prothrombin time (PT).
- The kaolin–cephalin clotting time (KCCT).
- The fibrinogen concentration (Table 22).

In an increasingly older surgical population, many of whom are being treated with drugs that affect coagulation or who have deranged hepatic function, abnormal coagulation is becoming more common. However, inherited abnormalities are very infrequent.

PLATELET ABNORMALITIES

Platelets may be altered in numbers or in behaviour. The normal concentration in the circulating blood is $150–350 \times 10^9$/L.

A deficiency of circulating platelets is **thrombocytopenia**. Insufficient mature platelets may be formed. They may mature abnormally or be destroyed in excess.

Alternatively, there may be increased platelet formation (**thrombocythaemia**) and/or abnormal platelet function (**thrombocytopathia**).

Platelets are destroyed in autoimmune diseases and their function is disturbed in a wide variety of conditions ranging from haemophilia and Christmas disease to other, even rarer, disorders.

Thrombocytopenia

Thrombocytopenia may be caused by a deficiency of bone-marrow megakaryocytes, by excessive destruction of platelets or by their haemorrhagic loss. Deficient production may be due to replacement of

Table 22 Alterations in haemostatic function in surgical patients (N = normal, ↑ = increased, ↓ = decreased)

Condition	Platelet count	Prothrombin time	KCTT	Fibrinogen concentration
Hepatic deficiency	N or ↓	↑	↑	↓
Warfarin therapy	N	↑	↑	N
Heparin therapy	N	N	↑	N
Fibrinolytic therapy	N	↑	↑	↓
DIC	N or ↓	↑	↑	↓
Haemophilia	N	N	↑	N
Christmas disease	N	N	↑	N
von Willebrand's disease	N or ↓	N	N or ↑	N

Table 23 Some causes of consumption coagulopathy

Amniotic fluid embolism	Septic abortion
Haemolytic transfusion reaction	Carcinoma, e.g. of lung, prostate
Gram-negative sepsis	Acute haemorrhagic pancreatitis
Heat stroke	Hepatic cirrhosis
Shock	

the bone marrow by metastases or leukaemia, or to the effect of a variety of chemicals and toxins, such as cytotoxic drugs, gold, poisons, uraemia and septicaemia. The maturation of megakaryocytes may be abnormal in patients with megaloblastic anaemia. There may be excessive destruction of circulating platelets in disseminated intravascular coagulation (DIC, p. 119), immune thrombocytopenic purpura and hypersplenism.

Thrombotic thrombocytopenic microangiopathy (TTMA) is characterised by the sudden development of petechiae and pallor. Paralysis, coma and death follow quickly. The syndrome is precipitated by the presence of large clusters (multimers) of von Willebrand (vWD) molecules in the plasma whence they become entangled in subendothelial connective tissue and accelerate platelet adhesion. In normal persons, vWD multimers are broken down by a metalloproteinase. When there is a deficiency of the activity of this enzyme, the dangerous TTMA syndrome results. It is provoked by the formation of anti-proteinase IgG antibodies, for reasons not yet known.

Thrombocythaemia

Thrombocythaemia is an increase in the number of circulating platelets. It is synonymous with thrombocytosis. Thrombocythaemia is a normal response to surgery: the platelet count reaches a zenith at ~10 days post-operatively.

Haemorrhagic thrombocythaemia occurs in **polycythaemia rubra vera**. Although the platelet concentration is grossly elevated, there may be defective platelet function, disturbing clot formation. Similar abnormalities occur in other myeloproliferative disorders, such as chronic myeloid leukaemia.

Thrombocytopathia

Platelet adhesiveness increases postoperatively. Platelet function may be affected by anti-inflammatory drugs such as salicylate, by vitamin K antagonists and by cytotoxic drugs. Platelet function is also defective in von Willebrand's disease (above).

Immune thrombocytopenic purpura is an auto-immune disease in which antiplatelet antibodies can be demonstrated in 50% of patients. There is excessive destruction of platelets in the spleen. The adult form is chronic. In infants the disease may be acute but does not recur after treatment by steroids and/or splenectomy.

CLOTTING ABNORMALITIES

Now read Coagulation (p. 95)

Haemophilia

There is an inherited deficiency of factor VIII (p. 97). The abnormal recessive gene is carried on the X chromosome. It is a disease of $100/10^6$ males and is transmitted through female carriers. The disease is said to be severe, moderate or mild when the plasma concentration of factor VIII or of factor IX is <1%, 1–5% or 5–20%, respectively.

Haemophilia can now be controlled effectively and safely by transfusions of antihaemophiliac globulin. Moreover, factors VIII and IX can be manufactured by recombinant genetic techniques, the products of which enable the risks of viral transmission to be avoided. Within the foreseeable future, gene therapy may eliminate the use of these older methods.

Although bleeding was often sufficiently severe to induce haemorrhagic shock, the principal causes of mortality and morbidity were cerebral haemorrhage and haemarthrosis, respectively. Before the routine testing of plasma extracts, many recipients contracted AIDS from blood given by infected donors. Many others became infected with the hepatitis C virus. Now, both virus infections are avoided by the testing of donor blood or of plasma extracts although the price of previous neglect means that chronic hepatitis C (p. 155) is still the most frequent, ultimate cause of death.

Christmas disease

This rare disorder was named after the first patient, a Canadian boy, in whom it was identified. There is an inherited deficiency of factor IX, transmitted in the same manner as haemophilia. It is often designated haemophilia B and affects 1: 60 000 ($17/10^6$) males.

von Willebrand's disease (vWD)

In vWD, there is a deficiency of a factor essential for the formation of factor VIII. The defect is transmitted as an autosomal dominant trait with partial penetration. Thus, the disease occurs in its fully expressed form in homozygotes. Unlike haemophilia, heterozygotes are affected to a lesser extent. Platelet function is also defective in both heterozygotes and homozygotes and there is a prolonged bleeding time. This associated defect may also explain why, in patients with von Willebrand's disease, there is bleeding into the skin and mucous membranes rather than into the joints.

Other clotting abnormalities

Other very rare deficiencies of factors II,V,VII, X, XI and XIII have been described. They cause haemophilia-like diseases.

ANTICOAGULANT THERAPY AND PROPHYLAXIS

When thrombosis is evident or anticipated, anticoagulant therapy may be required.

Now read Thrombosis (p. 320)

Heparin

Heparin is a naturally occurring glycosaminoglycan monomer. Parenteral heparin inhibits coagulation at several stages in the coagulation sequence. It appears to be particularly effective in preventing the activation of factors II, IX, X and XI, and probably that of factor VII. For acute anticoagulant therapy, heparin may be given intravenously. Subcutaneous heparin in low doses is now used routinely during the peri-operative period in order to lessen the risk of post-operative deep venous thrombosis (p. 320). Therapy is monitored by measuring the kaolin–cephalin clotting time, or the prothrombin time.

Vitamin K antagonists

Coumarin anticoagulants are employed for chronic oral anticoagulant therapy. Warfarin is the most frequently used agent. Vitamin K (p.352) is required for the hepatic synthesis of factors II,VII, IX and X. Warfarin induces a state analogous to vitamin K deficiency, delaying thrombin generation, and preventing the formation of thrombi. It impairs the biological activity of the prothrombin complex proteins. Its effect is monitored by measurements of the prothrombin time.

COLD

See Hypothermia (p. 162).

COLLOIDS AND CRYSTALLOIDS

Colloids

In physical chemistry, a colloidal solution, a sol, is one in which there are dispersed particles between 1 and 100 nm in diameter. The colloid (Gk: glue) is the disperse or discontinuous phase; and the medium in which the particles are dispersed is the dispersion medium or continuous phase. Because of their mass and large surface areas, the particles display properties like Brownian movement. They scatter light and can be measured by nephelometry. The particles can be brought out of the disperse phase by techniques such as high-speed centrifugation.

In an old, obsolete sense, the word colloid may be used to describe thyroid acinar colloid, colloid goitre and colloid carcinoma.

Crystalloids

A crystalloid is a soluble substance or solute, the particles of which, in solution, are less than 1 nm in diameter. In an older sense, the term defined a crystal-like material, distinct from the less readily soluble, glue-like colloids.

COLON AND RECTUM

Diseases of the large intestine are considered together.

Biopsy diagnosis of large intestinal disease

Biopsies may be obtained at proctoscopy, sigmoidoscopy or colonoscopy. In patients with inflammatory conditions, it is helpful to the pathologist if specimens are taken from apparently uninvolved tissue for comparison with samples from diseased parts. Similarly, in patients with recognisable tumours, biopsies from apparently healthy tissue may show dysplasia. Sometimes, a biopsy may be excisional and curative, for example when polyps are removed with a diathermy snare.

DEVELOPMENTAL AND CONGENITAL DISORDERS

Now read Anal canal (p. 11), Megacolon (p. 105)

DIVERTICULAR DISEASE

Diverticular disease of the colon is the presence of multiple diverticula in the wall of the affected portion of the large intestine (Fig. 20).

Causes

There is no demonstrable heritable factor. There are both geographical and chronological variations in prevalence. Diverticular disease is much more common in Western countries than in the Third World but there is a low frequency in vegetarians. In the UK, the prevalence has increased and diverticular disease can now be identified in more than 50% of individuals over 70 years of age, in 80% of those over 80. However, 20% are aged less than 50 years. Studies involving generations of immigrants indicate an environmental cause, the frequency of which appears to be inversely proportional to the intake of dietary fibre.

It is postulated that in patients who develop this condition, raised intra-colonic pressure is required to propel faecal streams that are low in residue. Repetitive, increased muscular contractions produce hypertrophy of the circular muscle and pulsion diverticula are pushed out at the sites where blood vessels pass through the bowel wall between the taenia. The rectum is not involved because it has two complete muscle layers, an inner circular and outer longitudinal.

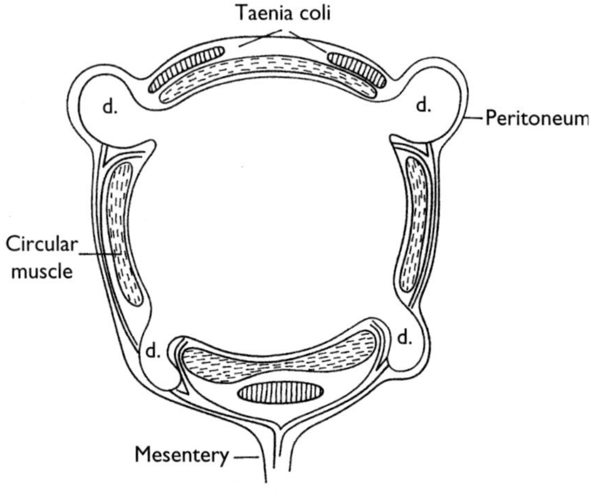

Figure 20 Diverticular disease of colon.
Diverticula develop in four rows, at sites (d) in circular, smooth muscle where blood vessels enter and leave. These are foci of relative structural weakness.

Structure

The longitudinal rows of diverticular sacs consist only of mucosa (Fig. 20). They are particularly common in the sigmoid colon and frequently contain faecoliths.

Behaviour and prognosis

Acute inflammation may develop within a diverticulum. The inflamed sac may perforate, with the formation of a localised abscess, or the development of diffuse peritonitis. The inflammatory process can be categorised as:

- Stage I: small, confined abscesses.
- Stage II: larger abscesses.
- Stage III: generalised suppurative peritonitis.
- Stage IV: faecal peritonitis.

If an abscess is not drained, it may perforate into other structures, such as the bladder, to produce a fistula (p. 132). If the inflammation resolves, there is likely to be residual fibrosis. Recurrent attacks of diverticulitis may produce stenosis of the colon, leading to intestinal obstruction. Another complication is haemorrhage attributable to erosion of one of the blood vessels at sites where diverticula form. The haemorrhage is sudden and is life-threatening in the elderly.

INFECTION

The large bowel may be infected by *Campylobacter jejuni*, Shigella spp., Salmonella spp. or *Clostridium difficile*. These acute, specific forms of colitis can be distinguished by rectal biopsy from chronic inflammation due to amoebic colitis, tuberculosis and inflammatory bowel disease (p. 165). Infection with *Chlamydia trachomatis* may follow anal intercourse. Toxic megacolon is a possible consequence of infection by any of these agents.

Pseudomembranous enterocolitis

Pseudomembranous enterocolitis (PMC), a potentially fatal disorder, is due to infection with *Clostridium difficile*. The macroscopic features of similar forms of colitis were described in the pre-antibiotic era.

The organism exerts its effects by means of two toxins, A (enterotoxin) and B (cytotoxin). PMC may follow treatment with any one of a range of broad-spectrum, beta-lactam antibiotics, particularly the cephalosporins, amoxicillin and co-amoxiclavilulanate. It was described originally after the use of lincosamides such as lincomycin and clindamycin. The sigmoidoscopic appearances are unmistakable, with scattered, yellow-white, membranous plaques of mucin, fibrin, leucocytes and epithelial debris lying upon the mucosa.

The stools of more than 90% of affected patients contain both *Cl. difficile* and its toxins. In diagnosis, it is convenient to test the stools for toxin rather than to attempt the difficult culture of the organism. Untreated, the acute disorder progresses to mucosal necrosis, perforation, peritonitis and death. However, *Cl. difficile* is sensitive to metronidazole and vancomycin and these antibiotics provide effective treatment.

Tuberculosis

Intestinal tuberculosis is increasingly rare in Western countries. The terminal ileum and, less often, the caecum, are the most frequent sites. Infection is primary, from ingested bovine bacilli, or secondary, from swallowed, infected sputum. In the West, pasteurisation of milk has eliminated the former source.

At first, transverse ulcers appear in the bowel. Later, there is fibrosis, with the development of strictures. Adhesions may lead to the drawing up of the caecum beneath the liver. Caseating granulomas are evident. Fibrosis accentuates the difficulty in distinguishing the infection from Crohn's disease.

Now read Tuberculosis (p. 332)

Amoebic dysentery

Amoebic dysentery is a consequence of infection with the protozoan *Entamoeba histolytica* (p. 282). Sigmoidoscopy reveals diffuse, small, yellow ulcers within a uniformly oedematous and inflamed mucosa. The ulcers, of characteristic flask shape, lie transversely across the colon and have overhanging edges (Fig. 53). The amoebae are usually evident upon biopsy. Perforation is uncommon. Occasionally, the infection may remain as a localised mass of granulation and fibrous tissue, an **amoeboma**, producing a stricture that can cause obstruction and which must be distinguished from carcinoma.

Now read Amoebiasis (p. 8)

INFLAMMATION

The term **inflammatory bowel disease** is used by common consent to distinguish Crohn's disease and ulcerative colitis from the many other specific forms of colitis and diverticular disease all of which are associated with degrees of inflammation.

Ulcerative colitis

Ulcerative colitis gives rise to debilitating, bloody diarrhoea with protein-losing enteropathy. In severe cases, there may be as many as 20 motions per day containing up to 20 g N, a loss equivalent to 600 g of hydrated muscle protein. Severe anaemia and malnutrition result. It is a disease of relapses and remissions.

Causes

In Western societies, ulcerative colitis is more frequent in early adult life than in the elderly. The aetiology is unknown. Like Crohn's disease, there is a genetic influence and relatives of affected patients have an increased risk of developing either form of inflammatory bowel disease. There have been many attempts to identify an infectious agent but none has been successful. Numerous alterations in cell-mediated and humoral immunity have been documented, changes thought to be secondary phenomena. The onset and relapses are frequent during times of psychological stress.

Structure

Inflammation with ulceration begins in the rectum and spreads proximally. In patients with total colitis, the severity of the inflammation is greater distally than proximally but occasionally the rectum is spared. In ~10% of patients there is inflammation in the distal 30–40 mm of the ileum but this 'backwash' ileitis is the result of an incompetent ileocaecal valve. The mucosa between ulcers is granular so that contact bleeding occurs during endoscopy.

Unlike Crohn's disease, granulation tissue and giant cells are not seen. Small 'crypt' abscesses are present due to blockage of the crypts of Lieberkühn. Polymorphs abound in the mucosa, lymphocytes, plasma cells and eosinophils in the submucosa. In severe, acute cases and in long-standing disease, the mucosa and submucosa may both be destroyed. Exudative inflammation extends into the submucosa only in severe cases. Crypt abscesses coalesce, producing longitudinal ulcers, between which the surviving mucous membrane is thrown up into inflammatory pseudopolyps. Fibrosis with shortening of the large bowel occurs only in chronic cases. Biopsy of an apparently normal mucosa inevitably reveals microscopic disease.

Behaviour and prognosis

In the young, protracted malnutrition leads to stunted growth and delayed puberty. In fulminating colitis, toxic dilatation of the colon and subsequent perforation are likely. Although late fibrosis is uncommon in chronic cases, strictures may be produced in the few patients in whom there is remission after long-standing disease.

Patients who have had total, symptomatic colitis for more than 10 years have a greatly increased risk of developing carcinoma of the colon. To anticipate this complication, colonoscopic surveillance has been recommended but its use is controversial. Compared with otherwise normal individuals who develop adenocarcinoma of the colon, patients with ulcerative colitis tend to develop tumours at a younger age; moreover, the cancers are more uniformly and widely distributed and less well-differentiated. They carry a poor prognosis.

Systemic disorders complicating ulcerative colitis include sclerosing cholangitis and hepatocellular fatty change. In a few patients, this liver disease progresses to biliary cirrhosis. Iridocyclitis, arthritis and a variety of dermatitides are recognised and amyloidosis (p. 9) may develop. A rare complication is a form of bronchiectasis in which mucosal inflammation typical of that found in the colon, is recognised in the bronchi or bronchioles.

Crohn's disease

The principal features of Crohn's disease (regional enteritis) are described on p. 165.

Crohn's disease is confined to the large bowel in 15% of instances. Like ulcerative colitis, but to a lesser degree, it results in protein-losing enteropathy. By contrast with ulcerative colitis, there is regional involvement of the colon. The mucosa between involved areas is often normal. Early in the disease, a few, small, punched-out aphthoid ulcers appear. They coalesce as the disease becomes more severe. The intervening, swollen mucosa remains in folds giving a 'cobblestone' appearance. Fibrosis is a major consequence of the inflammation and the bowel becomes shortened and strictured.

Inflammation extends throughout the layers of the bowel and the submucosa is particularly involved. Granulomas containing multinucleated giant cells are evident around fissures that penetrate deep into the submucosa. However, the depletion of goblet cells is not extensive. Toxic dilatation of the colon and, in severe cases, perforation, may occur but these complications are less frequent than in ulcerative colitis. Peri-anal abscesses, fissures and fistulas are much more common than in the latter condition. There is an increased risk of the development of adenocarcinoma but the hazard is less than in ulcerative colitis.

Pouchitis

This is an inflammatory condition of unknown aetiology arising in pouches of small intestine that have been created for continent ileostomies or for restorative proctocolectomy. Inflammation of previously healthy ileal tissue develops within a few weeks. The response is manifest in ~10% of those patients who have undergone restorative proctocolectomy for ulcerative colitis but it is a rare phenomenon after similar operations performed for familial adenomatous polyposis. Villous atrophy precedes the inflammatory reaction. There are increased numbers of anaerobic Bacteroides spp. in the pouch and some patients respond to treatment with metronidazole.

Proctitis

Inflammation of the rectum (p. 284) develops as a consequence of any inflammatory condition affecting the colon. The rectum tends to be more severely involved than the remainder of the large intestine. Occasionally, as in ulcerative colitis, it is the only part affected.

MECHANICAL DISORDERS

Megacolon

Megacolon is pathological dilatation of the colon. The disorder may be congenital or acquired. It is encountered in toxic megacolon, Hirschprung's disease (p. 372) and Chagas' disease (p. 370).

Toxic megacolon occurs in about 3% of patients with ulcerative colitis. The transverse colon is particularly involved. The condition is recognised less often in Crohn's disease and in infective colitides. If the diseased segment is not resected, there is a high risk of perforation and peritonitis.

Hirschsprung's disease

Hirschprung's disease (p. 372) is a congenital disorder arising in $50/10^6$ neonates. It is more common in males and there is a genetic predisposition. The grossly dilated colon terminates in a narrowed rectum, immediately above the anus. In this narrowed segment, there is an absence of the parasympathetic cells of Auerbach's and of Meissner's plexuses. Stimuli from the sympathetic system provoke contraction of the internal anal sphincter and inhibit propulsive contraction. Patients may not defecate for weeks and suffer repeated attacks of intestinal obstruction. Diagnosis requires full thickness rectal biopsy under general anaesthesia.

Abdominal compartment syndrome

Surgical attempts to replace the intestinal contents within the abdominal cavity may result in respiratory failure. The syndrome is due to displacement of the thoracic contents as a result of pressure on the diaphragm. There is impaired venous return to the heart and intestinal obstruction.

TUMOURS

Benign

Adenoma

Adenomas may be sessile and villous but most are polypoid, tubular structures (Fig. 49.1). They are often described as adenomatous polyps. As the name suggests, **tubular adenomas** comprise cylinders of epithelium separated by lamina propria. Although this appearance may mimic that of normal, colonic mucosa, the tubules are irregular in shape and size. The cells display hyperchromasia, pleomorphism and an increased proportion of mitotic figures. In ~20% there is a mixture of elements: they are tubulovillous adenomas. When the adenoma is polypoid, there is a stalk containing connective tissue separated from the proliferating epithelium by intact muscularis mucosae. If the component cells display the characteristics of malignant transformation, it is essential to ascertain whether the stalk has been invaded. A **villous adenoma** consists of finger-like projections of lamina propria covered with dysplastic epithelium (Fig. 49.2).

Familial adenomatous polyposis

Causes

Familial adenomatous polyposis (FAP) is an inherited autosomal dominant disease attributable to a deletion in the long arm of chromosome 5, at 5q21. The disease displays complete penetrance so that, untreated, colon cancer almost invariably results. The deleted *APC* gene has a tumour suppressor function. It encodes a large (APC) protein with a critical role in reducing the levels of E-cadherin, a protein that has important functions in cell adhesion and development (p. 88). β-Catenin regulates the expression of E-cadherin in mediating cell adhesion. The inherited *APC* gene mutation leads to a substantial increase in levels of free β-catenin some of which moves into the nucleus where it forms a protein complex. This complex binds DNA and induces the expression of genes that promote cell growth and proliferation. There is a link with nuclear hormone receptors.

Now read Carcinogenesis (p. 76)

Structure

In FAP, polyps are likely to be encountered throughout the gastro-intestinal tract. The affected sites include the stomach, small intestine, large intestine, gall bladder and pancreas. The most frequent and, in prognostic terms, the most serious site, is the large intestine. Affected adolescents have more than 100 and sometimes several thousand, minute polyps detectable by endoscopy. The adenomas are tubular. Most patients also have congenital hypertrophy of the retinal pigment epithelium (CHRPE) and this sign, together with DNA probes, is used to screen the relatives of those who have been found to have FAP.

Behaviour and prognosis

If the large bowel is not removed, one or more polyps undergoes malignant change in 10% of patients within 5 years, in 20% within 20 years. Panproctocolectomy with a permanent ileostomy eliminates the risk of large bowel cancer. Subtotal colectomy with ileorectal anastomosis allows diathermy or laser ablation of rectal polyps to be performed at required intervals. Subtotal colectomy with the creation of an ileal pouch and ileo-anal anastomosis almost entirely eradicates the polyp-bearing mucosa. In patients who undergo prophylactic colectomy, there is an increased risk of death from duodenal cancer or, less frequently, from gastric cancer. Bi-annual endoscopic surveillance of the stomach and duodenum is recommended. There is recent evidence to suggest that aspirin-like drugs reduce the frequency of colon cell apoptosis (p. 89) and decrease the rate of adenoma formation in individuals who have inherited the *FAP* gene. These drugs also suppress the development of colon cancer by preventing gene activation.

Gardner's syndrome

Gardner's syndrome is a variant of familial adenomatous polyposis (FAP) of the colon. The syndrome is accompanied by extracolonic manifestations. Polyposis coli is associated with skull and jaw osteomas and benign, soft tissue neoplasms that include desmoid tumours, cutaneous fibromas and tumours of sebaceous glands. There may also be desmoid tumours of the abdominal wall and mesentery, and epidermoid cysts.

The genetic abnormality comprises *APC* mutations in the germ line. The changes are very similar to those of *FAP*. They differ by only a few bases. The disease is transmitted as an autosomal dominant trait with a high degree of penetrance. There is a greatly increased risk of the development of carcinoma of the colon. Patients with Gardner's syndrome are likely to develop polypoidal tumours of the stomach, duodenum, biliary tract and small intestine. The papilla of Vater is particularly susceptible.

Juvenile polyps

The frequency of **single juvenile polyp** is greatest at 5 years of age but the lesion is still occasionally detected in adolescence. These hamartomas occur in the rectosigmoid and are a cause of insidious bleeding. Dilated glands lie within an extensive lamina propria but the epithelium is not dysplastic and the polyps do not have malignant potential. That they are solitary allows ready differentiation from the multiple polyps of the Peutz–Jegher syndrome (p. 256).

Dysplastic juvenile polyps form in the rare condition of **juvenile polyposis**, a condition associated with an increased risk of malignancy.

Malignant

Carcinoma

Each year, ~19 000 patients die from carcinoma of the large bowel in the UK. The incidence is $360/10^6$ population. Colon cancer is the second most frequent cause of death from malignant disease. There has been no improvement in survival during the last 50 years.

Causes

Familial adenomatous polyposis (FAP) cancer
This heritable form is discussed (above).

Heritable non-FAP cancer
Two per cent of Western populations but only 0.4% of the UK population, other than those with FAP, inherit a propensity to develop carcinoma of the colon (Tables 18, 24). The condition is hereditary non-polyposis colorectal cancer (HNPCC). The prevalence of HNPCC in the UK is 106×10^3 of those aged 30 to 70 years. In the general population,

the lifetime risk of colorectal cancer is 1 in 27. In HNPCC inheritance, if one first-degree relative is affected, the risk increases to 1 in 17 and if three such relatives are affected, the risk is as high as 1 in 3 individuals. Patients with HNPCC are also at increased risk of developing cancers of the ovary, endometrium, breast, stomach, small intestine and upper urinary tract. Much effort is being directed to the identification of individuals at risk. The present criteria for the referral of patients for genetic screening in the Greater Manchester area of the UK is shown in Table 24.

Screening by colonoscopy or virtual colonoscopy (computed tomographic colonography) of families in whom tumours occur before the age of 40 years, who have a predominance of proximal tumours or multiple growths, is beneficial but should only be offered to those with a mutant gene.

Non-heritable colon cancer

Many of the numerous, non-heritable forms of colon cancer display genetic mutations analogous to those of FAP. At least 20–40% of sporadic colon cancers are homozygous or hemizygous for chromosome 5 markers. The presence of the APC gene, dominant in FAP, is a mutant, recessive defect.

The geographical distribution indicates that colorectal cancer is at least partly attributable to environmental factors. Colorectal carcinoma is uncommon in African countries. Although the cancer was believed to be related to the intake of dietary fibre or animal-fat, recent studies of large numbers of Western female nurses have failed to confirm this influence. There is evidence to suggest that the majority of carcinomas of the colon arise from pre-existing adenomas. These benign tumours are more common in specimens resected for cancer than in those without cancer. Patients who have synchronous carcinomas or who develop metachronous carcinomas are more likely to have adenomas than patients with carcinoma alone. In patients with early carcinoma, residual adenomatous tissue can often be seen. Finally, the variation in the geographical incidence of carcinoma is similar to the geographical variation for adenoma.

There is also an increased incidence in those who have previously undergone surgery for peptic ulcer or who have been subjected to cholecystectomy. One explanation for the enhanced risk is a change in the content of bile acids distributed to the right side of the colon.

Table 24 Colorectal cancer – patients requiring genetic investigation

One first degree relative aged < 35 years
Two first degree relatives, same side of the family, aged < 60 years
Three first degree relatives, same side of family, any age
One colonic and one endometrial carcinoma, same side of family, one first degree relative and one second degree relative
One colonic and one endometrial carcinoma, same side of family, one aged < 50 years
FAP or Gardner's syndrome
HNPCC
Peutz–Jeghers' syndrome
Juvenile polyposis

Structure

Tumours of the large bowel are polypoidal, ulcerating or stenosing. The rectum is the most frequent site, followed by the sigmoid colon and the caecum. Up to 5% of patients have a synchronous tumour at presentation and as many as 10% may develop a metachronous tumour after presentation. It is often claimed that tumours in the caecum and ascending colon are polypoidal and bleed silently. Malignant tumours of the sigmoid colon, by contrast, are stenosing and provoke intestinal obstruction, while those of the rectum ulcerate and cause overt bleeding. Nevertheless, these individual forms may occur in any part of the large intestine.

The majority of carcinomas of the colon are glandular (adenocarcinoma) with varying degrees of differentiation. Some manufacture a relatively abundant connective tissue stroma. Mucin formation may be substantial so that the old description 'colloid carcinoma' can still be applied. Squamous carcinomas are rare.

Behaviour and prognosis

Carcinomas spread circumferentially rather than longitudinally. Peritoneal dissemination is uncommon but when it occurs the ovaries are often involved as they are, for example, in Krukenberg tumours (p. 260). Lymphatic spread is early and contiguous. Blood spread via the portal vein to the liver is late.

The prognosis is related to stage but is less

influenced by histological grade. The TNM staging system (p. 244) may be adopted but, in the UK, colonic tumours have usually been staged by Duke's system. The depth of invasion of the intestinal wall and the presence or absence of lymph node involvement are powerful predicators of whether a cancer will recur. The 5-year survival is shown in Fig. 44a (p. 245). One drawback of the original Duke system was that all tumours with lymphatic metastases were graded C, regardless of the extent of nodal involvement. Duke ultimately suggested dividing group C into C1 (locally involved nodes only) and C2 (involvement of mesenteric nodes). Other modified classifications have been proposed (Fig. 44b, p. 245). Their use has not added greatly to the possibility of predicting prognosis with accuracy. Resection of colorectal tumours should include 'en-bloc' excision of C1 and C2 nodes. The prognosis of rectal tumours is particularly influenced by the surgical technique. This requires total mesorectal excision with circumferential excision of a well-defined plane between the rectum and the pelvic viscera and side-walls.

Now read Tumour staging (p. 244)

Colonic carcinomas secrete carcino-embryonic antigen (CEA – p. 247). CEA is also secreted by other malignant tumours, in inflammatory bowel disease and in other non-neoplastic conditions such as bronchiectasis. Detection of CEA cannot be used as a diagnostic test but its assay can be employed in clinical management to detect recurrence and to assess response to chemotherapy.

VASCULAR DISEASE

Angiodysplasia

Angiodysplasia describes the occurrence of clusters of dilated, fragile venules in the mucosa and submucosa of the large intestine. The most frequent site is the ascending colon. The lesions are a cause of gastro-intestinal haemorrhage in the elderly. The haemorrhage may be acute and life-threatening or insidious and a cause of unexplained anaemia. It is thought to be due to obstruction of veins as they pass through the muscle wall.

Angiodysplasia may be difficult to visualise by endoscopy but can be demonstrated by selective angiography. After right hemicolectomy, the vascular lesions may only be identifiable in the laboratory if the vessels of the fresh, resected specimen are first injected with a coloured or radio-opaque medium.

Ischaemic colitis

Any form of sustained hypotension or impaired, local tissue perfusion may lead to ischaemic colitis. The causes include embolism, thrombosis *in-situ* or haemorrhage into an atheromatous plaque. Chronic ischaemia is attributable to proximal diseases such as obstruction of the lumen of a large artery by an atheromatous plaque sited near the origin. It may also be due to peripheral disease such as radiation-induced arteritis (p. 187).

Although the entire colon may be involved, there is a particular predilection for the splenic flexure where the peripheral arterial arcade depends upon an effective anastomosis between the superior and inferior mesenteric arteries. In severe cases, colonic necrosis and perforation may occur. In less severe cases, the mucosa undergoes infarction and there is haemorrhage into the lumen. Patchy submucosal oedema leads to the diagnostic 'thumb prints' sometimes seen in radiographs. If the bowel remains viable, complete recovery is possible, with no macroscopic or microscopic evidence of the episode. In most patients, however, ischaemic stricture is the end result.

COMPUTERS

A computer is an automatic, electronic machine for performing mathematical operations. In surgical practice, analogue information is usually converted into numbers, that is, it is digitised. The numerical information obtained in this way can then be manipulated electronically. To make this possible, two components are necessary: the hardware, the electronic device itself; and the software, the instructions or programme necessary to undertake the required functions. Computers are employed in three principal ways:

On-line computers control complex instruments and robots, and translate histopathological, chemical, haematological and immunological laboratory assays and measurements into displays of words and figures to aid diagnosis and treatment.

Off-line computer networks employing large

'server' computers lie at the heart of increasing numbers of hospital functions. In radiology and imaging, for example, the vast quantities of information derived from CT, MRI and isotopic scanning, can only be displayed and analysed by computer.

Personal computers (PCs) exploit word processing for education, graphics, photography and finance, letters, figures and pictures and for teaching. They also enable databases to be constructed that include patients' records and literature sources, and they facilitate the design of displays and images. They allow statistical programs to be used for the analysis of clinical trials, and they enable communication by e-mail. Finally, they make possible the 'surfing' of the World Wide Web and the use of the Internet.

Laptop and notebook computers are easily portable but costly. They are readily used with mobile telephones so that instant communication and the use of stored records are practicable at any distance from a hospital or office. Desktop computers are not portable; however, they are cheaper and can store and handle larger quantities of information rapidly.

Now read Telepathology (p. 234)

Searching the Internet

There is no single, 'correct' way to find what is wanted. These guidelines minimise the waste of time.

Search tools fall into two basic categories: **Web Indexes** which are held on large computers and are called Search Engines; and **Web Directories** which are lists of Titles of WebPages or Websites with an attached hyperlink to the appropriate universal resource locator (URL) (Table 25).

One example of a Web Directory is the Internet Gateway on the Royal College of Surgeons of Edinburgh Website at: http://www.rcsed.ac.uk/fmi/gateway.asp. Directories are also obtainable from the Royal College of Surgeons of England (www.rcseng.ac.uk), the Royal College of Physicians and Surgeons of Glasgow (www.rcpsglasg.ac.uk) and the Royal College of Surgeons in Ireland (www.rcsi.ie).

Web directories are valuable for browsing general topics. For specific information, use a Web Index (Search Engine). A good teaching programme on "Searching the World Wide Web (WWW)" can be found at http://inset.ul.ie/insetresources/Search%20 engines/index.htm.

When searching, focus specifically on the topic you want. Include as many descriptive words as possible in the search keywords. For instance, looking for infor-

Table 25 The active search engines commonly used in 2001

Search Engine or Web Directory (*)	Universal Resource Locator (URL)	Comments
Yahoo	http://uk.search.yahoo.com/	Widely used
Go	http://www.go.com/	Widely used
Lycos	http://www.lycos.co.uk/	Widely used
Mirago	http://www.mirago.co.uk/	Widely used
Excite	http://www.excite.co.uk/	Widely used
Virgin Net	http://www.virgin.net/search/	Good and UK orientated
Search Hawk	http://www.searchhawk.com/	
Alta Vista	http://www.altavista.com/	Comprehensive. US orientated
Ask Jeeves	http://www.ask.co.uk/	Very fast and comprehensive
All the Web, All the Time	http://www.ussc.alltheweb.com/	Very, very fast
Organising Medical Networked Information OMNI*	http://www.omni.ac.uk/	Medically orientated, very useful UK search engine
RCSEd Surgical Internet Gateway*	http://www.rcsed.ac.uk/fmi/gateway.asp	

mation on the 'cellular response' + injury yields the unwieldy result of 28 929 URLs.

A search is focused by using Plus (+) and Minus (–) or NOT preceding the key word or phrase. Therefore, narrowing the search to 'cellular response' + humans + injury + skin focuses the search to 779 documents. Unwanted items can then be excluded, for example, by entering 'cellular response' + humans + injury + skin NOT bone. This strategy yields the more manageable result of 352 documents.

Search terms, or keywords entered in lower case letters, are normally case-insensitive. The use of capitalized terms, or accented letters, may make a term case-sensitive. For example: 'Fat Embolus Syndrome' may not find a page displaying fat embolus syndrome. But 'fat embolus syndrome' will display Fat Embolus Syndrome. When looking for a specific condition with linked words, include the linked words in parenthesis. Advanced searching can be carried out by using the following full Boolean terms: OR, AND, NOT, NEAR. In some search engines you may also use the following symbols in place of the words: & (AND), | (OR), ~ (NEAR), ! (NOT).

CONGENITAL DISEASE

A disease or abnormality is said to be congenital when it is present at birth. Congenital diseases may be inherited or acquired. Many congenital defects such as syndactyly, oesophagotracheal fistula, cardiac malformation and spina bifida are apparent at or shortly after birth. Others, such as branchial cyst, bicuspid aortic valve or accessory rib, may not be identified until much later, perhaps in adult life.

The causes of inherited congenital disease are considered on p. 182. The causes of acquired congenital disease can be classified in two ways:

- As agents acting on the **gamete**. Among these agents are ionising radiation, viruses and chemical agents. All provoke genetic mutation.
- As agents acting on the **zygote, embryo or fetus**. One example is thalidomide, a tranquiliser taken by pregnant women that led to defective limb development. A further example is the rubella virus, acquired by the mother during the first trimester and acting directly on viscera such as the heart and eye to impair development. The administration of hydrocortisone or oestrogens acts similarly. Cigarette smoking is associated with an increased probability of the risk of the stillbirth of a malformed fetus. The smoke is believed to contain chemicals with a thalidomide-like action.

CONNECTIVE TISSUE

The connective tissues provide integral structural and mechanical support for the muscular and skeletal tissues and viscera. They form the microskeleton of all organs and tissues. Connective tissues are an essential part of granulation tissue, of scar tissue, and of many other abnormal tissues, including the stroma of tumours. The normal formation of connective tissue depends upon the availability of substances such as ascorbic acid, essential for the maturation and stability of collagen; and pyridoxine and copper, necessary for the synthesis and maturation of elastic tissue.

Assembled as composite materials, the connective tissues comprise cells and an extracellular matrix (ECM). When the organisation is dense, with a relatively low water content, a connective tissue is said to be **compact**. When the organisation is more open, it is **loose**.

Connective tissue cells are exemplified by fibroblasts. Chondrocytes, osteocytes and glial cells are among the many specialised forms. The relative quantity of the ECM varies from very large, as in articular cartilage, to small, as in synovia. The water content of the ECM varies widely from 70 to 80%. There are two principal solid components in addition to water: the structural, fibrous proteins – collagen and elastin – and the carbohydrate-rich, protein-containing macromolecules – the proteoglycans. However, an enormous spectrum of smaller molecules and ions penetrates the connective tissues. They are vulnerable to all the main categories of disease.

COLLAGENS AND ELASTIN

The main structural protein of the body is collagen. It comprises 15% of the wet weight but 50% of the dry weight of tissue such as hyaline articular cartilage. At least 18 genetically distinct types of collagen are known. Each has a different primary amino-acid composition. Type I and type X collagen are bone constituents. Type II is the main collagen of cartilage, type III of vascular and developing tissue, types IV and

VII of basement membranes. In tendons, ligaments, fascia and aponeuroses, collagens, organised in fibrils, resist tensile stress. In hyaline cartilage, labra and menisci, the collagens provide a microskeleton for tissues that resist compressive stress as they do in most forms of bone.

In ligaments, tendons and elastic cartilage the elastic material has two components: the protein elastin and a microfibrillar glycoprotein. 'Elastic' material is a misleading term. In a strict, physical sense an elastic material is non-deformable. Biological elastic material displays not non-deformability but reversible rubber-like deformability.

PROTEOGLYCANS

Proteoglycans (PGs) are large molecules with a protein core to which numerous glycosaminoglycan side chains are attached. The molecule is therefore shaped like a bottle-brush. The protein component represents less than 5% of the molecular mass. In turn, PGs are linked to hyaluronic acid to form macromolecules that give the connective tissues many of their characteristic properties, including high viscosity and the retention of water. PGs are located within a 3-D microskeleton of fibrillar collagen and expand to an extent determined by this meshwork. Held by electrostatic forces within the expanded PG, water provides resistance to compressive stress, the most important characteristic of hyaline articular cartilage.

CONNECTIVE TISSUE DISEASE

Connective tissue diseases are **primary**, local or systemic disorders of the connective tissue system. Many other conditions, such as hypo-adrenocorticalism, affect or involve the connective tissues **secondarily**. Primary connective tissue diseases are occasionally inherited but are more often acquired.

IMMUNE DISORDERS

Interest has centred on those connective tissue diseases in which a disturbance of the immunological mechanism is suspected. In systemic lupus erythematosus (SLE), for example, antibodies are formed against many constituents of the patient's own tissues and blood. They are auto-antibodies (p. 28). One of the most important is anti-ds (double stranded) DNA.

The role of an inherited predisposition is often suspected. In rheumatoid arthritis (RA), for example, the class II histocompatibility antigen HLA-DR4 (p. 330) occurs with greater frequency than in the normal population. In ankylosing spondylitis (AS), an association with HLA-B27 is extremely strong.

INFECTION AND INFLAMMATION

The connective tissues and their compartments are susceptible to a number of distinct, secondary infective processes.

Now read Joints (p. 190)

Acute

Cellulitis

Cellulitis is the rapid, diffuse spread of non-suppurative bacterial inflammation along connective tissue planes. The most frequently recognised causative micro-organism is *Streptococcus pyogenes* but other aerobic and anaerobic agents may be responsible. Of the latter, Clostridia spp. are the most important.

Streptococci (p. 311) produce exotoxins that include fibrinolysin, haemolysin and the enzyme, hyaluronidase. Hyaluronidase depolymerises the glycosaminoglycan chains of connective tissue matrix proteoglycans. It is this action, above all, which accounts for the nature of cellulitis. Formerly, hyaluronidase was called 'spreading factor' and the use of this old name serves to recall its essential role. The characteristic toxins and enzymes of the causative bacteria exert their actions in the connective tissue planes to create a rapidly extending, diffuse swelling with ill-defined, slightly raised margins. Lymphangitis and lymphadenitis co-exist. Tissue necrosis, the proliferation of other organisms and suppuration may occur. Streptococcal cellulitis responds early to high doses of parenteral benzyl penicillin.

Viral infection

A role for viral infection is proposed in systemic connective tissue diseases such as RA, SLE and polyarteritis nodosa. Patients with RA often have raised titres of antibody against Epstein–Barr virus.

It is suspected that the virus alters the regulatory functions of T lymphocytes.

Erysipelas

Erysipelas ('red skin') is a remorselessly spreading infection caused by *Streptococcus pyogenes*. The micro-organisms invade the dermis, leading to a painful, raised, red exanthem with a discrete margin. Surgical erysipelas develops at the site of wounds, for example after inguinal herniorrhaphy.

The infection advances very quickly. The involved skin is warm, slightly firmer than normal and reddened. There is often no obvious point at which the organisms can be seen to have gained access to the subcutaneous connective tissues and the infection is self-limiting. The red coloration of the skin is the result of intense vascular congestion. The clinical significance is not the local disease but the profound systemic effects on the patient of the streptococcal toxins. Haemolysis and hypotension are among the results. In treatment, penicillin is again the antibiotic of choice.

Fasciitis

Fasciitis is inflammation of any layer of fascia.

Now read Necrotising fasciitis (p. 137)

Chronic

Fibrosis is described on p. 131, fibromatosis on p. 130.

MECHANICAL DISORDERS

Fracture (p. 54), dislocation and laceration are among the numerous disorders of the connective tissues. Osteoarthritis (p. 192) may be regarded as a connective tissue syndrome mediated by mechanical changes.

TUMOURS

A very large range of tumours originates in the calcified and non-calcified connective tissues. Those of bone and cartilage are described on pp. 57 and 82, respectively. The remainder comprises the soft tissue tumours (p. 298).

Now read Sarcoma (p. 243), Soft tissue tumours (p. 298)

CONTRACTURE

A contracture is the irreversible replacement of part of the subcutaneous tissue, skeletal muscle or tendon by fibrous connective (scar) tissue, rich in collagen and of low vascularity. As the collagen matures, the fibrous tissue shrinks and deformity results. Contracture is a major feature of healing after severe burns (p. 71). When it occurs following injury to a tendon, a significant restriction of joint movement may result.

Dupuytren's contracture affects the ulnar aspect of the fascia of the palm of male caucasians. It is often bilateral and there is a familial tendency and an association with epilepsy. Alcoholic cirrhosis is thought to be one predisposing factor. An analogous but distinct process may develop after the prolonged occupational use of vibrating tools.

Volkmann's contracture, a result of the compartment syndrome (p. 188), typically involves the flexor muscles of the forearm.

Now read Fibrosis (p. 131)

CRYSTAL DEPOSITION

Crystals of normal body components, such as cholesterol, often form within the body. Other crystals grow when a normal constituent is present in excess. Insoluble crystals can excite inflammation and lead to crystal deposition diseases. The best known of these disorders is gout.

URATE DEPOSITION DISEASE (GOUT)

Gout (urate deposition disease) is a clinical syndrome in which inflammation of joints and connective tissue arises in certain individuals who have a persistently high serum concentration of urate. Insoluble, needle-shaped crystals of monosodium bi-urate form in the extracellular connective tissues. Crystal growth is likely in subcutaneous tissues, around synovial joints and in the connective tissues of the lobe of the ear, the arteries and the kidney. Some crystals are phagocytosed by polymorphs. They tend to disrupt the membranes of phagolysosomes so that lysosomal enzymes are released into the tissues. Crystals also bind protein and activate complement. Inflammation is provoked. It often becomes chronic, exciting a foreign body macrophage reaction and fibrosis. The granuloma that results is a **tophus**. Cartilage and bone can be destroyed.

Gout is usually **primary**. When there is excess formation of urate derived from nucleoprotein breakdown in chronic leukaemia or myeloproliferative disease, or during the chemotherapy of cancer, gout is **secondary**, as it is in chronic lead poisoning.

CALCIUM PYROPHOSPHATE DEPOSITION DISEASE – CHONDROCALCINOSIS

Chondrocalcinosis (pseudogout) is a clinical syndrome resembling gout. It is due to the formation in tissues of insoluble crystals of calcium pyrophosphate dihydrate.

The distinction between these two causes of acute arthritis is essential because of the availability of effective, specific prophylaxis and treatment for gout. The differentiation is made from synovial fluid or tissue sections by means of a polarising microscope. Urate crystals are negatively birefringent, pyrophosphate crystals positively birefringent.

CALCIUM HYDROXYAPATITE DEPOSITION DISEASE

Bone mineral includes calcium hydroxyapatite (p. 73). Crystals of this mineral are encountered in the soft tissues and may provoke inflammation. They are individually too small to be seen by the light microscope in body tissues and fluids but aggregates are readily detected with polarised light. They can be identified by electron microscopy.

Now read Calcinosis (p. 74)

OTHER CRYSTAL DEPOSITS

Cholesterol crystals, derived from red cell membrane lipoprotein, are common at sites of old haemorrhage. They may also develop from bile deposited in the wall of a chronically inflamed gall bladder. Biliary calculus is described on p. 37. Xanthine, hypoxanthine and cystine crystal deposits are rare. Urinary calculus is described on pp. 196, 338.

CYST

A cyst is a sac containing fluid that has been secreted by lining epithelial cells. Some cysts, such as those comprising ovarian cystadenoma (p. 260), are tumours. The majority of cysts are, however, not neoplastic and arise by the obstruction and dilatation of ducts or tubular structures.

CONGENITAL CYSTS

Congenital cysts be due to the persistence of embryonal tissue:

- **Branchial cysts** (p. 241) are lined by squamous epithelium.
- **Cystic hygroma** occurs in the region of the embryonic jugular lymph sac.
- **Dentigerous cysts** are developmental, odontogenic cysts.
- **Dermoid cysts** are due to imperfect fusion of embryonal skin flaps and are lined by squamous epithelium.
- **Lymphatic cysts** are found within the abdominal and thoracic cavities.
- **Para-ovarian and para-testicular cysts** are persistent remnants of the genital ducts.
- **Polycystic disease** of the kidneys (p. 197) and meningocele (p. 63) are examples of congenital cystic disease.
- **Thyroglossal cysts** (p. 323) are found in the midline of the neck, close to the hyoid bone.
- **Urachal cysts** are similar remnants that may be found anywhere between the dome of the bladder and the umbilicus.

ACQUIRED CYSTS

Acquired cysts are attributable to obstruction of a duct, a disorder that inevitably leads to the retention of secretions. Examples are sebaceous and pancreatic cysts. Dental cysts are acquired as a result of persistent inflammation around the apex of a tooth. A **ranula** is a cystic tumour of the under surface of the tongue or the floor of the mouth. Acquired cysts may also arise due to distension of natural cavities. Examples are ovarian cysts, hydrocoele (p. 290) and thyroid cysts. An **implantation cyst** is produced by translocation of the epidermis into subcutaneous tissues following injury; the cyst may contain hair follicles. **Hydatid cysts** (p. 357) are parasitic.

CYSTINURIA

In this disease, transmitted as an autosomal recessive trait, there is defective tubular re-absorption of the amino acids cystine, lysine, arginine and ornithine.

Although the urine of heterozygotes contains more cystine than that of normal subjects, the concentration does not usually exceed the limit of solubility. In homozygotes, the urine becomes saturated with cystine and calculi are formed. Cystine is more soluble in alkaline than in acid urine.

CYTODIAGNOSIS

Cytology is the knowledge or understanding of cells. Exfoliative cytology is the microscopic study of cells obtained as smears and by scraping, brushing, aspiration or lavage.

Now read Biopsy (p. 40)

Cytodiagnosis is a diagnosis made by these methods. In one commonly used procedure, part of an aspirate or exudate is spread evenly on a glass slide at the bedside, in the clinic or in the operating theatre. The smears are immediately fixed by means of an aerosol of alcohol. In a corresponding laboratory procedure, cells in suspension are spread uniformly and mechanically on a glass slide by means of a Cytospin centrifuge.

Before microscopy, it is necessary to stain a preparation. The Papanicolaou technique is still among the most widely used methods; it allows the ready differentiation of mature, keratinising cells from immature, dysplastic or malignant forms. The early recognition of potentially malignant disease of the uterine cervix is the aim of the most widely practised programme. Improved recognition of abnormal cells may come from the use of immunohistochemical methods. Suspect cells can be identified by labelling them with antibodies specific for the human proteins regulating DNA replication. The labelled cells are recognised by microscopy.

Screening programmes are maintained by skilled technical personnel working under close consultant supervision. The exclusion of false-positive and false-negative smears is of the utmost importance. The final interpretation of cell smears and sediments is a matter for expert pathological opinion. The identification of cells from a malignant tumour, for example, is determined on the basis of nuclear and cytoplasmic abnormalities. Whether screening for common diseases such as cervical cancer is cost-effective is debated. It is estimated that 1000 to 4000 cases of cervical cancer are prevented each year in the UK by the use of this procedure. However, no screening procedure can be 100% accurate.

- When women are erroneously informed that a smear is 'positive', further invasive tests are inevitable.
- When a test is erroneously reported as 'negative', the opportunity of early diagnosis and treatment has been missed. In ~90% of cervical smears, the result is negative. However, in ~10%, the sample is inadequate and an opinion cannot be given.

CYTOKINES

Cytokines (Table 26) are signalling molecules. They have endocrine (p. 126), autocrine and paracrine functions. Their actions are on cell growth and differentiation, on cell activation and on the promotion of chemotaxis. Cytokines play crucial parts in the immune response and in cell-mediated hypersensitivity. They contribute to the chronic inflammatory reaction, to repair and fibrosis, and to numerous other pathological processes.

Actions

Cytokines bind to cell surface receptors (p. 86). From the cell surface, signals are transmitted to mechanisms regulating gene expression. The energy driving these mechanisms is released by enzymes, kinases, some of which look 'outwards' to cytokine ligands while some look 'inwards' to the interior of the cell.

Many cells form particular cytokines. Interferon alpha (IFNα), for example, is made by all nucleated cells responding to a virus. However, each cell family liberates only certain cytokines. Numerous cell types have receptors for the same cytokine. Conversely, a single cytokine molecule can exert a distinctive variety of effects in different cell populations. Tumour necrosis factor alpha (TNFα), for example, catalyses the proliferation of B-cells but also activates macrophages and the production of nitric oxide (NO – p. 133).

There is a cytokine 'network' enabling different cell types to secrete a variety of cytokines to which a range of cells may respond simultaneously. Sometimes, the

Table 26 Cytokines of significance in surgery

Cytokine family	Examples	Examples of stimuli to formation	Properties
Interferons	Type I Interferon 1-alpha (IFNα)	Virus infection	Inhibit virus replication and cell proliferation Increase NK cell activity
	Type II Interferon gamma (IFNγ – immune interferon)	Modulates immunity in adaptive immune response	Activate macrophages and polymorphs Induce cytotoxic T-cell development
Chemokines	CXC RI	Infection Physical injury	Chemotaxis Regulation of leucocyte migration
Lymphokines Central role in immunity	Interleukin-2 (IL-2)	Produced by T-cells as antigen receptor interacts with peptide in MHC molecules on antigen-presenting cells	Growth factor for Th0 and Th1 cells and for cytotoxic lymphocytes
	Interleukin-3 (IL-3)	Produced by T-cells in response to required differentiation of haemopoietic cells	Synergistic actions with other cytokines in haemopoiesis
Monokines (pro-inflammatory cytokines)	Interleukin-1 (IL-1)	Ingestion of Gram-negative bacteria and activation by lipopolysaccharide	Many distinct systemic and local actions
Central role in immunity and inflammation	Interleukin-6 (IL-6) Tumour necrosis factor alpha (TNFα)	Inflammatory reactions	Activate lymphocytes Raise body temperature Activate phagocytes Activate endothelium
Others Development of myeloid cell series	Tumour growth factor beta (TGFβ)	Stimuli to inhibit cell growth	Restricts growth Inhibits inflammation
	Colony stimulating factors (CSF)	Demand to expand myeloid cell population in defence against micro-organisms	Promote expansion, development and differentiation of myeloid cells

actions of one cytokine, released in response to a stimulus, are opposed by another cytokine activated by the same stimulus. The final result therefore is the sum of the effects caused by all the cytokine molecules liberated in a particular situation.

Now read Cell division (p. 84)

Categories

It is convenient to group cytokines according to their properties and to the cells that produce them (Table 26).

- **Interferons** take part in innate defence against viruses.
- **Chemokines** activate and direct motile cells to sites of tissue injury.
- **Lymphokines** influence the immune response and stimulate lymphocyte proliferation.
- **Monokines** activate and mobilise macrophages, as well as influencing vascular endothelial cells.
- **Other** cytokines are less easy to categorise.

Regulation and use in treatment

There is a two-way relationship between cytokine secretion and gene function. Cytokine secretion is encoded by gene polymorphism. Conversely, cytokines influence gene activation and the expression of cell surface receptor molecules.

Monoclonal antibodies against cytokine molecules can be made, as can agents blocking cytokine receptors. Recombinant cytokines can be employed to stop or stimulate immune reactions. One such molecule is rIFN (recombinant interferon).

D

DEATH

Death is the cessation of vital function in an organism, tissue or cell. The clinical and pathological definitions of death express different viewpoints and excite controversy.

CLINICAL DEATH

The absence of electro-encephalographic (EEG) waves is definitive proof that there is irreversible cessation of cerebral function. The brain is dead and independent life is no longer possible. However, almost all body cells tolerate ischaemia (p. 187) better than those of the central nervous system. Consequently, the tissues of the kidney, liver, heart and lung can remain alive for varying periods after brain death has been established.

Bradycardia or circulatory arrest, hypothermia and the absence of breathing are not absolute indices of death. In one recent case, a woman recovered normal cerebral function after 1.5 hours immersion in water below an ice flow. Her breathing and cardiac contraction had ceased and her core temperature had sunk to 13°C.

Now read Transplantation (p. 329)

ORGAN AND TISSUE DEATH

The death of tissue is recognised when cell nuclei are irreversibly injured or lost, when membrane stability can no longer be maintained or when the activity of essential enzymes ceases. The vulnerability of cells is in inverse relationship to their metabolic activity.

Cell death

Cell death is presumed when microscopical changes such as the loss of stainable glycogen or of cardiac muscle cell striations are seen. Cerebral neurones reveal ultramicroscopical signs of irreversible damage within 2–4 minutes of permanent injury, heart muscle cells within 15 minutes, renal tubular cells within 60 minutes. By contrast, avascular tissues such as cornea and articular cartilage display the changes of apoptosis or death very slowly indeed.

Now read Cell death (p. 89)

DEATH RATE

The World Health Organization has shown that malnutrition, infection and trauma are the most frequent causes of death worldwide, in this order of frequency. On a global basis, cancer ranks tenth as a cause of mortality. In Western countries, the picture is different. Although starvation is very uncommon, infection remains a challenge and accident and injury are still frequent. The death rate in adults in the second and third decades from heart and respiratory disease has fallen by half and from cancer by a third but the mortality in young adults from drug abuse, suicide, accident and AIDS has increased by a much greater proportion.

DIABETES MELLITUS

Diabetes (flowing through) mellitus (sweet, sugar-like) is a state of hyperglycaemia and glycosuria due to a relative deficiency of circulating insulin.

There are two principal types:

- **Type 1. Childhood and adolescent onset diabetics** are prone to severe disease. They survive only by the repeated injection of insulin.
- **Type 2. Late, adult-onset diabetics** can be controlled by diet alone or with hypoglycaemic drugs such as glibenclamide. However, they may also require injections of insulin, particularly prior to surgery or during infection.

Causes

The deficient production of insulin by the pancreatic islets is recognised in ~1% individuals.

There are genetic and environmental causes.

- **Genetic**. A heritable predisposition can often be attributed to an autosomal recessive gene with incomplete penetrance. Diabetes mellitus complicates the rare heritable condition of haemochromatosis (p. 271).
- **Environmental**. Among the acquired causes of diabetes mellitus are the destruction of pancreatic tissue by neoplastic or inflammatory disease, and the loss of the islets of Langerhans (p. 373) at pancreatectomy.

Metabolic changes analogous to those of diabetes mellitus can be produced by the administration or secretion of excessive quantities of hormones with antagonistic effects to insulin. They include catecholamines, glucocorticoids, glucagon and somatotrophin. Thus, diabetes mellitus is a feature of Cushing's syndrome (p. 6) and of acromegaly (p. 272).

Structure

- **Pancreas**. The exocrine tissue of the pancreas is unaffected and the organ is not evidently reduced in size. The microskeleton of the pancreatic islets is retained but there is a reduction in the proportion of islet beta-cells or a hyalinisation of the islets.
- **Vascular disease**. Atheroma is very frequent and widespread hyaline arteriolar sclerosis is characteristic. The arteries and arterioles of the eyes, heart, kidneys, large bowel and limbs are vulnerable. Diabetic retinopathy remains the most frequent of all causes of blindness in Western countries. Coronary artery disease and limb ischaemia are commonplace. When limb amputation is necessary for the treatment of gangrene in a diabetic patient, the fact that the vascular disease is of small, peripheral arterioles may permit the operation to be confined to a finger or toe.
- **Peripheral nerve disease**. Peripheral neuropathy is common; it may be a consequence of arteriolar disease. Trophic ulcers result. Older individuals are prone to osteoarthritis as well as to neurogenic arthropathy. In males, ankylosing hyperostosis (p. 300) may affect the spine.

Behaviour and prognosis

Untreated, severe diabetes mellitus is characterised by polyuria; thirst and increased drinking (polydypsia); hunger and increased appetite (polyphagia); and paradoxical weight loss. The therapeutic control of carbohydrate metabolism prevents these changes and reduces morbidity due to secondary infection. In the same way, dietary recognition and the administration of insulin or insulin-like drugs can decrease the incidence and progression of microvascular disease.

Hyperglycaemia

There is hyperglycaemia and glycosuria. Keto-acidosis (p. 231) in uncontrolled diabetes is due to the increased oxidation of fat. The osmotic effects of excess renal tubular glucose cause polyuria and there is a constant hazard of disordered fluid balance. Muscle wasting is attributed to accelerated gluconeogenesis (p. 75): there is a diminished quantity of glycogen in both skeletal muscle and liver. The stress of surgery and anaesthesia accentuates these disturbances. In diabetic patients undergoing operation, the optimum procedure is therefore to:

- **Stop the administration of insulin** or oral hypoglycaemic preparations on the day of operation.
- **Infuse isotonic solutions of glucose** until a satisfactory oral intake can be re-established.
- **Inject amounts of insulin** indicated by measurements of the blood glucose concentrations.

There is a particular need to monitor plasma K^+ concentrations.

Infection

Diabetes mellitus greatly diminishes the capacity to resist infection. Patients are liable to develop many forms of bacterial and viral disease. They are particularly prone to cellulitis, carbuncles and wound infection the commonest cause of which is *Staphylococcus aureus*. This susceptibility is due to impaired immune responsiveness rather than to the relatively high glucose content of the tissues.

Transplantation

Although more than 300 diabetics have undergone islet cell allotransplantation (p. 265) and more than 9000 have received vascularised pancreatic transplants, the results have been poor.

DISINFECTION

Disinfection is the attempted destruction of pathogenic micro-organisms or their toxins or vectors by direct exposure to a chemical or physical agent.

Now read Antisepsis (p. 23), Sterilisation (p. 304)

The distinction between a disinfectant and an antiseptic (p. 23) is quantitative. Disinfecting agents can be viewed as powerful forms of antiseptic, suitable for application to inanimate structures. In surgical practice, two of the most valuable agents are very hot water and soap. In hospitals and laboratories, disinfectants are used to make safe instruments, containers, plates, dishes, tubes and jars in preparation for sterilisation, laundering and packaging.

The brief application of chemical disinfectants reduces many bacterial populations but even prolonged use does not guarantee sterility. In fact, continued use may lead to bacterial resistance or the overgrowth of resistant strains of which *Pseudomonas aeruginosa* is one example. Disinfectants destroy many other forms of pathogenic micro-organism although their value in the control of virus disease (p. 347) is very limited.

CHEMICAL DISINFECTANTS

Few disinfectants can bring about sterilisation reliably. Those that can kill bacterial spores must be used in proper conditions of temperature and moisture and in sufficient concentrations. Organic matter such as blood, pus and dirt decrease their effectiveness. In alphabetical order, those in use include:

- **Chlorhexidine**. Chlorhexidine ('Hibitane') is used as a 0.5% solution in 70% ethanol or in water. It is a halogenated compound as effective as 1% iodine in ethanol. There is a very slight risk of skin irritation and sensitisation. It is ineffective against *Mycobacterium tuberculosis* and against spores.
- **Chloroxylenols.** The chloroxylenols are weak disinfectants. They cause little irritation and are of low toxicity. One example is Dettol.
- **Ethanol**. From the time when Paré (p. 374) substituted wine for tar in the treatment of amputation stumps, ethyl alcohol has held a special place in surgical practice. It is a simple, safe but mild antiseptic used frequently in 50% or 70% dilution in wards and laboratories for cleaning and disinfection.
- **Ethylene oxide.** This gas is particularly valuable in disinfecting heat-labile instruments, plastics and polymers in apparatus such as renal dialysis and extra-corporeal circulatory machines. There are hazards: ethylene oxide in air is explosive. A non-explosive mixture prepared in carbon dioxide is a safe alternative.
- **Formaldehyde**. Formaldehyde is a toxic and carcinogenic chemical that kills bacterial spores as well as vegetative bacteria. It is used as a liquid or gas in a well-ventilated room. There are strict Health and Safety Regulations. Ten per cent aqueous formaldehyde disinfects contaminated surfaces quickly. Many heat-labile instruments such as cystoscopes can be sterilised by exposure to formaldehyde vapour at 80°C for 2 hours. Formaldehyde is also used to kill the bacteria employed to make some vaccines (p. 343).
- **Glutaraldehyde.** Solutions of gluteraldehyde are used to sterilise endoscopes and instruments containing plastic or rubber. Different exposure times are required for the destruction of different micro-organisms. In general, the inactivation of HIV

requires 5 minutes exposure, HBV not less than 30 minutes and *Mycobacterium tuberculosis* 60 minutes. However, gluteraldehyde may not destroy atypical mycobacteria associated with HIV and may cause contact dermatitis and lung disease in nurses subjected to frequent exposure.

- **Hexachlorophane**. Hexachlorophane is now rarely used.
- **Hypochlorite**. This simple molecule is of low toxicity and is easily removed by washing. However, it is ineffective in the presence of organic matter. It may be combined with a detergent and is the agent of choice in blood spillages. EUSOL (Edinburgh University Solution of Lime) is a mixture of calcium chloride and boric acid that yields hypochlorite.
- **Metal salts**. Inorganic and organic metal compounds constitute occupational hazards. They are therefore now used infrequently. Mercuric chloride exemplifies the former, methiolate the latter.
- **Phenols**. Lysol and cresol are effective in the presence of organic matter. However, they do not kill bacterial spores and have slight activity against viruses. Phenols are now little used.
- **Quarternary ammonium salts**. These compounds, of which cetrimide ('Cetavlon') is an example, are weak disinfectants with no action against *Pseudomonas aeruginosa*.

PHYSICAL DISINFECTANTS

Moist and dry heat and ultraviolet light are disinfectants. They are discussed on p. 305. Many other physical agents such as X-rays can also destroy microorganisms.

Pasteurisation

Biological materials that are easily damaged, and foodstuffs such as milk, can be disinfected but not sterilised by moist heat at temperatures below 100°C. The process is **pasteurisation** (p. 374). For example, milk is pasteurised at 63–66°C for 30 minutes. All non-spore-forming pathogenic bacteria, including *Mycobacterium tuberculosis*, *Brucella abortus*, salmonellae and streptococci, are killed. However, hepatitis B virus, CJD prions, *Coxiella burnetii*, Listeria spp., bacterial spores, and many protozoa are not destroyed.

DISSEMINATED INTRAVASCULAR COAGULATION (DIC)

In disseminated intravascular coagulation (DIC), the unregulated release of thrombin as a consequence of tissue damage (p. 96) leads to the formation of abnormal quantities of fibrin in the circulation.

DIC (Fig. 21) is common after severe injury; during cardiothoracic surgery; in patients with acute pancreatitis; in endotoxic shock; and following incompatible blood transfusion. Intravascular coagulation 'consumes' large quantities of the coagulation factors (p. 99). Afibrinogenaemia and thrombocytopenia result so that the alternative term, **consumptive coagulopathy**, is used. Excess fibrin obstructs small vessels, causing widespread, zonal infarction. Fibrinolysis is stimulated, removing some of the fibrin. However, the breakdown products have an anticoagulant action leading to severe, microscopic bleeding and anaemia (p. 11). The mortality rate is high. The cause of death is end organ failure due to microvascular thrombosis in the brain, lungs and kidneys.

Now read Coagulation and coagulopathies (p. 95)

DIVERTICULUM

A diverticulum is a pouch or cul-de-sac of an organ. Some diverticula are congenital; others are acquired later in life.

Meckel's diverticulum

Meckel's diverticulum is part of the residue of the vitello-intestinal duct. The mucosa often contains ectopic, gastric epithelium (p. 308) that may be a site for peptic ulceration and a rare source of gastrointestinal bleeding.

Pulsion diverticulum

Pulsion diverticula are encountered, for example, in the pharynx. They are caused by compressive forces that **push** part of the wall of the organ outwards at sites of weakness.

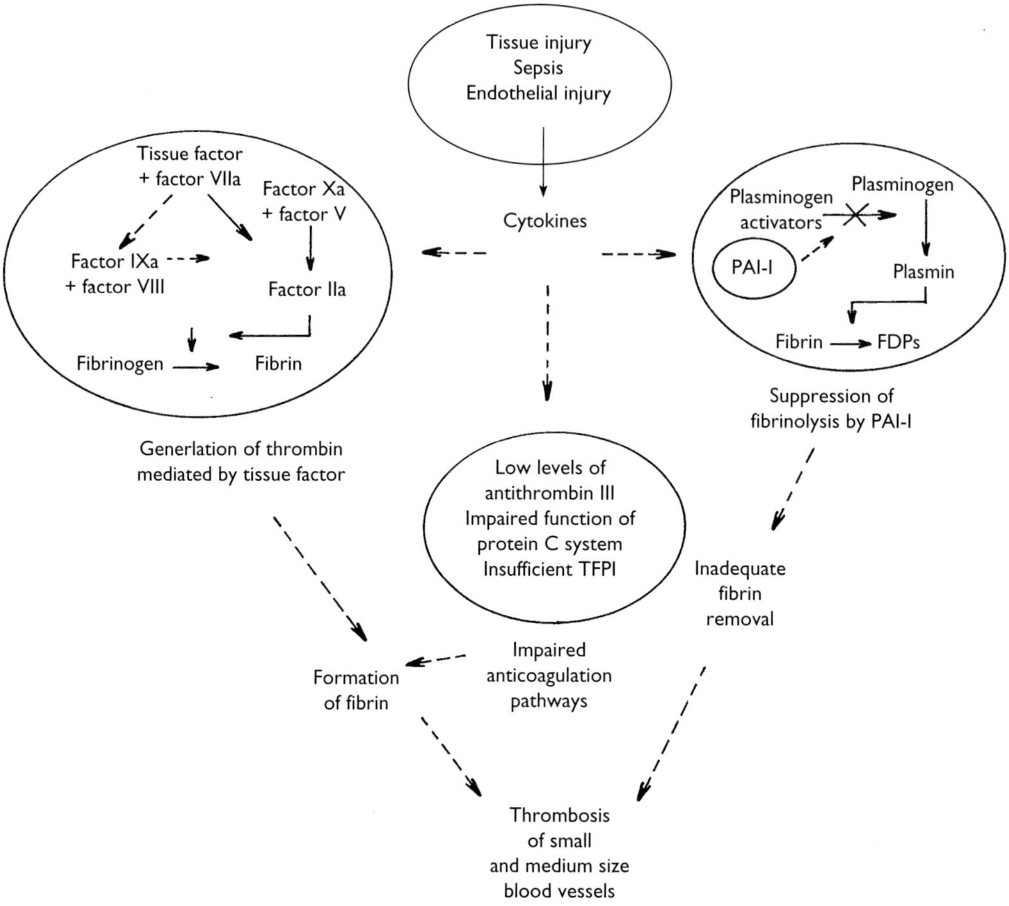

Figure 21 Disseminated intravascular coagulation (DIC).
Tissue injury, sepsis and endothelial injury (at top) are factors triggering DIC. Effects are mediated by cytokine activation. Thromboplastic substances are released and coagulation cascade (p. 95) is activated. Excess generation of thrombin (left) leads to fibrin formation and thrombosis of small blood vessels. Suppression of fibrinolysis (right) results in inadequate fibrin removal. Intravascular thrombosis, end-stage of DIC, is terminal event in sequence provoked, for example, by Gram-negative bacteriaemic shock. FDPs: Fibrin degradation products; PAI-I: Plasminogen activator I-I; TFPI: Tissue factor protein inhibitor.

Traction diverticulum

Traction diverticula are recognised in the pharynx and oesophagus. They are created by tensile forces that **pull** the wall of the viscus outwards. They result from the contraction of scar tissue (p. 290).

False diverticulum

False diverticula form by the **protrusion** of a mucosa through a defect in the muscle coat of a hollow organ such as the colon.

DIVERTICULITIS

Diverticulitis is inflammation of the wall of a diverticulum. It is a sequel to obstruction.

Now read Diverticular disease (p. 102)

DUCT OBSTRUCTION

Ducts such as those of the salivary glands and pancreas, the bile duct, ureters and Eustachian tubes are often obstructed. Lesions causing obstruction may lie:

- Outside the duct.
- Within the duct wall.
- In the lumen of the duct.

The effects are specific to each organ or gland. They lead to malfunction and loss of tissue. In the kidney, for example, cortical atrophy results from the hydronephrosis caused by prolonged ureteric obstruction. In the gall bladder, fibrosis is a consequence of the mucocoele that occasionally follows longstanding bile duct obstruction.

The most important and most common result of duct obstruction is infection. Bacteria may ascend in a retrograde direction within the lumen of the duct or within adjacent lymphatics. Alternatively, blood-borne organisms can lodge in tissue proximal to an obstructed duct. Cholangitis (p. 38) and some cases of pyelonephritis (p. 198) are examples of the secondary syndromes that result.

DUODENUM

Biopsy diagnosis of duodenal and small intestinal disease

Biopsies of the duodenum are obtained readily by endoscopy. The specimens contain mucosa and sometimes a small quantity of submucosa. Biopsies distal to the duodenum may be taken 'blindly', by means of a Crosby capsule. In centres with facilities for enteroscopy, target biopsies may also be obtained endoscopically; they permit the diagnosis of diffuse small intestinal disorders such as giardiasis, regional enteritis and coeliac disease.

DEVELOPMENTAL AND CONGENITAL DISORDERS

Duplication of the duodenum is a rare defect. The duodenum may also be implicated in congenital anomalies of other structures. Thus, ectopic pancreatic tissue is a common finding upon endoscopic examination of the duodenum. It is usually symptomless. Annular pancreas (p. 262) may produce duodenal obstruction.

Diverticulum

Diverticula are often found on the medial wall of the second part of the duodenum, adjacent to the papilla of Vater. There appears to be an association between the formation of these diverticula and choledocholithiasis. However, the precise mechanism of their formation remains obscure. Rarely, they lead to obstruction of the common bile duct.

INFECTION AND INFLAMMATION

Ulcer

Although the prevalence of duodenal ulceration has declined steadily in Western countries, it remains a common cause of dyspepsia. Duodenal ulcer is now no more frequent in men than in women. Those who develop the condition are more often of blood group O, and of non-secretor status, than normal individuals. Ulceration is three times more likely to occur in first-degree relatives of sufferers than in the general population.

Causes

Duodenal ulcer is a form of autodigestion. It is due to the actions of pepsin, an acid protease. It is usually, but not always, associated with excess acid secretion by gastric parietal cells of which there is an increased number.

The principal, normal defence against peptic autodigestion is the production of mucus and bicarbonate ions by the epithelial glands. Hyperacidity alone, in the absence of pepsin, does not cause ulceration but duodenal ulceration rarely develops in subjects with achlorhydria. In the Zollinger–Ellison syndrome (p. 377), duodenal ulcers are unusually frequent, often multiple and resistant to conventional treatment. Hypersecretion of acid contributes to the increased incidence of duodenal ulcer in hyperparathyroidism.

Bicarbonate secretion, mucus secretion and mucosal blood flow are stimulated by the endogenous secretion of prostaglandins. Aspirin and other non-steroidal anti-inflammatory drugs (NSAIDs) inhibit prostaglandin production and peptic ulceration is common in patients consuming these compounds. There is an increased incidence of duodenal ulceration in smokers and an impaired response to treatment. However, cigarette smoking does not raise the levels of gastric acid secretion but may contribute to the rapid emptying of the stomach.

The role of *Helicobacter pylori* in the aetiology of duodenal ulceration remains uncertain. Some 95% of patients with duodenal ulcers and ~80% of those with gastric ulcers are infected with this bacillus (p. 308). Eradication increases the rate of healing and diminishes the frequency of ulcer recurrence. The majority of those infected do not develop peptic ulceration. Bacterial virulence and strain, the age of the host, susceptibility and environmental factors all influence the outcome. In patients with duodenal ulceration, inflammation is mainly confined to the antral mucosa. The inflammatory process interferes with the feedback mechanism controlling gastrin-induced acid production. *H. pylori* may also induce subtle changes in mucin, reducing duodenal protection against pepsin.

Now read *Helicobacter pylori* (p. 151)

Structure

- **Acute**. An acute duodenal ulcer is a very small, superficial lesion with a clearly defined, hyperaemic margin.
- **Chronic**. Chronic ulcers (Fig. 53) are round or oval with shelving margins and an irregular and indurated fibrotic base that is covered by an inflammatory and necrotic exudate. From the base, the partly digested, thrombosed branches of the gastroduodenal artery may project.

Ninety-five per cent of chronic duodenal ulcers are found in the first part of the duodenum. Of these, the majority lie within 30 mm of the gastroduodenal, mucosal junction. Occasionally, the ulcers are paired and lie on opposing walls of the duodenum as so-called 'kissing ulcers'. Silent ulceration is recognised in patients treated for long periods with corticosteroids and NSAIDs. Very large ulcers, as much as 50 mm in diameter and of equal depth, occasionally penetrate the pancreas.

Behaviour and prognosis

Chronic duodenal ulcer may be complicated by perforation; haemorrhage; or pyloric stenosis. Perforation may lead to the development of localised abscess or to diffuse peritonitis. Whereas perforation is more common in anterior ulcers, haemorrhage is a feature of posterior ulcers.

In earlier times, surgical treatment was by highly selective vagotomy; truncal vagotomy together with either pyloroplasty or gastrojejunostomy; or partial gastrectomy. The late complications of these operations are still recognised. Stomal ulcer is one example.

Most patients in the West are now treated with H_2 receptor antagonists or proton pump inhibitors. In spite of the widespread use of these costly drugs, there has been no reduction in the mortality rate. Approximately 5000 patients die annually in the UK. Many of these deaths result from haemorrhage or perforation in elderly patients treated with NSAIDs for arthritis.

TUMOURS

Benign and malignant tumours may originate at any point within the duodenal mucosa. They are most likely to arise from the epithelium covering the papilla of Vater. The diagnosis of tumours forming within the ampulla may only be possible by biopsy after endoscopic sphincterotomy.

Benign

Adenoma

Adenomas tend to be villous. They display varying degrees of dysplasia. Malignant change is relatively common. Multiple duodenal adenomas are found in more than 90% of patients who have familial adenomatous polyposis (p. 105).

Malignant

Carcinoma

Carcinoma is rare. It usually develops in the first or second parts of the duodenum. The prognosis is poor compared with that of other parts of the gastrointestinal tract. However it is much better than that of carcinoma of the head of the pancreas from which this tumour is necessarily distinguished.

Other tumours

A variety of neuro-endocrine tumours (p. 126) can be identified. Many are non-functioning but some secrete gastrin, glucagon, vaso-intestinal polypeptide or somatostatin. Leiomyomas and leiomyosarcomas (p. 235) are uncommon and usually occur in the third or fourth part of the duodenum. Their behaviour varies. Many grow slowly to a large size without metastasis. They are difficult to extirpate and local recurrence frequently follows attempted surgical excision.

DYSENTERY

Dysentery is inflammation of the colon. There is diarrhoea of varying severity with blood, pus and mucus in the stools. The ileum may be implicated. Two principal forms of dysentery are distinguished: bacillary and amoebic.

BACILLARY DYSENTERY

Bacillary dysentery, shigellosis, can be caused by several species of shigella which differ widely in pathogenicity. In Europe, schoolchildren suffer mild attacks due to *Shigella sonnei*. More severe episodes are caused by *Shigella flexneri*, an agent encountered frequently in the Middle East and in South-East Europe. Infection attributable to *Shigella dysenteriae* is largely confined to the Far East.

The abrupt, febrile presentation and the appearances of the stools, avoid confusion with non-infective forms of diarrhoeal disease such as ulcerative colitis. When differential diagnosis is demanded, culture and the techniques employed for bacterial identification are combined with histological examination of a biopsy. Like ulcerative colitis, chronic bacterial dysentery can produce pseudopolyp formation with fibrous scarring and intestinal stenosis. An illness indistinguishable from shigellosis may be caused by some toxigenic strains of *Escherichia coli* (p. 32).

Now read Bacteria (p. 30)

AMOEBIC DYSENTERY

Now read Amoebiasis (p. 8)

E

ECTOPIA AND HETEROTOPIA

- **Ectopia** is the abnormal, congenital or acquired site of an organ or part of an organ. Retrosternal thyroid and the pancreatic tissue of Meckel's diverticulum are examples of abnormal congenital disposition; the fragments of skin found in tissues at compound fracture sites exemplify abnormal acquired location. Hormones secreted inappropriately from some cancers are described as ectopic.
- **Heterotopia** has essentially the same significance as ectopia. It is the development and growth, in an organ or part, of a tissue that does not normally exist in that situation. It is a variety of malformation or deformity.
- **Sequestration** describes a particular variety of ectopia and is applied, for example, to the rare location of fetal lung tissue within the abdomen.

ELASTOSIS

Elastosis is any degeneration of elastic tissue. It is a common feature of ageing and is recognised in the wrinkled, thinned skin of the elderly (p. 8). There is an excess of weak, fragmented, dermal elastic material. **Solar elastosis** is the basophilic change in dermal collagen and the degeneration of elastic material that develops after prolonged exposure to sunlight. Irradiation of the skin by X- or gamma-ray sources leads to a similar defect.

EMBOLISM

Embolism is the process by which a solid, liquid or gas enters and lodges within blood or lymphatic vessels during life. The majority of symptomatic emboli are venous but arterial embolism is an important cause of life-threatening disease.

SOLID

Solid emboli are often formed of an individual's tissues, of cells or of their components, but may be composed of foreign substances or materials.

Venous

Pulmonary embolism

Pulmonary embolism occurs annually in ~0.001% of all Western populations, a figure indicating 1810 cases annually in the UK. However, the incidence of embolism is greatly raised in surgical patients. The mortality from pulmonary embolism is high in those with right ventricular dysfunction.

Causes
Venous thrombi are by far the most important sources of pulmonary emboli. Other solid objects that act as emboli include bone marrow; arthroplasty cement; tumour cells; plastic cannulas; talc; metal objects including bullets and shrapnel; and micro-organisms. An episode of pulmonary embolism may be the first sign of an occult cancer.

Now read Thrombus (p. 320)

Structure
The anatomical effects of pulmonary embolism range from the trivial to the disastrous. A portion of thrombus, detached from a leg, pelvic or arm vein, is carried in the venous circulation, enters the right side of the heart and lodges in a pulmonary artery. If the pulmonary artery itself or a main branch is obstructed, immediate death is usual. The only change observed *post-mortem* is the presence of the thrombus within the obstructed vessel. If the obstruction is to a smaller branch, survival is often possible. The passage of time then allows the changes of pulmonary infarction to develop.

Now read Lung infarct (p. 178)

Behaviour and prognosis
The measurement in plasma of the D-dimer fibrin degradation product, together with leg venous compression ultrasonography and isotopic lung scanning, permit the non-invasive diagnosis of suspected thrombo-embolism.

Effects
In those who survive a pulmonary embolus, serotonin is released from platelets, raising pulmonary arterial resistance. The exchange of gases is impaired. There is increased alveolar dead space and a redistributed blood flow. Reflex bronchoconstriction and airway resistance result in lung oedema. Tension rises in the right ventricular wall leading to dysfunction and right ventricular ischaemia. There is a higher fatality rate in the elderly than in the young and in men than in women.

Prevention
To prevent deep vein thrombosis, early ambulation after surgery is advisable. Many patients are given small doses of heparin peri-operatively. Attempts have been made to prevent pulmonary embolism in high-risk patients with recurrent deep venous thrombosis by placing filters in the lumen of the inferior vena cava. There is not yet evidence that the benefits outweigh the risks. Survivors, particularly those who have suffered multiple, small emboli, frequently suffer permanent pulmonary fibrosis and may develop cor pulmonale (p. 150).

To prevent pulmonary embolism, the prompt recognition of deep vein thrombosis is essential.

Arterial

- **Small emboli**. Tumour cell micro-emboli are often carried in the arterial blood stream. The cells of breast carcinoma, for example, are conveyed to the brain, bones and adrenal glands.

- **Large emboli**. Larger, embolic thrombi are commonly borne in the systemic arterial circulation from the internal surface of a cardiac infarct or an atherosclerotic plaque, to lodge in the renal, carotid, popliteal or other arteries.
- **Paradoxical embolism**. When a direct communication such as patent interatrial septum (p. 147) exists between the venous and arterial circulations, a post-operative rise in blood pressure in the right atrium permits paradoxical embolism. In this condition, an embolus from the right, venous side of the circulation lodges in the end arteries of the left, arterial side. Infarcts of a limb or of the brain are among the often fatal results.

FLUID AND GAS

Fluid

Fluid emboli are formed of substances such as fat that are fluid at body temperature but differ from plasma in viscosity, density and solubility. Amniotic fluid is a source of microscopic pulmonary embolism in difficult labour.

Fat

Fat embolism is the obstruction of pulmonary and systemic capillaries by micelles of lipid that enter or form within venules or sinusoids.

Characteristically, fat embolism follows severe injury, in particular bone fracture (p. 54). The time interval between injury and fat embolism is ~2 days. Fat embolism succeeds ~2% of fractures. In the majority of cases, no clinical signs are recognised. The onset of fat embolism may occasionally be detected after trauma to non-osseous, adipose tissue.

Lodging haphazardly within the vessels of the lungs, brain, kidneys and skin, scattered fat droplets cause foci of tissue ischaemia and hypoxia. The tissue injuries of fat embolism may be the result of local anoxia. Alternatively, they have been attributed to the actions of lipoprotein lipase. Fatty acids freed within injured tissues are themselves irritant. There is respiratory distress and defective arterial oxygenation, disturbed cerebral function, petechial skin haemorrhages and the presence of fat micelles in the urine and in the sputum. Cerebral hypoxia is due to a defect in oxygen exchange in the lungs. Death may occur.

The immediate causes of fat embolism are disputed. Fat may be liberated directly from the marrow of fractured bone into the circulation. When metal rods or prostheses are inserted into marrow cavities it is easy to envisage the release of fat droplets. It is less simple to explain fat embolism in the absence of bone injury or manipulation. An acute disorder of the system regulating fat solubilisation has been considered: plasma lipids may coalesce in the plasma because of a defect in the mechanism that keeps them in solution so that micelles of phospholipid join to form droplets.

Gas

Under special circumstances, bubbles of gas may obstruct small blood vessels. Caisson disease is one example.

Caisson disease is a syndrome of multiple infarcts caused by gaseous emboli in those who have worked under high atmospheric pressures. In the building of underwater foundations of bridges and in deep-sea diving, men necessarily work in pressure chambers. The gases of the air pass into solution in the body fluids. When decompression occurs quickly, nitrogen, which comprises ~80% of the dissolved air, comes out of solution and forms small bubbles that act as gaseous emboli. The bubbles lodge in capillaries, terminal arterioles or end-arteries, in territories such as the brain and spinal cord. Ischaemia results and foci of necrosis cause permanent injury. Within the CNS, damage may result in death or paralysis. In bone, aseptic necrosis predisposes to osteoarthritis, particularly of the femoral head.

A comparable form of embolism can be caused by the accidental release of air into the circulation during surgery or in the course of blood transfusion. The introduction of as little as 50 mL may be rapidly fatal: in this rare event, the right atrium is occluded, venous return is impeded and cardiac output ceases.

Much more commonly, air embolism is encountered during the measurement of central venous pressure; during abortion, and in operations on the neck. Continuous ultrasonic monitoring of the neck veins minimises the risk during this latter form of surgery, allowing emboli to be identified quickly.

EMPYEMA

Empyema is the collection of pus in a cavity bounded by mesothelium or epithelium. It is a form of abscess (p. 1). Empyema thoracis is mentioned on p. 217 and 275, empyema of the gall bladder on p. 38.

ENDOCRINE SYSTEM

The endocrine system is of two parts:

- The **classical endocrine system** comprises the anterior and posterior pituitary glands, the pineal, the thyroid and parathyroid glands, the adrenals, the pancreatic islets and the gonads.
- The **diffuse endocrine system** comprises cells or clusters of cells widely dispersed throughout the gastro-intestinal tract, the lungs, the bronchi and the skin.

Endocrine glands secrete hormones and other molecules directly into the vascular system, into the cellular environment or into a cell itself. The cells of the endocrine system are therefore endocrine, paracrine or autocrine.

- **Endocrine cells**. The cells of the classical endocrine system are typified by those of the islets of Langerhans. Their secretory product, the polypeptide hormone insulin (p. 117), is passed directly into islet capillaries.
- **Paracrine cells**. Some chemical messengers are released locally and act only in the immediate environment of the parent cell, properties characteristic of the diffuse endocrine system.
- **Autocrine cells**. These cells secrete chemical agents that bind to receptors on their own surface.

HORMONES

Hormones are agents of chemical signalling systems that exist to provide intercellular communication in the classical endocrine system. They are formed by an endocrine glandular cell in one part of the body and transmitted by a portal or systemic blood circulation, to another site where a specific effect is exerted.

Many hormones, such as prolactin and thyroid-stimulating hormone (TSH) are glycoproteins. Some, such as adrenocorticotrophin (ACTH) and parathormone (PTH), are polypeptides. Others, such as the adrenal corticosteroids and the sex hormones, are steroids while a few, such as the adrenal medullary catecholamines, are phenols.

Hormones may be synthesised and secreted by ectopic endocrine tissue and by neoplasms of endocrine organs. Occasionally, as in the multiple endocrine neoplasia (MEN) syndromes, several tumours secrete an excess of a number of different hormones simultaneously. Cells of neoplasms arising from non-endocrine tissues may secrete hormones **inappropriately** and **paradoxically**. The cells of a small cell carcinoma of the bronchus, for example, may secrete excess corticotrophin leading to Cushing's syndrome (p. 6).

Technical, laboratory advances now facilitate the distinction between endocrine and non-endocrine cells and the identification of tumours thought to be of endocrine origin. The methods include immunolocalisation with monoclonal antibodies, electron microscopy and *in-situ* hybridisation.

- Immunolocalisation identifies sites of hormone storage so that the somatotrophs and lactotrophs of an adenoma of the anterior pituitary gland, for example, can be differentiated.
- Electron microscopy recognises and identifies the hormonal and non-hormonal components of a suspect tumour. Hormonal microstructures include the neurosecretory granules found in functioning tumours such as insulinoma and glucagonoma. They are distinguished from non-hormonal organelles that include the chromogranins.
- *In-situ* hybridisation enables hormonal peptide mRNA to be identified in neoplastic cells.

Disorders of the individual glands of the classical endocrine system are described separately.

Now read Adrenal (p. 5), Ovary (p. 259), Pancreas (p. 262), Parathyroid (p. 267), Pituitary (p. 272), Testis (p. 316), Thyroid (p. 322)

MULTIPLE ENDOCRINE NEOPLASIA (MEN)

MEN 1

Patients with this hereditary syndrome develop parathyroid, pancreatic or pituitary adenomas or hyperplasia (Wermer, p. 377). The abnormal gene is located on chromosome 11. The pancreatic islet cell tumours are multiple and secrete insulin, glucagon, gastrin, or pancreatic polypeptide. The most frequent manifestation is hyperparathyroidism (p. 267).

MEN 2

This heritable disorder comprises parathyroid hyperplasia, phaeochromocytoma and medullary carcinoma of the thyroid. The abnormal tumour suppressor gene occurs on chromosome 10, at 10q11. There are two variants. MEN 2a phenotypes (Sipple) display a normal appearance but MEN 2b individuals suffer from the Marfan syndrome (p. 190) and have submucosal neuromas.

DIFFUSE ENDOCRINE SYSTEM

The term diffuse endocrine system is applied to families of single or grouped endocrine cells widely distributed throughout the gastro-intestinal tract and present in other epithelial structures such as the prostate and bronchus. Microscopy shows that they bind silver (Ag).

- The location of Ag is revealed only when a reducing agent is added, the property of **argyrophilia**.
- Some cells, such as those of the small intestine, reduce Ag from solution spontaneously: they are **argentaffin**.

The cells of the diffuse endocrine system arise from the embryonic ectoderm. They share common properties with cells derived from the neural crest. The endocrine properties of the argentaffin cells include the ability to synthesise and secrete amines such as 5-hydroxytryptamine and polypeptides such as insulin, glucagon and gastrin (pancreatic islets), gastrin and enteroglucagon (stomach), secretin and gastric inhibitory polypeptide (duodenum), enteroglucagon (intestine), and calcitonin (thyroid C cells). Some cells synthesise and secrete more than one hormone.

Now read Carcinoid (p. 82)

The cells of diffuse endocrine system tumours secrete the hormone characteristic of the parent cell. The tumours are therefore functional and each may cause a clinical syndrome reflecting the nature of the hormone released.

ENDOTOXIC SHOCK

Endotoxic shock results from the entry into the blood of large numbers of dead Gram-negative bacteria, particularly *Escherichia coli*, *Proteus vulgaris*, *Pseudomonas aeruginosa* and *Klebsiella aerogenes*. Bacterial lipopolysaccharide endotoxin (p. 327) is released. Endotoxic shock is particularly likely after gastro-intestinal surgery or intestinal perforation. It is also a complication of urological and gynaecological sepsis and of infected burns and is increasingly probable in immunosuppressed patients.

Now read Bacteria (p. 30), Shock (p. 290), SIRS (p. 293)

ENTERIC FEVER

Enteric fever, **typhoid**, is a frequent diagnostic challenge in many countries. This insidious and often life-threatening disease is caused by *Salmonella typhi* or by *Salm. paratyphi* A, B and C. Worldwide, *Salmonella typhi* remains the greatest challenge. *Salm. paratyphi* B is the most common cause of enteric fever in the UK. *Salm. paratyphi* C is prevalent in Eastern countries.

Enteric fever is spread between individuals, under conditions where poor hygiene prevails. Contaminated food or water convey infection. The micro-organisms survive in symptomless **carriers**. Faecal carriage may be due to the persistence of *Salmonella typhi* in the gall bladder; the organisms thrive in the presence of bile salts. Faecal carriers can cause epidemics in populations with good sanitation if an individual is a food-handler. Not all such carriers are cured by cholecystectomy. Urinary carriers are much less common but much more dangerous because of the ease with which urine can spread infection.

In a preliminary incubation phase, *Salmonella typhi* multiplies in the lymphoid tissues of the gut and enters the blood stream. The phase of incubation coincides with anti-Salmonella antibody formation. Febrile illness is accompanied by bacteraemia. The organisms are disseminated widely but small intestinal infection is dominant. Longitudinal ileal ulcers form within Peyer's patches. Intestinal **haemorrhage** and **perforation** may follow; they are important causes of death. With recovery, healing is complicated neither by fibrosis nor by intestinal obstruction, characteristics that distinguish typhoid ulcers from those of tuberculosis.

Definitive diagnosis cannot be confirmed by clinical means alone. Diagnosis is made by early blood culture (2 weeks), later culture of the urine and stools (2–4 weeks), using modern techniques of bacterial identification. In Western countries, the time-consuming Widal agglutination test for antibodies formed against these bacteria is no longer employed: the results are ambiguous without a knowledge of whether a patient has been immunised previously. The test may be seriously misleading. However, this form of agglutination test is still the best means of identifying brucellosis, another cause of pyrexia of uncertain origin.

F

FALLOPIAN TUBES

Many of the diseases of the Fallopian tubes are related to the pathology of pregnancy and are not considered in this work.

INFECTION AND INFLAMMATION

Salpingitis

In the majority of cases, no cause of salpingitis is demonstrable but in a minority, infection follows abortion or delivery. Pathogenic bacteria reach the Fallopian tubes via the uterine cavity or, occasionally, by the bloodstream. The causative organisms are those of the intestinal tract, including *Escherichia coli*, *Bacterioides fragilis*, *Enterococcus faecalis* and *Pseudomonas aeruginosa*. Salpingitis is now seldom a direct result of gonococcal infection but the frequency of disease attributable to Mycoplasma and Chlamydia is increasing.

- **Acute**. The tubes appear red, swollen and oedematous and a purulent exudate escapes from the fimbrial ostia. Occlusion of the ostia leads to **pyosalpinx**. In this condition, the tubes remain distended with pus.
- **Chronic**. Following acute, bacterial salpingitis, low-grade, chronic inflammation may persist with a plasma cell and lymphocytic infiltrate and an increasing proliferation of vascular fibrous tissue. Infertility results. The tubes remain obstructed and may fill with clear fluid, the condition of **hydrosalpinx**.

Very occasionally, tuberculosis (p. 332) leads to caseating, granulomatous salpingitis.

TUMOURS

Metastatic

Metastatic tumours are very uncommon.

Primary

Among the infrequent primary, benign tumours are fibroma, adenoma and leiomyoma. Carcinoma is rare. It is poorly differentiated and may be bilateral.

FAT

The word 'fat' is used in a number of ways. It describes adipose tissue and is synonymous with 'obesity'. A

70 kg man has ~15 kg of fat as adipose tissue, 6 kg of protein and 0.2 kg of glycogen. Adipose tissue is solid at room temperature.

The word 'fat' is also employed loosely to describe a greasy, semi-solid material, found both in animals and plants, and composed of a mixture of glycerol esters. In the present context, 'fat' is used to mean the acylglycerols.

Now read Lipids (p. 207), Obesity (p. 250)

FAT DEFICIENCY

Although surgical patients are often deprived of food for substantial periods of time, deficiency of fat is uncommon and individuals possess sufficient depot fat (adipose tissue) to allow survival for months. Injuries or surgical operations impose large, additional metabolic demands but the principal reason for nutritional support is the need for glucose which is not obtainable from fat.

Within a few hours of withdrawing food, or following severe injury, insulin levels fall and glucose transport and metabolism are depressed. There is consequently a decrease in the synthesis of fatty acids and tri-acylglycerol. Raised catecholamine levels activate hormone-sensitive lipase with the hydrolysis of stored tri-acylglycerol. Fatty acids are released into the blood. There is a rapid, consequential increase in the plasma concentration of free fatty acids. The fatty acids are bound to albumin and transported to target tissues to be used as fuel. The breakdown of tri-acylglycerol produces glycerol which enters the Embden–Meyerhof pathway as triose phosphate and is oxidised ultimately in the tricarboxylic acid (Krebs) cycle.

In the face of the greatly increased fatty acid and pyruvate oxidation that follows the onset of starvation, the liver manufactures excess aceto-acetate, β-hydroxybutyrate and acetone. These are the 'ketone bodies'. Their excretion begins. As starvation continues, these substances (p. 195) are themselves used in growing amounts as energy sources, a process of **keto-adaptation**. Increasingly, ketones replace glucose as the source of energy for the cells of the cerebral cortex, bone marrow and other vulnerable tissues. During starvation, glucose can only be provided by gluconeogenesis (p. 75). Keto-adaptation is therefore an important mechanism for survival.

Signs of deficiency of the essential, long-chain, polyunsaturated fatty acids do not become apparent until starvation has been enforced for many days. This state can be reversed by the intravenous infusion of fat emulsions. Short- and medium-chain fatty acids can be absorbed from the intestinal mucosa without the assistance of micelle formation. However, their use is restricted by nausea and diarrhoea.

FAT NECROSIS

Necrosis of fat is particularly associated with trauma and with pancreatitis.

Traumatic

Traumatic fat necrosis is encountered in the breast tissues of middle-aged women. The established lesion is painless but there is often a history of trivial injury. Reaction to the injury results in a *peau d'orange* (orange peel) appearance which may simulate carcinoma. There is a characteristic inflammatory reaction. Many plasma cells are present. The injured tissue is infiltrated by macrophages containing lipid and haemosiderin. Ultimately, foreign body giant cells are found and the lesion becomes circumscribed by granulation tissue.

Pancreatic

In patients with acute pancreatitis, the release of lipases catalyses the de-esterification of the acylglycerols to fatty acids and glycerol. The fatty acids combine with calcium in a process of saponification. Where this has occurred, white flecks appear in the fat of the omentum and other intraperitoneal structures and in sites such as the adipose synovia. Arthritis may develop.

Fatty change

Fatty change is a microscopic phenomenon. It is common in the liver. Fatty change describes the abnormal accumulation of fat by cells that, in health, contain little or none. Ultramicroscopic fat droplets are seen in cells as varied as chondrocytes and macrophages. In the latter, myelinoid bodies, the remnants of lipoproteins, lie within single, membrane-bounded vacuoles.

Fatty change is an indication of severe cell injury. The disorder is frequently caused by starvation, hypoxia, ischaemia or cell poisons. It is recognised, for example, in heart muscle cells in severe anaemia, in hepatocytes during cardiac failure and ethanol poisoning, and in skeletal muscle cells as a result of the action of the alpha-toxin of *Clostridium perfringens* (p. 93).

FIBRINOLYSIS

Fibrinolysis is the dissolution of a fibrin clot or coagulum. In the cascade of molecular events characterising fibrinolysis, inactive plasminogen, a plasma protein synthesised in the liver, is converted to the active fibrinolytic enzyme, plasmin, by intrinsic and extrinsic activators. Kinases are liberated from precursors in the blood or damaged tissues.

A dynamic equilibrium normally balances blood coagulation and fibrinolysis. A systemic imbalance in the factors regulating this state may lead to inappropriate coagulation such as disseminated intravascular coagulation (DIC) (p. 119) or to hypofibrinogenaemia.

The fibrinolytic system (Fig. 22) is activated following injury, haemorrhage, anaphylaxis and other forms of shock and, to a much lesser extent, after exercise. Both thrombus dissolution (fibrinolysis) and coagulation are brought about by the activation of inert precursors. Fibrinolysis is a feature of the later stages of wound healing (p. 358) and the resolution of inflammatory exudation. In zones of trauma, fibrinolysis confines coagulation to the injured zone. It limits thrombus deposition and extension, and aids the organisation of thrombus. Fibrinolysis can also be initiated by bacterial enzymes such as streptokinase and staphylokinase that convert inert blood pro-activator into activator.

The restoration of blood flow in vessels such as end arteries occluded by recently formed thrombi often requires the dissolution of thrombus. Streptokinase, urokinase and tissue plasminogen activator can be infused for this purpose. Lysis can sometimes be achieved within 3 hours. In other instances, the surgical removal of thrombi may be quicker and more certain.

Now read Coagulation (p. 95), Thrombus (p. 320)

FIBROMATOSIS

Fibromatosis is a local or diffuse, non-neoplastic, non-inflammatory proliferation of collagenous connective

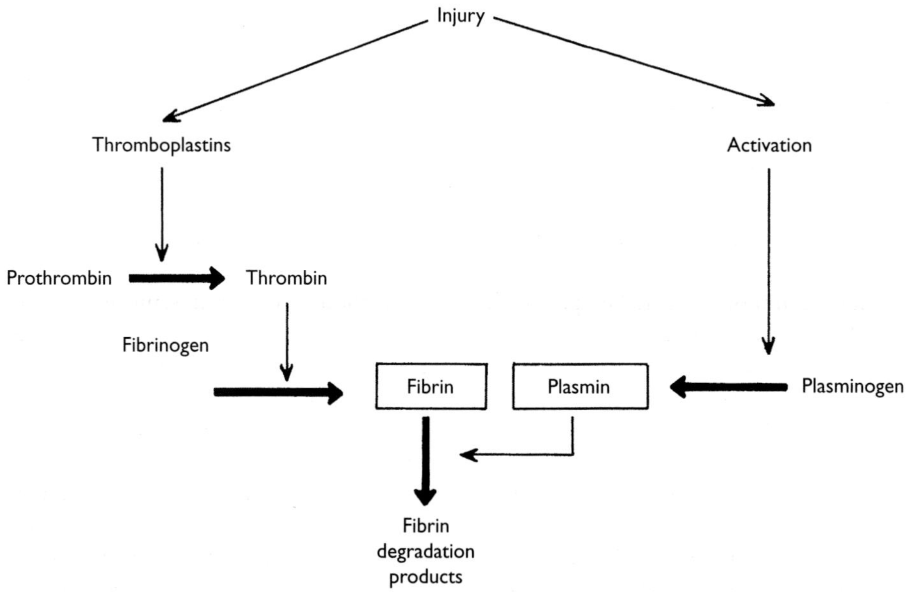

Figure 22 Fibrinolytic system.
Dynamic equilibrium between coagulation (p. 95) and fibrinolysis. Both systems are activated by injury, often trivial.

tissue. The causes are genetic and environmental. For example, ethanol, beta-blockers or injury may contribute to the onset of the disorder.

PALMAR AND PLANTAR FIBROMATOSIS

- **Palmar fibromatosis**, Dupuytren's contracture (p. 371), is an insidious process of excess new collagen formation commencing as a localised island of fibrous tissue sited in the palm of older persons. The cells responsible for the process are myofibroblasts. Continued collagen formation leads to the development of cords of tissue stretching across the palm in the distribution of the flexor tendons of the fourth and fifth fingers. Alcoholic cirrhosis and diabetes mellitus are predisposing factors and there is a genetic predisposition.
- **Plantar fibromatosis** is a similar but much less common process developing in the foot.

PEYRONIE'S DISEASE

Peyronie's disease (penile fibromatosis) is a condition analogous to palmar fibromatosis. The cause is uncertain but there may be a disorder of tolerance leading to auto-immunity (p. 28). Plaques and nodules of fibrous tissue form in the corpora cavernosa. They are followed by hyaline degeneration, calcification and ossification.

RETROPERITONEAL FIBROSIS

Retroperitoneal fibrosis describes the insidious formation of excess, retroperitoneal collagenous tissue. It is a form of fibromatosis. There are two varieties:

- **Primary (idiopathic)**. Primary retroperitoneal fibrosis is more common in middle-aged males than in females. It is associated with mediastinal fibrosis, sclerosing cholangitis, inflammatory bowel disease and Riedel's thyroiditis, all conditions linked to disorders of the immune mechanism.
- **Secondary**. Secondary retroperitoneal fibrosis was first recognised to be a consequence of the prolonged intake of methysergide. The syndrome was associated with the use of beta-blocking drugs. The signs of the disease centre on ureteric obstruction and impairment of renal function. A comparable disorder is recognised as a complication of prolonged peritoneal dialysis.

FIBROSIS

Fibrosis is a process of repair by **substitution**, by means of which tissues and organs restore anatomical continuity when reconstitution of the part by regeneration is prevented or is not possible. Fibrosis is also a common, late consequence of infection; of aseptic inflammation; of prolonged or repetitive mechanical irritation; or of X- and gamma irradiation.

In spite of the vascularity of the tissues, cardiac muscle and arteries frequently repair by fibrosis. In hyaline articular cartilage, an avascular tissue in which regeneration is not possible, limited repair may take place by the formation of fibrocartilage or by fibrosis. In the central nervous system, repair is by gliosis (p. 61).

Fibrosis is a response of fibroblasts and myofibroblasts. The cells are activated and form new collagens. The collagens mature and the fibrous tissue becomes denser, stronger and less vascular.

Now read Contracture (p. 112), Regeneration (p. 285)

ADHESIONS

Persistent inflammation within the abdominal cavity, for example after infection or in the course of Crohn's disease, often results in excess fibrous tissue. Adhesions form. The consequences include intestinal obstruction and intestinal stenosis.

A potent stimulus to adhesion formation is intraperitoneal haemorrhage. Intestinal perforation, with or without local or disseminated sepsis, is another cause. The formation of adhesions is particularly likely after gynaecological surgery, when more than half of women may be affected, and following operations on the colon and rectum. There is a high risk after appendicectomy.

Preventative measures include avoiding the use of talc, starch powder or cellulose fluff and lint, in or near a wound. The application of tissue plasminogen activator has been tested in prophylaxis. Bioresorbable membranes applied to wound surfaces can prevent adhesions forming. The administration of anti-integrin (p. 88) antibodies may offer a possible way of minimising the extent of the adhesions.

FISTULA

A fistula (L: a pipe) is an abnormal communication between two epithelial surfaces. It may be congenital or acquired.

Developmental defects can persist as fistulas. A failure of the urachus or of the vitello-intestinal duct to atrophy are examples.

Acquired fistulas commonly involve the gastrointestinal tract. They may form between the stomach and transverse colon because of chronic peptic ulceration, or between the gall bladder and the duodenum, as a result of chronic cholecystitis. Choledochoduodenal fistula allows the passage of a calculus from the gall bladder to the small intestine. Gallstone ileus is a rare complication of this sequence (p. 37). Fistulas may develop between different parts of the small and large intestine because of a combination of infection and local ischaemia. This is particularly likely in Crohn's disease; intestinal tuberculosis; in diverticular disease of the colon; and following therapeutic, ionising irradiation. Fistulas that develop between loops of small intestine may produce blind loops (p. 165) with bacterial proliferation in the stagnant contents of the loop. Fistulous communications between the trachea and oesophagus, and between the colon and urinary bladder, are common results of tissue destruction by cancer. Bronchopleural fistulas arise in tuberculosis and lead to empyema thoracis. Fistulas form between blood vessels but these channels are better described as arteriovenous aneurysms (p. 14).

Fistulas (Fig. 23) are:

- **Simple** when there is a single track, **complex** (complicated) when there is more than one track or an associated abscess.
- **Internal** when they connect hollow viscera without a communication with the skin.
- **External** when they communicate with the skin; the majority are enterocutaneous. The presence of obstruction distal to an external fistula is important since it prevents healing or closure.

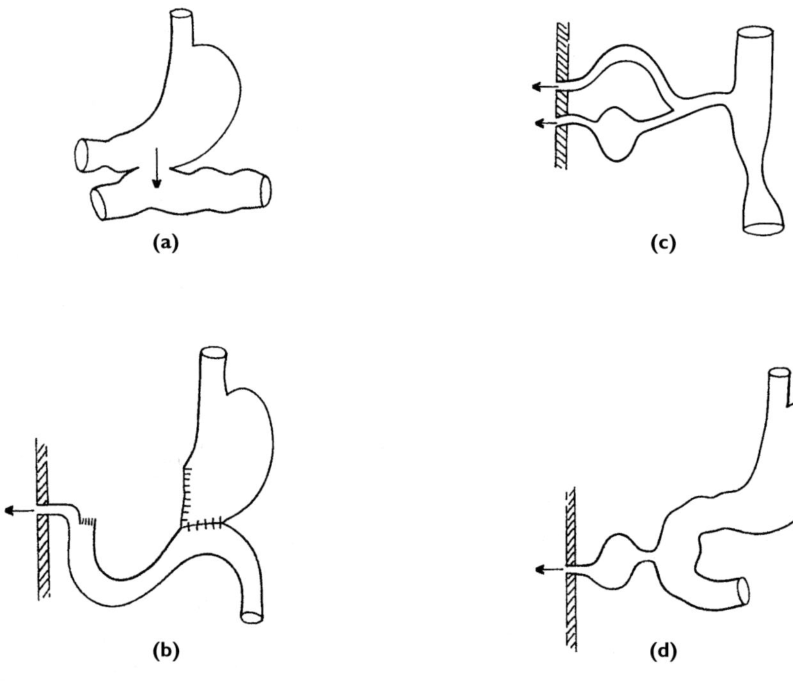

Figure 23 Fistula.
(a) Simple, internal, gastro-colic fistula; (b) Simple, end duodeno-cutaneous fistula; (c) Complex, external fistula with distal stenosis; (d) Complex, lateral duodeno-cutaneous fistula with abscess.

- **End fistulas** for example, those that occur at the duodenal stump following partial gastrectomy.
- **Lateral fistulas** for example, those formed at the site of duodenal closure after transduodenal sphincterotomy of the sphincter of Oddi.

The nature and quantity of the fluid flowing through a fistula depends upon the site. In internal fistulas, there is no loss of fluid from the body, provided absorption can take place distal to the opening. The volume of fluid escaping from external fistulas may be very large as it is in the case of high, enterocutaneous fistulas of the duodenum or jejunum. Fistulas of this kind are described as **high output**. As much as 1500 mL/day fluid may be lost. The result is serious dehydration, electrolyte disturbances and malnutrition. Fistulas of the colon are usually **low output**.

FOREIGN BODIES

Foreign bodies are materials that are physically, chemically or immunologically distinct from the native tissues of a host.

Materials of an immense variety are introduced accidentally or deliberately into the body tissues or spaces. The response that follows the introduction of a sterile foreign body varies in intensity according to the degree of physical and chemical irritation provoked. There is often an initial, acute inflammatory reaction, with subsequent migration of mononuclear phagocytes from the blood. Endeavouring to phagocytose the foreign material, these macrophages tend to fuse to form multinucleated, foreign body giant cells (p. 142). Unless the foreign material can be digested or destroyed, the inflammatory and cellular reaction persists. Granuloma formation (p. 143), sinus (p. 294) or fistula (p. 132) are possible results.

The reaction to a foreign body is strongly influenced by its size and form, particularly according to whether it is smooth or rough, and finely or coarsely particulate. The identity, and therefore the reactivity, of a foreign body may be suggested by its microscopic appearances and proven by methods such as electron probe X-ray micro-analysis, by histochemical or by immunocytochemical tests. Individual foreign bodies such as particles of silicate, fragments of cobalt–chrome steel, or pieces of suture material display highly characteristic properties.

Foreign bodies evoke other responses according to their biocompatibility. Thus, materials that are apparently smooth and devoid of immunoreactivity may still provoke inflammation, predisposing to infection. This form of foreign body response is important surgically in the selection of inert metals and plastics for use in orthopaedics and the choice of plastic mesh for tissue repair. Very large fragments of high-density polyethylene tend to become covered by large, multinucleate cells whereas fine, metallic fragments, such as those of titanium, invoke an entirely different, inflammatory reaction to which the immune mechanism may contribute.

When host tissue such as kidney, bone or myocardium undergoes infarction, the residual dead, sterile tissues become antigenically distinct from those of the host. Active inflammation is characteristic of the margins of infarcts and the response is comparable with the reaction to a foreign body.

FREE RADICALS

A **radical** is an element passing intact from one compound to another. Some radicals have a brief existence as **free radicals**, atoms each of which contains an unpaired electron. Important forms of free radical include:

- **Oxygen free radicals** often derive from molecular oxygen (O_2). Oxygen free radicals ($O_2^{\bullet}$) are termed **superoxide**.
- **Hydroxyl free radicals** ($OH^{\bullet}$) are highly reactive. They are responsible for cell injuries such as those occurring after ionising radiation (p. 185).
- **Nitric oxide free radicals** ($NO^{\bullet}$) are described below.

Whether originating from molecular oxygen or from other sources, $O_2^{\bullet}$ is much less reactive than $OH^{\bullet}$ but is formed in a wide variety of circumstances, either by accident or deliberately. $O_2^{\bullet}$ plays an important part in phagocytosis (p. 270), and in bacterial killing (p. 231).

FREE RADICAL INJURY

Free radicals form naturally as a result of normal metabolic processes. **Excess** free-radical formation incites damage to the lipids of cell membranes, increasing permeability, and provoking genetic mutations. Normally, iron and copper are conveyed and stored as inert molecules such as caeruloplasmin and ferritin. In the free state, they are powerful promoters of free radical damage. The cumulative effects of excess free radicals comprise a syndrome of **oxidative stress**.

Defence against free radicals is provided by enzymes such as superoxide dismutase. Other free radical scavengers are plasma proteins like albumin, and dietary components such as vitamins C and E (Table 27).

Table 27 Causes and prevention of $O_2^{\cdot}$-induced oxidative stress

Oxidative stress: $O_2^{\cdot}$-induced disease	Protection against $O_2^{\cdot}$-induced disease
Traumatic and reperfusion injury	
Excess exercise, heat or cold	Diet: vitamins C, E, beta-carotene
Systemic infection	Enzymes e.g. superoxide dismutase
Heart disease	
Smoking-related lung disease	
Ultraviolet radiation injury	

Nitric oxide

Nitric oxide (NO) is a universal, super-messenger. It is a gas, a free radical with a capacity to bind to haem-containing compounds. $NO^{\cdot}$, nitric oxide free radicals, can be made by many mammalian tissue cells. They are short-lived and not stored. NO, is of great importance in inflammatory reactions and in many cardiovascular, osteo-articular, traumatic and immunological disorders.

NO is formed through the actions of the enzyme nitric acid synthase (NOS) acting on the amino acid arginine. There are three forms of the enzyme. Two, endothelial cell and neuronal, are naturally present (**constitutive**). The third is **induced** in response to stimuli that include the cytokines and other molecules that initiate the inflammatory cascade (p. 180). NO generation is also provoked by hydrodynamic factors such as increased blood flow and physical factors such as shear stress. In smooth muscle cells, NO production is controlled by lipopolysaccharide, by IF-γ and by TNFα. However, the action of the enzyme, and thus NO production, is inhibited by anti-inflammatory compounds such as glucocorticoids (p. 6) and also by a series of growth factors and proteins (Table 28).

Table 28 Factors opposing the activation of inducible NOS

Transforming growth factor beta (TGFβ)
Interleukins 4, 8, 10 and 13 (IL-4, -8, -10 and -13)
Macrophage inflammatory protein 1 alpha (MIP-1α)
Epidermal growth factor (EGF)
Platelet derived growth factor (PDGF)
Fibroblast growth factor (FGF)

Now read Antibacterial agents (p. 17, 231)

Reperfusion injury

Cell and tissue injury caused by short periods of hypoxia (p. 261) or arterial insufficiency (p. 187) are followed by recovery, although the degree of recovery varies very greatly.

The effects of hypoxia or ischaemia are to deprive cells of the metabolic pathways necessary to synthesise the high-energy phosphate (ATP) essential for the preservation of the integrity of plasma and other cell membranes. After a more prolonged period of hypoxia or ischaemia, restoration of the oxygen supply or of arterial blood flow is likely to be followed not by recovery but a further cell and tissue injury. This disorder, a consequence of free radical formation, is a contributory factor in the tissue damage sustained in the crush (p. 236); compartment (p. 188); and adult respiratory distress (p. 219) syndromes.

Chronic granulomatous disease

Deficient free radical formation by phagocytes is a cause of inefficient bacterial destruction (p. 236). It is a factor in the pathogenesis of **chronic granulomatous disease**. In this quickly fatal disorder, there is prolonged and recurrent infection with granulomatous lesions in bone, liver and skin. The underlying fault is deficiency of hydrogen peroxide formation and thus a defect in the capacity to kill bacteria such as *Staphylococcus aureus* (p. 303).

FUNCTIONING TUMOURS

Functioning tumours secrete hormones, enzymes and/or pharmacologically active substances. There are two categories:

- In a first category, tumours secrete hormones natural and appropriate to the parent tissue although the secretions may be produced in excess. Thus, an islet-cell tumour of the pancreas, for example, may secrete excess insulin (insulinoma) or glucagon (glucagonoma). Other examples include the multiple endocrine neoplasia (MEN) syndromes (p. 126).
- In a second category, hormones or other substances are secreted by cells that do not normally form these substances. The formation is ectopic (p. 242), inappropriate, and may be excessive. Thus, small cell lung carcinoma (p. 70) often secretes ACTH. In 10% of instances, this leads to Cushing's syndrome (p. 6). Such tumours may liberate ectopic hormones that are only detectable microscopically, as granules within the cytoplasm of the cancer cells. The cells of small cell lung carcinoma may also secrete other humoral substances such as vasopressin and oxytocin. Renal cell carcinomas periodically liberate parathyroid hormone and hepatocarcinoma may synthesise gonadotrophin.

The mechanism and reasons by which the cells of a non-endocrine tumour synthesise and secrete large amounts of a hormone are not known. It is assumed that all such cells are genetically programmed to manufacture all human proteins. If the latent ability to express endocrine polypeptides is de-repressed, for example by the lack of a protective agent such as the p53 protein (p. 78), or by the action on the cell of an exogenous carcinogenic agent such as virus, then the neoplastic cells may become autonomous.

FUNGI

Fungi are members of a group of non-vascular plants that have no chlorophyll. They are excluded from the algae and from the higher plant orders because of their reproductive and vegetative structures. Some are sources of antibiotics (p. 17). Others are saprophytes. A few cause human disease.

MYCOSES

Mycoses are specific superficial or invasive fungal infections.

Superficial mycoses

Superficial mycoses such as candidiasis (candidosis), caused by *Candida albicans*, are opportunistic. The organism thrives when mucosal pH is altered or mucus secretion is impaired. Any patient to whom an antibiotic has been administered is threatened with an overgrowth of *C. albicans*. The fungus proliferates in the throat, in urine, in the blood and in wounds, and when AIDS, immunosuppression or cytotoxic therapy have prejudiced host defence mechanisms. For diagnosis, brushings or biopsies taken from sites such as the oesophagus are placed in Sabouraud's medium.

Invasive mycoses

Invasive mycoses are much more frequent in subtropical or tropical countries than in temperate regions. Some are systemic and air-borne. They may be endemic (histoplasmosis: *Histoplasma capsulatum*) or epidemic (coccidioidomycosis: *Coccidioides imitis*). Others, of particular dermatological and surgical importance, are locally invasive. They include South American blastomycosis (*Blastomyces dermatiditis*) and maduramycosis (*Madurella mycetomatis* or Allescheria spp.).

Invasive fungi such as *Aspergillus fumigatus* or Mucor widely infiltrate tissues that have been injured by ischaemia or neoplastic growth. They also invade the tissues of immunosuppressed individuals and patients given cytotoxic agents. Aspergillus poses a particular risk for patients in bone marrow transplant units, especially if there is any nearby building work from which spores may originate.

Mycetoma

Mycetoma is a term for a chronic, localised mycosis of the subcutaneous and underlying tissues. The lower limb is often affected, leading to a deforming and disabling disorder termed 'Madura foot'. There is gross swelling, destruction of tissue and the formation of sinuses through which coloured particles and granules, the fungal colonies, are discharged.

Mycetoma may be caused by one of a considerable number of organisms that are of two main groups: true filamentous fungi such as *Madurella mycetomatis* and bacteria, including Nocardia and Streptomyces spp.

MYCETISM

Mycetism is an illness due to the ingestion of fungi such as mushrooms.

MYCOTOXICOSIS

Mycotoxicosis is the intoxication produced by the ingestion of food contaminated by the toxins of poisonous fungi. Ergot and aflatoxin poisoning are examples.

G

GALL BLADDER

The biliary tract is discussed on p. 36.

GANGRENE

Gangrene is an ancient term that describes a sequence of degradative changes that follow death of part of the body. It is synonymous with **putrefaction**. The provocative factor is a loss of blood supply, for example, to a limb or a segment of gut. Vegetative, saprophytic bacteria are already present on or in the limb just as micro-aerophilic or anaerobic bacteria commonly inhabit the bowel. The organisms multiply, breaking down the ischaemic tissues by proteolysis. The result is a mass of discoloured, softened, foul-smelling material, the high water content of which accounts for the description 'wet gangrene'.

Mummification

Extensive tissue death is not always followed by gangrene. For example, causative organisms may not be present, or their growth may be prevented by antibiotics. When the environmental humidity is low and the temperature high, dead tissue is likely to dry slowly, retaining its form. The effects are identical with those seen when a body mummifies in the hot, dry atmosphere of a desert. Mummification is encountered in the legs of patients with slowly advancing occlusion of limb arteries. The description 'dry gangrene' has been employed but is self-contradictory.

Fournier's gangrene

Fournier (p. 374) described the spontaneous onset of rapidly progressive gangrene of the scrotum in otherwise healthy young men. King Herod, who probably suffered from diabetes mellitus, is believed to have been afflicted by this condition. Vascular thrombosis, subcutaneous tissue necrosis and skin gangrene develop in sequence.

Meleney's gangrene and necrotising fasciitis (p. 374) may be the same condition. They produce a rapidly spreading gangrene of the groin, perineal, genital or peri-anal regions in males and females although the disorder is much more common in the former.

Since the introduction of antibiotics, the pattern

has changed. Many of those persons affected are, indeed, older diabetics. Contributory factors such as urinary, perineal or retroperitoneal infection, or recent groin or perineal surgery, are often implicated. The cause is synergism between faecal bacteria, including micro-aerophilic streptococci, and anaerobes such as *Clostridium perfringens* or peptostreptococci.

Necrotising fasciitis

Necrotising fasciitis is a potentially lethal form of local infection that very occasionally succeeds group A streptococcal cellulitis. Following an otherwise simple and uncomplicated operation, for example the repair of an inguinal hernia, fulminating inflammation of the skin accompanies rapidly spreading gangrene of subcutaneous, fascial, muscular and associated tissues. There is an accompanying severe, systemic, toxic state. The infection is more likely in a patient who is immunocompromised or in whom diabetes mellitus or cancer already exist, than in normal persons.

In many instances, *Streptococcus pyogenes* can be recovered from the affected tissues but there may be a mixed bacterial flora. Small blood vessels are occluded by microthrombi and the destruction of tissues is very rapid. In spite of treatment with large doses of penicillin combined with small, intravenous doses of gentamicin, the explosive progression of this unusual form of gangrene is so dramatic that extensive surgical procedures, including amputation, may be required to arrest its spread and prevent death.

Gas gangrene

This dangerous form of spreading, tissue necrosis is liable to occur when the spores of Clostridia spp. gain access to a wound in which there is extensive soft-tissue or muscle injury. Clinical diagnosis is suspected when a foul smell and wound crepitus are detected. Dirty wounds contaminated by soil are particularly at risk. Within the injured parts, where oxygen tension is low, the spores of *Clostridium septicum, Cl. perfringens* and other anaerobes enter a vegetative phase and multiply. The micro-organisms form potent exotoxins which themselves break down tissue. For example, the important α-toxin of *Cl. perfringens*, a haemolysin, kills muscle cells and destroys fat. A vicious circle is established. Proteolysis and saccharolysis in the injured tissues, with gas production, are caused by enzymes that are among the toxins liberated by anaerobes such as *Cl. histolyticum*, *Cl. novyi* and *Cl. sordelli*. In spite of treatment by radical debridement and antibiotics, the mortality is ~20%. The media refer to 'flesh-eating bacteria'.

Orofacial gangrene

Orofacial gangrene may develop at sites of ulceration and is the result of trauma or infection. Two bacterial species, *Borrelia vincenti* and fusiform bacteria of the Bacterioides and Fusobacterium spp., are parasites of man and live in symbiosis in sites such as the normal gum. When the resistance of this tissue to invasion is lessened, for example as a result of immunosuppression, granulocytopenia or nutritional deficiency, the host–parasite relationship is disturbed, the micro-organisms proliferate and progressive local tissue destruction results. Massive orofacial gangrene (**noma** or **cancrum oris**) may develop under these circumstances.

Now read Ischaemia (p. 187)

GASTRO-ENTERITIS

Gastro-enteritis is acute mucosal inflammation of the small intestine, accompanied by signs of gastric disease.

The causes of gastro-enteritis are viral, bacterial and protozoal. Rotaviruses and Norwalk viruses are among the agents of infantile disease in which enteropathogenic strains of *Escherichia coli* often provoke epidemic diarrhoea. In the UK, many cases of infective diarrhoea are due to infection with Campylobacter. Old people are particularly susceptible to Norwalk or small round structured viral gastro-enteritis in winter. Adult travellers to Third World countries and infants in the tropics are also prone to infections with Salmonella or Shigella spp. The protozoal causes of gastro-enteritis include *Giardia lamblia* and Cryptosporidium. The tissue changes of gastro-enteritis are those of acute inflammation. An intestinal, polymorph exudate is usual although, in rare instances, eosinophil polymorphs accumulate.

Mesenteric adenitis, the enlargement of mesenteric lymph nodes in children, is usually due to infection with adenoviruses. There is often associated pharyngitis and cervical lymphadenitis. One bacterial cause is Yersinia (p. 362).

Now read Colon (p. 101), Ileum and Jejunum (p. 164)

GENES

Genes, the units of heredity, are segments of the macromolecule DNA (p. 139).

Genes are transmitted from parent to offspring in the gametes, usually as part of a chromosome. Each gene is capable of controlling or determining a single heritable characteristic. Every human somatic cell contains approximately 2 million molecules of DNA, representing between 40 000 and 100 000 genes. Together, they comprise the **genome**. Each cell nucleus includes a coded programme of instructions, the **codon**, designed to ensure the exact reproduction of the form and behaviour of the parent cell when division takes place.

Those segments of the DNA molecule that transcribe genetic information are **exons**. However, the coding sequences comprise only 5% of the molecule. They are interrupted by very large, non-coding segments, **introns**. The functions of the non-coding parts of the nuclear DNA are not fully understood. There are additional non-coding regions at each end of the gene, the **telomeres** (p. 91). Non-coding DNA exhibits great variability between individuals and is the basis of the DNA fingerprinting test used in forensic pathology.

The **Human Genome Project** has analysed, sequenced and recorded the entire human genome. The project, centred on cells obtained from 12 volunteers, has been completed recently. There is no perfect, single sequence since individual human genomes are only 99.9% identical. With the exception of identical twins, each human genome therefore differs by 0.1% from every other. The variation is largely due to single nucleotide polymorphisms; they affect ~1 in every 1000 bases. The sequencing of the human genome may prove to be as important a step for medical science as the periodic table was for inorganic chemistry. However, determining the nature and location of genes associated with a disorder such as trisomy 21 (p. 92) does not guarantee an understanding of the mechanisms by which the disorder comes about.

GenBank is the database of all cloned genes from all the kingdoms of life. It is accessible on the Internet.

Now read Chromosomes (p. 90)

UNDERSTANDING GENES AND THEIR PRODUCTS

There have been rapid advances in the understanding of gene structure and of the relationship between identified genes and clinical disease. One delicate and widely used technique that has played a large part in this progress is restriction fragment length polymorphism (RFLP). Another is the polymerase chain reaction (PCR). These and other methods have facilitated the identification of genes enabling selected parts of the DNA of normal genes to be inserted into abnormal cells.

Restriction enzyme fragment length polymorphism (RFLP)

RFLP centres on enzymes called endonucleases that recognise short sequences of base pairs within dsDNA and subsequently cut the DNA at an exact distance from the recognised site.

Using these enzymes, DNA can be divided into different sized fragments. The slight variation in fragment length is used to locate ('map') genes to specific chromosomes. Restriction endonucleases exist in many bacteria. They 'recognise' specific sets of DNA sequences in dsDNA and cut both strands at or near these sequences. Sometimes, the enzymes cut at a single point: this generates blunt ended molecules. With others, the cuts are at precisely spaced points along the two strands. This generates overlapping ('sticky' or overhanging) ends.

With these methods, unrelated DNA molecules can be joined (ligated). This is especially useful for propagating human gene sequences within cells such as those of bacteria or yeasts, a method that allows the production of bacterial or yeast artificial chromosomes (p. 90). In the same way, the entire genetic information from a human chromosome can be joined to bacteriophage DNA. This gives a 'library' of human DNA. From the 'library', homogeneous clones can be isolated, amplified, and manipulated further.

Polymerase chain reaction (PCR)

There are three components in this widely used and delicate reaction: (1) An enzyme, polymerase; (2) an excess of the nucleotides A, T, C and G (p. 140); and (3) DNA with one or two short lengths of bases, oligonucleotides that are only 15 to 25 bases long and which constitute the 'primer' for the reaction.

When the reaction is started, polymerase copies the sequence of bases next to this identified primer which acts as a template, creating a length of double-stranded DNA. The process is repeated many times so that thousands of copies of the base sequence adjacent to the primer are harvested. The 'reagent' obtained in this way enormously increases the sensitivity with which minute markers called minisatellites and microsatellites can be identified in cells obtained from patients under investigation.

FAMILY STUDIES

A first step in recognising the inherited basis of a disease is a study of family data. Dominant and recessive characteristics may become apparent. A second step is the preparation of low resolution maps by the chromosomal analysis (p. 91) of members of the family. The location and identification of a gene determining susceptibility to a disease is then greatly helped by finding a marker gene, sited close to the candidate gene. The identification of marker genes has been made possible by restriction fragment length polymorphism (RFLP) (p. 138) and by the polymerase chain reaction (PCR).

Now read Inheritance (p. 182)

DEOXYRIBONUCLEIC ACID (DNA) AND HEREDITY

DNA is the chemical basis of heredity. The greater part of all DNA exists within cell nuclei but some is present in mitochondria; DNA also plays an essential part in cell metabolism and division. Within a nucleus, the long threads of DNA are coiled around proteins to form larger clumps that are assembled as chromosomes (Fig. 16 and p. 90).

DNA is a double helix (Fig. 24) composed of two extended, molecular threads or strands. The backbone of each thread is a long chain formed of two elements: the sugar deoxyribose linked to phosphate by strong, covalent bonds. By contrast, weak, hydrogen bonds link the opposing strands of DNA. They readily break so that the strands can easily separate as they do prior to cell division (Fig. 14). The arrangement of the phosphate radicals, substituted through hydroxyl groups, is directional and determines that

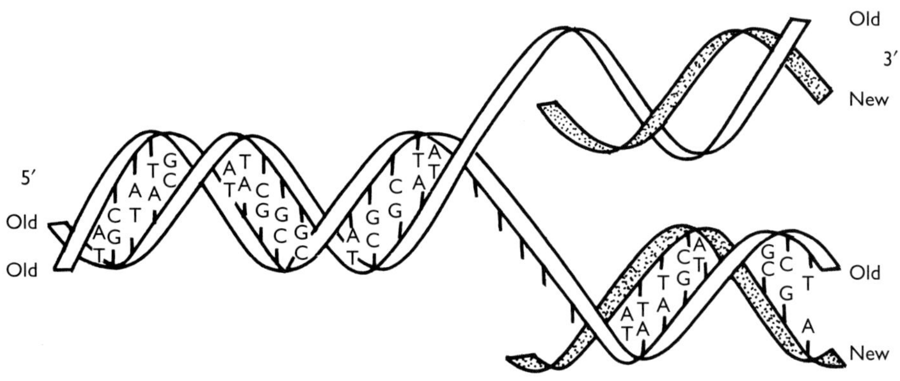

Figure 24 DNA.
Nuclear DNA comprises pair of strands assembled as double helix. Order of bases forming one strand is complementary to the other. Each DNA strand is formed of backbone of deoxyribose sugar linked by phosphate groups. Terminations of strands define beginning (5′) and end (3′) of the DNA macromolecule. At these sites, translation and division commence. There are 64 base triplets so that several may code for a single one of the 20 amino acids found commonly in man. ACA = cystine; AGC = serine; CGT = alanine; CTT = glutamine; GAA = leucine; GCA = arginine; GAT = leucine. ATC is a stop codon.

each thread has two identifiable ends, 5′ and 3′. Any process or change passing along a thread is orientated similarly but in a complementary manner so that 'forwards' in one thread equates with 'backwards' in the other. The arrangement is that of an **antiparallel double helix**.

The genetic code carried by DNA is a precisely defined sequence of bases attached to the deoxyribose units of the DNA double helix. Every strand of DNA comprises 6×10^9 pairs of bases. Two of these bases, adenine (A) and guanine (G), are purines; the remaining two, thymine (T) and cytosine (C), are pyrimidines. The two strands of the double helix of DNA 'face' each other (Fig. 24). Chemically, adenine always pairs with thymine (A-T), cytosine with guanine (C-G). The order in which the bases are arranged on each strand is complementary to that of the other, so that GAC on one strand necessarily opposes CTG on the other. A **codon** comprises three adjacent bases. Each triplet codes for an individual amino acid. Thus, the amino acid arginine is coded by AGA. There are also codons that instruct protein synthesis to start and to stop.

Separation, a process of 'unpeeling' that extends from one end of the DNA double helix to the other, starts at the onset of each cell division (Fig. 14). Unpeeling always takes place in the 5′ to 3′ direction. The separated strands then act as templates for new strands of DNA that are synthesised during the formation of each daughter cell. The order in which the bases are assembled in this process precisely mirrors that of the original template. Each new strand is therefore identical with that of the parent cell so that the genetic code is perpetuated. A mechanism exists for the repair of DNA damaged by extraneous factors such as sunlight and ionising radiation (p. 185).

In the case of the enzymic and some other proteins, two or more independent genes may code for different parts of the same molecule. Usually, these different regions lie close together but, occasionally, as in the case of the regions coding for the α- and β-chains of haemoglobin, the genes are on different chromosomes. Genes on the same chromosome may be linked. Moreover, separated genes may recombine. Genes vary in the degree to which they express their influence on the phenotype so that there is complete or incomplete **penetrance** (p. 183). They exert their effects at different phases of embryonic and postnatal development. A single gene may influence a variety of characteristics (pleiotropy) or multiple genes may regulate one characteristic (polygenic inheritance).

Now read Cell division (p. 84)

PROTEIN SYNTHESIS AND RIBONUCLEIC ACID (RNA)

When a gene enables the synthesis of a protein, it is said to **express** this product. The control of gene expression is not well understood but is probably a result of a change in the configuration of the DNA coils. Alternatively, it can be brought about by proteins with binding sites for metals such as zinc. Much human DNA is non-coding ('junk' DNA) and does not specify genes but may regulate gene expression.

Within the cell nucleus, the coded information carried by DNA is **transcribed** to messenger RNA (mRNA) (Fig. 25). RNA is a very long, thin, chain-like molecule, closely resembling DNA but with the sugar ribose taking the place of deoxyribose. The nucleotide sequences of DNA and RNA are complementary. Like DNA, three of the bases that form the core of the RNA molecule are adenine, guanine and cytosine but the fourth base is uracil, not thymine.

RNA exists in several forms of which the most important are **messenger RNA** (mRNA) and **transfer RNA** (tRNA). Both play essential parts in the exact synthesis of all enzymic and structural proteins. One of the two strands of nuclear DNA acts as a template for the synthesis of the mRNA and all inherited information is conveyed from the nucleus to the cytoplasm by this molecule. There is a co-linear relationship between DNA, RNA and the protein for which they code. Thus, the gene bearing the 'antisense' version of information contained in DNA is faithfully copied into a complementary 'sense' version of mRNA.

In the cytoplasm, the information carried by mRNA is **translated** by means of the second form of ribonucleic acid, tRNA, into the proteins necessary for cell structure and function. Mobile packets of RNA, **ribosomes**, bring individual amino acids to assembly points on the cytoplasmic RNA of the endoplasmic reticulum. Peptide bonds form between adjacent amino acids. Protein synthesis begins and continues until a stop codon on the mRNA is reached. The assembly of proteins into their normal, three-dimensional structures (p. 281) then takes place.

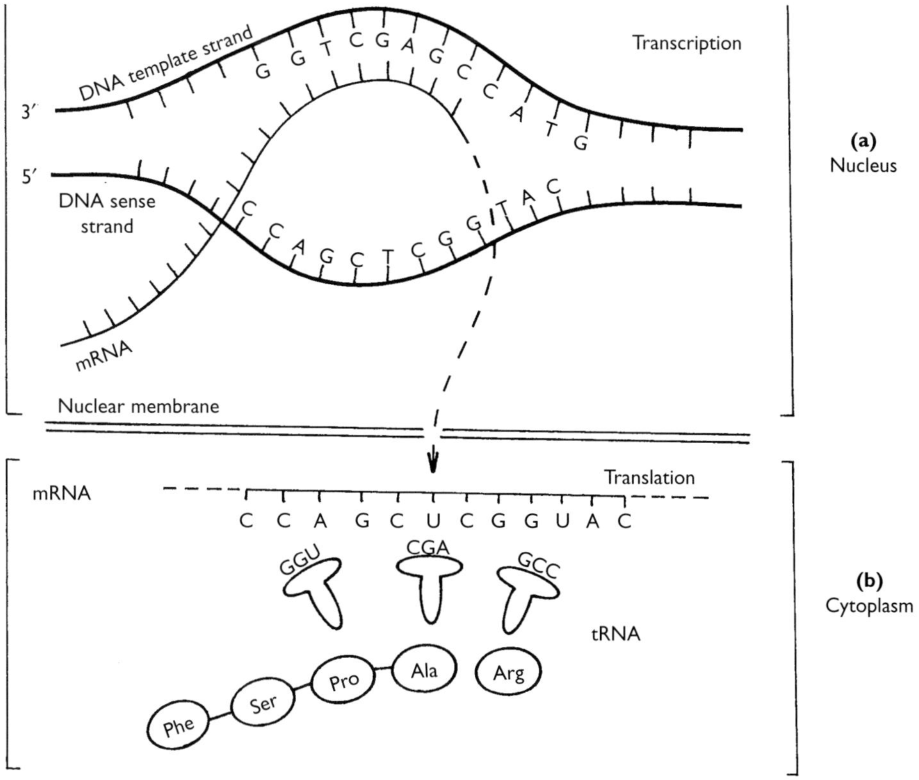

Figure 25 Transcription and translation of genetic information.
(a) In cell nucleus (top), genetic instructions carried as part of DNA molecule, are transcribed to messenger RNA (mRNA). Introns are cut out and exons spliced together to manufacture mature RNA.
(b) In cytoplasm (bottom), amino acids, bound to transfer RNA (tRNA), are aligned on ribosomes in order prescribed by mRNA which translates coded information into sequence of amino acids required to assemble individual polypeptides and proteins.
Ala = alanine; Arg = arginine; Phe = phenylalanine; Pro = proline; Ser = serine.

The protein molecules accumulate in the Golgi apparatus of the cell before export into the extracellular matrix. The three-dimensional organisation of many proteins is often finalised within the cell but the assembly of some common macromolecules, such as collagen, is only completed in the extracellular matrix where maturation and cross-linking enable the proteins to assume a mature form and function.

Now read Protein (p. 281)

Mitochondrial DNA

Mitochondria (p. 84) produce cellular energy and control apoptosis (p. 89). They contain their own, limited amount of DNA, supporting the idea that these organelles may be the residues of ancient bacteria. The mitochondrial genome is a relatively small, circular molecule of 16 569 bp encoding 13 mitochondrial proteins, 22 types of transfer RNA (tRNA) and two types of ribosomal RNA (rRNA).

Mitochondrial DNA is transmitted to a child only by the mother. Mutations in this genome are responsible for many clinical syndromes including occasional types of cancer and forms of neuropathy, myopathy, and cardiomyopathy; retinal degeneration; diabetes mellitus; and hearing loss.

DNA damage

The integrity of DNA is constantly threatened by natural and pathological mechanisms. Damage is readily caused, for example, by sunlight, chemicals and ionising radiation. There are 'built-in' DNA repair mechanisms. If these are defective, even the mild hydrolytic action of cellular water is a threat to the accurate retention of genetic information. In rare disorders, such as xeroderma pigmentosum (pp. 295, 362), defective repair is precancerous (p. 76).

Mutation

A mutation is a change, such as the altered sequence of a base pair, in the chemical structure of a gene. Mutations are perpetuated in subsequent divisions of the cell in which they occur.

Transgenic therapy

As a consequence of these many advances, it is now practicable to undertake transgenic therapy, the delivery of replacement genes or gene segments. Trials of this form of treatment began with single-gene disorders such as cystic fibrosis but the correction of a wide range of defects including cancer, AIDS and atherosclerosis is now contemplated. It is also possible, for example, that the administration of genes coding for insulin in diabetes mellitus; for erythropoietin in some anaemias; and for factor VIII in haemophilia, may initiate the sustained *in vivo* production of the deficient proteins or polypeptides.

Cells do not normally assimilate foreign DNA. To allow the new DNA to be integrated into the defective nuclei of a patient, the replacement material must therefore be incorporated into a delivery vehicle. The delivery system may be a non-viral agent such as a collection of liposomes or a conjugate with DNA virus protein. Alternatively, the new DNA may be carried by a non-pathogenic virus vector. Among the vectors under test are retroviruses. They have the advantage that the foreign DNA is directly integrated into the host cells but the disadvantage that they require dividing cells as targets. Adenoviruses may be used in a comparable way. They readily infect a large number of host cells but their effects may be short-lived and there is the uncertainty of toxic effects.

The administration of replacement DNA to patients may be *ex vivo* or *in vivo*. As an example of the former approach, a replacement gene segment can be introduced into bone marrow stem cells before they are restored to a patient. In the latter, a replacement gene is conveyed to a patient parenterally either by aerosol or by intravenous injection. The criterion by which gene therapy is judged is 'transfection efficiency'. This index measures the proportion of cells within the defective tissue that show evidence of the expression of the new gene.

The important ethical issues raised by gene therapy are under active discussion.

GIANT CELLS

Giant cells are very large cells. They may have single nuclei but osteoclasts, skeletal muscle cells, cardiac muscle cells and those of the cytotrophoblast, are often multilobed or multinucleate.

The **largest** normal cells in the human body are those of skeletal muscle. They are often called muscle 'fibres'. The **longest** cells are the neurones transmitting impulses between the spinal cord and the foot.

The presence of many nuclei in a large cell is an indication of abnormal nuclear division during mitosis or a sign of cell fusion. Thus, the multinucleated giant cells encountered in viral infections such as measles demonstrate that the virus has impaired nuclear division; the multinucleated (Langhans, p. 373) giant cells of tuberculosis indicate that macrophages have fused in their efforts to phagocytose mycobacteria.

Abnormal multinucleate giant cells are further typified by the foreign body giant cells that phagocytose particulate debris in injured tissues (p. 270); the 'mulberry' (Warthin–Finkeldy) giant cells of viral infections such as measles; and the mirror-image, twin nucleus Reed–Sternberg cell of Hodgkin's lymphoma (p. 223). The giant cell of the xanthomas is the Touton cell.

GLOVES

The wearing of sterile gloves is an inescapable responsibility of any surgeon endeavouring to avoid sepsis.

Gloves (Halsted, p. 372) reduce but do not eliminate the possibility of transferring pathogenic bacteria such as *Staphylococcus aureus* from a surgeon's hands to a sterile surgical wound. Gloves cannot be donned with unwashed hands without adding skin-borne bacteria to the external surface and hands should be washed thoroughly before gloving. Sterile gloves should also be worn for procedures in which asepsis is necessary such as the insertion of urinary catheters and lumbar puncture. The likelihood of cross-infection in a ward is reduced if nursing staff is instructed to use disposable, clean gloves for each dressing.

Surgical gloves must be sufficiently thin to be flexible and allow tactile sensation but sufficiently thick and strong to prevent organisms from being transferred to the surgical field. The likelihood of glove perforation increases with the duration and scale of surgery. Double gloving has therefore received much recent attention. A coloured marker associated with the inner glove may allow penetration of the outer glove to be detected easily. Additional protection may occasionally be necessary so that stainless steel, mesh gloves can be donned to cover conventional gloves.

Modern gloves are made of latex. Previously, lubrication was necessary before they could be worn. The adverse tissue responses to some earlier lubricants are described on p. 133. The granulomas that resulted from the use of talc as a glove powder are described on p. 315. Talc was replaced by starch or more soluble powders made from *Lycopodium clavatum* spores that also proved irritant. A non-inflammatory, soluble potassium bitartrate powder was substituted. Modern gloves require no lubricant.

Now read Hospital acquired infection (p. 159); Needle-stick injury (p. 362)

GRANULATION TISSUE

Granulation tissue is the young, vascular connective tissue that forms when healing occurs by repair rather than by regeneration. As inflammation subsides and healing begins, phagocytic leucocytes digest cell debris. Vascular, endothelial buds extend into the injured part and capillaries form. Fibroblasts divide and a matrix of proteoglycan and young collagen is deposited between the blood vessels. With time, vascularity diminishes and the residual collagen constitutes a scar (p. 290).

Granulation tissue is characteristic of healing **'by second intention'** (p. 360). The healing surface is punctuated by small, pink dots or granules, the appearance of which is due to the presence of arcades of young blood vessels seen at the healing surface before it is covered by regenerating epithelium.

GRANULOMA

A granuloma is an aggregate of macrophages (p. 225).

With time, organisation occurs and the granuloma becomes an island of fibrous connective tissue with many small, thin-walled blood vessels. There is a close resemblance to granulation tissue. Granulomas, in spite of their name, are not tumours. The macrophages of granulomas were thought to resemble the cells of some epithelia and are often still called 'epithelioid' cells. In many types of granuloma, macrophages are accompanied by activated mononuclear phagocytes and by lymphocytes. In some instances, small numbers of neutrophil and eosinophil polymorphs are seen.

Many granulomas are the result of chronic staphylococcal, tuberculous or leprous infection. Others follow protozoal (leishmanial), fungal (coccidioidal) or parasitic (filarial) infestation. Granulomas also result from immunological reactions or auto-immune disease (p. 28) when they may be spermatic, pulmonary or rheumatoid. Physical agents such as retained oil, suture material and foreign bodies elicit granulomas, as do chemical agents like beryllium. Some granulomas, such as those of Crohn's disease (p. 165) and sarcoidosis (p. 289), do not yet have a known cause.

GROWTH

Growth is the progressive development and increase in size of part or the whole of an organism. The ancient word growth is used in common speech as a synonym for a tumour.

Now read Cell growth (p. 84)

Growth of the whole body takes place during the period from fertilisation to maturity but individual tissues grow in response to functional demand or to compensate for structural loss. The rate of fetal growth, indicated by the body length, stature, is highest midway through pregnancy. The rate slows late in pregnancy and accelerates briefly after birth. The rate of growth in childhood declines until puberty when it accelerates again. The long bones cease growing at the age of ~16 years in girls and

~18 years in boys although the closure of some epiphyseal plates may not take place for a further 5–7 years.

Factors affecting growth of stature are both genetic and environmental. Growth is closely controlled by the growth hormone of the anterior pituitary. It is influenced by thyroid hormone and by adrenal and testicular androgens. Malnutrition slows growth, as does any severe systemic disease. The body tissues and organs have growth patterns that are regulated differentially. The growth processes and the factors that control them also influence tissue and organ maintenance, regeneration (p. 285) and repair (p. 147).

Atrophy

Atrophy, wasting, a decrease in the size of a tissue, organ or part, is described on p. 28.

Hypertrophy

Hypertrophy is an increase in the size of the individual cells of an organ or tissue, often resulting from increased work demand, or from an endocrine stimulus. It leads to an overall increase in size of the part relative to that of other normal organs and tissue.

Now read Abnormal growth (p. 85); Atrophy (p. 28)

GROWTH FACTORS

Growth factors are polypeptides and small proteins that regulate cell proliferation locally. They are present in tissues and occasionally, in very small quantities, in the circulation. Growth factors have other important properties including the control of cell survival, differentiation, migration and function. A cell responds to a growth factor only when an appropriate **receptor** is present at the cell surface. The specific response initiated in this way generates second messenger molecules within the cell. In turn, these messenger molecules provoke the sequence of cellular events that culminate in cell division.

Many growth factors have a broad range of specific activities, others a very narrow range. In this respect, growth factors resemble cytokines (p. 114). **Platelet-derived growth factor** (PDGF) exemplifies the former: it acts on fibroblasts, smooth-muscle cells and neuroglial cells. **Erythropoietin** is an example of the latter: it exerts its influence only on red blood cell precursors. Growth factors often act in combination to influence particular cell changes. Sometimes, a growth factor that stimulates cell division at one concentration is inhibitory in another.

There are now many examples of the *in vitro* isolation of segments of DNA encoding particular growth factor proteins. The DNA fragments are used for the biosynthesis of these factors by recombinant gene technology (p. 138). Although very costly, the factors, or the monoclonal antibodies prepared against them, are becoming available for clinical use in circumstances such as delayed wound healing or fracture repair.

- **Insulin-like growth factors (IGF-1 and 2)**. IGF-1 promotes postnatal cell proliferation and is a paracrine growth factor in healing. IGF-2 is present in plasma and is a growth-promoting agent during embryonic development.
- **Fibroblast growth factor beta (FGFβ)**. FGFβ exists as at least seven members of a large family of related proteins. They provoke cell proliferation in a variety of different tissues.
- **Transforming growth factor beta (TGFβ)**. TGFβ is secreted by macrophages and many other mesenchymal cells. It is present in the alpha particles of platelets and released during blood clotting and thrombosis. It plays an important part in cell division (p. 84) and wound healing.
- **Platelet derived growth factor (PDGF)**. PDGF is released from the alpha granules of platelets during wound healing. It is chemotactic for smooth muscle cells and causes them to proliferate by mitotic division.
- **Epidermal growth factor (EGF)**. EGF and transforming growth factor alpha (TGFα) are related molecules. They stimulate the proliferation of many cell types, such as those of the ascending limb of the loop of Henlé in acute renal tubular necrosis, and act in embryonic development. TGFα is manufactured by epithelial cells at an increased rate in response to injury.

H

HAEMATOMA

An haematoma is an ill-defined swelling composed of blood, resulting from injury, vascular disease or a disorder of coagulation.

Haematocoele

A haematocoele is a collection of blood confined within a cavity. The effusion may be parametric, pelvic, pudendal, retro-uterine or scrotal. The term is sometimes restricted to mean an effusion of blood into the tunica vaginalis of the testis.

HAEMATURIA

Haematuria, the presence of blood in the urine, may be 'frank' (overt) or microscopic. The presence of red blood cells can be detected by the *naked eye* only when a large number of cells is present. In diagnosis, microscopy is essential as well as urinalysis by 'stick'. Among the significant surgical causes of haematuria are urinary calculi; renal and bladder carcinoma; papilloma; and urinary bladder tuberculosis. Infection must always be sought.

HAEMOLYSIS

Haemolysis is the breaking down of red blood cells with the release of haemoglobin. It is the normal fate of ageing erythrocytes captured by the reticulo-endothelial cells of the spleen. Large-scale, rapid haemolysis may lead to **haemoglobinaemia** and **haemoglobinuria**.

Red blood cell survival can be measured *in vivo* by labelling a sample of cells with radioactive chromium (^{51}Cr) and re-introducing them into the circulation. Abnormal haemolysis can be recognised *in vitro* by suspending red blood cells in serial dilutions of saline. Healthy red cells begin to break down in 0.5% saline. Abnormal cells show a much greater osmotic fragility and begin to break down at concentrations of saline nearer to the normal plasma concentration of 0.9%.

Excessive haemolysis is characteristic of:

- Mismatched blood transfusion (p. 46).
- Haemolytic anaemias of which spherocytosis is one example.
- Haemoglobinopathies such as sickle-cell disease.
- Splenomegaly.
- *Plasmodium falciparum* malaria.

Haemolysis of red blood cells that have been damaged in burnt tissue (p. 71) can induce anaemia sufficiently severe to necessitate blood transfusion. In the laboratory, haemolysis has been used as an end-point in the complement fixation reaction (p. 232). It is an undesirable change in blood collected carelessly for haematological or serological tests and may occur if blood is left standing at ambient temperatures before it is centrifuged.

Now read Jaundice (p. 189)

HAEMOPOIESIS

Haemopoiesis is the production of blood cells.

The erythrocytes, leucocytes and platelets develop from **stem cells**. These precursors are of great replacement value when it is necessary to irradiate or suppress (ablate) the bone marrow completely in the treatment of leukaemia and other cancers.

- In the **fetus**, red and white blood cells and platelets are formed in the bone marrow, spleen and liver. The marrow location is said to be medullary, the spleen and liver sites extramedullary.
- In the **newborn**, haemopoiesis is still recognisable in the liver.
- In the **adult**, zones of red, haemopoietic marrow

remain only in the axial skeleton, ribs and skull and in the proximal thirds of the humerus and femur.

The bone marrow cells that are erythrocyte precursors are large **erythroblasts**. As they mature, they become smaller and acquire cytoplasmic haemoglobin before losing their nuclei. Mature red blood cells survive for 80–120 days in the circulation before undergoing destruction in the spleen. The regulation of red blood cell production is by the renal hormone **erythropoietin**, a polypeptide available commercially as recombinant human erythropoietin and used for the treatment of severe anaemia of renal origin.

White-cell precursors, **myeloblasts**, are at first undifferentiated. They acquire characteristic granules to become **myelocytes** before maturing as neutrophil, eosinophil and basophil **granulocytes**.

Platelets are derived from **megakaryocytes**, each of which breaks up to form as many as 3000 of these small, freely-movable, anucleate cells.

Now read Anaemia (p. 10), Leucocytes (p. 206), Platelets (p. 273)

HAEMOSIDEROSIS

Haemosiderosis is the accumulation of excess iron-containing haemosiderin in the cells of the mononuclear macrophage system. So much iron may be present that organs like the liver and spleen come to have a deep brown colour. The clinical abnormality originates because a small number of patients with persistent blood loss or a failure of red blood cell production require repeated blood transfusion over many months or years. The cells of the transfused blood are haemolysed more quickly than normal, liberating large quantities of iron-containing pigment.

Haemosiderosis is distinguished from the heritable condition of haemochromatosis.

Now read Iron (p. 271)

HAEMOSTASIS

Following injury, haemorrhage (p. 42) is diminished by arterial vasoconstriction, a process mediated by the sympathetic nervous system. The vascular response is induced by the release of adrenaline from blood platelets. Haemostasis and vasoconstriction begin to arrest bleeding simultaneously. The process has two components, primary and secondary.

PRIMARY HAEMOSTASIS

Within seconds of injury, there is the formation of a platelet plug, the function of which is to prevent bleeding from capillaries, arterioles and venules. When a blood vessel is damaged, von Willebrand factor (vWF) is bound to the damaged endothelium, promoting platelet adhesion. A plug of platelets accumulates and reduces or arrests the loss of blood. The poor formation of a platelet plug makes excessive haemorrhage clinically evident immediately after operation or injury.

Now read Bleeding, Blood loss (p. 42)

SECONDARY HAEMOSTASIS

Secondary haemostasis, the coagulation of blood *in vivo*, begins some minutes after vascular injury. The process comprises activation of the coagulation cascade (p. 95), the function of which is to prevent subsequent, delayed bleeding, hours or days after the initial trauma. This is achieved by the deposition of fibrin over the fragile platelet plug.

von Willebrand factor (p. 100) and platelets (p. 273) are also important in secondary haemostasis. Disorders of vWF (p. 100) or of platelets (p. 99) produce abnormalities of both primary and secondary haemostasis.

Now read Coagulation (p. 95), Thrombosis (p. 320)

HAMARTOMA

A hamartoma is a congenital malformation. It is a tumour-like mass or nodule. Many hamartomas are formed of a conglomerate of tissues but one tissue usually predominates. Unlike a tumour, a hamartoma grows at the same rate and in the same proportions as the tissue in which it arises. There is no capsule. The tissues of which a hamartoma is formed are often vascular, but, as in the case of pulmonary hamartoma, the lesion is sometimes composed of hyaline cartilage or of other mesenchymal or epithelial tissues. Although arising *in utero* and present at birth, hamartomas may only be recognised in later life. They atrophy with advancing age.

HEALING

In a **general** sense, to heal is to cure a disease, or to restore to health.

In a **specific**, surgical sense, the term 'healing' is applied to the restoration of the tissues of a wound to normal. Healing of tissues that retain a capacity for cell division is by regeneration. Thus, the epidermal cells of the skin and those of the liver, renal tubules, bone and adrenal cortex regenerate by mitotic division. By contrast, the central nervous system and heart muscle heal by repair. This process is the substitution of glial or fibrous tissue for a defect.

Now read Fibrosis (p. 131), Repair (p. 285)

HEART

Biopsy diagnosis of cardiac disease

Repetitive biopsy of the atrial musculature plays a central part in assessing the response to cardiac transplantation (p. 149). Needle biopsy of the ventricular muscle can be used to identify cardiac metastases, amyloidosis and parasitic disease.

DEVELOPMENTAL AND CONGENITAL DISORDERS

Fewer than 10% of congenital abnormalities of cardiac development arise on the basis of genetic mutation. Some, such as the tetralogy of Fallot, are polygenic; others such as atrioventricular septal defect, are attributable to a single gene defect. An even smaller proportion has a demonstrable, environmental cause. The majority remain unexplained. Among the known causal agents are rubella virus and compounds such as thalidomide, anticonvulsants, drugs of addiction and alcohol. Many of the developmental cardiac defects compatible with independent existence are recognisable shortly after birth or in infancy. A substantial number can be corrected either by open heart surgery or, as in the case of persistent ductus arteriosus, by the intra-arterial introduction of an occluding umbrella or other device. In many instances, emergency or preliminary surgical treatment is effected at the time of diagnosis, to be followed by definitive surgery later in childhood.

Congenital cardiac defects can be categorised:

- **anatomically** according to their nature and location;
- **functionally** according to the presence (cyanotic) or absence (acyanotic) of cyanosis.

The functional effects of developmental cardiac disease are principally those of shunts. Blood ejected from the heart may be diverted by a left-to-right shunt leading to heart failure. Among the complications are bacterial endocarditis, pulmonary hypertension with reversal of the shunt and paradoxical embolism. Alternatively, blood may be diverted by a right-to-left shunt. In other instances of congenital cardiac defect, however, no shunt is present.

Acyanotic congenital cardiac defects

The presence of a defect may not be recognised until adult life.

With left-to-right shunt

- **Patent interatrial septum** is the most common defect. Unless an excessive rise occurs in right atrial blood pressure, simple valvular patency, persistent ostium primum and persistent ostium secundum are symptomless. Paradoxical arterial embolism may occur without warning in an otherwise healthy individual, or following surgery (p. 125).
- **Isolated interventricular septal defect** is usually detected high within the interventricular septum. The abnormality often exists as part of **Fallot's tetralogy**.
- **Patency of the ductus arteriosus** is a consequence of defective closure which normally takes place soon after birth. The onset of pulmonary hypertension determines that the flow of blood through a patent ductus may be reversed. Cyanosis is then recognisable.

Without left-to-right shunt

Right-sided lesions

- **Uncomplicated pulmonary valve stenosis**. In this defect, cyanosis is not evident unless further change leads to pulmonary artery hypertension with outflow obstruction. The effects of stenosis of the pulmonary artery and of the infundibulum of the right ventricle are similar.

- **Ebstein's anomaly**. In this rare defect, a more complex situation exists. A raised right atrial blood pressure is attributable to tricuspid valve incompetence with right ventricular hypoplasia. The high right atrial blood pressure is relieved by the co-existence of an atrial septal defect but, under these circumstances, mycotic or sterile paradoxical embolism may ensue.

Left-sided lesions

- **Aortic valve stenosis**. In this condition, the valve, which may be bicuspid, may be affected by stenotic lesions occurring above, at, or below the valve.
- **Mitral valve stenosis** may also be recognised congenitally.
- **Coarctation of the aorta** is a narrowing of the aorta between the origin of the left subclavian artery and the ductus arteriosus. The narrowing may be proximal (infantile) or distal (adult) to the opening of the ductus.
  - The adult form may be asymptomatic until maturity. By this time, the defect may have allowed the development of a collateral circulation, diverting blood from the carotid and subclavian arteries to aortic branches below the obstruction. One consequence is hypertension restricted to the upper limbs and proximal vessels.
  - In the infantile form, the pulmonary artery blood pressure is higher than that of the aorta beyond the coarctation. Since non-oxygenated blood enters the aorta distal to the subclavian artery, there is selective cyanosis and failure of growth of the lower limbs only.

Cyanotic congenital cardiac defects

- **Tetralogy of Fallot** is the most common cyanotic syndrome. There are four inter-related defects: pulmonary artery stenosis; consequential right ventricular hypertrophy; interventricular septal defect; and transposition of the aorta which overrides the septal defect. The aorta receives both oxygenated blood from the left ventricle and non-oxygenated blood from the hypertrophic right ventricle. Central cyanosis results from the passage of blood from the hypertrophic right ventricle to the left ventricle.
- **Eisenmenger's complex**. In an analogous situation, there is no pulmonary stenosis and little or no right-to-left shunting of blood.
- **Transposition of the great vessels**. In this uncommon syndrome, the pulmonary artery arises from the left ventricle, the aorta from the right. The pulmonary and systemic circulations are therefore separate. Blood cannot be oxygenated. Survival is therefore only possible if a septal defect or patent ductus co-exists or if a communication can be made surgically. In corrected transposition, there is inversion of the ventricles so that the left ventricle receives blood from the right atrium, the right ventricle blood from the left atrium. When pulmonary stenosis accompanies patency of the interatrial septum, the venous blood is directed to the left rather than to the right atrium.
- **Persistent truncus arteriosus**. There is defective formation of the spiral septum of the truncus arteriosus, determining that a common truncus arises from both ventricles. Few children survive infancy unless the defect is corrected surgically.
- **Tricuspid atresia**. When the tricuspid valve is absent, there is no connection between the right atrium and the hypoplastic right ventricle. Blood is shunted from the right to the left atrium and the child is cyanotic.

METABOLIC DISORDERS

Amyloidosis

Primary amyloidosis (p. 9) of the heart cannot be reversed. It is inevitably fatal unless treated by cardiac transplantation.

Now read Amyloid (p. 9)

INFECTION AND INFLAMMATION

Endocarditis

Acute bacterial endocarditis – inflammation of the endocardial surfaces of the heart, including the valves – occasionally results from the presence of a central 'line' or cannula. It is a complication of immunosuppression. The infection may be bacterial or fungal but the causative organisms are often coagulase-negative *Staphylococcus epidermidis* and faecal streptococci.

When endocarditis develops in the absence of a central 'line', there are two main causes:

- The first is the presence of an abnormal cardiac valve or other defect. Viridans streptococci are liberated into the bloodstream during dental manipulation; they colonise the valve and lead to its destruction.
- The second cause is drug addiction. In those taking 'hard' drugs intravenously, bacteria grow on the previously normal tricuspid valve. *Staphylococcus aureus* is a particular problem However, coagulase-negative staphylococci are increasingly implicated in infections associated with foreign bodies such as heart-valve prostheses.

Myocarditis

Myocardial muscle may be parasitised by virus, bacteria and protozoa and injured by immune complexes or, directly, by chemical and physical irritants. Coxsackie B virus and the toxin of the diphtheria bacillus, *Corynebacterium diphtheriae*, are potent agents causing myocardial cell injury. Chagas' disease infects ~8% of the populations of Brazil and the Argentine. Heart muscle is one of its principal targets.

TRANSPLANTATION

With improved immunosuppression, the transplanted heart may survive long periods (p. 369). Nevertheless, the organ is just as liable to develop coronary artery atheroma as the original organ. In countries where the surgical skills are available, the operation is now restricted by the supply of donor hearts, raising new and difficult ethical considerations. More than 40 000 heart transplants have been completed worldwide and the demand is increasing. Because of secondary damage to the lungs, many patients formerly treated by cardiac transplantation alone now undergo simultaneous, combined heart–lung transplantation.

Episodes of rejection occur most frequently during the first year after transplantation. The frequency of these episodes decreases thereafter but persists throughout life. The diagnosis of rejection is made by repetitive transatrial myocardial biopsy. A grading system is used to assess rejection. It centres on recognising lymphocytic infiltration and myocyte necrosis.

Now read Transplantation (p. 329)

MECHANICAL AND HYDRODYNAMIC DISORDERS

Heart failure

Heart failure exists when the organ is unable to maintain a circulation sufficient for the needs of the body, in spite of an adequate venous filling pressure. In patients unsuitable for cardiac transplantation, tests are being made of large, intracorporeal or perivascular, mechanical pumps, and of small intracardiac pumps, that can maintain a circulation artificially.

Acute

Acute heart failure occurs in shock, of which many instances are cardiogenic. Missiles such as rubber bullets and objects like cricket balls can injure the myocardium directly, resulting in ventricular fibrillation and immediate heart failure. Sudden death among young athletes and footballers may result from the long QT syndrome (LQTS) or other unrecognised congenital heart disease. In LQTS, ion channels function poorly, either because of a genetic mutation, or because of acquired metabolic abnormalities such as hypokalaemia. A considerable number of drugs including quinidine, citrate and some antibiotics may have this effect. Ventricular polarisation is impaired, resulting in a ventricular arrhythmia. Acute heart failure may also be a complication of virus or bacterial infection. Diphtheria is one cause, Coxsackie virus infection another.

Chronic

Heart failure poses problems for surgeons and anaesthetists. There may be defective metabolism of anaesthetic agents and drugs; defective tissue perfusion with impaired regulation of water balance, gaseous exchange, pH and electrolytes; inadequate cardiovascular response to haemorrhage; and an increased susceptibility to venous thrombosis and its complications.

Mechanisms

The heart fails either because of an overwhelming load of work or because the cardiac muscle is abnormal. These factors frequently co-exist. An increased load is imposed by either a demand to expel a higher volume of blood per unit time than normal (**volume load)** or because of increased resistance to the expulsion of blood from the heart (**pressure load)**.

Examples of failure due to volume load include anaemia and thyrotoxicosis, in which a high cardiac output is required to become increasingly higher; and mitral and aortic valve incompetence, in which the heart attempts to expel both the normal ventricular volume of blood and that which regurgitates through the abnormal valve.

Examples of failure due to pressure load are systemic hypertension and aortic stenosis. Impaired cardiac muscle function is usually the result of coronary artery insufficiency but cardiomyopathy and amyloidosis are other causes.

Effects

As the heart responds to an increased workload, the ventricle dilates and cardiac muscle hypertrophies. Cardiac output then becomes inadequate and there is a progressive retention of Na^+, and thus of water. This is in part due to impaired glomerular filtration but is largely attributable to increased renal tubular Na^+ reabsorption. Hyperaldosteronism (p. 6) is characteristic of advanced cardiac failure. These changes together culminate in rising venous pressure and in capillary and venous stagnation ('congestion') in the viscera.

Left heart failure

In left heart failure, resulting from defective function of the left ventricle or atrium, there is engorgement of the pulmonary veins and capillaries and ultimately pulmonary oedema. The causes include systemic hypertension; aortic and mitral valvular disease; myocardial infarction; and cardiomyopathy.

Right heart failure

In right heart failure, due to defective function of the right ventricle or atrium, there is engorgement of the liver, kidneys and other organs, and of the systemic veins, together with oedema (p. 251). The common causes include pulmonary diseases such as chronic bronchitis and emphysema. Right heart failure commonly follows left heart failure.

CARDIOMYOPATHY

The cardiomyopathies are a complex series of diseases that affect the myocardium directly. They are not the result of hypertension or of congenital, valvular, coronary arterial or pericardial abnormality. There are two categories. In the first, the cause is often uncertain. Some cases may be familial. Fifteen per cent of these cases can be explained by mutations in the gene for cardiac myosin-binding protein C. In the second, the causes range from metabolic deficiency, connective tissue and storage disorders, to hypersensitivity and neuromuscular disease. The possibility exists of replacing myopathic left ventricular muscle with grafts of skeletal muscle.

TUMOURS

Metastases to the heart are rarely detected clinically but can be found microscopically in more than 10% of cases of metastatic carcinomatosis. The heart is seldom the site of primary benign or malignant neoplasms but atrial myxoma and rhabdomyosarcoma are occasionally identified.

DISORDERS OF THE CARDIAC VASCULATURE

Acute myocardial ischaemia

The sudden loss of, or obstruction to, the arterial blood supply to part of the left or, less commonly, the right ventricular myocardium leads quickly to irreversible injury to heart muscle cells. A significant fall in blood pressure during or after surgery may be a precipitating factor. Cardiac muscle cells sustain such injury within 5–15 minutes of the onset of ischaemia. The result is myocardial infarction, the anatomical distribution of which is determined by the extent of the tissue supplied by the affected artery.

The most common cause of acute cardiac ischaemia is thrombosis of the proximal part of the anterior descending branch of the left coronary artery or vasospasm of this vessel. There is often an underlying atheromatous plaque. The resulting infarct is of the anterolateral wall of the left ventricle, although more extensive infarcts include the anterior part of the interventricular septum.

Now read Ischaemia (p. 187)

Chronic myocardial ischaemia

Cardiac muscle cells, like those of the arteries, do not regenerate. Following recovery from an episode of acute ischaemia, a zone of myocardial necrosis persists. It is often of a left ventricular or septal distribution and of varying extent. In time, the infarct is replaced by fibrous tissue. The mechanical properties of the ischaemic zone are impaired and arrhythmias, heart failure and ventricular aneurysm are among the possible consequences. In older patients, the recognition of electrocardiographic abnormalities is a warning of possible surgical catastrophe.

CARDIAC TAMPONADE

The escape of blood at arterial pressure into the pericardial sac quickly fills this cavity, leading to obstruction of the venous return to the right atrium. Cardiac output falls and, unless the tamponade is quickly relieved, death occurs. The cause is commonly rupture of a transmural myocardial infarct. The second most frequent explanation of tamponade is as a complication of acute aortic dissection. Other causes include surgical operations upon the heart; deliberate or accidental injury by sharp objects; bleeding during the course of diseases of the blood and bone marrow; uraemia; or the presence of local inflammatory or auto-immune disease.

HEAT EXCESS

LOCAL

The local effects of heat on a tissue depend upon the temperature attained. Tissue can be irreversibly injured at temperatures exceeding 45°C. Up to a temperature of 50°C, there is profuse vasodilatation, with an increase in vascular permeability and the formation of a protein-rich exudate. Above 50°C, there is denaturation of protein and inactivation of intracellular enzymes. Sludging of blood and intravascular haemolysis are recognised.

Diathermy

The heat used to coagulate tissue by diathermy is generated by high-frequency electric currents. Temperatures in excess of 1000°C can be produced. By altering the frequency and current, the same apparatus can cut (high temperature) or coagulate (low temperature) tissue.

SYSTEMIC

Heat stroke

Heat stroke is a body temperature greater than 40.6°C accompanied by anhidrosis and delirium, coma or seizures. The principal cause of 'heat stroke' is inadequate loss of heat because of deficient cutaneous evaporation, a situation that may develop when there is exposure of the unacclimatised body to excessive temperature and high humidity. Heat stroke occurs when there is thermoregulatory failure. The systemic, pathological effects of heat show similarities to septic shock. In fever, thermoregulation is usually intact.

Now read Burns (p. 71), Shock (p. 290)

HELICOBACTER PYLORI

Spiral organisms such as *Helicobacter pylori* were first identified in the human stomach in the nineteenth century but the significance of such an infection has only been recognised during the last two decades. *H. pylori* is a well-adapted parasite, occupying a specialised ecological niche: it lives only in the human stomach and, possibly, the duodenum.

In humans, the organism is carried by at least 50% of persons over the age of 50 years. Compared with healthy individuals, there is a greatly raised prevalence in patients with gastric (p. 308) and duodenal ulceration (p. 121); in patients with acute or chronic gastritis; in those with carcinoma of the stomach (p. 309); and in patients with intestinal lymphoma (p. 168). In adults, the frequency of infection is particularly high among subjects in regular contact with infected individuals. Those at risk include endoscopists and school teachers. The incidence of infection is high within families. However, the frequency of infection in the West has been decreasing spontaneously and rapidly.

This decline has been attributed to improved nutrition, including the consumption by children of fresh fruit and vegetables; and to the refrigeration of food. The benefits of small family size; improved standards of hygiene; and of the judicious use of antibiotics, have been recorded.

The organisms can be identified rapidly in endoscopic biopsies. They express a potent urease. Ammonia, released by the enzyme, induces a change in colour in a pH indicator. The procedure is described inaccurately as a CLO test since *Helicobacter pylori* was at first categorised as a Campylobacter-like organism (CLO). Urease is also the basis of a breath test. Serological tests employing the ELISA technique demonstrate circulating antibodies and are used in diagnostic and epidemiological studies.

The genome sequence of *Helicobacter pylori* has been identified. Mutations are frequent and there are many strains with differing pathogenicity and antibiotic sensitivity. Some strains possess a cytotoxin associated gene (*Cag*). The cytotoxin is highly antigenic and may be related to pathogenicity, particularly with regard to the development of gastric cancer (p. 309). The toxin can be detected in the serum of infected patients. The identification of the *Cag* gene may allow the development of an effective vaccine.

HEPATITIS

Hepatitis is inflammation of the liver. The inflammation may be focal or diffuse, acute or chronic. Acute hepatitis of surgical significance is usually viral although inflammation of the liver can be bacterial (as in abscess), protozoal (as in amoebiasis) or metazoal (as in hydatid disease).

ACUTE VIRAL HEPATITIS

Acute viral hepatitis is a result of liver-cell injury caused by the hepatitis viruses (Table 29). It may also be provoked by other agents, including the Coxsackie B and herpes simplex viruses in neonates; the virus of yellow fever; cytomegalovirus; rubella virus in the embryo or adult; the Epstein–Barr (EB) virus in glandular fever; and herpes simplex and varicella zoster viruses in immunosuppressed subjects.

Now read Virus (p. 347)

HEPATITIS VIRUSES

There are at least eight different viruses (Table 29). The clinical features they cause have many similarities. Some, at least, may be transmitted by sexual contact. Hepatitis A (HA) and E (HE) are transmitted by the faecal–oral route. They are largely of medical interest and are not considered further. Hepatitis B (HB), C (HC), D (HD) and G (HG) are transmitted by blood and blood products and they are therefore of high significance in the practice of surgery.

Hepatitis B

Hepatitis B (HB) (Fig. 55b) is caused by a DNA virus, a member of the Hepadna group.

Virus structure

The virion or Dane particle (Fig. 55b), a 42 nm diameter icosahedron, has an inner 27 nm diameter core containing DNA, and an outer envelope. The very small amount of DNA of the viral genome is circular and, in part, double-stranded. Three viral antigens are recognised. In infection, each gives rise to corresponding antibodies.

- **Hepatitis B surface antigen (HBsAg)** exists on the outer surface of the HBV virion. It is present in the blood as numerous small particles. Their presence indicates infectivity. Anti-HBsAg antibody (HBsAb) provides immunity to hepatitis B but appears late. It is not formed in carriers.
- **Core antigen (HBcAg)** encloses the DNA core. Antibody to HBcAg (HBcAb) appears early in the disease.
- **Antigen derived from the HB virus core, HBeAg**. This antigen is formed from the breakdown of HBcAg released from infected liver cells. The appearance of e antigen in the serum is correlated with viral replication and its presence indicates heightened transmissibility. Anti-HBeAg antibody (HBeAb) forms.

Transmission

HB virus present in the circulating blood can be conveyed by extremely small quantities of blood or blood products, or other body fluids, by means of direct contact. Patients with acute hepatitis and carriers of virus bearing the e antigen are particular hazards for the transmission of infection by inoculation injury; by

Table 29 The hepatitis viruses and their properties

	HA	HB	HC	HD	HE	HF	HG
Nature of virus	Enterovirus 72 ssRNA	Hepadnavirus dsDNA	Togavirus ssRNA	Very small ssRNA	Calicivirus ssRNA	Not yet known	Not yet known – the 'orphan' virus
Route of transmission	Faecal–oral	Blood Sexual contact	Blood ?Sexual contact	Blood	Faecal–oral	Blood	Blood Transplacental Drug abuse Associated with carriage of HC
Incubation period	2–4 weeks	~ 100 days	8 weeks	2–12 weeks	6–8 weeks	Not known	Not known
Diagnosis by detecting serum	Anti-HA-specific IgM	HBsAg in incubation period; later, anti-HBsAb Presence of serum HBeAg indicates transmissibility	Presence of anti-HBcAg suggests virus may also be present and patient may be infectious Polymerase chain reaction	HDdAg (delta Ag) or anti-HBdAg Ab	Tests not yet available	Tests not yet available	Test not yet available
Carriage of virus long-term	–	+	±	+	–	Not known	+
Treatment	Passive or active (vaccine) immunisation No antiviral drug yet effective	Active (vaccine) immunisation or specific gammaglobulin No specific antiviral drug available Interferons alpha and beta may clear virus	No vaccine Interferon alpha and ribavirin may be effective	No vaccine Anti-HB vaccination prevents hepatitis D	?Passive immunisation	Not yet possible	May not be necessary – benign outcome
					Largely in Asia, especially India		

perinatal infection in pregnant women; and by sexual contact. Spread also takes place between those who abuse intravenous drugs of addiction; male homosexuals; and during ear-piercing, tattooing or acupuncture. Particularly in South-East Asia, vertical transmission between mother and child is frequent. The infection may be intra-uterine; perinatal; or post-natal, in breast milk.

Incubation

HB has a mean incubation period of ~100 days (Fig. 26). Virus replicates in lymphoid tissue before entering the blood and passing to the liver. Inflammation is provoked and liver cells undergo necrosis. Clinical signs of disease appear. Liver-cell injury is not direct but is mediated by cytotoxic T-cells (p. 173). Immune complexes are formed. They lodge in the joints, skin and arteries, and may cause transient arthritis, skin rashes and vasculitis.

Antibody formation

Following infection, antibodies are formed against all three of the viral antigens but the significance of their identification differs in an important sense.

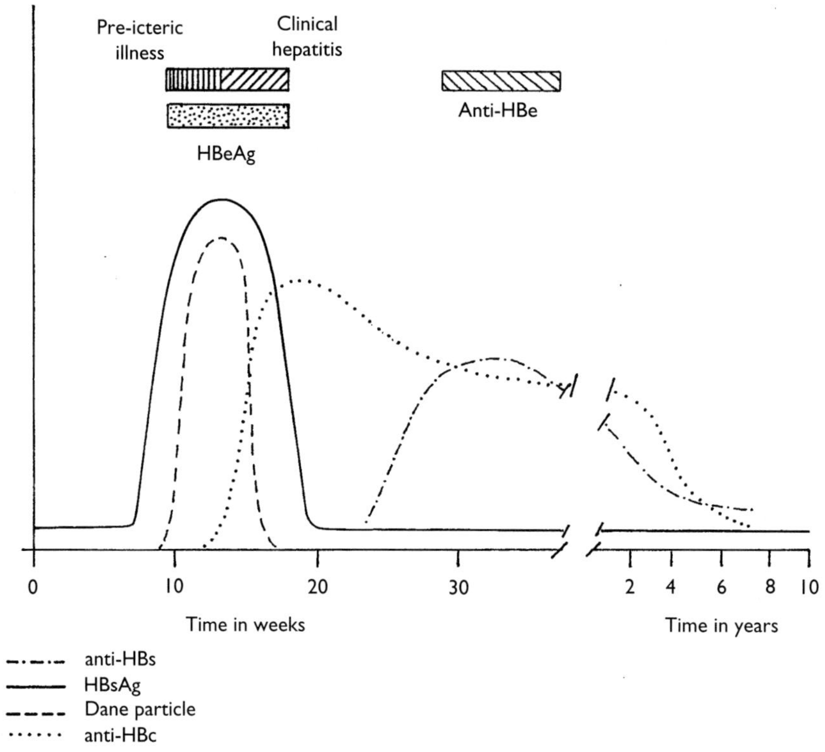

Figure 26 Pathogenesis of hepatitis B.
Diagram indicates time scale of events in self-limiting disease, with clinical and virological course and sequence of events. Following infection, virus replicates in lymphoid tissue before passing to blood stream and liver. As specific antibodies form, immune complexes may provoke arthralgia and skin rashes. Liver injury, caused mainly by virus-specific T-cells, increases. Clinical signs of hepatitis appear. Subsequently, immunity increases, fewer virions are formed, and signs of clinical disease decline. Ultimately, blood may become non-infective. However 10% of infected individuals, particularly infected infants, become carriers. HBc, HBe and HBs are viral antigens.

- Infected persons and carriers have HBsAg and anti-HBcAg but lack anti-HBsAg in their blood.
- On recovery from infection, HBsAg disappears from the blood. Anti-HBsAg is demonstrable later, together with anti-HBcAg.

Clinical manifestations

Raised serum levels of enzymes such as aspartate aminotransferase (AST) (Appendix Tables) precede the insidious onset of jaundice which may persist for 4–12 weeks. Fifty per cent of infections are subclinical. Those who have had the infection, clinically or subclinically, may survive as symptomless carriers.

Carriers

A carrier is a person shown to have had HBsAg for not less than 6 months.

Between 7% and 10% of survivors in Western Europe become carriers. World-wide, this amounts to ~3×10^6 individuals. Most have had an anicteric infection. Patients who have become jaundiced usually recover. Carriers are very frequent among drug addicts (50%), those who have been tattooed, and male homosexuals. There is also a high incidence of HB among the populations of South-East Asia and in other places where the liver is prone to injury because of malnutrition or other co-incidental disease. A large proportion of the infections in South-East Asia is among neonates. The carrier rate in these populations can vary from 10 to 30%. Predisposition to infection may be racial as it is among the Chinese.

Many patients contract infection and become carriers as a result of perinatal infection transmitted by carrier mothers at the time of birth. Others who have a high chance of becoming symptomless carriers, if exposed to HB infection, are individuals with chronic uraemia; those treated with immunosuppressive drugs; and those with heritable disorders such as Down's syndrome. There is increased hazard in institutions and among patients with mental disease.

Chronic hepatitis B

The continued presence of hepatitis virus infection may lead to chronic hepatitis that may become either persistent or active (p. 211). The former is a self-limiting process and is innocuous. The latter, in which a disturbance of the immune mechanism has been provoked, is progressively damaging. It is likely to lead to hepatic cirrhosis (p. 211) and its consequences.

Now read Liver infection (p. 210)

Hazards in surgery

The chances of seroconversion to HBV-positivity are 100 times greater than to HIV-positivity (p. 2).

Infective virus may survive in blood and body fluids for many years after the acute infection has subsided. Affected surgeons constitute a hazard to all patients. The presence of HBsAb is of no significance but the persistence in the blood of infective virus in the form of circulating HBeAg particles precludes the safe practice of surgery.

- **Patients**. Patients with normal immune systems who require great quantities of blood or blood products such as factor VIII, prepared from large pools of plasma, have an increased likelihood of contracting HB but no increased tendency to become carriers.
- **Surgeons and other staff**. There is an increased risk of infection among staff working in units where blood and blood products are frequently used in treatment and in laboratories dealing with blood, blood products or unfixed tissues. The amount of blood constituting a hazard may be microscopic. Vaccination minimises this risk provided that circulating antibody levels remain adequate. Consequently, periodic tests for HBsAb are required and booster doses of recombinant vaccine given when necessary. All hospital staff in the UK have a legal obligation to inform management if they become infected with HBV.

Vaccination

Active protection against HB is provided by a vaccine made from genetically engineered HBsAg. Partial protection after accidental inoculation injury or sexual contact can be given by the **passive** administration of hyperimmune globulin prepared from the plasma of donors such as haemophiliacs who have acquired high titres of anti-HBsAg antibody. Combined active and passive immunisation may be highly effective if given within 48 hours of exposure, for example after needle-stick injury (p. 362).

Pathogenesis

Liver injury in hepatitis B is due to cell-mediated hypersensitivity associated with anti-HBc. The identification of HBeAg confirms that the HB virus is actively replicating within hepatocytes. Complexes of HBe and anti-HBe may cause arteritis, glomerulonephritis and synovitis as well as exacerbating liver injury.

Carcinogenesis

Long-standing hepatitis B infection is closely associated with a high incidence of hepatocellular carcinoma (p. 213). The carrier state, chronic hepatitis and cirrhosis precede neoplasia. Multiple copies of hepatitis B viral DNA are integrated into the liver-cell genome within 1–2 years of infection. Cancer develops 20–30 years later and HB virus can be identified in the tumour cells.

Hepatitis C

The hepatitis C virus (HCV) is the cause of more than 90% of cases of post-transfusion hepatitis (p. 47). Fifty per cent of drug abusers are HCV-positive and the virus is thought to be transmissable sexually. Blood donors are now always tested for the presence of anti-HCV antibody. Following infection, more than 50% of those infected develop chronic active hepatitis. The risk to health is much greater than with hepatitis B. Post-hepatic cirrhosis is common and there is a predisposition to hepatocellular carcinoma. The hepatitis G virus is associated with the carriage of HCV.

Hepatitis D

A further hepatitis virus, hepatitis D virus (HDV), is transmitted by blood and blood products. The disease is common in South America and Africa but uncommon in the UK and the USA. The virus is 'defective' and can only multiply within a liver cell if the cell is already infected by HBV. When HDV buds from the surface of a hepatocyte, it acquires an envelope of HBs that renders HDV infectious. The clinical syndrome caused by HDV infection is more severe than that of hepatitis B alone. Infected blood contains very large amounts of the infective agent.

Hepatitis F

The cause of 10% of cases of post-blood-transfusion hepatitis is attributed to an agent designated hepatitis F virus (HFV).

Hepatitis G

The nature of this transfusion-related virus is not yet known.

HEPATORENAL SYNDROME

This term has been used to describe the condition of patients dying from liver failure with concurrent evidence of renal failure. There is no microscopical evidence of tubular necrosis. The association between hepatic and renal failure is observed following operations for long-standing obstructive jaundice. Renal damage may therefore be caused by bacterial endotoxins liberated from Gram-negative micro-organisms in the bile. If liver transplantation is effected, kidney function recovers.

HERNIA

Hernia is a protrusion of a structure beyond the cavity in which it is normally confined. The orifice through which a hernia protrudes may be a natural opening, such as the oesophageal hiatus, or an acquired opening, such as an incision. When a hernial sac can be returned to its original site, the hernia is **reducible**. If an abdominal hernia becomes **irreducible**, there is a risk of strangulation, that is, an obstruction to the flow of blood through the tissues contained within the hernia. The consequences are gangrene of the hernial sac contents; intestinal perforation; and peritonitis. Strangulation is most frequent with femoral, umbilical and para-oesophageal herniation.

ABDOMINAL HERNIA

The majority of hernias are associated with the abdominal cavity. The hernial sac is derived from the peritoneum and may contain bowel. Most abdominal hernias are external: they are inguinal, femoral, umbilical, ventral or lumbar. A few are internal: hiatus hernia is one example (p. 254).

External abdominal hernia

Inguinal hernia

Inguinal hernias are much the most common and occur predominantly in males because of the congenital weakness of the inguinal canal caused by the descent of the testes *in utero*.

Femoral hernia

Femoral hernias are more frequent in females than males. The female pelvis is wider than that of the male, the diameter of the femoral canal greater.

Obturator hernia

Obturator hernias are rare. The symptoms may mimic hip joint disease.

Internal abdominal hernia

The only common variety is hiatus hernia (p. 254). Herniation may follow traumatic rupture of the diaphragm, an injury associated with road-traffic or aircraft accidents. Rarely, internal herniation takes place into the paraduodenal and para-appendiceal fossas.

Incisional hernia

These common hernias are protrusions of the peritoneum through a weak scar after an operation or following a penetrating wound. Many are asymptomatic. Careful post-operative review shows an increase in incidence to >10% after 10 years, suggesting a failure of collagen formation and maturation.

Some of the many factors associated with an increased risk of incisional hernia are indicated in Table 30.

Table 30 Some factors associated with the development of incisional hernia

Cancer
Diabetes mellitus
Immunosuppression
Jaundice
Malnutrition
Obesity
Old age
Poor surgical technique
Wound haematoma
Wound sepsis

CEREBRAL HERNIA

Cerebral hernia is one result of raised intracranial pressure (p. 62).

Now read Intracranial disease (p. 61)

HISTOLOGY

Histology is the study of tissues. Histopathology is the study of diseased tissues. Histological preparations and their microscopic investigation are of crucial importance in surgical diagnosis and management.

Most histopathological diagnoses are made with microscopes that transmit light through thin tissue preparations. Conventional light cannot penetrate thick samples so that images sufficiently clear to allow surgical diagnosis cannot be obtained from specimens more than ~10–12 μm in thickness. It is therefore necessary to cut biopsy specimens into thin sections. To allow this to be done expeditiously, it is generally necessary first to harden the specimen by fixation or freezing (p. 41). Fixation has the additional value of ensuring sterility and of preventing autolysis and putrefaction.

Fixation

For most purposes, a specimen to be preserved should be placed in ten times its own volume of fixative. The solutions used for this purpose are neutral buffered formalin or formal saline, ethanol or glutaraldehyde.

Now read Biopsy (p. 40)

Processing

Blocks of tissue, often about 15 × 15 × 4 mm in size, are cut carefully from a fixed specimen. Compression of tissue by forceps and scissors is avoided since it distorts the material and obscures the subsequent microscopic interpretation of sections. The blocks are placed in the labelled, plastic casettes of a processing system. In large laboratories, these machines are computer-controlled and operate on increasingly brief schedules. The blocks are passed through a sequence of ethanols or other alcohols of increasing concentration, into xylol from which the tissue is impregnated in molten paraffin wax. A wax is chosen that has a melting point high enough to remain solid on the warmest days. The plastic cassette with its tissue block is brought out of the paraffin bath on to a warm plate. The tissue is orientated in a metal mould, the cassette replaced on top and filled with wax which is allowed to cool and harden.

Sectioning

Sections for microscopy are often 3 to 5 μm thick. They are cut from a solidified wax block by means of a microtome – a strong, heavy, metal machine in which the tissue is moved across the blade of a disposable steel-alloy or glass knife. For special purposes, such as the cutting of very hard tissues, horizontal sledge microtomes with tungsten steel knives are used. The cut sections are floated on to glass slides in a water bath. They adhere to the glass as they dry, a process made more effective by coating the glass with an agent such as albumin or poly-l-lysine.

Frozen sections are commonly made in a cryostat, a chamber containing a microtome and chilled to –25°C.

In preparation for electron microscopy, use is made of thinner 0.5 to 1.0 μm sections cut from tissue embedded in high-density polymers.

When bone and calcified tissues are to be examined, undecalcified specimens are prepared on a specialised bone microtome or the calcium is removed after fixation but before processing.

Staining

Stains (Table 31) are dyes and chemicals used to create optical contrast by colouring cells, tissues and micro-organisms to make them visible. Without stains, tissue sections remain transparent. Before staining, the paraffin wax is removed from a section with xylol. In surgical diagnosis, the classical haematoxylin and eosin (HE) method is still widely employed. Eosin colours cytoplasm, haematoxylin nuclei. The further identification of surgical disorders is made by applying a variety of stains or reagents specific for individual tissue structures or molecules.

Table 31 Some staining techniques used in surgical histopathological diagnosis

Material demonstrated	Staining method
Amyloid	Congo red + polarised light
Bacteria	Gram Ziehl-Neelsen
Bone and calcified tissues	Goldner Masson von Kossa
Collagen	picro Sirius red van Gieson
Elastic tissue	Weigert's
Lipid	oil red O Sudan III
Mucin	Alcian blue–periodic acid Schiff (PAS)
Proteoglycan	toluidine blue

Histochemical methods

Histochemical methods offer the possibility of demonstrating a very wide range of inorganic and organic molecules in tissue preparations. Elements such as iron and copper can be identified and enzyme reaction products shown. In enzyme histochemistry, the fresh tissue is exposed to a substrate that yields a characteristic colour at the sites of activity of particular enzymes. Prostatic acid phosphatase (prostatic cancer) is one example, glucose-6-phosphate dehydrogenase (skeletal muscle disorders) another.

Immunohistochemical methods

Surgical diagnosis has been revolutionised by the introduction of a large and increasing range of commercially available antibodies. Many are monoclonal (p. 234) and individual antibodies for special requirements can be made to order. Immunocytochemical techniques form an indispensable part of routines for categorising a great range of surgical disorders. The techniques of immunohistochemistry can demonstrate, for example, tumour antigens (p. 247); human leucocyte antigens; immunoglobulins; complement; fibrin; hormones; growth factors; and cytokines. The methods are sensitive and precise. However, fresh, frozen sections may sometimes be required.

Fluorescent methods

Fluorescent techniques form an indispensable part of routines for identifying surgical abnormalities. The use of ultraviolet or laser light enables a wide range of large molecules to be located with sensitivity and precision. Fresh, frozen sections may be needed. Moreover, fluorescent labels can be destroyed ('quenched') quickly by the high-energy, short-wavelength light that is used. Indeed, paradoxically, the higher the magnification of the lens chosen to identify cell detail, the more rapid the loss of fluorescence.

Many antigens can be shown by an indirect, sandwich method. A small quantity of costly, diluted, monoclonal antibody is applied to a section. The specific antigen–antibody binding site is then displayed at the reaction site by the application of a second, cheaper polyclonal anti-antibody. Laser confocal microscopes allow two, three or more binding sites to be located simultaneously.

Non-fluorescent methods

For reasons of convenience, non-fluorescent methods have been adopted. The avidin-biotin method is a favoured procedure. In this method, a primary antibody is used to identify a cell component, tumour marker or other putative antigen. A second, anti-antibody is then applied to the same tissue section. This secondary antibody has been labelled with biotin, part of the vitamin B_2 complex. Biotin has a high affinity for the egg white glycoprotein, avidin. Avidin, labelled with inactive horseradish peroxidase or alkaline phosphatase, binds to sites where biotin-labelled primary antibody has identified the cell component, tumour marker or antigen that is sought. The labelled enzyme product appears microscopically as a brown–red reaction product.

In-situ hybridisation

In a search for a diagnostic marker antigen, virus or other protein, RNA (p. 140) is used to 'hybridise' cells or tissues. A RNA probe is applied to the tissue section and the site of binding to the target shown by incorporating a radio-active isotope as label. The method allows the identification of viral and other antigens not only in frozen material but in fixed, paraffin-embedded, tissue blocks. The technique can be used to search for genes and gene products in archival material, retrospectively. In one recent example, extensive efforts have been made to identify the strain of influenza virus that caused the 1919 pandemic.

HOSPITAL ACQUIRED INFECTION

Diseases contracted in hospital are **nosocomial**: they are often infections. In the UK, 14% of new patients contract a new infection when they enter a hospital (Fig. 27). The frequency, morbidity and mortality of these bacterial infections are therefore much greater than in the general population. Infections are a major cause of morbidity in patients undergoing operation and may arise in the wound itself; in the abdominal and thoracic cavities and their organs; in bones; and in the brain.

Although conditions have improved since pre-Listerian times, hospitals can still be viewed as 'cauldrons of fermenting bacteria'. Bacteria are carried on white coats; on instruments in daily use such as stethoscopes; on auroscopes; on tendon hammers; and on sphygmomanometers. To minimise such infections, antiseptic care includes regular cleaning of the walls and floors of wards and operating theatres and the use of surgical dressing rooms on wards. Isolation units segregate patients infected with pathogenic or highly contagious organisms, such as methicillin-resistant *Staphylococcus aureus* (MRSA), *Mycobacterium tuberculosis* and Salmonellae spp., and individuals who are at particular risk. Among the latter are immunosuppressed patients awaiting bone marrow transplantation.

The bacteria that cause these infections are often of low virulence towards the general population, in whom they may be carried unnoticed. The organisms assume higher pathogenicity due to the depressed immunity of the aged and ill. The consequence is **opportunistic** infection. Ten per cent of hospital acquired infections are caused by *Pseudomonas aeruginosa*. Other organisms often implicated are Enterococcus spp., coagulase-negative staphylococci, and *Candida albicans*.

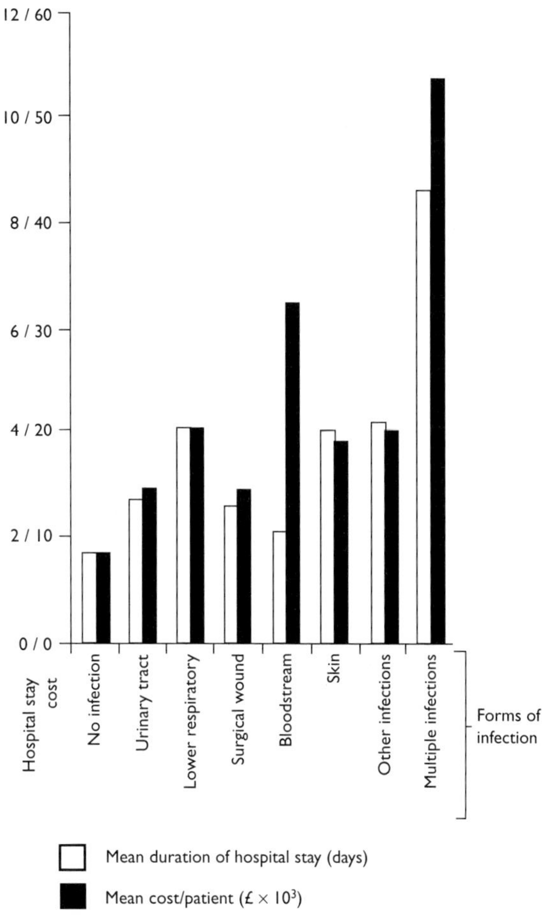

Figure 27 Hospital acquired infection.
Influence of nature of infection shown on the horizontal, x-axis, on duration of hospitalisation (left column) and cost of treatment (right column) both shown on the vertical, y-axis.

It is impossible to eliminate all hospital infection. Respiratory disease following anaesthesia is caused largely by a patient's own nasopharyngeal or gastric micro-organisms. Most men and women harbour microbes in their urethra. During urinary bladder catheterisation, organisms are inevitably inoculated. Once the catheter is inserted, infective agents pass between the catheter and the walls of the urethra. A similar form of transmission may follow the insertion of abdominal drains but this risk has been reduced by the use of closed drainage systems.

AUTO-INFECTION

Normal skin is colonised by skin commensals and by intestinal bacteria. Self (auto)-infection of wounds is therefore anticipated. One example is gas gangrene of an amputation stump. Another is *Staphylococcus aureus* infection of an intravenous line site in a nasal carrier of this organism.

CROSS-INFECTION

Cross-infection describes microbial infection from a source other than the patient. The origin may be another patient; a member of staff who may be an asymptomatic carrier; contaminated equipment and instruments; or the environment. Cross-infection becomes an **outbreak** if two or more individuals are infected with an identical strain of organism.

Organisms associated with particular equipment may be the source of an outbreak. When identified, such a focus may be disinfected rapidly. Appropriate policies are then pursued to safeguard patients who may require the use of the same equipment in the future. Cross-infections, or even outbreaks originating from a more general source such as the hospital floor, are more difficult to control. They may not even be recognised because of the sporadic nature of the responsible organism or the small numbers of infecting bacteria. Ultimately, such organisms may become endemic. Examples include *Clostridium difficile*, MRSA and coliforms resistant to multiple antibiotics. The source of an outbreak or its mode of dissemination may not be identifiable.

Factors involved in outbreaks of infection

Many factors may be implicated. They include:

- Carriage by staff of micro-organisms.
- Defective environmental hygiene.
- Poor hand-washing practice.
- Inappropriate choice and use of antibiotics.
- Sub-optimal laundry and cleaning practices.
- Insufficient ventilation.
- Absence of facilities for isolation.

In some hospitals, one surgeon in three may be a nasal and/or perineal carrier of *Staphylococcus aureus*. Organisms carried in this way often develop resistance to the commonly used antibiotics. Gentamicin-resistant coliforms, *Pseudomonas aeruginosa* and methicillin-resistant *Staphylococcus aureus* (MRSA) are common examples.

Isolation units are used to segregate patients infected with these organisms, those with *Mycobacterium tuberculosis* and *Salmonellae* spp., and individuals at particular risk. Among the latter are immunosuppressed patients awaiting bone marrow transplantation. Patients with organisms such as *Clostridium difficile*, *Mycobacterium tuberculosis*, Salmonella spp. and beta-haemolytic streptococci of groups A, C and G should also be isolated. Because of space constraints, those with MRSA (p. 304) or *Cl. difficile* may have to be grouped within a single ward.

Isolation rooms or units create physical barriers between patients colonised by hazardous bacteria and other patients. The rooms protect immunosuppressed patients from the microbial traffic of other patients and staff. The use of long-sleeved gowns, disposable gloves and aprons is obligatory. Medical and nursing staff should leave their coats and aprons outside and wear disposable gloves when examining any patient. Hands are washed on leaving.

Now read Antibiotics (p. 17)

HYPERSENSITIVITY

Hypersensitivity is a condition in which undesirable tissue damage follows the development of humoral or cell-mediated immunity. Hypersensitivity is particularly likely when foreign antigen persists while antibody formation is occurring. Individuals sensitised by first exposure to foreign antigen develop a beneficial or at least harmless primary immune state. Subsequent exposure to the same antigen enhances this immunity. Hypersensitivity represents an exaggeration or perversion of this secondary reaction.

There are four forms of hypersensitivity: types I, II and III hypersensitivity are 'immediate' and expressed by reactions between antigen and antibody; type IV hypersensitivity is 'delayed' and mediated by T lymphocytes.

Now read Antigens and antibodies (p. 19), Immunity (p. 171)

TYPE I HYPERSENSITIVITY

Type I hypersensitivity is **anaphylaxis**. It is a harmful condition, the opposite of **prophylaxis** that is protective and beneficial. The responses of type I hypersensitivity may be generalised or localised, depending on how antigen reaches the sensitised tissues. Some individuals exposed to certain foreign antigens are prone to form IgE antibodies. The Fc non-antigen-binding parts of IgE molecules bind to Fc receptors on the surface of mast cells and basophil leucocytes. These antibodies are **reagins**. When there is further contact with the original sensitising antigen, the antigen molecules link the free, Fab (antigen-binding fragment) parts of the IgE molecules. Mast cells or basophil leucocytes degranulate and release histamine; heparin; the leukotrienes, and other factors into nearby tissues or the circulation.

Local anaphylaxis

Local anaphylactic reactions in man include hay fever, extrinsic asthma and urticarial responses to foods.

Generalised anaphylaxis

Generalised anaphylaxis in man is rare but life-threatening. The injection of anti-tetanus horse serum in passive immunisation (p. 94) was one ancient cause but the use of human immunoglobulin concentrates has minimised this hazard. Insect or arthropod stings and the systemic administration of penicillin are examples of agents that may lead to this acute condition.

TYPE II HYPERSENSITIVITY – CYTOTOXIC/CYTOLYTIC

Cytotoxic and cytolytic hypersensitivity is directed against cells by antibody molecules bound to cell surfaces. One result is to facilitate phagocytosis; contact with macrophages is promoted. Cytotoxic hypersensitivity is often allo-immune. It is exemplified by the haemolytic reactions of incompatible blood transfusion (p. 46) and by the antibodies formed against organ transplants. Analogous reactions are observed in auto-immune haemolytic anaemia (p. 11) and in Hashimoto's thyroiditis (p. 324). Some drugs elicit cell-mediated hypersensitivity when they behave as haptens binding to tissue proteins to form antigenic complexes.

TYPE III HYPERSENSITIVITY – IMMUNE-COMPLEX-MEDIATED

Free, soluble antigen and antibody, present in the circulation in appropriate (optimal) proportions, can combine to form immune complexes, the presence of which is shown by laboratory tests. Immune complexes can be identified in tissue sections by the application of labelled anti-immunoglobulin and anticomplement antibodies. In the blood, they are recognised by precipitation with polyethylene glycol or by determining the extent to which they bind to the walls of complement-coated plastic tubes. Soluble immune complexes lodge in or pass through blood vessel walls, bind complement and initiate inflammatory, tissue-damaging reactions. Polymorphs are attracted by chemotaxis. In turn, these cells release enzymes such as elastase and neutral collagenases. Platelets aggregate and thrombus formation is encouraged.

Systemic immune complex disease

Lodging in the small, terminal blood vessels of the joints, kidneys, heart and skin, these complexes cause a potentially fatal syndrome (serum sickness) comprising arthritis, glomerulonephritis, oedema, cutaneous vasculitis and carditis.

Local immune complex disease

If antigen persists at a site of injection or administration, for example because of indolent infection or auto-immune response, immune complex deposition may be recurrent and the resulting disease long-lasting. Rheumatoid arthritis (p. 191) and polyarteritis nodosa are examples of conditions in which this mechanism is active.

TYPE IV HYPERSENSITIVITY – CELL-MEDIATED

Cell-mediated, type IV delayed hypersensitivity is of crucial importance in determining the cell injuries and tissue lesions of infection by bacteria such as *Mycobacterium tuberculosis*; by fungi; and by some viruses, for example the measles virus. Type IV hypersensitivity is responsible for many examples of transplant rejection (p. 329) and for skin reactions to important, small molecules such as neomycin; paraphenylenediamine (in hair dyes); nickel, and chromate metals that act as haptens. The Mantoux reaction (p. 229) is one example of type IV hypersensitivity, the tissue reaction to BCG vaccination (p. 333) another.

The state of cell-mediated hypersensitivity can be transferred passively by T lymphocytes or by a lymphocyte transfer factor extracted from them, but not by the transfer of antibody. Macrophages are activated by the specific behaviour of the antigen that has sensitised the T lymphocytes. Advantage has been taken of this behaviour in the attempted treatment of some cancers by BCG vaccination (p. 248).

HYPERTENSION

Hypertension is a state in which there is either sustained raised blood pressure or frequent periods when the pressure is significantly elevated. Hypertension may be demonstrated in the systemic, pulmonary or portal circulations. Pressures may be recorded directly in the arterial, capillary or venous parts of a circulation. Indirect measurements, by manual or electronic devices, may be of the systolic, diastolic, or mean blood pressures. In terms of the systemic circulation, an individual is hypertensive when the blood pressure, measured under basal conditions, exceeds two standard deviations above the norm for a given race, sex and age. Alternatively, continuous recordings are taken over a 24-hour period. Important distinctions are made between changes in the mean levels of the systolic and diastolic pressures, and in the diurnal patterns of raised pressures.

The significance of persistently raised, mean blood pressure is the irrefutable evidence of an increased susceptibility to stroke and myocardial ischaemia. There is a diminished life expectation.

HYPERVOLAEMIA AND HYPOVOLAEMIA

HYPERVOLAEMIA

Hypervolaemia describes an abnormally increased circulating blood volume. In surgical practice, the most common cause is the intravenous infusion of excessive volumes of blood or other oncotic fluids. An increase in plasma volume can be produced by an excess of sodium in the plasma as a consequence of the raised secretion of aldosterone (p. 6). An abnormally high blood volume may also be due to an increase in the red blood cell volume, polycythaemia (p. 275).

Now read Oedema (p. 251), Water (p. 355)

HYPOVOLAEMIA

Hypovolaemia is an abnormal reduction in blood volume. In surgical practice, the most frequent explanation is abnormal fluid loss combined with decreased or absent oral fluid intake in a patient who has received an inadequate intravenous infusion (pp. 44, 355).

A low total blood volume can follow haemorrhage or the loss of plasma or total body water. The kidneys, and to a lesser extent the brain and heart, are the organs most at risk. The body responds quickly by increasing catecholamine secretion. The consequence is peripheral and splanchnic vasoconstriction. The reduction in the volume of the circulation brought about in this way maintains blood pressure. Antidiuretic hormone and aldosterone are secreted to conserve water and sodium and total blood volume is restored. Ultimately, any residual reduction in red blood cell volume is corrected by accelerated haemopoiesis.

Now read Anaemia (p. 10), Blood loss (p. 42), Shock (p. 290)

HYPOTHERMIA

Man is warm-blooded and loses heat to the environment continually. Hypothermia, a reduction in body temperature, is usually harmful but can be used with benefit to protect tissues against metabolic or hypoxic injury.

SYSTEMIC (GENERALISED) HYPOTHERMIA

Generalised hypothermia exists when the internal or core body temperature falls below 35°C. The fall in core temperature may be the result of excessive heat loss, for example in extreme, Arctic environmental conditions. It may also be caused by decreased heat production, as in prolonged immobility or in hypothyroidism. By contrast with normal individuals in whom muscular activity can generate heat, the surgical patient is often unconscious.

Physiological thermoregulatory responses to low body temperatures, such as shivering, are inactive during general anaesthesia. Warming blankets containing circulating hot air are now commonly used to prevent hypothermia during long surgical operations. The systemic response to cold is influenced by the degree of hypothermia. As the temperature falls to 35°C, the body attempts to conserve heat by peripheral vasoconstriction and to maintain vital centres at normal temperature by increased cardiac output. Below 32°C, metabolic activity is depressed and cardiac output is reduced. Below 24°C, all thermoregulation is lost and the body loses heat uncontrollably to the environment.

Now read Death (p. 116)

Patients with hypothermia are often old, malnourished and have low core temperatures. Newborn infants are also particularly at risk. Death is due to ventricular fibrillation, which may occur at 30°C. However, young, otherwise healthy people can survive prolonged hypothermia with no or little cerebral damage, even when comatose, if they are quickly re-warmed by cardiopulmonary bypass.

In peri-operative situations, hypothermia impairs immune function and decreases subcutaneous oxygen tension. Hypothermia promotes wound infection and dehiscence. In earlier years, generalised hypothermia was used frequently in patients undergoing cardiac surgery. The purpose was to reduce tissue metabolism and the requirement for oxygen, particularly by the brain. Profound hypothermia with temperatures less than 20°C has been employed allowing circulatory arrest of up to 40 minutes. However, with more-efficient extracorporeal systems, this use of hypothermia is now uncommon.

LOCAL HYPOTHERMIA

The severity of the adverse, local effects of cold are in proportion to the rate and degree of heat loss. They also vary according to the nature and mass of the exposed tissue.

- Brief cooling to a low temperature, or prolonged mild cooling, injures the endothelium of capillaries and results in oedema and superficial vesication. The skin and subcutaneous tissues of the periphery of the limbs are the most vulnerable but the ears and nose are susceptible. Raynaud's phenomenon is one consequence.
- Very rapid and extreme chilling causes slowing and cessation of cell metabolism. Ultimately, there is intracellular ice-crystal formation. The clinical effects of cold are, however, dominated by vascular changes.

Chilblain

The mildest hypothermic injury is a chilblain, a tender, erythematous swelling with inflammatory changes in subcutaneous fat. Spontaneous resolution occurs at normal temperatures.

Cold injury with ischaemia

When chilling is both rapid and severe, there is vascular occlusion by masses of red blood cells. There may be no overt evidence of ischaemia until the temperature rises and the circulation is re-established. Serious injuries of this kind occur in mountaineers when vascular occlusion leads to tissue infarction and the subsequent loss of digits.

Frostbite

Frostbite is the formation of ice in tissues. Subsequent thawing destroys cells by the breakdown of osmoregulation. Gangrene or mummification, result. In 'trench' or immersion foot, prolonged exposure to cold water causes similar extensive injury.

Local anaesthesia

Local hypothermia may be induced for therapeutic reasons or to permit the conduct of limited, surgical procedures. Local anaesthesia can be produced by spraying the skin with ethyl chloride.

Cryosurgery

This destructive procedure can be performed using probes cooled by liquid nitrogen at −196°C or, more commonly, by decompressing pressurised, gaseous nitrous oxide. Using the latter, rapid freezing of tissue to temperatures lower than −20°C is sufficient to produce intracellular ice crystals. The probes also possess a mechanism for rewarming, a process that destroys the frozen cells. The procedure is repeated when a maximum effect is sought. Capillaries and small vessels in the 'ice ball' are eradicated. Blood in large arteries may freeze but does not coagulate. Neither the blood nor the arterial walls show evidence of injury when thawing is allowed. A normal circulation can be restored. Since nerve endings are ablated, cryosurgery is relatively painless.

I

ILEUM AND JEJUNUM

Biopsy diagnosis of small intestinal disease

See p. 40.

DEVELOPMENTAL AND CONGENITAL DISORDERS

The most frequent sites of atresia or stenosis are the distal ileum and the duodenum adjoining the papilla of Vater. There may be an association with Down's syndrome (p. 92). Malrotation of the small intestine *in utero* is occasionally recognised. The caecum lies in the left iliac fossa with the entire small intestine to the right of the midline. There is a long, narrow mesentery so that the intestine is prone to torsion and volvulus. Duplications and enterogenous cysts are common. Although symptomless, haemorrhage, obstruction or intussusception are recognised complications.

Meckel's diverticulum

Meckel's diverticulum is the most common congenital abnormality of the small intestine. The diverticulum is the persisting, proximal end of the vitello-intestinal duct. It is situated on the anti-mesenteric border of the ileum and is present in ~2% of people. The defect lies within 1 m of the ileo-caecal valve and is ~50 mm in length. The diverticulum is usually free but may be connected to the umbilicus by a fibrous cord, the residue of the vitello-intestinal duct.

Several categories of disorder complicate Meckel's diverticulum. The lining mucosa is of a small-intestinal, mucin-secreting form but an island of ectopic gastric epithelium is sometimes present. When this is the case, a peptic ulcer may form and be complicated by bleeding and perforation. Neuro-endocrine tumours and carcinoma occasionally develop. Infection and intestinal obstruction are encountered. Acute inflammation of Meckel's diverticulum simulates acute appendicitis. Obstruction of the intestine itself is attributable either to intussusception or to volvulus around the fibrous cord.

Peutz–Jegher syndrome

The syndrome, inherited as an autosomal dominant characteristic, comprises deep brown-black spots on the lips and within the mouth together with multiple hamartomatous polyps throughout the gastro-intestinal tract. Polyps are especially frequent in the small intestine. They may ulcerate and bleed. Iron deficiency anaemia is one result. Malignant transformation of this form of polyp is rare but there is an increased risk of neoplasia at sites external to the intestine.

Angiodysplasia

Angiodysplasia is much less common than in the large intestine (p. 108) but may cause massive and life-threatening, occult or overt haemorrhage.

INFECTION

Cholera

This infamous, life-threatening epidemic disease results from water-borne infection by *Vibrio cholerae*. The micro-organism is a motile, Gram-negative comma-shaped bacillus. Infection begins when organisms are ingested by refugees or pilgrims living under conditions of poor hygiene and sanitation, especially where drinking water is not purified. Cholera is the partner of poverty and of natural and man-made disasters and is a hazard during large population movements. In cities, cholera remained a threat until central, clean water supplies were constructed.

The organism secretes an enzyme that destroys mucin. An exotoxin is formed that binds to receptors on the cells of the intestinal epithelium. The toxin blocks molecules regulating the production of cyclic AMP (adenosine monophosphate) so that the normal Na^+/Cl^- flux across the intestinal cell membrane is deranged. There is an enormous, rapid loss of water. The result is a catastrophic and profuse watery diarrhoea with so-called 'rice-water' stools. Untreated, the disease is rapidly fatal. Death may take place within 2 to 3 hours of the onset.

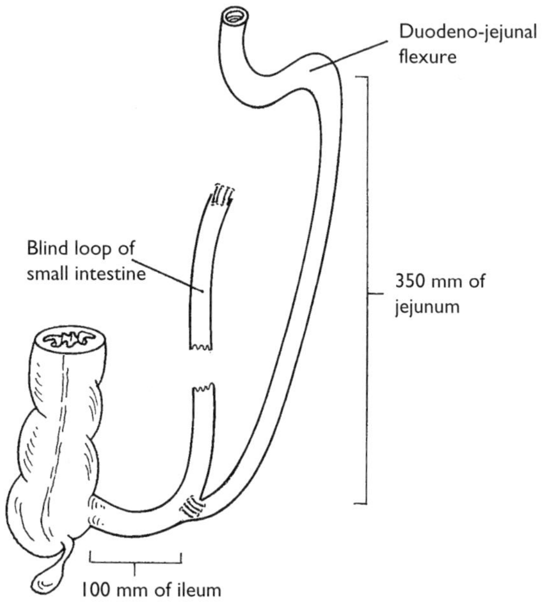

Figure 28 Blind loop in jejuno-ileal bypass. Formerly, operation of jejuno-ileal bypass was performed to assist weight reduction in morbidly obese individuals. Extensive portions of the jejunum and ileum were taken out of the intestinal circuit in order to restrict intestinal absorption of digested foods. However, this procedure created very large, blind loops.

Other infections

Actinomycosis (p. 5), amoebiasis (p. 8), dysentery (p. 123), enteric fever (p. 127) and tuberculosis (p. 332) are described on other pages.

Enteritis necroticans (pibel) is a life-threatening illness characterised by haemorrhage, inflammation, and ischaemic necrosis of the jejunum. It occurs in developing countries but, in the West, is restricted to adults with underlying, chronic illness. The cause is *Clostridium perfringens* type C.

Blind loops

A variety of surgical operations create blind-ended loops of intestine (Fig. 28). The contents of the new cavities become static. Stagnation frequently results in abnormal bacterial proliferation. The changed bacterial flora interferes with the absorption of fat and the lipid-soluble vitamins (p. 351), particularly vitamin B_{12}. Within the loop, there is a high concentration of non-deconjugated bile acids. A comparable change in the intestinal flora may result from jejunal diverticulosis or chronic, subacute intestinal obstruction, conditions often attributable to strictures or to external constriction caused by adhesions.

INFLAMMATORY BOWEL DISEASE

Strictly, the term 'inflammatory bowel disease' describes all forms of inflammation and infection of the entire gut. In practice, the description is confined to Crohn's disease and ulcerative colitis (p. 103).

Crohn's disease (regional enteritis)

Crohn and his colleagues (p. 370) are credited with the definitive description of regional enteritis but earlier accounts have been recognised.

Causes

The cause(s) remain uncertain. There is a genetic predisposition and siblings of affected individuals have a 30-fold increased probability of developing the condition. There is a particularly high incidence in

Ashkenazy Jews. The condition is more common in smokers than non-smokers. The similarity of the structural abnormalities to those of tuberculosis has led to speculation about the aetiological role of infection. *Mycobacterium pseudotuberculosis* and virus have been invoked as causal agents. Recent suggestions of an increased incidence of Crohn's disease following measles vaccination have been discounted.

Structure

Any part of the gastro-intestinal tract from the lips to the anus may be involved. The terminal ileum is the usual site. Mucosal ulcers develop into fissures that penetrate deeply into the wall of the gut. They are separated by zones of less severely diseased, oedematous mucosa. The intestinal wall is thickened, the serosa inflamed. The disease process is discontinuous so that normal epithelium intervenes between diseased segments to form 'skip' lesions. Ulceration of the skin has been observed. It is indistinguishable histologically from the changes seen in the bowel. The gall bladder may be similarly affected.

Microscopically, there is early involvement of all layers of the intestine. The pathognomonic change is the presence of non-caseating granulomas, with multinucleated giant cells and epithelioid cells (macrophages) in the intestinal wall and within nearby lymph nodes. The large bowel only is affected in ~20% of cases. Unlike ulcerative colitis, in which the microscopic changes are confined initially to the mucosa, inflammation implicates all intestinal coats. Endarteritis of intestinal blood vessels is common, particularly in the elderly. There is a perivascular infiltrate of lymphocytes. Peri-anal fissures, abscesses and fistulas occur in the majority of patients who have either small or large bowel disease. They are more common in the latter.

Behaviour and prognosis

Fibrotic, intestinal stricture is a characteristic complication. The strictures are multiple, particularly in the terminal ileum. Intestinal obstruction is common. Sudden, acute or insidious, chronic bleeding may take place. Crohn's disease is a frequent cause of intestinal fistulas: they form between the loops of diseased intestine; between the intestine and the abdominal wall; or between the intestine and other viscera. Acute ('toxic') dilatation of the colon (p. 104) may occur. **Perforation of the colon** may follow with generalised or localised peritonitis and abscess formation. However, the colon may perforate in the absence of dilatation. **Perforation of the small bowel** is uncommon because the diseased segment of intestine usually adheres to another structure. However, fistulas arise. When the small bowel is extensively involved, malabsorption and malnutrition become severe. Megaloblastic anaemia develops; it is attributable to a deficiency of either vitamin B_{12} or folic acid.

Systemic disorders are chacteristically associated with Crohn's disease. The incidence of cirrhosis; sclerosing cholangitis; ankylosing spondylitis; arthritis; erythema nodosum; pyoderma gangrenosum; and iritis is higher than in the general population. Amyloidosis may ensue.

Now read Inflammatory bowel disease (p. 103), Crohn's disease (p. 104)

MECHANICAL DISORDERS

Intussusception

Intussusception is the invagination of a proximal part of the intestine into an adjacent, distal part. The former is designated the intussusceptum, the latter the intussuscipiens. Intussusception is usually prograde but retrograde intussusception has been described.

Ileocolic intussusception is the form encountered most frequently. It is more common in infancy and early childhood than in later life. There is a relationship to season so that, in Northern Europe, the disorder is more prevalent in the spring and autumn than in the summer and winter.

The apex of the invaginated part is usually a hypertrophied Peyer's patch, swollen as a result of viral infection. In adults, the apex is often a polyp. Obstruction of the intestine may be a consequence of the invagination. An almost inevitable result is that the blood vessels of the intussusceptum are also obstructed leading, in sequence, to intestinal haemorrhage, ischaemia and infarction, and gangrene, followed by perforation and generalised peritonitis.

Paralytic ileus

Paralytic ileus describes the onset of impaired intestinal motility in the absence of physical obstruction. It is liable to occur following laparotomy as a consequence both of the effects of anaesthesia and of the handling of the bowel. The development of ileus reflects the duration and severity of an operation. It is an occasional complication of lumbar, pelvic and rib fracture. Persistent ileus, a common result of peritonitis or generalised toxaemia, is aggravated by hypokalaemia (p. 276).

Volvulus

Volvulus is the obstruction of a hollow abdominal viscus by torsion. **Small intestinal volvulus** occurs when the intestine rotates about the axis of the mesentery and the afferent vascular supply. The mesentery, in relation to which this process takes place, is often found to have undergone prior contraction because of fibrous adhesions. The terminal ileum may be involved in **caecal volvulus**.

Strangulation

In the context of small intestinal disease, strangulation ('choking') describes the constriction of the neck of a hernial sac. The contents are deprived of a vascular circulation.

MALABSORPTION

Intestinal malabsorption is the deficient absorption of the products of digestion. It is almost exclusively a consequence of subacute or chronic disease of the small intestine but an exact cause is not always demonstrable. In Western societies, the most frequent agencies are coeliac disease and Crohn's disease. The disorder may also follow extensive resection of the small intestine.

The identity and extent of a small intestinal disorder determine which nutrients are affected by malnutrition and the degree to which absorption is disordered. Hypo-albuminaemia, anaemia and vitamin deficiencies are common sequelae. Duodenal disease leads to iron deficiency anaemia since this element is mainly absorbed at this site. Many nutrients are absorbed in the jejunum. A wide variety of deficiency states may accompany prolonged disease. Some molecules such as vitamin B_{12} (cyanocobalamin) are absorbed specifically from the distal ileum so that chronic ileal disease may culminate in megaloblastic anaemia.

Steatorrhoea, the presence of excess fat in the faeces, and **creatorrhoea,** the presence of excess protein, are features of severe malabsorption.

Coeliac disease

Gluten is that part of wheat and other grains that contains the insoluble protein gliadin. In coeliac disease, there is a genetically determined hypersensitivity to gluten. An affected individual is compelled to conform to a diet in which gluten is absent. The intestinal disorder that results from gluten hypersensitivity is a form of malabsorption attributable to a reduction in the surface area of the small intestinal mucosa. The characteristic histological change is mucosal villous atrophy. There is an 80-fold increased risk of the development of carcinoma of the small intestine and a link with enteropathy-associated T-cell lymphoma (EATL). The risk of developing oesophageal carcinoma is also increased.

Tropical sprue

This disorder is largely confined to defined geographical regions such as South-East Asia. There is intestinal villous atrophy. Bacterial overgrowth may be the initiating change, a view supported by evidence that the condition may respond well to treatment with broad-spectrum antibiotics.

Other causes of malabsorption

Regional enteritis; exposure to ionising radiation; tuberculosis; amyloidosis; bacterial overgrowth; and Whipple's disease, are further causes of malabsorption.

Whipple's disease is an uncommon disorder of middle-aged, white males. There is steatorrhoea. The condition results in arthralgia; generalised lymphadenopathy; skin pigmentation; and abdominal pain. It may be caused by the bacterium *Tropheryma whippelii* but this observation has not been confirmed and does not explain the racial, gender and age incidence of the condition.

RADIATION ENTERITIS

The most frequent cause of radiation damage to the small intestine is radiotherapy for cancer of the female genital system. During treatment, loops of ileum within the pelvis are inevitably exposed to sources of ionising radiation. In an early, acute response, there is an inflammatory reaction in the mucosa leading to diarrhoea with blood and mucus. The villi are stunted, absorption defective. In severe cases, there is ulceration and perforation. Complete recovery is possible within 4–6 months. In a later, chronic phase of response, there is progression to an obliterative vasculitis. The disorder culminates in intestinal fibrosis and stricture. Intestinal obstruction, bacterial overgrowth and malabsorption are consequences.

Now read Irradiation (p. 185)

TUMOURS

In spite of the large surface area of the small intestinal mucosa, tumours are exceedingly rare.

Benign

Adenoma

The frequency of small intestinal adenoma is conspicuously less than that of the large bowel. Small intestinal adenomas are more often encountered in the proximal part than in the distal. Adenomas are premalignant as they are in the large intestine and villous adenomas are more common than tubular. There may be more than 1000 of these tumours in the small intestine of a patient with familial adenomatous polyposis (FAP – p. 105) but the malignant potential of these tumours is very much less than in those of the large intestine.

Haemangioma

Haemangiomas are single or multiple. They develop in the small or large intestine but may co-exist in either territory. Haemangioma is frequently complicated by occult or overt haemorrhage. Large haemangiomas provoke intussusception or intestinal obstruction.

Leiomyoma

Intestinal leiomyoma is difficult to distinguish from leiomyosarcoma (p. 235). Leiomyomas tend to ulcerate and bleed. Microscopically, these smooth-muscle tumours are formed of elongated, spindle-shaped leiomyocytes. When nuclear pleomorphism and vascular invasion are identified, a tumour is assumed to be malignant. Distant metastasis is infrequent but local recurrence after excision is relatively common.

Neuro-endocrine neoplasms

Neuro-endocrine neoplasms (carcinoid tumours – p. 82) are small, yellow, slow-growing and often ulcerating. Islands or cords of closely-packed, uniform cells contain darkly-staining nuclei. Within the cytoplasm are argentaffin-positive granules from which 5-hydroxytryptamine (5-HT) is derived although not all these cells have potential for secretion. Even small carcinoid tumours may metastasise to the liver. Under these circumstances, much 5-HT is liberated into the systemic venous circulation, from extending hepatic deposits. The carcinoid syndrome (p. 82) results. Haemorrhage and intestinal obstruction, with or without intussusception, are other complications.

Now read Carcinoid (p. 82)

Lymphoma

Small-bowel lymphomas arise spontaneously. Occasionally, they develop in association with coeliac disease or AIDS. In the West, most small-intestinal lymphomas form in the terminal ileum. In the Middle East, where they are frequent in young adults, they are more common in the jejunum than the ileum. Lymphomas occurring *de novo* are of B-cell origin as are those complicating AIDS. Lymphomas in patients with coeliac disease are of T-cell origin. The tumours predispose to intestinal obstruction. Bleeding and perforation are less frequent. MALToma is described on p. 224.

Malignant

Carcinoma

Carcinoma is very uncommon. The greater number of the tumours arise in pre-existing adenomas. There is an increased risk of cancer in patients with coeliac or with Crohn's disease. Most carcinomas have undergone metastasis by the time they are identified clinically. Among the indirect consequences are anaemia and intestinal obstruction.

VASCULAR DISEASE

Vascular insufficiency is acute or chronic, arterial or venous. It may be due to embolism or local thrombosis and is recognised in large vessels such as the superior mesenteric artery or in small vessels such as those arising from a marginal artery. The consequences depend upon the anatomical distribution of the vascular tree and the duration and severity of the ischaemia.

Arterial disease

Atheroma of the superior mesenteric artery is an occasional cause of **abdominal angina** and malabsorption. Acute obstruction is followed by haemorrhagic infarction of much of the small intestine. There is a poor collateral circulation and an anastomosis with other vessels that is insufficient to permit recovery. Individuals with diabetes mellitus are especially susceptible to the focal ischaemic changes produced by atheroma. Disease of the smaller intestinal vessels occurs in rheumatoid arthritis, systemic lupus erythematosus and polyarteritis nodosa.

Venous disease

Mesenteric venous occlusion is an uncommon cause of intestinal ischaemia. Thrombosis may complicate diseases of the blood such as polycythaemia. Localised vascular obstruction may be due to compression by tumours or to strangulation within a hernial sac. Complete occlusion inevitably provokes intestinal infarction. The clinical signs cannot be differentiated from those of arterial infarction but the anatomical and histological changes are distinctive.

IMAGING

It is often possible to obtain reliable, indirect evidence of the nature and extent of a disease process by non-invasive imaging. Sufficient understanding of a suspected pathological process may be gained without the need for biopsy (p. 40) or autopsy (p. 29). The principal techniques employed in imaging are ultrasonography (HFS); computerised axial tomography (CT); magnetic resonance imaging (MRI); and isotopic scanning.

ULTRASOUND

Low-intensity sound waves have no effect upon the material through which they pass and can be used for the non-invasive imaging of tissues, particularly for differentiating solid and cystic masses. Ultrasound is employed to identify gallstones; intra-abdominal abscesses; ovarian and thyroid masses; and to demonstrate the tissues of the growing fetus. Using ultrasonography to guide a needle, it is possible to obtain fluid for cytology and tissue for histology.

The higher the frequency of the sound waves, the better the image resolution, but the less the penetration of the ultrasound beam into tissues. Thus, the greatest diagnostic precision is obtained by placing the source of the waves as close as possible to the tissues to be imaged. Pelvic tissues can be displayed using vaginal and rectal probes. Other abdominal and thoracic structures can be imaged by endoscopic and laparoscopic instrumentation. Exploiting the Doppler technique of change in frequency induced by motion, ultrasonic vibrations can be applied to measure the rate of blood flow.

There are theoretical disadvantages. DNA may be degraded by high-intensity ultrasound, but there is no evidence that this change occurs in the range of frequencies selected for diagnostic purposes.

Therapeutic ultrasound is described on p. 336.

COMPUTED AXIAL TOMOGRAPHY (CT)

In CT scanning, the patient lies upon a table and an X-ray tube rotates around the table, at right angles to its long axis. The arm supporting the X-ray tube is therefore a radius of the circle subtended by the movement of the tube. The tube moves within a surrounding ring of X-ray detectors. At each of many thousands of positions, an X-ray image of the patient's tissues is recorded. With the aid of a computer program, reconstructed axial images are produced from these many records. These composite images embrace horizontal slices of the body of varying, selected thicknesses. They are often 1.5 to 10 mm apart. The stored data can then be employed to reconstruct 'secondary' images in any desired plane. Series of these coronal and sagittal pictures can be displayed, saved and analysed. The technique is of especial value in constructing 3-D views of structures such as bone, rich in elements like Ca^{++} of high atomic number.

SPIRAL CT

Image resolution in a circumferential, axial plane is constrained by movements such as those of respiration. Improved resolution and very rapid, accurate imaging can therefore be obtained by increasing the speed of imaging during a single, suspended breath. The procedure, spiral CT, is accomplished by passing a patient rapidly through the radial, X-ray beam. It is accomplished by continuous rotation of the X-ray tube combined with a continuous, rotary movement of the table on which the patient is lying.

MULTI-SLICE CT

The use of four X-ray detectors rather than one offers further advantages. Four spiral images can be obtained simultaneously. In this way, even more rapid scanning can be performed, embracing yet greater volumes of tissue. Both spiral and multi-slice CT permit the retrospective reconstruction of thin tissue slices without exposing a patient to unnecessary, further irradiation.

CONTRAST ENHANCEMENT

The resolution of almost all spiral and multi-slice CT scans can be enhanced by the injection into the vascular system of soluble agents that enhance contrast. These injections are made rapidly, at a rate, for example, of 3 mL/second.

MAGNETIC RESONANCE IMAGING (MRI)

MR imaging takes advantage of pulsed, radio frequency signals to create images of signals emitted by protons in water after perturbation of hydrogen atoms, within a high magnetic field. The final images are generated by computer.

New methods now take advantage of all aspects of the emitted signals. The range and quality of MR images is enhanced by the use of an intravenous contrast medium, gadolinium. A variety of magnetic field strengths is available. The versatility of MR imaging allows a large range of different types of image to be produced, in any plane. The imaging of complex vessels and ducts is possible. Magnetic resonance cholangiography is one example of what can be achieved.

POSITRON EMISSION TOMOGRAPHY (PET)

Because of cost, PET scanning is not yet widely used. It has great potential. The value of PET scanning is explained by the observation that whereas all normal cells metabolise glucose, cancer cells may use a five times greater amount.

The radio-isotope ^{18}FDG (fluoro-2-deoxy-D-glucose) is taken up into cells in the same way as normal glucose. It emits positrons spontaneously. These positrons can be detected in the same manner as they are when a gamma camera images technetium ^{18}fluorine. Images of 'hot spots' are produced, sites where the isotope, and therefore the label, have become concentrated. The most promising use of PET is in oncology. The technique detects many primary and metastatic cancers with high sensitivity.

IMMOBILISATION

It is dangerous to lie in bed in hospital. Immobilisation confers a series of hazards.

SYSTEMIC EFFECTS

The **immediate systemic effects** of bed rest include disturbances of fluid balance, nutrition and intestinal function. Dehydration, weight loss and constipation soon follow. There is a tendency to deep venous thrombosis. Pulmonary embolism is a common consequence. *Streptococcus pneumoniae* bronchopneumonia (p. 216) may develop and may prove fatal: it is called the 'old man's friend'. The same sequence is not uncommon in elderly patients following fracture of the neck of the femur.

The **late systemic effects** include the cumulative influences of insidious malnutrition. There is anaemia and osteoporosis. The loss of skeletal calcium can result in the formation of renal calculi.

LOCAL EFFECTS

In prolonged immobilisation, the development of gravitational ulcers is anticipated. Regional osteoporosis; the formation of fibrous adhesions; ankylosis of limb joints; localised oedema; and epidermal atrophy are other changes.

IMMUNITY

Immunity is a state of resistance to the harmful effects of foreign antigens, particularly those causing infection. Immunity may be innate or acquired (Fig. 29), active or passive. In the course of a lifetime, every normal person interacts with a very large number and variety of pathogenic micro-organisms. In surgery, the body is protected against these agents in three ways:

- First, viruses, bacteria, protozoa and metazoa are denied access by the physical and chemical barriers of skin and mucosal surfaces.
- Second, there is a system of inborn but **non-specific immunity** (p. 231).
- Third, the individual acquires **specific immunity** on exposure to a pathogen or its components or products.

The mechanisms of active immunity appear less effective in premature or small infants and the aged than in younger adults. Resistance to infection is impaired when two or more infections coincide; when the immune mechanism is imperfect or is compromised; and when dehydration, shock, tissue injury and mechanical factors contribute to abnormal organ function.

SPECIFIC IMMUNITY

There are two, mutually supportive systems of specific, acquired immunity. They centre on the

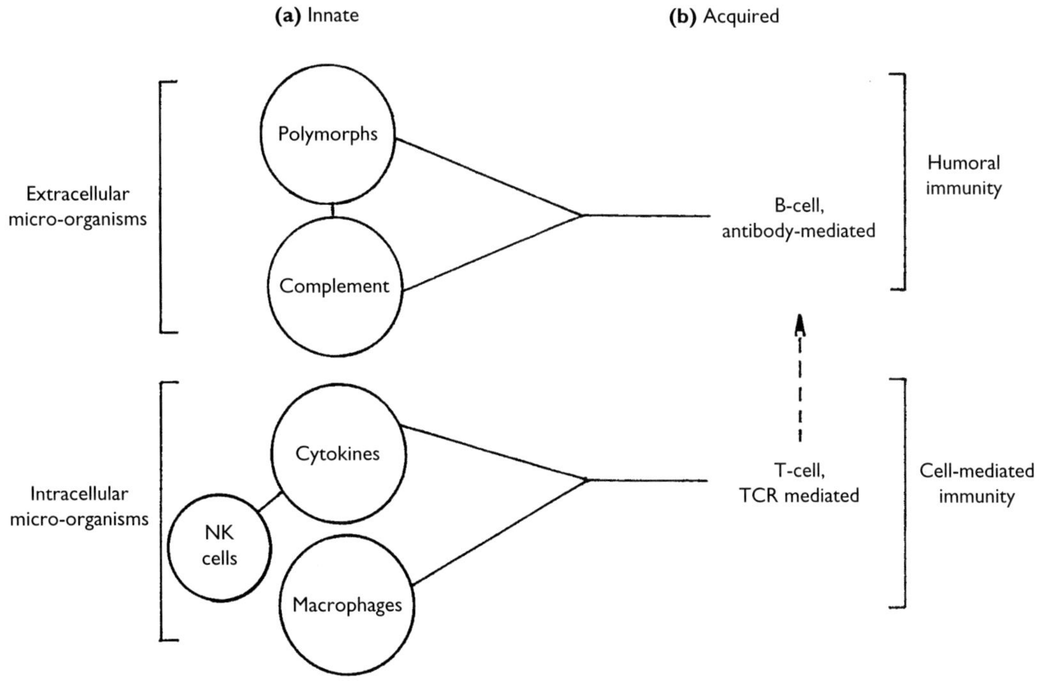

Figure 29 Relationship between innate and acquired immunity.

(a) Innate immunity. Irrespective of any specific response to predatory micro-organisms, each normal person inherits a natural capacity for defence. This innate system takes advantage of (i) phagocytic polymorphs and the alternative complement pathway for protection against extracellular micro-organisms such as streptococci, and on (ii) natural killer (NK) cells, cytokines and macrophages for protection against intracellular agents, particularly viruses.

(b) Acquired immunity. When specific defence mechanisms come into play, B-cells and T-cells add powerfully to defence. However, vast range of T-cell receptor and of antibodies generated by somatic mutation, requires 5 or more days to be initiated.

properties of two populations of lymphocytes that are identified by their reaction with monoclonal antibodies (p. 234).

- **B lymphocytes (B-cells)**. The first population, identified by CD 19, 21 and 40 (p. 205), is derived from **B**one marrow precursors. These B-cells comprise 65 to 80% of all circulating lymphocytes and bear immunoglobulin molecules as antigen receptors. Their function is the synthesis and secretion of antibodies that give specific, **humoral** protection against the **extracellular** antigens of microbial pathogens such as those of *Staphylococcus aureus*, *Streptococcus pneumoniae* and *Haemophilus influenzae*. Humoral immunity also neutralises bacterial exotoxins such as those of the Clostridia and *Corynebacterium diphtheriae*.
- **T lymphocytes**. The second population, identified by CD4, 8 and 28, also originates in the bone marrow but must traverse the **T**hymus in order to mature. These T-cells comprise 20 to 35% of circulating blood lymphocytes. They bear surface receptors that resemble immunoglobulins. T lymphocytes **support** B lymphocytes in antibody production. They also confer **cell-mediated** immunity, which offers specific protection against proliferating **intracellular** pathogens like *Mycobacterium tuberculosis* and *Leishmania donovani*.

Specific protection against extracellular micro-organisms

By the time of birth, circulating lymphocytes begin to be able to distinguish between foreign antigens such as those of micro-organisms, and the antigens of the body itself (p. 174). B lymphocyte reactions are the basis for humoral immunity and lead to the manufacture of the immunoglobulins that are called antibodies.

Now read Antigens and antibodies (p. 19)

B-lymphocyte cell surface receptors

The variety of foreign, microbial antigens to which the normal individual is exposed in the course of a lifetime is very large indeed. Yet the specific defence mechanisms are so effective, their flexibility so great, that they are able to respond precisely to any of this multitude of threats.

The defensive process begins when antigens on the surfaces of predatory micro-organisms are recognised by specific receptors on the surfaces of continuously circulating B lymphocytes. The receptors are immunoglobulin (antibody) molecules. The antigens of predatory microbes bind to and 'select' B lymphocytes with surface receptors specific to and complementary to their own shape. Each cell has ~10^5 of these identical receptor molecules. The receptors cross-link in a process that stimulates the B lymphocyte to proliferate, differentiate and to synthesise many more of the antibody molecules specific to the invader.

Clonal expansion

To deal with the continuing microbial threat, it is necessary for a large number of antibody molecules to be made. Activated B lymphocytes are therefore driven to divide. Each cell in this rapidly enlarging population forms part of a clone with identical antibody specificity. The process is **clonal expansion**. The new and expanded cell population matures into **plasma cells**.

Plasma cells are easily recognised. They are relatively large, 15 to 20 μm in diameter and have eccentric nuclei and 'cartwheel' clumps of chromatin. However, not all B lymphocytes that have encountered antigen differentiate in this way. Some persist in the circulation as **memory** B-cells.

The initial process by which the immune system counters a microbial threat, is a **primary** immune response. When there is continued or repeated exposure to the same antigen, a memory of the first reaction kick-starts a **secondary** response. This is much quicker and more vigorous than the primary response so that there is an accelerated production of much higher levels of antibody.

Now read Immunisation (p. 175)

Destruction of micro-organisms

Specific antibodies bind to pathogenic micro-organisms via the Fab part of the IgG antibody molecule (p. 19), preparing them, first, for phagocytosis (p. 270), second for intracellular destruction. This preliminary binding of antibody is **opsonisation.** The Fc end of the antibody molecule bound to the microbe surface links to Fc receptors on the plasma membrane of macrophages and other phagocytes. The C3 component of complement is activated ('fixed') and a dual process of active phagocytosis and inflammation is promoted. Micro-organisms that have not been bound to antibody are engulfed (endocytosed) slowly and inefficiently. Antibodies that promote phagocytosis are opsonins: those that simply 'fix' complement are not necessarily opsonins. Immunoglobulin G (IgG) molecules (p. 19) are particularly effective against pyogenic micro-organisms, especially those such as *Streptococcus pneumoniae* that are encapsulated.

The specific destructive effects of antimicrobial antibodies are mediated via the **classical pathway** of the complement system (Fig. 42; p. 232). The classical pathway is activated when one IgM or two adjacent IgG antibody molecules bind to microbial antigen. Component C3 is split. The early C1 complex is proteolytic; it acts on C2 and C4 to form an enzyme that splits C3. The cascade shares this purpose with the alternative pathway, part of the non-specific defence mechanism (p. 231). From this point onwards, the cascade of enzymatic and other process in the classical and alternative pathways (p. 232) is identical.

Now read Microbial defence (p. 231)

Some bacteria possess mechanisms to counter opsonisation. Thus, the opsonisation of *Staphylococcus aureus* can be prevented by a bacterial wall component, protein A, that blocks the free Fc end of the antibody molecule (p. 19).

Complement fixation was the basis of sensitive and specific serological tests used to search for antibody against viruses such as rubella. The principle is still applied to the identification of foreign proteins and cells such as those of malignant tumours and tissue transplants.

Specific protection against intracellular micro-organisms

T lymphocytes circulate continually from the blood to the lymph, returning from lymphoid tissue to the blood via the thoracic duct.

T lymphocyte receptors

Each T lymphocyte has an array of cell-surface receptors (TCR) that bind antigen specifically. These receptors are the essential recognition elements of cell-mediated immunity. Two types of signal initiate a T lymphocyte response, one via an interaction of T-cell receptors with antigen-derived peptides presented with molecules of the major histocompatability complex (MHC), the other via an interaction of CD28 with costimulatory molecules such as B7.

Although some functions of the TCR are analogous to those of antibodies, there is a structural difference. Unlike antibodies, the TCR is never secreted from the cell. The T-cell receptor is a transmembrane heterodimer (Fig. 30) that reaches across the cell wall, providing communication between the inside and the outside of the cell. T-cells recognise antigen only when antigen peptide is associated with MHC molecules on the surface of another cell (Fig. 30).

In response to antigen recognition and co-stimulation, the T lymphocyte is activated. The cell enlarges, becomes a lymphoblast and undergoes clonal expansion so that an increasing number of identical cells is created by mitotic division, a process that occupies several days.

T-helper (Th) cells

This sub-population of T lymphocytes recognises antigen only when antigenic peptides are presented at the surface of an antigen presenting cell (APC) in association with **class II MHC molecules** (Fig. 30). There are two subdivisions of Th lymphocytes:

- Th 1 lymphocytes are implicated in inflammatory processes and delayed, type IV hypersensitivity reactions. These cells promote macrophage activity by aiding the killing of intracellular pathogens, using the varied microbicidal mechanisms inherent in all such cells. They also activate cytotoxic T lymphocytes.
- Th 2 cells release cytokines that support B lymphocyte antibody manufacture.

T-cytotoxic (Tc) cells

A second population of T lymphocytes recognises antigen only when extraneous peptides are presented in association with **MHC class I molecules**. They have particular significance in viral infection: peptides of endogenous viral origin reach the cell surface in these molecules. The resulting T-cell responses enable viruses to be killed before they replicate. Simultaneously, Tc-cells release gamma interferon (pp. 23, 115) so that nearby tissue cells acquire resistance to viruses before they can spread.

T-regulatory cells

A poorly understood mechanism suppresses both humoral and cell-mediated immune responses. The processes of delayed hypersensitivity, cytotoxicity and antigen specific T-cell proliferation can be ablated.

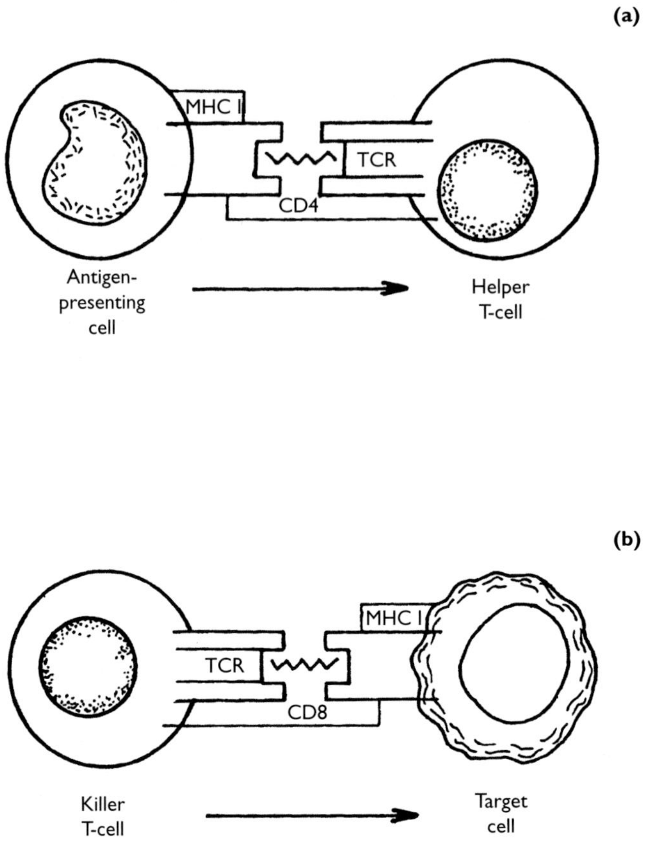

Figure 30 Presentation of antigen to T lymphocytes.

(a) Role of T helper (Th) cells in facilitating cell-mediated immune response. In presence of class II MHC, macrophages present antigenic peptides at cell surface. Here, interaction of peptide with T-cell receptor (TCR) on surface of Th cell is made possible by CD4.

(b) Role of T cytotoxic/cytolytic (Tc) cells. Target cell infected with virus is attacked by Tc cell. In presence of CD8, T-cell receptor binds to foreign, viral antigen presented at surface of infected cell together with class I MHC.

Whether there is a distinct population of T-cells with these properties remains uncertain.

RECOGNISING SELF ANTIGENS

No system of defence can be effective unless friend is distinguished from foe. The tissues of the individual him/herself must be differentiated clearly lest they be attacked by the immune mechanisms. Some tissues, such as the lipoproteins of the central nervous system; the cornea; the lens; and the colloid of thyroid follicles, contain effective antigens but do not establish contact with the immune mechanism because there is a blood–brain barrier or because they lack a vascular supply or lymphatic drainage. In the majority of tissues, however, antigens of the individual self ('self' antigens) are continuously available. To enable 'self' to be identified, a process comes into play very early in life that permits T and B lymphocytes to identify the antigens of the individual but then prevents them from undergoing the clonal expansion that is the prelude to the development of cell- or antibody-mediated immunity.

This state of non-reactivity is **tolerance**. It is of crucial importance in regard to tissue transplantation (p. 329). Very young, immunologically immature animals can be made tolerant of foreign antigens readily, that is, they can be **tolerised**. The newborn, for example, can be induced to tolerate skin grafts from foreign donors. The young are also susceptible to agents such as rubella virus that cause malformations and to tumour viruses. Tolerance is specific, that is, confined to a single antigen. It persists into adult life.

Adult animals can be **artificially tolerised** by suppressing or depleting the lymphocyte population when antigen is given or by giving antigen that cannot be processed effectively by macrophages. In particular circumstances, protein antigens can be tolerated when they are given in very low or very high doses or when they are administered intranasally or orally.

T-cell tolerance

A first step is negative selection. In infancy, self antigens are continuously presented by the macrophages of the corticomedullary region of the developing lymph nodes and by dendritic cells. Although there are relatively small numbers of circulating T lymphocytes in early life, any of the cells that has encountered a self antigen is deleted within the neonatal thymus by a process termed **clonal deletion**. The destruction is by apoptosis (p. 89). A second prophylactic step is signal suppression. As described above, when an antigen-presenting cell (APC) processes any antigen, and offers it to T-cell receptors in association with class II MHC molecules, the T-cell responds only if it receives a simultaneous, second, co-stimulatory signal. This second signal is not sent when the antigen is part of the 'self'. The result is **clonal anergy**.

B-cell tolerance

The processes of tolerance by B lymphocytes are closely similar to those that deal with T-cells. However, clonal deletion and clonal anergy are complemented by receptor editing and by a state of B lymphocyte 'helplessness'. In the former, genetic changes alter B-cell specificity. In the latter, an absence of T-cells prevents B lymphocytes from responding to self-antigens.

Now read Auto-immune disease (p. 28)

IMMUNISATION

Immunity to pathogenic micro-organisms can be brought about by short-term passive, or by long-term active, immunisation, a process that takes advantage of the accelerated secondary response to antigen (p. 19) (Fig. 31). In surgery, the choice of active immunisation against, for example, hepatitis B virus, is preferred to the expedient of passive immunisation.

- **Active immunity** is attained naturally, but to a varying degree, during recovery from infection. Microbial antigen reaches lymphoid tissues and is phagocytosed and degraded by phagocytic, dendritic cells. It is prepared for presentation to lymphoid cells that 'recognise' foreign antigen.
- **Passive immunity** is provided in post-neonatal life by the parenteral injection of purified preparations of preformed antibody. The use of anti-measles antibody is one example. The threat of anaphylaxis or serum sickness, because of the use of animal serum, has long been avoided by the use of purified human gamma-globulin. In surgery, passive immunity is largely confined to prophylactic treatment against hepatitis B, tetanus and gas gangrene.

Immunity is conferred on the newborn by the transplacental transfer of maternal IgG but not by IgM antibody molecules that do not pass the placental barrier. They are not recognised by the Fc receptors that specifically bind IgG to placental endothelium.

Now read Hypersensitivity (p. 160), Vaccination (p. 343)

IMMUNODEFICIENCY

Immunodeficiency may be a primary congenital or heritable defect, or a secondary result of disease; drugs; infections; irradiation; and other causes. The patient is said to be immunocompromised. **Anergy** describes an inability to generate an immune response against a substance expected to be antigenic.

Primary immunodeficiency

Primary immunodeficiency is classified, first, according to whether T-cells, B-cells, or both, are defective or absent; and, second, according to the phase of T-cell or B-cell development and function that is affected. There are many categories of more or less

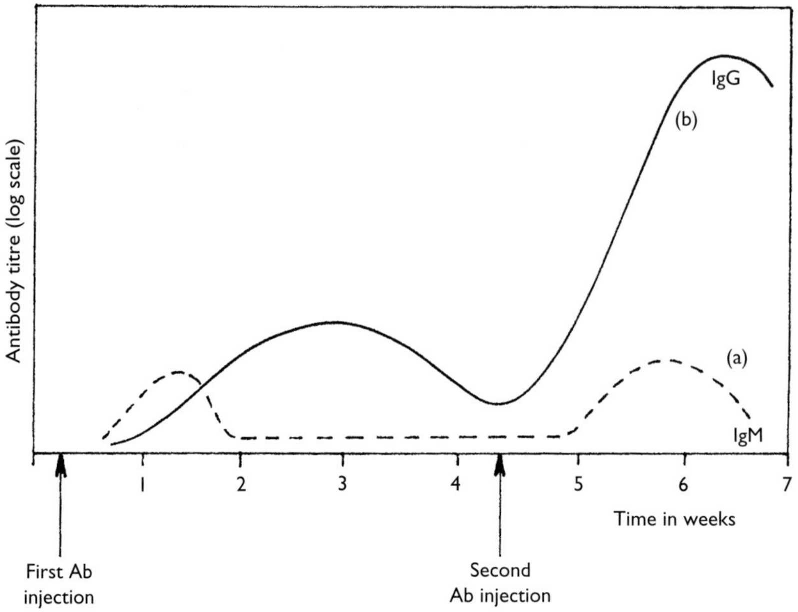

Figure 31 Primary and secondary immune responses.

(a) Primary response. Initial response of patient to challenge by foreign antigen is secretion of modest quantities of IgM antibody. Secretion of IgG is slower and later.

(b) Secondary response. When individual who has been immunised is re-challenged by same antigen, for example at the time of injection of a second dose of antiviral or antibacterial vaccine, additional secretion of IgM is delayed and of limited degree whereas formation of IgG is both accelerated and greatly increased. Heightened response is mainly due to clonal expansion of B-cells.

severe primary immunodeficiency disease (Fig. 32). They are rare conditions of which some examples are given below.

A complete lack of B-cells

In the absence of B-cells, there is a lack of antibody synthesis. The affected infants in Bruton-type agammaglobulinaemia are highly susceptible to bacterial infection but have a normal degree of immunity to viral, mycotic and mycobacterial disease.

A complete lack of T-cells

An absence of T-cells, and thus of cell-mediated immune responses, is encountered in the rare Di George syndrome. The thymus does not form. Affected individuals have normal humoral immune responses to pyogenic bacterial infections but display little resistance to viral infections, such as measles and chickenpox and to mycobacterial infection. The local injection of attenuated *Mycobacterium tuberculosis* in BCG vaccination is followed by progressive local and even systemic infection.

Combined immunodeficiency

In severe forms of combined immunodeficiency, both B-cell and T-cell formation are defective and there is a lack of both humoral and cell-mediated immune responses. Consequently, an extreme defect of resistance to all forms of infection prevails.

Secondary immunodeficiency

Disease of the lymphoreticular tissues may lead to secondary immunodeficiency. Although the numerous cells of myeloma usually secrete large quantities of monoclonal immunoglobulin, there is an overall deficiency in B-cell diversity resulting in a defect of humoral immunity. Hodgkin's lymphoma, with a neoplastic proliferation of mononuclear macrophage-type cells, is associated with a deficiency of T-cells and

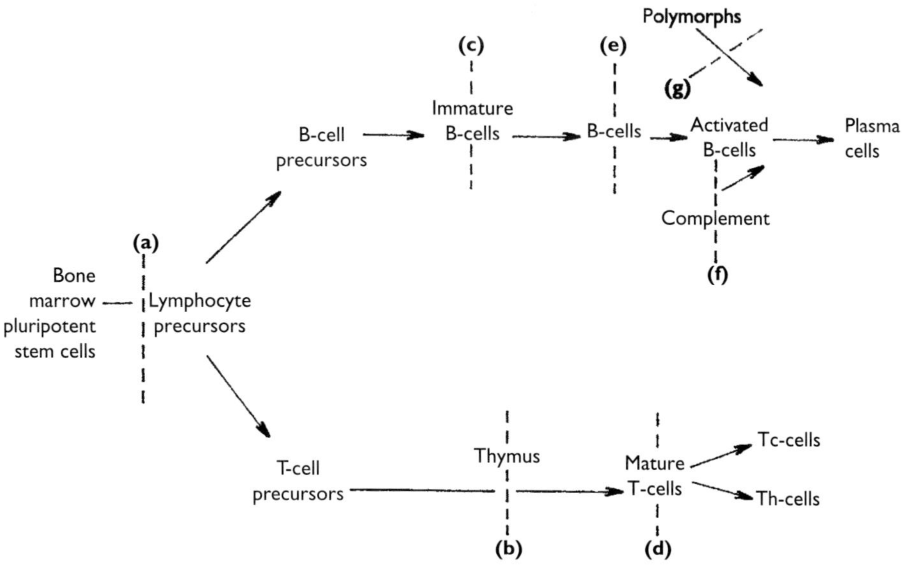

Figure 32 Causes and varieties of immunodeficiency.
(top) Prejudiced defence against extracellular, bacterial infections (c, e, f, g).
(bottom) Prejudiced defence against intracellular viral, protozoal and fungal infections (b, d).
Varieties of deficiency are: (a) combined immunodeficiency; (b) thymic aplasia (di George); (c) agammaglobulinaemia (Bruton); (d) secondary T-cell deficiency (for example in Hodgkin's disease); (e) secondary B-cell deficiency (for example, in multiple myeloma); (f) primary or secondary complement deficiency; (g) chronic granulomatous disease.

lowered resistance to viral, mycobacterial and fungal infections. HIV infection (p. 2) may lead to AIDS.

Immune suppression and immunodeficiency are associated with an increased frequency of cancers, such as leukaemia, lymphoma and malignant melanoma. Sometimes these cancers are caused by oncogenic agents such as EB virus that may be latent within the B-cells of normal adults. Cytotoxic T-cells normally regulate the transformation of EB virus-infected cells and suppression or lack of T-cell activity allows infected B-cells to behave without this constraint.

IMMUNOSUPPRESSION

Suppression of the T-cell immune reaction against a graft is required to permit prolonged survival of the transplanted organ or tissue. It is of interest that several important immunosuppressive drugs (Table 32) were first employed as cytotoxic drugs in the therapy of cancer. A common bond between these drugs is a similarity to bases of the DNA molecule (p. 23). A number of other immunosuppressive compounds are carcinogens. A hazard of prolonged immunosuppression is the emergence of an unexpectedly high incidence of neoplasms, particularly lymphomas. The mechanism of neoplasia may be a failure of T-cells to suppress the multiplication of B-cells bearing tumour-promoting agents such as the Epstein–Barr virus.

IMPLANTATION

Implantation is the act of setting a piece of tissue from one part of the body into another site. To flourish, tissue implants require particular environments and stimuli. Implantation also describes the insertion of foreign bodies, such as radio-active needles, in the treatment of cancer, and the implantation of avalon sponges in the treatment of rectal prolapse.

Implantation dermoid cysts are usually found on the fingers but may occur at any site at which squamous epithelium is driven beneath the skin by a penetrating wound. Other epithelia undergo similar displacement. Thus, implantation cysts may form in the lower rectum following haemorrhoidectomy or polypectomy, and neoplastic cells may be implanted in wounds or suture lines.

Table 32 Some effective immunosuppressive agents

Immunosuppressive agent	Properties
Analogues of DNA bases	These agents compete in DNA synthesis. Azathioprine and 6-mercaptopurine are important examples.
Alkylating agents	Cyclophosphamide is one example.
Antibiotics	Cyclosporin A suppresses T- but not B-cells and may permit virtually permanent tolerance of a graft. It has allowed successful renal allografting without the need for donor matching. Its use has led to increasing success in liver and multi-organ transplantation. Actinomycin blocks protein synthesis.
Anti-lymphocytic serum	Serum may be used in the form of purified antilymphocytic IgG.
Corticosteroids	The properties of the corticosteroids are given on p. 6.

Theoretically, the implantation of neoplastic cells might be anticipated at many sites of needle biopsy. In practice, this hazard is very rare but has occurred sufficiently often in patients with hepatocellular carcinoma for the use of this technique in diagnosis to be questioned. The implantation of neoplastic cells at sites of trocars inserted during laparoscopy is more frequent and may have serious consequences.

Now read Transplantation (p. 329)

INFARCT

An infarct is the dead tissue remaining when the oxygen, nutrition or blood supply to, or drainage from, a tissue or organ is reduced below a critical level. Infarction is often ischaemic necrosis. Infarcts may be arterial or venous.

The sensitivity of tissues to ischaemia varies widely and is described on p. 187. Infarcts are said to be as red or white (pale). When afferent vessels are end-arteries, as in the case of the spleen or kidney, the infarcted tissue remains pale. In the lung, blood continues to flow through the bronchial arteries and the ischaemic tissue becomes 'stuffed' (infarcted) with blood and appears red or purple.

INFECTION

Infection is the invasion of the body by pathogenic or potentially pathogenic micro-organisms and their subsequent multiplication. Infections may be direct, for example after contact, or indirect, when the causative agents are transmitted by an intermediary such as food, fomites or by insect or arthropod vectors. Sepsis describes infection with pyogenic, that is, pus-forming, bacteria.

Now read Bacteria (p. 30), Fungi (p. 135) Protozoa (p. 282), Virus (p. 347), Worms (p. 356)

OVERGROWTH

This term, also described as 'superinfection', is used to describe two situations.

In the first, there is infection with an organism that supersedes a different agent ('secondary infection'). In one example, superinfection with *Pseudomonas aeruginosa* is common in infected burns and in the lungs of patients requiring prolonged ventilation; in another, superinfection with *Candida albicans* is increasingly common in patients surviving septicaemia. Overwhelming infections of this kind may result from impaired immunity following initial infection by other organisms. The infection can then be considered to be 'opportunistic'.

In the second, there is infection with an organism that is a normal commensal but which expresses its latent pathogenicity due to a change in its environment. Thus, *Clostridium difficile* causes pseudomembranous enterocolitis when the other gastro-intestinal organisms that predominate are eradicated by oral antibiotics (p. 17). In the same way, *Staphylococcus epidermidis* colonising central lines may become invasive.

Now read Abscess (p. 1), Immunity (p. 171), Microbial defence (p. 231)

INFLAMMATION

Inflammation is the response of living, vascularised tissues to injury caused by chemical, physical, immunological, infective or other agents. It is usually beneficial and protective but may, nevertheless, exert damaging effects upon the tissues in which it develops. Inflammation may be acute or chronic.

ACUTE INFLAMMATION

There are five clinical (cardinal) signs: redness, swelling, pain, heat and loss of function. These signs reflect a complex series of molecular and microscopic changes centred upon the arterioles, capillaries and venules. The changes of inflammation cannot develop in avascular tissue: the inflammatory responses at sites of infarction, for example, are confined to the surrounding zones where vascular perfusion continues.

The phenomena of acute inflammation depend upon the formation and activation of a cascade of mediators. There are important secondary alterations in the behaviour of the circulating leucocytes, tissue mononuclear phagocytes and mast cells.

Vascular changes

Three of the five clinical signs of inflammation can be simulated by drawing the head of a pin firmly across the surface of the living skin. The flexor surface of the forearm is a convenient site to observe. A **triple response** (p. 373) results. The reaction comprises an immediate dull red flush in and around the site of injury; a wider zone of reddening, the flare; and a more slowly developing weal along the track of the pin-head. The flush is due to the dilatation of venules. It results from the rapid activation locally of chemical mediators, particularly histamine. The flare is caused by arteriolar dilatation which results from an axon reflex and which leads to a rise in local temperature. The weal is a form of local oedema, a result of the action of agents such as histamine.

The increased vascularity of sites of inflammation enables foci of infection and sites of abscess to be identified after the injection of radio-active isotopes such as ^{67}Ga-citrate. Radio-active indium (^{111}In)-labelled leucocytes can be employed in a similar way.

Oedema

One effect of histamine is to cause the endothelial cells of the venules to separate. Fluid rich in protein escapes from the plasma through these gaps. Among the proteins are fibrinogen and the immunoglobulins. Fibrinogen polymerises to form fibrin (p. 97), the accumulation of which is commonplace in inflammatory foci. Fluid containing only smaller molecules crosses the endothelial cells by pinocytosis. The volume of fluid leaving the venules in inflammation exceeds that returning by osmosis. Oedema results; the fluid is an exudate (p. 252).

The flow of lymph from an inflamed part increases as extravascular tissue fluid accumulates. The inflammatory agents and the products of tissue injury are conveyed to local and thence to regional lymph nodes. Lymphadenopathy develops.

Cellular phenomena

At inflammatory foci, axial blood flow in post-capillary venules slows. The central column of red cells and leucocytes is dispersed. Within a few minutes, the most numerous white cells, the polymorphs, adhere to the 'sticky' endothelium. Inserting cytoplasmic processes between the endothelial cells, the polymorphs move actively to the extravascular tissue spaces; they are followed slowly by mononuclear macrophages and passively by red blood cells. Chemotactic influences draw the leucocytes towards the inflammatory focus. Reactions between the defensive white cells and the damaging agent initiate processes such as antibody production and phagocytosis. Lymphocytes migrate through the blood and lymph nodes and are sequestered at sites of inflammation where they mediate immune responses to infective agents such as mycobacteria.

Mediators and modulators

As the inflammatory reaction begins, a complex series of interrelated and interactive molecular responses is triggered. There are three groups of mediators corresponding to three phases of acute inflammation:

- Early (histamine).
- Intermediate (kinins).
- Prolonged (prostaglandins and leukotrienes).

The mediators can be categorised according to whether they originate in precursor molecules in the blood plasma or are derived from component molecules of tissue plasma membranes.

Plasma-derived

There are four important systems: the kinin cascade, the complement cascade, the coagulation cascade and the fibrinolytic system (Fig. 33). The four systems are interlinked. The kinins, polypeptides made by the action of enzymes (kallikreins) on plasma precursors (kininogens), increase vascular permeability and aid leucocyte margination and migration. Kallikreins are activated by Hageman factor (factor XII). The coagulation cascade is described on p. 95, the complement system on p. 232. Fibrin degradation products (Fig. 22) increase vascular permeability and potentiate the action of bradykinin. Proteinase inhibitors are activated: they include alpha 2-macroglobulin (α_2-macroglobulin) and alpha 1-anti-trypsin (α_1AT – p. 209).

Tissue-derived

There are at least four further systems of interacting molecules:

- The most abundant comprises products of arachidonic acid, a component of cell wall phospholipids (Fig. 34). In the delayed, later phase of acute inflammation, prostaglandins are quickly manufactured from arachidonic acid as they are needed. The phospholipase of neutrophil polymorph lysosomes is one source. However, arachidonic acid is also the precursor of the leukotrienes, formed by neutrophil polymorphs and mast cells. Leukotrienes are potent chemotactic agents for neutrophil polymorphs; they increase endothelial 'stickiness'.
- A second group comprises the vaso-active amines. These molecules include histamine and 5-hydroxytryptamine. Histamine is responsible for the immediate, transient changes in vessel permeability. It is manufactured in and released from mast-cells (p. 229) near blood vessels.

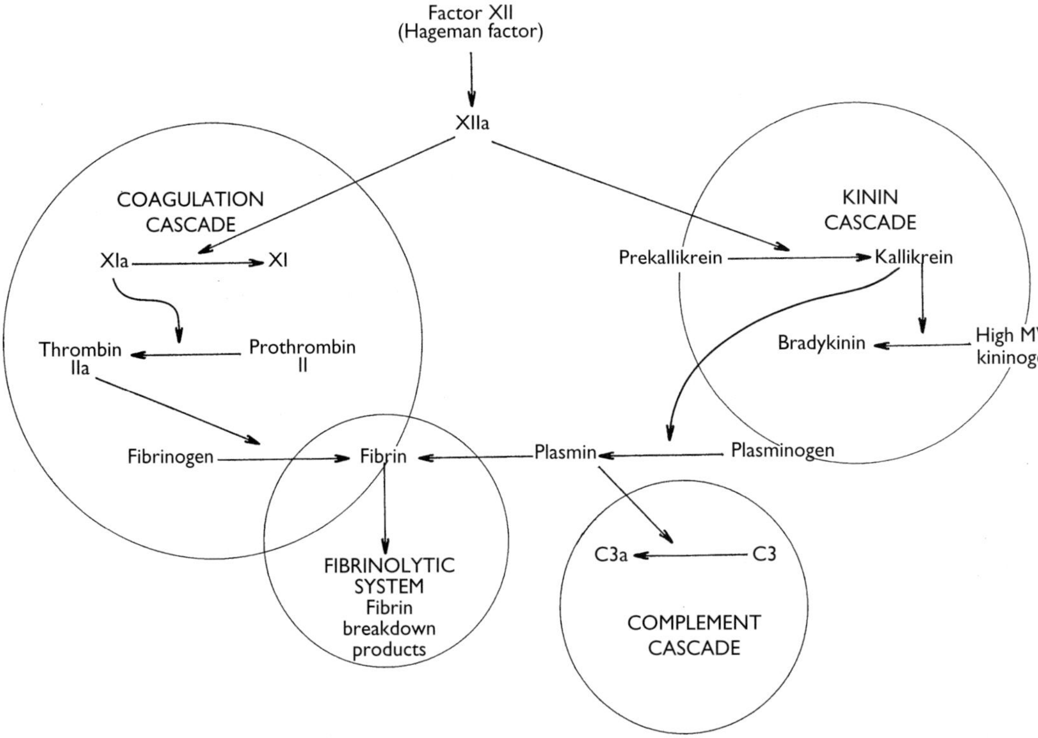

Figure 33 Plasma-derived mediators. Relations of coagulation, fibrinolytic, kinin, and complement cascades. Hageman factor (Factor XII) plays key role in activating four cascades: clotting; fibrinolytic; kinin; and complement. Diagram indicates their mutual relationships. (Redrawn from Mitchell RN and Cotran RS: In *Basic Pathology*, 6th edition, Kumar V, Cotran RS, Robbins SL (eds). Philadelphia, London: WB Saunders Company, 1997).

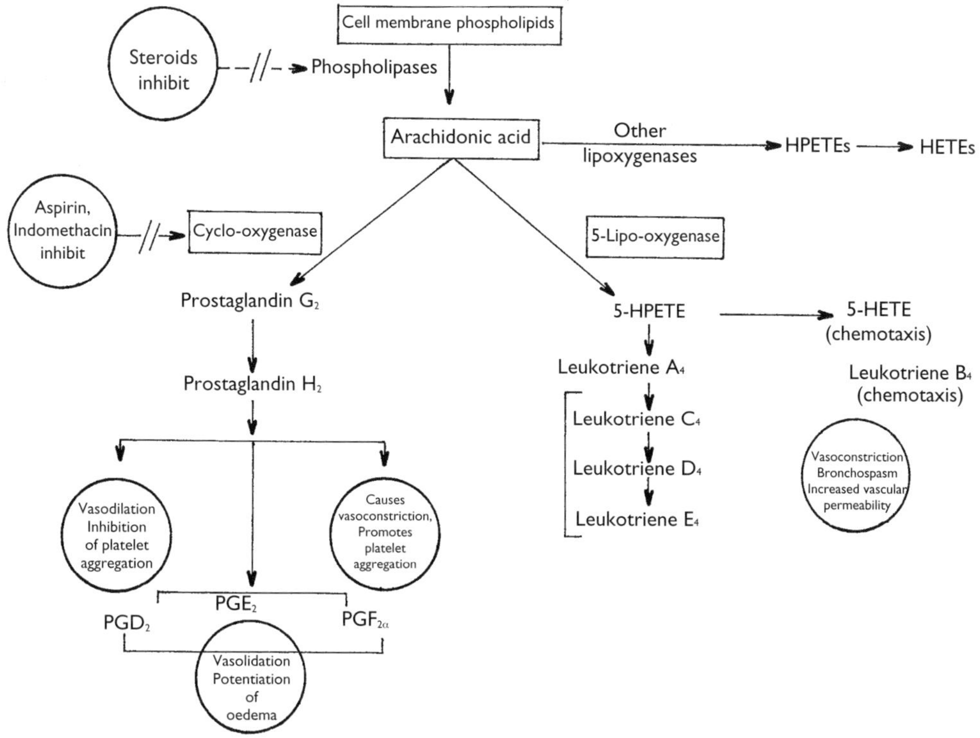

Figure 34 Tissue-derived mediators. Formation of metabolites of arachidonic acid.
Numerous effects of inflammatory process originate through liberation of arachidonic acid from cell membrane phospholipids by action of phospholipases. Enzymes are activated by physical, chemical and mechanical stimuli that cause inflammation. Following its liberation, metabolism of arachidonic acid pursues one of two alternative pathways. The first, catalysed by cyclo-oxygenase, leads to the formation of the prostaglandins (PGA). The second, catalysed by the lipo-oxygenase of polymorphs, results in formation of leukotrienes. Two forms of cyclo-oxygenase are COX-1 and COX-2. Circles indicate actions of prostaglandins and leukotrienes, and sites at which some anti-inflammatory drugs take effect. PG = prostaglandin; HPETE = unstable hydroxy derivative of arachidonic acid; HETE = reduction product of HPETE. (Redrawn from Mitchell RN and Cotran RS: In *Basic Pathology*, 6th edition, Kumar V, Cotran RS, Robbins SL (eds). Philadelphia, London: WB Saunders Company, 1997).

- The third category is that of the cytokines (p. 114). Those of importance in acute inflammation include interleukins-1 and 2 (IL-1 and IL-2).
- At the onset of acute inflammation and during other pyrexial illnesses, further populations of molecules appear in the plasma. These are the acute phase reactants; they include precursors of amyloid. Free radicals also play a part in the inflammatory response. Superoxide ($O_2^{\bullet}$ – p. 133), for example, exerts an early and important influence and the significance of nitric oxide $O_2^{\bullet}$ is increasingly recognised.

Nitric oxide

Inflammatory mediators stimulate the generation of nitric oxide (NO – p. 134). They include bradykinin, thrombin, histamine, acetylcholine and 5-hydroxytryptamine. NO also interacts with the prostaglandins. In early inflammation, NO causes vasodilatation leading to erythema and heightened local temperature. It may also lead to oedema. NO reduces the adhesion of polymorphs to vascular endothelium, partly by scavenging the reactive oxygen intermediates (p. 133) that enhance adhesion.

Now read Free radicals (p. 133), Microbial defence (p. 231)

Cytokines in inflammation

Cytokines make an important contribution in inflammation. They enhance host defence mechanisms, but may also cause tissue destruction.

Antibacterial and antiparasitic cytokines

Distinct subsets of cytokines are secreted by CD4 T lymphocytes. T-helper 1 (Th 1) lymphocytes drive antibacterial immune responses, Th 2 -cells promote antiviral and antiparasitic responses.

Chemokines

Chemokines are a special group of cytokines. Their function is the attraction of leucocytes to foci of inflammation. They also have other properties including cell activation and angiogenesis. Chemokines comprise more than 40 closely related 8 to 10-kDa proteins. There are four families. Some receptors are restricted to particular cells; others are more widely expressed. CXCR1 is largely restricted to neutrophil polymorphs. CCR1 and CCR2 are constitutively expressed on monocytes.

Now read Cytokines (p. 114)

CHRONIC INFLAMMATION

Active inflammation may persist for very long periods. Among the numerous causes of chronic inflammation are:

- Persistent infection by organisms resistant to or inaccessible to antibiotics.
- The formation of granulation and fibrous tissue in the wall of an abscess.
- The presence of foreign bodies ranging from non-absorbable suture material to particles of dirt and bullet fragments.
- The local extension of malignant neoplasms.
- Recurrent mechanical abrasion or ulceration.

Chronic inflammation is characteristic of the granulomatous infections: tuberculosis, syphilis and leprosy. Mycobacteria survive within macrophages. Foci of ischaemic necrosis defeat attempts at resolution and repair and caseous, necrotic tissue debris persists for long periods. Where particles of metal, dirt or crystals are present, macrophages unite in a common purpose, fusing to form foreign body giant-cells (p. 142). Fibrosis (p. 131) is the ultimate fate of chronic inflammatory foci. The persistence of infection in chronic osteomyelitis, bronchiectasis or tuberculosis is a basis for the development of amyloidosis.

INHALATION

The inhalation of nasopharyngeal secretions or vomit is a possible complication of impaired consciousness from any cause. It may occur after surgical procedures, particularly in patients allowed to remain supine. Intense bronchial irritation and excess mucus secretion are followed by peptic digestion of the bronchial tree and subsequent bronchopneumonia. One or more pulmonary lobes collapse, but sudden, early death due to anoxia or vagal cardiac stimulation is commonplace. A further, frequent cause of death is the inhalation of food and teeth or dental appliances, a particular hazard in unconscious accident cases. In fires and explosions, noxious and hot gases are often inhaled, damaging the trachea and bronchi directly. The onset of pulmonary oedema may then lead to death from respiratory failure.

INHERITANCE

Inheritance is the natural derivation of characters from parents and ancestors and their expression in the progeny. It is a function of the genetic information exchanged after two gametes unite at fertilisation. The zygote obtains half its genetic information from each parent; the information is transmitted by the coding units of DNA (p. 139).

Now read Chromosomes (p. 90), Genes (p. 138)

Mutation

A mutation is a change in the structure of DNA. There are many different kinds. A point mutation is the replacement of one base (nucleotide) in the DNA of the gene by another base. A classical example of point mutation is the sickle-cell trait (Fig. 35). The original gene and the new, mutant form are alleles, that is, they are alternative genes at a single locus. There may also be deletions, insertions, re-arrangements and duplications of parts of the DNA molecule.

Among the known causes of mutations of genes located on either somatic or sex chromosomes are ionising radiation; virus infection; chemical agents; or hormones acting on the gonads or on germ cells prior to fertilisation.

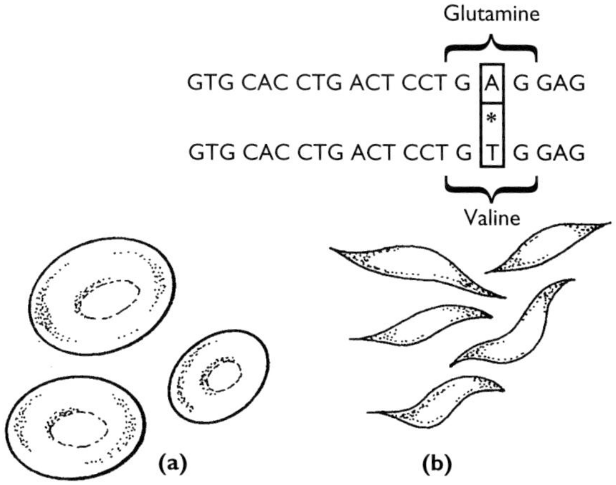

Figure 35 Inheritance of single gene defect – sickle cell anaemia.
Disease results from mutation at specific point in DNA that codes for β chain of haemoglobin molecule. Sequence of bases at this point* is changed from GAG to GTG. Valine is therefore formed instead of glutamic acid. Consequence is reduced solubility of abnormal haemoglobin which forms fibrous precipitates, changing shape of red blood cells, particularly under conditions of low oxygen partial pressures, and increasing fragility of affected cells.

Individuals with mutation in only one of the two genes coding for β haemoglobin have sickle cell trait. Those inheriting two mutant β haemoglobin genes have sickle cell disease.

a. Normal red blood cells; b. Sickled red blood cells.

Mechanisms of inheritance

Individuals vary in weight, height, colour, intelligence, behaviour and every other bodily characteristic. The genetic constitution delineating these characteristics is the **genotype**. The physical and mental features themselves constitute the **phenotype**. Under similar circumstances, the inheritance of a genetic abnormality may or may not affect two related individuals to an identical degree. The genetic defect is said to exhibit different **penetrance**.

At least 4000 uncommon or rare disorders are now known, in which the condition is entirely explicable by the inheritance of a defect of a single gene (Fig. 35). These are single gene defects. In a rapidly growing number of these single gene defects, the identity of the mutant gene has been established, raising the possibility of transgenic therapy (p. 142). Cystic fibrosis; muscular dystrophy; and alkaptonuria are examples.

Many other disorders result from the action of multiple genes. Their inheritance is complex (multifactorial).

In a large number of further common disorders, heredity contributes to the onset or severity of a disease but is not solely responsible, so that, in peptic ulcer; cholelithiasis; Crohn's disease; and many cancers, both genetic and environmental factors play important roles.

Mendelian inheritance

In Mendelian inheritance, the appearance of characters in the offspring or progeny follows the laws first established by Mendel (p. 374). The actions of a single mutant gene are responsible for an inherited defect which may be dominant or recessive in the manner of its expression.

Abnormal autosomal inheritance

- **Autosomal dominant**. In abnormal autosomal dominant inheritance, for example familial adenomatous polyposis, the affected parents are heterozygous for the mutant gene: one parent is normal, the other carries the dominant allele. Males and females are equally affected. The severity of the disorder varies due to differing degrees of gene penetrance. Half of the children suffer from the disease but may remain asymptomatic until adult life. The remaining children are normal. Since young persons may not know whether they have inherited the dominant gene, a search for the inherited defect is required to permit family planning.
- **Autosomal recessive**. In abnormal autosomal recessive inheritance, for example cystic fibrosis, both healthy parents carry the same recessive, mutant gene. There is usually no family history of disease. The inherited abnormality appears in 25% of the offspring. If the parents are consanguineous, the risk of disease is increased. The rarer the disorder, the more likely is it that the parents of an affected child are related. There is an increased risk in some ethnic groups in which particular genes may be frequent. When there is no detectable defect, the mutant gene is 'silent' and the inherited abnormality can only be recognised by molecular analysis.

Abnormal sex-linked inheritance

The pattern of abnormal sex-linked inheritance is determined by whether the single mutant gene is located upon the X or Y chromosome and whether the trait is recessive or dominant.

- **Y-linked**. Y-linked faults may include web toes, porcupine skin and the 'hairy ear' trait. They are transmitted from father to son.
- **X-linked**. In abnormal X-linked recessive inheritance, for example haemophilia or colour blindness, the mutant gene is carried by females but they rarely suffer from the abnormal state. Half of the sons develop the disease and half of the daughters are carriers. In abnormal X-linked dominant inheritance, for example vitamin D resistant rickets, all the daughters of affected men have the disease but none of the sons. All children of affected homozygous females and 50% of the children of heterozygous, affected females suffer from the defect.

Multifactorial inheritance

In many disorders, there is no evidence of Mendelian inheritance, yet a familial predisposition or a relatively high frequency among identical twins suggests that genetic factors are operative. Under these circumstances, the disorder is inherited on a polygenic basis, with the actions of several genes combining. The majority of instances of carcinoma of the breast, and rheumatoid arthritis are examples. Alternatively, there may be non-penetrance, or the condition may arise as a consequence of an environmental influence acting upon a genetically determined abnormality.

In a further category of cases, a mutation is unstable so that the effects of the mutant gene vary in successive generations. There may also be functional differences in the expression of a mutant.

INTERVERTEBRAL DISC

The fibrocartilage of the 23 intervertebral discs is inevitably affected by hereditary, spinal disorders such as achondroplasia and by congenital deformities such as scoliosis. The discs are also implicated in common traumatic, infective and neoplastic diseases including compression fracture; tuberculosis; metastatic carcinoma of the bronchus, breast and prostate; and multiple myeloma.

INTERVERTEBRAL DISC PROTRUSION AND PROLAPSE

The collagenous connective tissue of the discs becomes progressively less hydrated with age and its mechanical properties change. As a result, large forces applied across the interspinous joints are liable to cause, first, protrusion and then prolapse of the nuclei pulposus of the discs. The forces most likely to have this effect are those created by lifting heavy objects with the spine angled postero-anteriorly. The discs most susceptible to this fault are those of the mid- and lower lumbar region. Consequently, prolapsed disc tissue is likely to compress the nerve roots of the cauda equina. The most frequent result is nerve root pain affecting L5 and S1 segments and referred in the distribution of the sciatic nerve. However, other segments including L3 and L4, are periodically affected when the pain is of a femoral nerve distribution. The degeneration and protrusion of cervical intervertebral discs is a potent cause of the common condition of cervical spondylo-arthropathy.

Now read Spine (p. 300)

INVASION

Invasion is the aggressive intrusion of living cells or micro-organisms into tissues or organs. The word is used in several ways. Degradative enzyme activity is always the responsible mechanism.

Bacterial invasion

Pathogenic bacteria such as *Streptococcus pyogenes* penetrate tissue planes quickly, causing disorders such as cellulitis (p. 111).

Invasion by cancer cells

Malignant neoplasms invade tissues directly, by lymphatic or blood vascular permeation, or by metastasis. Collagenase, hyaluronidase and lysosomal proteases degrade connective tissue molecules and catalyse the invasive process.

Invasion in systemic connective tissue disease

In inflammatory connective tissue diseases such as rheumatoid arthritis, activated macrophages release neutral proteases, elastase and cathepsins. Cartilage matrix is degraded. Macrophages, lymphocytes, capillary endothelial cells and young fibroblasts extend into the cartilage, replacing it with granulation tissue.

IRRADIATION

Organs, tissues or the whole body may be exposed accidentally or deliberately to electromagnetic or particulate radiation (Tables 33 and 34). Some terms employed in nuclear medicine are defined in Table 35. Some units of measurement are given in Tables 36 and 37.

Ionising radiation is particulate or electromagnetic radiation with an energy sufficient to ionise the irradiated tissues or cells. Small quantities of ionising radiation are emitted from television tubes and other domestic equipment but the sources are carefully screened and are safe. Exposure to ionising X-rays and gamma-radiation is a potential occupational hazard among radiographers; workers in nuclear reactors; and space travellers, but they also are guarded from these sources.

Non-ionising radiation is of lower energy and includes visible, white light; invisible, ultraviolet and infrared light; and radio waves. Exposure to ultraviolet irradiation in the form of sunlight is a

Table 33 Forms of electromagnetic irradiation

Energy increases as wavelength decreases	
Form	**Wavelength**
Radio	1500 to 10 m
Infrared	700 to 600 nm
Visible	600 to 400 nm
Ultraviolet	400 to 250 nm
X-ray	1.0 nm
Gamma	0.1 nm
Cosmic	Very short

Table 34 Characteristics of some forms of particulate radiation

Particle	Tissue penetration	Mass	Charge
Beta-particles			
β^- (electron)	5 mm	1/100 H nucleus	–
β^+ (positron)	5 mm	1/100 H nucleus	+
Proton	Short	1	+
Neutron	~50 μm	1	Nil
Alpha-particle	Short	4	++
Heavy nuclei			–

Table 35 Some definitions of terms used in nuclear physics

Nuclide	A nuclide is a species of atomic nucleus as characterised by charge, mass number and quantum state, capable of existing for a measurable life time
Daughter nuclide	A daughter nuclide originates from a nuclide by radio-active decay
Nuclear isomer	Nuclear isomers are separate nuclides. However, transient excited nuclear states and unstable intermediates in nuclear reactions are not described in this way
Half-life	The half-life of a radio-active material is the time during which half the original nuclei disintegrate
Specific activity	The specific activity of a compound is proportional to the number of radio-active atoms present

Table 36 Old (CGS) units of ionising radiation

Unit	Definition
röntgen (R)	A röntgen (p. 375) was a measure of the radiation source, equivalent to the ionisation produced in air by X- or γ-radiation (p. 186). 1 R was the quantity of radiation such that the associated corpuscular emission in 1 cc of air produced 1 electrostatic unit of charge
rad	A rad was a measure of absorption. 1 rad was the deposition of 100 ergs/g material, at the point of interest, by ionising radiation
curie (Ci)	A curie (p. 370) was a measure of radioactivity, originally related to the activity of radium (^{226}Ra). 1 Ci was 3.7 × 10^{10} disintegrations/second
rem	A rem was a unit of radiation dose that expressed, on a common scale for all ionising radiations, the presumed biological damage incurred by exposed persons. It was obtained by applying a correction factor to the absorbed dose in rads

Table 37 New (SI) units of ionising radiation. The joule (J) is the SI unit of energy. It ≡ 10^7 ergs and is intended to replace the calorie which ≡ 4.184 J

gray (Gy)	A gray (p. 371) is the measure of absorbed radiation dose as J/kg. It is equivalent to 100 rad
becquerel (Bq)	A becquerel (p. 369) is a measure of radioactivity as disintegrations per second; it is equivalent to 2.703×10^{11} Ci
sievert (Sv)	A sievert (p. 376) is a measure of dose equivalence as J/kg. One sievert corresponds to 100 rem

universal experience from which protection is highly desirable.

Now read Malignant melanoma (p. 227)

ELECTROMAGNETIC RADIATION

X-rays (röntgen rays) are emitted from cathode ray tubes through which a high voltage current is passed. X-rays are also emitted incidentally from high voltage apparatus such as electron microscopes and, in nature, from stellar sources.

The wavelength of X-rays varies considerably. The short wavelength, 'harder' X-rays used in radiotherapy penetrate tissues to a much greater extent than do the longer wavelength, 'softer' X-rays used in radiodiagnosis. The damaging effects of diagnostic X-rays are diminished by combining low doses with image video-amplification. Computed axial tomography (p. 169) has the advantage of minimising radiation hazards while offering high-resolution scanning. In the laboratory, the X-rays used to identify and measure very small amounts of elements such as iron, calcium or lead in tissue are employed under safe conditions.

Gamma-rays

Gamma-rays are of very short wavelength and high energy. They are emitted spontaneously by many natural and some artificial radio-active isotopes. Radium, discovered by Marie and Pierre Curie (p. 370) was the first known source. Stellar gamma-rays reach the earth as cosmic rays and therefore comprise part of the background radiation to which all living creatures are continuously exposed.

Ultrasonic and laser radiations

Ultrasonic and laser radiations are described on pp. 169, 335 and 203, respectively. Other uses for electromagnetic radiation include microwave ovens, TV monitors and radar.

PARTICULATE IRRADIATION

Tissues may be exposed to alpha-particles (nuclei of helium atoms), beta-particles (electrons), deuterons, protons and other particles, depending on the source. Many radio-active isotopes used safely in diagnosis are rapidly decaying beta-emitters with short half-lives. Phosphorus (^{32}P), yttrium (^{90}Y) and tritium (^{3}H) are examples. Alpha-particle emitters such as thorium (^{232}Th) have extremely long half-lives and are potent carcinogens. Thorium was employed in the form of colloidal thorium dioxide (thorotrast) as a contrast medium for angiography. Many individuals subjected to the effects of this material developed malignant tumours after a latent period of 20 or more years.

ISOTOPES

An isotope is a nuclide (Table 35) of a particular chemical element which has the same atomic number (of protons) but a different mass number (protons + neutrons) from other nuclides of the same element. Thus, an isotope is an element that has the same atomic number as another element but a different atomic weight. Some elements consist of several isotopes and the atomic weight is the mean of these weights.

When the nuclear composition of an element is unstable, the nuclei may undergo spontaneous disintegration with the emission of alpha- or beta-particles, or gamma-radiation. The isotope is said to be radio-active. Some radio-active isotopes exist naturally but many others now used in diagnosis are prepared artificially by bombarding a stable element in a nuclear reactor or cyclotron.

BIOLOGICAL EFFECTS OF IONISING RADIATION

The biological effects of any form of radiation (Tables 33 and 34) depend on the frequency of exposure, the intensity (that is, the energy of the radiation), the duration of exposure, and the nature of the tissue. The tissue effects are cumulative and damaging. They are due to the absorption of energy by cells, particularly cell nuclei. Electromagnetic radiations such as short-wavelength X-rays and gamma-rays have the highest energy (Table 33), penetrate furthest and produce severe tissue disturbance by the transfer of much energy. Large particles such as helium nuclei (alpha-particles) possess similar properties (Table 34).

Cells are injured by ionising radiation and may be killed. Both the cytoplasm and the nucleus are damaged. Large doses of radiation produce ionisation of water in the cytoplasm. The hydroxyl ions denature protein and cell membranes. Organelles and enzyme systems are disorganised and the cell dies rapidly. Lower doses are sufficient to damage DNA. Major chromosomal injury can prevent cell replication. Even smaller doses can lead to mutations that are usually recessive.

Short-term effects

The short-term effects of ionising radiation are recognised in tissues in which there is rapid cell turnover (Table 38). The nucleus is particularly vulnerable during division. The cells of the lymphoid tissues and bone marrow; the spermatogonia and oogonia; and those of the gastro-intestinal tract, are most readily injured. Lymphoid tissue quickly atrophies and the bone marrow becomes acellular. Externally, the skin may desquamate. The intestinal effects, with diarrhoea and fluid loss, are those of radiation enteropathy. Following treatment for abdominal and cervical cancer, signs resembling those of gastro-enteritis may develop within a few days of exposure to ionising radiation.

Now read Radiation enteritis (p. 167)

Table 38 Relative radiosensitivity of different tissues

High (radiosensitive)	Lymphocytes; immature blood-cell precursors; intestinal epithelium; thymocytes; spermatogonia; oogonia
Intermediate	Endothelium; hair follicles; fibroblasts; lens; growing cartilage; parenchyma of liver, pancreas, kidney, endocrine glands, glandular epithelium, breast, skin
Low (radioresistant)	Blood; skeletal muscle; mature connective tissue; bone; mature cartilage; nervous tissue

Long-term effects

The long-term effects of excessive exposure to ionising radiation include keratosis and local neoplasia, particularly of the skin (squamous carcinoma). Bone marrow becomes aplastic and leukaemia may follow. The frequency of congenital defects in the progeny is increased. Many long-term effects result from occlusion of small blood vessels. According to the mass of tissue irradiated and the nature of the exposed tissue, a series of post-irradiation syndromes can be defined (Table 39).

ISCHAEMIA

Ischaemia is the partial or complete reduction of blood flow to a tissue or organ. It is frequently initiated by vascular diseases such as atheroma or thrombosis; by arterial obstruction in trauma or surgery; by irradiation – a potent cause of necrosis of skin flaps after mastectomy; or by the action of vaso-active drugs such as the catecholamines. All of these agencies lead to reduced arterial blood flow. Incomplete or

Table 39 Clinical syndromes following excessive whole-body irradiation

Syndrome	Dose in röntgen needed to cause onset	Signs	Death
Bone marrow	275 to 500 R	Bone marrow aplasia	~30 days
Intestinal	700 to 1000 R	Anorexia and diarrhoea	15 to 7 days
Central nervous	10 000 R	Convulsions	A few days to a few hours

Table 40 Sensitivity of tissues to ischaemia

Moderate	Low	High
Bone	Hyaline cartilage	Spinal cord
Tendon	Intervertebral disc	Brain
Skeletal muscle	Cornea	Liver
Small intestine		Heart muscle
Skin		Adrenal cortex
Renal glomeruli		Pituitary
		Renal cortex

slowly developing ischaemia cause tissue atrophy but sudden, complete ischaemia results in infarction or gangrene.

The organs and tissues of the body display wide differences in susceptibility to the effects of ischaemia (Table 40). They can be arranged in three groups: of high, medium and low sensitivity. The vulnerability of a part to ischaemia is in proportion to the rate of aerobic respiration of the component cells. One index of this respiratory activity is the size and number of the mitochondria. Another indication of sensitivity is the number of capillaries per unit mass of tissue. Cardiac muscle and brain cells are highly sensitive, skeletal muscle of modest sensitivity. Hyaline cartilage and cornea, both avascular, are tolerant of ischaemia. A hypoxia-inducible factor 1 (HIF-1) initiates the cardiac cellular response to hypoxia. It is a transcriptional activator of vascular endothelial growth factor (VEGF).

The effects of ischaemia on a tissue or part are modified by the existence of an alternative, collateral circulation, and by temperature. Thus, the sudden lodging of an embolus in the femoral artery, where there is a collateral circulation, is much less likely to cause infarction than an embolus entering the arcuate artery of a kidney, an end-artery. Equally, tissues cooled during the interruption of arterial blood flow in cardiovascular surgery are less likely to sustain ischaemic injury than are tissues maintained at normal body temperature.

ANGINA

Angina is an oppressive sensation or pain in the throat. The autonomic innervation of the heart centres on cervical segments C3 and C4. Myocardial ischaemia therefore results characteristically in a constricting sensation in the chest but also in pain referred to the throat. The term **angina pectoris** is applied to this common symptom, a complaint encountered in oesophageal as well as cardiac surgery. Abdominal angina is pain following eating. It is attributable to stenoses of the coeliac axis, superior mesenteric and inferior mesenteric arteries (p. 24).

COMPARTMENT SYNDROME

On rare occasions, unusually strenuous or prolonged exercise may cause painful swelling of the connective tissue compartment within which the anterior tibial muscle is contained. After thrombolysis, a similar condition may complicate revascularisation of the lower limb. An analogous complication is associated with tibial fracture and requires urgent surgical relief. In severe cases, if the swollen compartment is not opened, muscle ischaemia follows. If prolonged, this may culminate in muscle necrosis, one consequence of which is myoglobinaemia with myoglobinuria. Contractures (p. 112) and deformity are late results of the untreated syndrome.

INTERMITTENT CLAUDICATION

Incomplete obstruction to the arterial blood supply to the legs leads eventually to the formation of a collateral circulation. Nevertheless, the circulation may be insufficient to sustain vigorous exercise and cramp-like pain develops in the gluteal, thigh or calf muscles, depending on the level of arterial obstruction. The pain is characteristically relieved by rest.

Lériche syndrome

The Lériche syndrome results from occlusion of the aorta, at or near the bifurcation, by embolus or saddle thrombus. There is buttock claudication, coldness and weakness of the legs, sexual impotence and skeletal muscle wasting.

ISCHAEMIC ENTEROCOLITIS

When the arterial circulation of the mesenteric arteries is compromised by atheroma or aneurysm, a fall in blood pressure or obstruction to small vessels may induce foci of necrosis of both the small and of the large intestine. The syndrome may be caused by disseminated intravascular coagulation (DIC); by shock; by renal failure with uremia; or by congestive cardiac failure. The splenic flexure of the colon is particularly susceptible: it is the zone where the superior and inferior mesenteric arterial supplies anastomose. In severe, acute cases, necrosis and perforation occur. The development of a fibrous stricture is one late consequence.

J

JAUNDICE

Jaundice is a yellow discoloration (p. 271) of the tissues, the body fluids and the glandular secretions due to an excess of bilirubin (p. 36). The yellow coloration of jaundice is not recognisable clinically until the serum bilirubin concentration reaches levels of 50 to 150 μmol/L. These values are greatly in excess of the upper limit of normal, ~20 μmol/L. The circulating bilirubin is either insoluble, unconjugated bilirubin; water-soluble, conjugated bilirubin; or a mixture of both.

Now read Bile pigments (p. 36)

There are four categories of jaundice, depending on whether there is:

- Excess production of bilirubin.
- Decreased liver uptake of bilirubin.
- Decreased liver conjugation of bilirubin.
- Decreased excretion of bilirubin into the bile.

In practice, it is convenient to group these disorders according to the sites of dysfunction so that there are prehepatic, hepatic and posthepatic categories. However, in some cases, two or more abnormalities of bilirubin metabolism may co-exist. In hepatic jaundice due to viral hepatitis, for example, the jaundice is initially hepatic: it is due to cellular dysfunction. Ultimately, the jaundice becomes posthepatic since tissue swelling leads to obstruction of intrahepatic biliary canaliculi.

PREHEPATIC (HAEMOLYTIC) JAUNDICE

There is increased production of bilirubin due to heightened destruction of circulating red blood cells. One example is familial spherocytosis (p. 11). The excess of unconjugated plasma bilirubin cannot pass through the glomerular capillary basement membrane. The jaundice is therefore 'acholuric'. However, the excretion of an increased quantity of bile pigment into the intestine results in raised faecal stercobilinogen levels. Absorbed into the blood and excreted by the kidney, the molecule appears as excess urinary urobilinogen.

Now read Haemolytic anaemia (p. 11)

HEPATIC (HEPATOCELLULAR) JAUNDICE

Abnormal liver cell function results in defective bilirubin conjugation. The serum consequently contains excess unconjugated bilirubin. Re-absorbed faecal urobilinogen is incompletely excreted in the bile and excess urobilinogen is detected in the urine.

The causes may be heritable or acquired. They include:

- **Inherited**. Decreased conjugation is noted in the rare Crigler–Najjar syndrome, an autosomal recessive characteristic, and to a lesser degree in Gilbert's disease, a familial condition (p. 182);

- **Infective**. HBV infection (p. 152) is a frequent, viral cause of impaired hepatocyte function. In leptospirosis, bacterial infection has a similar impact.
- **Chemical**. Organic solvents like ethanol; chemotherapeutic agents such as methotrexate; and analgesics such as paracetamol, also impair liver cell actions.
- **Toxic**. The toxins of some fungi are hepatotoxic. Aflatoxin is one example.
- **Antibody-mediated**. Liver cell damage may be induced by hypersensitivity to anaesthetic agents such as halothane, and by antibiotics including para-amino salicylic acid (PAS).

Now read Hepatitis (p. 152)

POST-HEPATIC (OBSTRUCTIVE) JAUNDICE

There is either failure to transport conjugated bilirubin or obstruction to the excretion of this molecule. The obstruction may be at any point between the intrahepatic canaliculi and the ampulla of Vater. Conjugated bilirubin fails to reach the gut. Bilirubin and bile salts appear in the urine but urinary urobilinogen disappears. More than one factor is often operative, particularly if the disease is prolonged.

The albumen-free, conjugated bilirubin that accumulates in obstructive jaundice is highly soluble and readily escapes through the glomerular basement membrane. The urine is therefore dark. However, the bilirubin does not reach the lumen of the intestine. The stools are therefore pale since they lack stercobilinogen. Bile salts are also absent and the stools contain increased quantities of fat.

The causes of post-hepatic jaundice may be heritable or acquired. They include:

- **Inherited**. The Dubin–Johnson and Rotor syndromes are caused by genetic abnormalities of bilirubin transport from hepatocyte microsomes to the biliary canaliculi. Both conditions are inherited as autosomal, recessive characteristics.
- **Acquired**. Obstruction to bilirubin excretion within liver biliary canaliculi is frequently due to hepatic tumours or to the late stages of viral hepatitis. The resulting jaundice is cholestatic. Obstruction to the extrahepatic biliary system is commonly caused by tumours (p. 39); calculi (p. 37); or, less frequently, abscesses (p. 1).

Now read Biliary tract (p. 36)

JOINTS

SYNOVIAL

Although articular cartilage has neither blood vessels nor lymphatics, the 264 freely moving, synovial joints have a large blood supply. They are therefore susceptible to all forms of inflammatory disease, particularly those caused by immunological disorders; the deposition of crystals; and infection. They are prone to trauma and to the non-inflammatory syndrome, osteoarthritis.

Biopsy diagnosis of synovial joints

Needle biopsy provides sufficient fluid for bacterial culture and for a search for cells and crystals. Fibre-optic arthroscopy enables small samples of synovial or cartilaginous tissue to be taken. Larger pieces may be obtained at open, exploratory arthrotomy and during procedures such as arthroplasty and other forms of joint reconstruction. Blocks of soft or of hard tissue are provided by methods similar to those adopted during bone biopsy (p. 50).

The less numerous fixed, fibrous and fibrocartilaginous joints have no synovium and few blood vessels. They also are susceptible to injury, infection and metabolic disorder but, because of the limited vasculature, are not sites for primary inflammatory diseases. They are often destroyed by the invasive properties of metastatic tumours and by trauma, but are tolerant of the pulsatile, compressive stress imposed by enlarging aneurysm (p. 14).

Now read Spine (p. 300)

DEVELOPMENTAL DEFECTS

Synovial joints are affected by rare heritable disorders such as the Marfan and Ehlers–Danlos syndromes (p. 111). In the former, there is an inherited defect in the gene coding for the microfibril fibrillin. Affected individuals are tall and have long, spidery fingers and toes, characteristics of the 'Harlem Globetrotters'. There is hyperextensibility of the joints and soft connective tissues; patellar dislocation; and prolapse of the lenses of the eyes. Dissecting aortic aneurysm may prove fatal. In the Ehlers–Danlos syndrome, autosomal dominant defects in the genes coding for collagens I and III are recognised.

NON-INFECTIVE INFLAMMATORY DISEASE

The synovial joints are the main targets for the auto-immune disorders rheumatoid arthritis and systemic lupus erythematosus (p. 28). They are also implicated in allergic and metabolic disorders and are frequently subject to closed, sterile injuries such as those that accompany ligamentous, tendinous or meniscal tears.

Rheumatoid arthritis

This non-infective, symmetrical polyarthritis, nearly three times more common in women than men, affects 1% of the entire world population. Rheumatoid arthritis (RA) is a systemic disease, often complicated by secondary infection. It affects the skin, the lymphoreticular tissues, the blood vessels and the lungs. Rheumatoid arthritis shortens life and is responsible for many articular and soft tissue disorders that require surgical correction.

Causes

There is a genetic predisposition associated with female sex and the inheritance of the MHA class I antigens HLA-DRB1 and 4 (p. 330, Fig. 52). Little is known of the provocative factors. Parvovirus infection has been implicated. A role for physical and mental stress is suggested.

Now read Auto-immunity (p. 28), Immunity (p. 171)

Structure

Any or all of the freely moving, synovial joints may be affected (Fig. 36). The disease begins in the small joints of the hands and toes but, eventually, any of the synovial joints, including those of the cervical spine, larynx and ear, may be affected. The onset is insidious

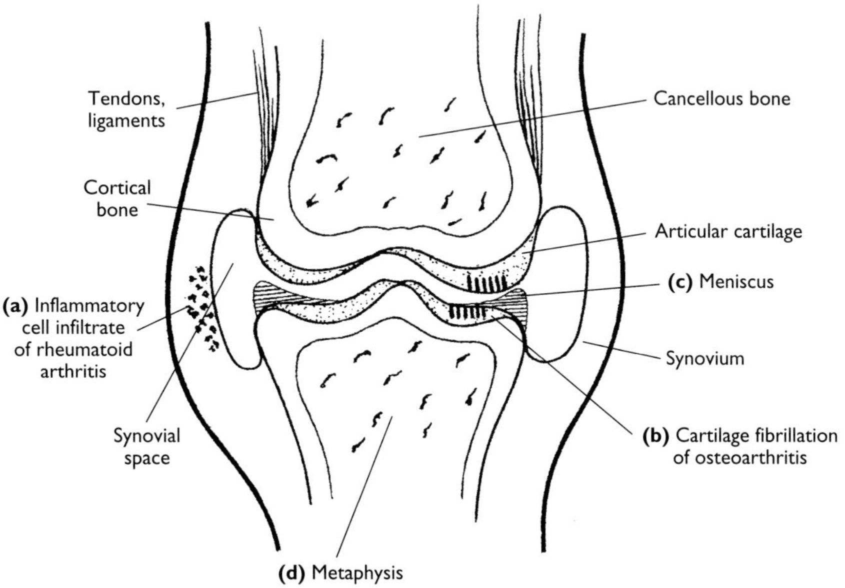

Figure 36 Inflammatory and degenerative synovial joint disease.
Diagram of adult knee joint with femur (at top), tibia (at bottom). Synovial fluid-filled space separates bearing surfaces of articular cartilages (stippled). Parts of surfaces of tibial condyles are covered by fibrocartilaginous menisci.

(a) Inflammatory joint diseases such as rheumatoid arthritis begin in vascular synovium and degrade cartilage secondarily.
(b) Non-inflammatory diseases such as osteoarthritis begin in main bearing surfaces formed by articular cartilage and degrade cartilage primarily.
(c) Some metabolic diseases such as chondrocalcinosis are first recognised in avascular menisci.
(d) Bacterial arthritis may be blood-borne or may originate in vascular bone of metaphysis.

with early morning inflammation, particularly of the affected finger and toe joints.

Inflammation begins at the chondrosynovial margins where the arcades of synovial capillaries terminate. The swollen, red synovium constitutes a **pannus** (cloth) that induces centripetal destruction of articular cartilage. Circumferential, osteoclastic bone reabsorption takes place, leading to marginal **erosions** recognisable radiologically. Tendinous synovia are implicated and tendon rupture is an important feature of hand disease just as the cruciate ligaments and menisci are subject to inflammation and disruption.

As joint disease advances, the weakening of muscles and the destruction of tendons and ligaments permit articular **subluxation** and, eventually, **dislocation**. Within the soft, subcutaneous tissues of parts like the ischium, occiput and elbow, sterile, rheumatoid nodules often form. They have a necrotic centre and an array of marginal, pallisaded macrophages. Their structure distantly recalls that of the tuberculous granuloma (p. 332).

Vasculitis is frequent. One variety of arterial disease is a necrotising arteritis that may lead to intestinal or limb infarction. Interstitial lung disease accompanies pleuritis.

Behaviour and prognosis

Secondary osteoarthritis of the large, limb joints is frequent. Regional and generalised osteoporosis is commonplace.

The most severe, destructive form of RA is associated with the inheritance of HLA-DRW4. The resistance of patients with rheumatoid arthritis to infection is lowered and this may influence adversely the outcome of surgical operations, particularly arthroplasty. In the most severe, chronic cases, in whom life expectancy is abbreviated, secondary amyloidosis is found in 1 case in 6. It is one reason for the renal excretory failure that is a well-recognised cause of death.

INFECTION

Infection of synovial joints may result from local or systemic sources.

Local infection is one consequence of penetrating injuries; it is a frequent complication of hip and knee joint arthroplasty. Because the freely moving joints adjoin the ends of the metaphyses of long bones, they are the secondary targets for many acute viral, bacterial, mycotic and parasitic infections, and for infestations of bone.

Now read Osteomyelitis (p. 53)

Systemic infection frequently results in purulent arthritis. The causative organisms include *Staphylococcus aureus*, *Streptococcus pyogenes* and *Pseudomonas aeruginosa*. *Neisseria gonorrhoeae* provokes an acute arthritis in which hypersensitivity plays a part. In the Eastern USA, *Borrelia burgdorferi* is a common cause of Lyme disease, a spirochaetal infection transmitted by a tick. Acute and chronic arthritis are among the consequences. In Western countries, *Mycobacterium tuberculosis* was a frequent cause of arthritis. The disease, prevalent in Third World countries, is now less common in Western Europe. Its recognition is high among immigrants from some African and Asian countries and among those with AIDS. *Mycobacterium tuberculosis* reaches the joints from synovial or metaphyseal sites. The hip, knee and main intervertebral joints are prone to infection. Many viruses provoke arthritis: they include the rubi- and parvoviruses. Metastatic joint infection is a feature of fungal diseases such as histoplasmosis.

POST-INFECTIVE AND REACTIVE ARTHRITIS

Post-infective or reactive arthritis occur in epidemic or sporadic forms following Shigella dysentery or Salmonella or Yersinia enteritis. The pathological changes mimic those of rheumatoid arthritis but rheumatoid factor is absent from the serum. The diseases are therefore **'seronegative'**. In some, no prior infection is recognisable. The arthritis is 'reactive' and the insidious onset resembles that of the spondylo-arthropathies. These poorly understood conditions (p. 301) include ankylosing spondylitis with which the HLA-B27 antigen is closely associated.

DEGENERATIVE DISEASE

Osteoarthritis

Osteoarthritis (OA) is a common syndrome of degenerative, osteo-articular disorder. The condition is confined to the freely moving, synovial joints and does not disorganise the fixed, fibrous joints. It is a syndrome, not a single disease. The tissue changes are superimposed upon those of ageing. The early features are asymptomatic. Whatever the primary cause, the end stage abnormalities affect articular cartilage, bone and adjoining synovial tissues.

Causes

Heritable

Rarely, individuals with inherited chondrodystrophy have a genetic disorder of the type II collagen gene that predisposes to the late onset of OA. In most cases of sporadic OA, no such predisposition is detectable although a subset of OA is encountered in post-menopausal, anaemic women who develop a systemic disease and have osteophytes of the distal interphalangeal joints (Heberden's nodes).

Environmental

The development of OA in later life is often attributable to repetitive, severe dynamic loading in earlier years. The risk is highest in occupations such as coalmining or football playing, and after injury, infection or inflammatory disorders such as RA. Osteoarthritis is also commonplace when the length of the legs has been unequal, in diabetes mellitus, or after fracture. Wearing high-heeled shoes presents an increased risk. Loss of sensory innervation to a leg, for example as a result of intervertebral disc prolapse, may initiate OA and accelerate its progression.

Structure

The structural changes at load-bearing surfaces, in order of increasing severity, are:

- Roughening and loss of articular cartilage (Fig. 36).
- Exposure of bone.
- Bone excoriation and osteophytosis.
- Secondary synovitis.

Osteoarthritis begins at an early age and at a preclinical, molecular level. Articular cartilage cells synthesise and export defective matrix molecules that cannot sustain the loads to which articular tissue is subjected during movements like walking. The earliest visible, microscopical abnormality is a roughening of the articular cartilage, **fibrillation**. Cartilage degradation then extends more deeply. The exposed surface of the thickened bone becomes the load-bearing surface; it is excoriated and fissured. Exposed, subchondral bone tolerates compressive and shear stress much less well than normal articular cartilage. Pain results. It is persistent and deep-seated. New bone forms at the joint margins and a secondary synovitis accompanies the release of fragments of cartilage and bone into the joint space.

Behaviour and prognosis

There is insidious progression. The femoral head, the femoral condyles, the patellar surface of the femur and the central parts of the medial tibial condyles are sites particularly affected but the temporomandibular, acromioclavicular and other small joints, including those of the middle ear, are vulnerable. OA is the most common reason for knee and hip joint arthroplasty.

Synovial chondromatosis

As an occasional result of injury, cartilage cells lodge in the synovial tissues and grow as small cartilaginous islands. Chondrosarcoma is a rare complication.

Neuropathic arthropathy

In diabetes mellitus, in syringomyelia and in tabes dorsalis, a loss of sensory innervation to large joints of the upper or lower limbs leads to synovial joint destruction. The pathological changes are due to a failure of the reflex mechanisms, particularly of postural sensation, that protect synovial joints against the repetitive minor injuries of day-to-day movements. In tabetic disease, the designation Charcot's arthropathy is still used.

MECHANICAL INJURY AND TRAUMA

Trauma to synovial joints may be direct or indirect.

Direct

Road traffic, aeroplane and many other forms of accident may result in disabling, articular injury. Among the most severe examples are dislocation of the knee, avulsion of the shoulder joint and fracture dislocation of the hip joint. Injuries caused by explosions, missiles (p. 358) or sharp weapons have become frequent.

Indirect

Indirect injuries are very common. They include the tears of the medial, knee joint meniscus in footballers and skiers that complicate sudden, rotational movements. Synovial joints are frequently damaged secondarily in the traumatic lesions of bone and connective tissue resulting from accidents.

Subluxation and dislocation

When injury or arthritis destroy intra- or para-articular ligaments, normal joint alignment is lost (**subluxation**). When articular components are completely separated, either by injury or in the course of surgery, the joint is **dislocated**.

Arthroplasty

Surgery offers the chance of replacing the whole or parts of many synovial joints with prostheses (p. 280). The common operations are on knee and hip but the shoulder, elbow, finger and temporomandibular joints are among the others that can be re-constructed.

Now read Prostheses (p. 280)

Some operations for arthroplasty may employ bone cements such as polymethylmethacrylate.. This polymer elicits an inflammatory reaction that can contribute to loosening of a prosthesis. Many operations are therefore now cementless. Soft tissue adhesives are more recent. Fibrin glues, made from human sources, have been developed for this purpose but the risk of possible contamination from viral sources has resulted in the introduction of chemical glues. One agent is butyl-2-cyanoacrylate (Indermil). It has also been used for the repair of inguinal hernia and to close skin incisions.

METABOLIC DISORDERS

The metacarpophalangeal, knee and finger joints are affected by crystal deposition diseases such as gout (p. 112) and chondrocalcinosis (p. 113). Synovial joint function is impaired in diabetes mellitus, hyperpituitarism and hyperparathyroidism.

TUMOURS

Cancer cells rarely lodge in synovial joints but the articulations may be infiltrated by osteosarcoma.

Benign

Haemangioma

Haemangioma (p. 49) of a knee is a rare cause of intra-articular bleeding.

Lipoma

Lipoma (p. 298) is occasionally identified by fibre-optic arthroscopy.

Malignant

Synovial sarcoma

So-called synovial sarcoma is a misnomer. It is described on p. 299.

TUMOUR-LIKE CONDITIONS

Pigmented villonodular synovitis (PVNS)

The cause of this uncommon, non-neoplastic disorder of synovial joints is not clear. The knee joint synovia are susceptible. Villonodular synovitis is a benign proliferation of synovial tissue that has some of the characteristics of neoplasia. There is a population of myofibroblasts. Much collagen is present and the many macrophages are laden with haemosiderin some of which is extracellular.

Ganglion

This common, painless, soft and fluctuant swelling arises in relation to the tendon sheaths of the posterior aspect of the hand. The swelling is lined by attenuated cells of synovial origin and filled with a viscous, gelatinous fluid.

K

KELOID

A keloid is a firm or hard, irregular-shaped but smooth-surfaced, raised, erythematous mass that develops in the skin. The formation of keloids is more common in black races than in Caucasian. In some populations, keloids are encouraged for cosmetic reasons. Keloids are particularly likely to occur after burns, following wounds about the ear and neck, or after tattooing. It has been suggested that they are due to the implantation of keratin and hair into the dermis since they can be produced experimentally by this means.

The mechanism of keloid formation is not fully understood. Abnormal cell migration and proliferation; the enhanced synthesis and secretion of extracellular matrix proteins, in particular, of the collagens; and a remodelling of the wound matrix, are described. The deposition and maturation of collagen is essential for the healing of wounds but, in keloids, collagen is formed continually and in excess. The collagen fibre bundles become hyalinised. There is increased and exaggerated activity of the fibrogenic cytokines (p. 114) including TGF-β1, IGF-1, and IL-1. A mutation of the tumour suppressor gene *p53* (p. 78) may also play a part.

After each excision, keloid is liable to recur. Treatment by the local injection of corticosteroids or by ionising radiation is often attempted but is usually ineffective.

HYPERTROPHIC SCAR

Keloids are distinct from the transient condition of hypertrophic scar. During the first 2 or 3 months of post-operative healing, any dermal scar may hypertrophy (p. 144). The majority regress. Within a year, the residual tissue becomes pale and shrunken.

Now read Scar (p. 290)

KETOSIS

The excessive oxidation of fatty acids results in an increase in the plasma concentration and urinary excretion of the harmless substances aceto-acetate and beta-hydroxybutyrate. Traditionally, the phrase 'ketone bodies' has been used to describe these metabolites although neither is a ketone; beta-hydroxybutyrate is not a keto acid.

The term 'ketosis' is applied when 'ketone bodies' are found in abnormal concentration. This usage arose because acetone, which is a true ketone, can be detected in the breath and urine of diabetics and of fasting or fat-fed subjects. Ketosis is an important sign that a patient may be starving. In starvation, aceto-acetate and hydroxybutyrate act as substrates for the provision of energy, an important homeostatic response that diminishes the requirement for gluconeogenesis.

Now read Carbohydrate (p. 75), Diabetes mellitus (p. 117), Lipids (p. 207), Metabolic response to trauma (p. 230)

KIDNEY

Many methods exist for the identification of the causes of kidney disease. The techniques range from urine analysis and biochemical assays to renal function studies, angiography and those of nuclear medicine.

Biopsy diagnosis of renal disease

The identity of many renal lesions can now be deduced from the study of CT and MRI scans (p. 169). Nevertheless, biopsy is often necessary to confirm the precise identity of renal masses and to ascertain the causes of haematuria, proteinuria and renal failure. In the majority of cases, tissue is obtained percutaneously by an ultrasonically guided, core-cutting needle. In most successful biopsies, a cylinder of renal tissue can be obtained corresponding to a volume of cortex containing 15 to 30 glomeruli. When a renal disorder is focal or of limited extent, the sample, however, may not include abnormal tissue.

The procedure of renal needle biopsy is not without risk and should not be performed in patients with coagulation disorders, particularly if tissue is to be taken from a single functioning kidney. No more than three passes with a needle should be made, at the lower pole of the kidney. Other contra-indications include perinephric abscess, hydronephrosis, pyonephrosis and large renal cysts. Haematuria develops in 5 to 10% of cases and blood transfusion is necessary in 2%. As a precaution, blood is cross-matched before biopsy.

DEVELOPMENTAL AND CONGENITAL DISORDERS

Either, or both, kidneys may be subject to congenital defects in size, shape, site or number.

Agenesis and hypoplasia

Agenesis

Unilateral agenesis, the absence of a single kidney, is a characteristic of ~0.1% of apparently normal individuals. However, the defect often coincides with the presence of other congenital abnormalities. It is more common in males than females. In accident and emergency surgery, where one kidney is severely injured (p. 199), it is essential to ensure that a second kidney is present before nephrectomy is undertaken. Rarely, bilateral agenesis is recognised. The failure to form both kidneys is the most significant abnormality in Potter's syndrome in which there is renal agenesis; a characteristic facies; and pulmonary hypoplasia. The syndrome is incompatible with postnatal life.

Hypoplasia

Unilateral renal hypoplasia is much more common than bilateral. In unilateral hypoplasia, only a rudimentary renal structure remains. There is a reduction in the size of the kidney but no malformation. Renal hypoplasia predisposes to infection and may be followed by systemic hypertension. If an affected child survives infancy, the chronic failure of renal tubular function may lead to stunting of growth and to renal rickets.

Horseshoe and supernumerary kidney

A single ectopic kidney may lie at any point in the path of either ureter. In 1 in 500 individuals, the embryonic kidneys remain united across the midline. The structures are joined by fibrous tissue, constituting a **'horseshoe'** kidney. The pelvi-ureteric junctions are anterior. Like many of the other defects of urinary tract development, horseshoe kidney predisposes to infection, calculus formation and hydronephrosis. The abnormal organ is prone to injury and susceptible to neoplasia.

CALCULUS

Calculi may form at any point in the urinary tract but the majority arise in the kidneys. Renal calculi tend to damage the urothelium, producing ulceration and haematuria. Calculi may be primary or secondary.

Now read Calculus (p. 75), Urinary bladder calculus (p. 338)

Primary

Primary calculi form because there is a persistently high local concentration of a metabolite or other molecule. The responsible substance may be present in the urine because of a heritable or acquired disorder.

Genetic

- **Cystine** is poorly soluble. Pale yellow or white calculi frequently appear in patients suffering from cystinuria.
- **Xanthine** is also poorly soluble and, in persistent xanthinuria, reddish brown calculi develop.
- **Oxalate** calculi form in patients suffering from oxalosis. In their presence, however, no metabolic disorder can usually be identified. The calculi are hard, dark-brown in colour and have an irregular surface particularly likely to produce urothelial damage. Their pathogenesis is unclear.

Cystine and oxalate calculi form in acid urine.

Acquired

Urate calculi are common in patients with persistent hyperuricaemia of which one result is gout (p. 112). The calculi are firm, brown and smooth-surfaced.

Secondary

Secondary calculi form at the site of a pre-existing nidus of bacteria, around a foreign body. They are commonplace when urinary tract infection is prolonged. Calcium is a constant component. The calculi are friable, white, smooth-surfaced mixtures of calcium and magnesium ammonium phosphates with calcium carbonate. In many patients, the provocative cause is the urinary excretion of an excess of calcium. Hypercalciuria is recognised after prolonged immobilisation; in hyperparathyroidism; with renal tubular acidosis; in sarcoidosis; as a result of chronic pyelonephritis; or because of increased calcium absorption due to hypervitaminosis D.

Now read Hyperparathyroidism (p. 267)

Randall's plaques are zones of dystrophic calcification in the renal papillae. They arise because of the high calcium concentrations at these sites. The foci of calcification can lacerate through the pelvic mucosa where they sometimes act as niduses for calculus formation. The calcium phosphates of secondary calculi are deposited in an alkaline urine, particularly in infection due to *Proteus mirabilis*. This micro-organism splits urea and liberates ammonia. In a reciprocal manner, infection is likely to follow calculus formation, especially when there is urinary stasis due to an obstruction.

Staghorn calculus is a very large, mixed stone that forms within, and assumes the shape of, the renal pelvic calyceal system. It is a result of chronic or recurrent infection.

CYSTS

Single renal cysts are present in half of all adults over the age of 50 years. They are asymptomatic and rarely of functional significance. **Multiple renal cysts** are encountered in infants, children and adults. Their presence underlies a number of well-defined, heritable and congenital syndromes. A particular form of cystic kidney develops in patients maintained on renal dialysis.

Polycystic disease

There are two forms: childhood and adult. The severity of the disease and the rate of progression to renal failure are inversely proportional to the age of the patient.

Childhood disease

- In perinatal disease, the child is stillborn or dies soon after birth.
- In neonatal disease, death is usual within 1 year.
- In infantile disease, the enlarged kidneys are recognised within 3 to 6 months of birth. Hepatosplenomegaly co-exists and death is the result of renal failure complicated by systemic and portal hypertension.
- In juvenile disease, the consequences are similar but the onset is in the second decade of life.

Adult disease

This is the most frequent form of the disorder. The defect is inherited as an autosomal dominant characteristic. The mutant gene is located on the short arm of somatic chromosome 16. Adult polycystic disease is recognised in middle-age, earlier in females than males. Renal excretory failure and secondary hypertension are frequent consequences. Untreated, the mean age at death is ~59 years.

An adult polycystic kidney may weigh as much as 1.0 kg and measure up to 220 mm in length. Great numbers of thin-walled cysts cover the renal surface and enlarge throughout life. They contain clear, serous or orange–brown fluid and compress the intervening renal tissue that subsequently undergoes fibrosis. Liver, pancreatic and lung cysts often coexist. Rarely, the hepatic changes lead to portal hypertension and liver failure. Ten per cent of patients suffer subarachnoid haemorrhage (p. 65).

Medullary sponge kidney

In this uncommon, congenital disorder, renal papillae of one or, more often, both kidneys are affected by dilatation of the collecting ducts. There are numerous small cysts.

INFECTION

The kidneys, ureters, urinary bladder and urethra form a single tract within which pathogenic micro-organisms spread readily. Infection is usually from the exterior, precipitated by the introduction of instruments into the urinary bladder (p. 338). Virtually all urinary catheters become colonised by bacteria within 3 days of insertion but, particularly in females, urinary infections are frequent without such provocation. Occasionally, infection is blood-borne.

Now read Bacteriuria (p. 34)

Causes

The micro-organisms responsible are bacteria resident in the large intestine. The most common is *Escherichia coli*. *Proteus mirabilis* is particularly associated with calculi; the organism renders the urine alkaline. Klebsiella, Enterobacter, Serratia spp. and *Pseudomonas aeruginosa* are encountered in hospital infections. Antibiotic treatment favours their growth and spread. In blood-borne infection, *Staphylococcus aureus* lodge in the glomeruli during bacteraemia or septicaemia.

The single most important factor predisposing to infection is mechanical obstruction to urinary outflow. Pregnancy; congenital malformation; benign prostatic hyperplasia; calculi; stricture; and benign and malignant tumours, are encountered with varying frequency. In infants and children, the role of vesicoureteral reflux is important.

Structure

Pyelonephritis

Pyelonephritis is unilateral or bilateral bacterial infection of the renal pelvis, calyces and parenchyma. The micro-organisms frequently reach the renal pelvis from the lower urinary tract but they may lodge in the kidney from the arterial bloodstream.

Acute. The inflamed kidney is large, swollen and hyperaemic. Linear aggregates of polymorphs extend within the collecting ducts and tubules to the outer parts of the renal cortex where discrete abscesses form. The leucocyte-laden ducts and tubules are seen as conspicuous, linear, radial streaks.

Chronic. Chronic pyelonephritis causes progressive destruction of the renal parenchyma and culminates in renal excretory failure. It is the underlying disorder in one in seven of those patients requiring renal dialysis or transplantation.

Either or both kidneys is small, shrunken and scarred. The epithelium of the renal pelvic mucosa is thickened and the pyramids and calyces distorted. There are microscopic signs of continuing, active inflammation. The renal tubules are atrophic. Many include a protein-rich, eosinophilic material that gives them a resemblance to the colloid-containing acini of the thyroid gland. The glomeruli are fibrotic and hyalinised.

Pyonephrosis

In a small proportion of cases where severe, urinary tract infection complicates obstruction to urinary flow, pus accumulates within the dilated renal pelvis. The pelvis comprises a sac bounded by fibrotic, compressed renal tissue.

Tuberculosis

In the West, tuberculosis of the urinary tract remains a problem in migrant populations and in those with AIDS-related disease. *Mycobacteria tuberculosis* enter the circulation from the lungs and lodge in the renal glomeruli. Sterile pyuria is a result. Less often, the initial focus is in the epididymis. Renal cortical granulomas form (p. 143). As the disease progresses, the destruction of renal tissue becomes extensive. Large zones of caseous necrosis appear. They may calcify, a process enhanced by antibiotic treatment and chemotherapy.

The infection is liable to involve, in turn, the ureters; urinary bladder; prostate gland; and associated tissues. Fibrosis of the renal calyces predisposes to hydronephrosis and calculus formation. The urine, sterile on conventional culture, contains small numbers of leucocytes. Microscopic searches for urinary *Mycobacteria tuberculosis* are not reliable since other, non-pathogenic Mycobacteria (p. 237) are often present. Microbiological diagnosis is then by the prolonged culture of decontaminated deposits obtained from early morning specimens of urine.

MECHANICAL AND HYDRODYNAMIC DISORDERS

Hydronephrosis

Hydronephrosis is dilatation of the renal pelvis and calyces of one or both kidneys. It is the result of an obstruction to the outflow of urine. According to the site of the obstruction, there may also be **hydro-ureter**. Occasionally, superadded infection leads to pyonephrosis.

Hydronephrosis is most probable when urinary obstruction develops gradually over a prolonged period. It may be a complication of primary obstructive mega-ureter but any condition prejudicing urinary outflow may be responsible. Congenital obstruction is due to valve-like folds of mucosa at the pelvi-ureteric or the vesico-urethral junctions, in the ureter or in the urethra. In adults, common causes include carcinoma of the colon, urinary bladder, prostate gland or uterine cervix; calculi; sustained mechanical pressure, exerted, for example by an abnormally located renal artery; injury; or ureteric transplantation. Retroperitoneal fibrosis is an uncommon cause.

Hypertrophy

After nephrectomy for unilateral renal disease, the remaining, normal kidney quickly undergoes compensatory hypertrophy by the mitotic division of renal tubular cells.

TRAUMA

The kidneys are protected by their position near the posterior wall of the abdomen, by the ribs that cover their upper half, and by the surrounding viscera and musculature. Nevertheless, missile injuries; stab wounds; explosions; and accidents of a wide variety may lead to severe disruption of renal tissue, to local haemorrhage and to renal failure.

TUMOURS

Metastatic deposits from carcinomas of the bronchus, colon and breast are frequent. Primary benign renal tumours are extremely common and malignant tumours very frequent.

Benign

Renal cortical adenoma

Renal cortical adenomas are often present. They are symptomless, small, circumscribed, yellow nodules derived from clones of cells resembling those of the proximal convoluted tubules. Renal cell carcinoma may evolve from adenoma so that, when an adenoma is recognised, it is excised on the assumption that it is premalignant.

Oncocytoma

Oncocytoma is a circumscribed tumour formed of eosinophilic, granular cells that show no tendency to invade. In the salivary gland, a comparable tumour is the oxyphil adenoma.

Malignant

Renal cell carcinoma

Renal cell carcinoma comprises 90% of all malignant tumours of the kidney and ~2% of all cancers. In adults, the annual incidence of renal cancer in England and Wales is rising and is currently ~$80/10^6$ population. The tumour is twice as common in men as in women. Painless haematuria is an early clinical sign. The sporadic form of the tumour appears in individuals aged 40 to 60 years. The mean age at diagnosis is, however, 60 years.

Causes

Little is known of any predisposing or initiating factors. An origin from renal cortical cell adenoma has been suggested. The aberrant chromosomes recognisable in renal cell carcinoma cells include deletions affecting chromosomes 14 and 17. There is a familial form (p. 76).

Structure

The tumour arises towards one pole of a kidney and forms a variegated, yellow–red, haemorrhagic, partly necrotic mass, incompletely bounded by a 'false' capsule of compressed renal tissue. Microscopically, renal cell carcinoma comprises clear cells laden with glycogen that resemble proximal convoluted tubules. Although the tumour may be a uniform, solid mass, the component cells are often arranged in alveolar, trabecular or spindle cell patterns. The cancer permeates nearby lymph nodes and spreads directly to the adjacent adrenal gland, spleen, colon and liver.

Behaviour and prognosis

Renal cell carcinoma displays a number of unique behavioural characteristics. In a very small proportion of cases metastases may regress after resection of the primary tumour. Endocrine and metabolic effects induced by the tumour include hypertension, polycythaemia (erythropoietin), hypercalcaemia (parathormone-like substance) and neuromuscular abnormalities. There may be excess or aberrant secretion of ACTH; chorionic gonadotrophin; enteroglucagon; and insulin.

The direct extension of cancer cells into venous channels results in the propagation of thrombosis within the renal vein itself, a process often extending into the inferior vena cava and, periodically, to the right atrium. Metastases are the presenting feature in 25 to 30% of cases and take place via the bloodstream to the lungs; bones; liver; opposite kidney; and brain. Lung metastases often display a round, 'cannon ball' appearance on X-ray. Thyroid metastases are very common. They are asymptomatic but occasionally provoke hyperthyroidism.

The prognosis of renal cell carcinoma is poor. In treatment, embolisation of the renal artery may be performed before nephrectomy, changing much of the tumour to necrotic tissue. The mean survival rate after nephrectomy is 40% but this figure ranges from as little as 30% to as much as 80% depending on the degree of histological differentiation. Interleukin-2 has been used in treatment but leads to complete, long-term remission in only 4% of cases. If resection cannot be complete, relentless progression occurs and the median survival is no more than 12 to 18 months.

Transitional cell carcinoma

Transitional cell carcinoma is an uncommon tumour arising from the urothelium of the renal pelvis. The presence of large calculi and chronic infection encourage dysplasia of the pelvic epithelial cells. The structure and microscopic characteristics of the tumour closely resemble those of transitional cell carcinoma of the urinary bladder (p. 338).

Squamous carcinoma

Squamous metaplasia of the renal pelvic urothelium is a frequent result of chronic infection, particularly in the presence of a single, large calculus. Malignant transformation is an occasional result. The structure and behaviour of the tumour closely resemble those of squamous carcinoma of the urinary bladder (p. 339).

Spindle cell carcinoma

Spindle cell carcinoma is a rare form of renal carcinoma. It accounts for only 1% of all renal neoplasms. The tumour behaves aggressively and may be mistaken for sarcoma.

Wilms' tumour

Wilms' tumour, nephroblastoma, is an important malignant neoplasm of childhood (p. 77). It affects $10/10^6$ children in the age range 2–5 years.

Causes

The majority of tumours are sporadic. Only 1 to 2% of cases are familial and no more than 2% arise as part of a predisposing syndrome. Several genes associated with Wilms' tumour have been cloned and in 95% of cases, there are mutations in these genes. The genes include *WT1* at 11p13 and *WT2* at 11p15. *WT1* codes for a transcription factor. Like many childhood tumours, the tumour is often recognised with other congenital malformations. In this instance, the urinary tract and eye (aniridia) are implicated and there may be hemi-hypertrophy of the body. Regions of primitive nephrogenic tissue persist in nearby tissue in 40% of cases.

Structure

Wilms' tumour forms an increasingly large, painful, abdominal mass, often associated with hypertension. The tumours are sometimes bilateral. The microscopic structure of Wilms' tumour mimics nephrogenesis, a process normally ceasing at 36 weeks of intra-uterine development.

The neoplasm comprises three elements: embryonic foci of poorly formed renal tubules and glomeruli; sheets of compact, darkly staining cells; and mesenchymal connective tissue that may include smooth muscle, striated muscle, cartilage and bone.

Behaviour and prognosis

Wilms' tumour grows quickly and spreads both directly and via the renal vein to the lungs, liver and brain. The prognosis after appropriate treatment is related closely to the stage of the tumour and its histological features. Anaplasia, meticulously defined, indicates an unfavourable outlook; differentiation indicates a favourable response. In stage I tumours, a combination of pre-operative chemotherapy followed by surgery yields a 2-year survival rate of more than 90%. By contrast, stage IV cases treated with radiotherapy and chemotherapy give a 2-year survival rate of only 40%.

RADIATION INJURY

The kidney is susceptible to the long-term, damaging effects of ionising radiation (p. 186). There is tubular loss; collagenous connective tissue formation; glomerular ischaemia; and secondary hypertension.

Now read Irradiation (p. 185)

TRANSPLANTATION

Although the first successful renal transplants were made with organs from identical twins, the transplantation of a kidney from an unrelated donor, an allograft, has now become a highly effective treatment for non-neoplastic, end-stage renal disease. As techniques improved and problems of rejection lessened, the 1-year survival for grafts from living donors increased from 89 to 94% for the years 1988 to 1996. For cadaveric grafts, the figures were 76 and 88% respectively.

Now read Transplantation (p. 329)

VASCULAR DISEASE

Arterial

Acute

Renal infarction occurs when the renal artery, or one or more of its main branches, is obstructed. The causes include dissecting aneurysm of the aorta; embolus originating in the left ventricle; and renal artery thrombosis.

Renal cortical necrosis

In a small group of patients who die in shock, the kidneys show a dramatic change in colour. Each cortex is intensely pale and has undergone massive infarction. The medullae are spared and appear normal. There is an association with Gram-negative bacterial infection. Renal cortical necrosis is also encountered in the haemolytic uraemic syndrome and in septic shock. The appearances are distinct from the ill-defined pallor of acute renal tubular necrosis. An analogous lesion develops in uncontrolled **eclampsia** in which the small renal veins are blocked by fibrin plugs.

Chronic

A gradual and incomplete reduction of renal arterial blood flow leads to progressive loss of cortical tubular cells and results in renal atrophy. Ultimately, the little renal tissue that remains undergoes fibrosis and dystrophic calcification, changes resembling those seen in unilateral renal hypoplasia.

The most common cause of slowly advancing renal ischaemia in elderly persons is atheroma affecting the aorta near the mouths of the renal arteries. In younger individuals, renal artery stenosis is attributable to medial fibromuscular dysplasia of the middle or distal part of the vessel. Both lesions lead to renal artery stenosis and insufficiency but can be corrected surgically. Sustained renal ischaemia is a classical and potent factor promoting secondary hypertension.

Venous

Thrombosis

The renal veins are prone to thrombosis and are frequently invaded by malignant tumours. The sudden obstruction of venous return from a kidney results in venous infarction.

RENAL FAILURE

Acute

Viewed in terms of excretory function, acute renal failure arises as a result of:

- **Pre-renal** disorders affecting the arterial supply to the kidney.
- **Renal** disorders that operate within or beyond the kidney.
- **Post-renal** disorders that disturb the venous drainage or the urinary tract.

When body temperature is within the normal range and the urinary outflow is unobstructed, the preservation of normal renal function requires an arterial blood supply of approximately 1.0 L/minute.

If the renal arterial blood supply is reduced, on account of local disorders such as renal artery thrombosis or embolism, or by systemic disturbance including any form of shock (p. 290), renal function may fail abruptly. Acute renal failure is an occasional result of inflammatory diseases including acute glomerulonephritis or urinary tract infection. Urinary outflow may be blocked at any point between the distal urethra and the renal calyceal system. The failure of renal function that results may be sudden or insidious.

Now read Multi-organ failure (p. 292)

Chronic

Chronic renal failure often succeeds postrenal obstruction due, for example, to prostatic hypertrophy. It is also a consequence of glomerular destruction, the causes of which include chronic glomerulonephritis; diabetes mellitus; and chronic pyelonephritis. Inevitably, there is renal tubular atrophy and loss. The syndrome of failure may culminate in uraemia; the nephrotic syndrome; renal bone disease; or accelerated hypertension, depending on the degree to which different vascular, glomerular or tubular functions are disorganised.

KOCH'S POSTULATES

Koch (p. 373) established strict criteria by which the causal relationship between a bacterial species and a disease could be irrefutably confirmed. The criteria, Koch's postulates, were:

- That a bacterium should be detected in the body in all cases of a disease.
- That the bacterium isolated from a case of the disease should be capable of growth in pure culture.
- That the isolated bacterium should then be shown to cause the original disease when inoculated from pure culture into a susceptible animal.

Koch's requirements have not always been easy to satisfy. The aetiological association between *Mycobacterium leprae* and leprosy was not questioned during the first 100 years after the discovery of the microorganism, in spite of the fact that the bacillus was not grown until 1974. The requirement that a virus be isolated from a disease, grown in pure culture and then used to reproduce the disease experimentally has not been met in the case of very many common, human, viral pathogens.

L

LARYNX AND TRACHEA

In all forms of surgery requiring general anaesthesia, the integrity of the larynx and trachea is crucial.

Biopsy diagnosis of laryngeal disease

The most frequent reason for laryngeal biopsy is the presence of a localised area of epithelial roughness, irregularity or ulceration, suspected of being either carcinoma *in-situ* or overt cancer. The procedure is usually endoscopic.

INFECTION AND INFLAMMATION

Bacterial and viral infection

Influenza, measles and other forms of viral laryngitis are encountered in surgical patients as they are in the non-surgical population. Laryngotracheobronchitis is one sequel. Bacterial infection by *Streptococcus pneumoniae* may supervene and *Haemophilus influenzae* can provoke epiglottitis.

Other forms of inflammatory disease

The small synovial joints of the larynx are affected by rheumatoid arthritis (p. 191). The **ankylosis** of the intrinsic joints of the larynx that often results is one cause of difficulty in intubation. An **inflammatory polyp** appears as a small, neoplastic-like nodule on a vocal cord. The lesion is formed of fibrous and myxoid connective tissue and may contain amyloid.

MECHANICAL AND TRAUMATIC DISORDERS

The larynx and trachea can be injured during resuscitation or tracheostomy. Oedema is one effect of mild injury and a possible cause of airway obstruction. Flames, hot gases or irritant chemicals reach the larynx and trachea, in fires, explosions, and occupational accidents. Tracheal compression may occur in patients with large goitres.

TUMOURS

Benign

Squamous papilloma

The most frequent benign tumour is squamous papilloma. The lesion is a small, circumscribed nodule originating on a vocal cord or at the commissure. It may recur. Among other tumours of the larynx are **granular cell tumour** and **angioma** (p. 49).

Malignant

Carcinoma

Carcinoma of the larynx, the most common cancer of the upper respiratory and upper alimentary tracts, represents 1.0% of malignant tumours in men but only 0.2% in women. The annual incidence in England and Wales is ~$40/10^6$ population. Co-existent, second primary tumours are frequent. Nearly half are bronchial.

Causes

Smoking and alcohol consumption are synergistic, predisposing factors.

Structure

Ninety per cent of laryngeal cancers are squamous. They occur in the glottis, the region of the true vocal cords and less often in the supraglottis, the region extending from the false vocal cords to the laryngeal inlet. They are seldom present below the glottis.

Behaviour and prognosis

At first, the lesion is a small, indurated nodule. Ulceration then occurs. Unless the tumour is excised or irradiated, it invades local tissue directly, destroying the vocal cords. Prognosis is closely related to TNM staging (p. 244). Laryngeal carcinoma extends by lymphatic permeation to the cervical lymph nodes. At the time of diagnosis, 40% of supraglottic tumours, but only 5% of glottic tumours, are found to have behaved in this way. Distant metastasis is rare.

TRANSPLANTATION

It has proved possible to transplant the entire larynx together with the nearby, associated tissues.

LASER

A laser is a device containing a medium which, when stimulated by light energy of sufficient intensity, emits a beam of light that is coherent, monochromatic and highly directional. The word LASER is an acronym for **L**ight **A**mplification by **S**timulated **E**mission of **R**adiation.

Care is necessary in any application of lasers since they are potential sources of thermal eye injury: the lens of the eye can focus a beam of laser light onto an area of the retina as small as 10 μm^2. Advantage is taken of this property in ophthalmology where lasers are used to treat retinal and choroidal disease. Lasers are also frequently employed in vascular, plastic and dental surgery; and in cancer therapy. Laser light can be delivered through fibres inserted in endoscopes and is exploited in the ablation of gastro-intestinal, urological and gynaecological tumours, and of atheromatous plaques in peripheral and coronary arteries. Multiple lasers can be employed in scanning light microscopes, enabling simultaneous identification of three or more labelled antibodies in tissue blocks or sections.

specific, azurophilic granules. There is a circulating pool of these cells. Some are constantly marginated, others free. However, the largest number constitutes a reserve, bone marrow pool that is called upon in response to infection and other stimuli.

Neutrophil polymorphs move very quickly to sites of inflammation (p. 179), attracted by chemotaxis. Adhering to endothelial surfaces, they pass through blood vessel walls within 20 to 30 minutes of a stimulus and surround and phagocytose foreign material or bacteria. The half-life of circulating polymorphs is only 6 to 8 hours. In an abscess (p. 1), the activated proteolytic enzymes from dead cells are released, digesting surrounding tissue components, fibrin and cell debris. The residual products constitute pus.

Lymphocytes

Lymphocytes are the class of white blood cells responsible for all specific immune reactions (p. 171). They comprise ~16–35% of the leucocyte population. The peripheral blood normally contains 1.5 to 4.0 × 10^9/L. Lymphocytes are small cells with relatively large, round nuclei, little cytoplasm and few organelles. They originate from stem cells in the bone marrow and move in large numbers in the bloodstream to the spleen, lymph nodes, gut, tonsils and thymus. There is a continual recirculation. They can migrate through the blood and lymph nodes and are sequestered at foci of inflammation.

Now read Immunity (p. 171)

Monocytes

Monocytes are circulating, mononuclear phagocytes. Their properties and behaviour are essentially the same as those of the other mononuclear phagocytes (p. 225). Monocytes represent ~3–7% of the circulating white blood cells. The mean number in the peripheral blood is 0.2–0.8 × 10^9/L.

Eosinophils

Approximately 5 to 10% of the granular series is eosinophil. The mean number in the blood is ~0.04–0.4 × 10^9/L. The cytoplasm contains large granules of rhomboidal shape. Eosinophil polymorphs accumulate in inflammatory reactions caused by immediate hypersensitivity (p. 161), in response to parasitic and protozoal antigens, and in anaphylaxis (p. 161). They also aggregate in tissues implicated in infections with helminths; pneumonitis and asthma; inflammatory bowel disease, gastro-enteritis and allergic colitis; allergic rhinoconjunctivitis and eczema; idiopathic hypereosinophilic vasculitis; drug reactions; lymphoma; and colon carcinoma. They are the predominant cell type in the rare eosinophilic granuloma.

Basophils

Less than 1% of the granular series is basophil. The mean number in the blood is ~0.01–0.1 × 10^9/L. The cytoplasm contains large, blue-staining granules closely resembling those of mast cells with which they have comparable functions. The granules contain histamine, leukotrienes and other mediators of acute inflammation and anaphylaxis and play a role in reactions, such as asthma, initiated by immediate hypersensitivity (p. 161). They also release a platelet-activating factor and the anticoagulant, heparin.

Leucocytosis

Leucocytosis is a significant increase in the total number of leucocytes in the circulating blood (Table 42), characteristically in response to acute bacterial infection.

An increase in the total number of neutrophil granulocytes is **neutrophil granulocytosis**; in the number of lymphocytes, **lymphocytosis**; and so on. When a change occurs in the total white cell count, it is important to distinguish whether there is a relative alteration in the proportions of the individual leucocyte populations. Thus, in sepsis, both a relative and an absolute increase in the numbers of neutrophil granulocytes are usual.

Leucopenia

Leucopenia is a significant diminution in the total number of leucocytes present in the circulating blood (Table 42). Owing to the effects of bacterial toxins upon the bone marrow, leucopenia may develop in patients with overwhelming sepsis. Bacterial infections caused by *Salmonella typhi*, Brucella spp. and *Legionella pneumophila* also have this result. Old people may not respond to infection by leucocytosis: there is relative leucopenia. A paradoxical reaction may be recognised in chronic lymphocytic leukaemic patients in whom bacterial infection may cause the total white blood cell count to fall.

A deficiency of neutrophil granulocytes is **granulocytopenia**. It may result from the action of drugs such as cytotoxic agents and some antibiotics. The total absence of granulocytes from the blood is **agranulocytosis**. In many virus infections, a relative and an absolute lymphocytosis is common but there may be **lymphopenia**, a significant decrease in the number of circulating lymphocytes.

LEUCOPLAKIA

Leucoplakia is a clinical, not an histopathological term. It describes a local lesion of the mouth; vulva; penis; or bladder in which smooth, dry, white, thickened patches result from a multiplicity of causes ranging from chronic irritation to squamous carcinoma. There is no single, microscopic disorder but rather a series of epithelial abnormalities, expressed to different degrees in different parts of a single lesion. The variegated nature and extent of the changes may demand multiple biopsies. Because many of the factors evoking leucoplakia initiate epithelial dysplasia, it is not surprising that patients with untreated disease are frequently found to have a malignant, epithelial tumour.

Erythroplasia, a term analogous to leucoplakia, describes red, papular eruptions of the penis (Queyrat's erythroplasia – p. 268) or mouth. Erythroplasia is synonymous with **erythroplakia**.

LEUKAEMIA

Leukaemia, literally 'white blood' (pp. 204, 243), is a potentially fatal neoplastic disease of the leucocytic precursor cells of the bone marrow. There is a characteristic and premature release, from the bone marrow into the circulating blood, of an excess of one or other of the precursors of the granulocytic, lymphocytic or mononuclear series. The features of leukaemia were first described by Bennett (p. 369) and by Virchow (p. 377). The annual incidence of leukaemia in England and Wales is ~$90/10^6$ persons.

One known cause of leukaemia is exposure to ionising radiation in accidents at nuclear reactors. Leukaemia was a characteristic complication of Second World War atomic bomb explosions. Other agencies are genetic and the role of the *c-abl* gene has been invoked. A retrovirus leads to leukaemia in cats.

Leukaemia may be acute or chronic. The acute leukaemias are disorders of the young; the chronic leukaemias, particularly chronic lymphocytic leukaemia, affect the elderly. In chronic leukaemia, the enormous excess of leucocytes can readily be seen as a large buffy coat. There are other, poorly understood leukaemia-like disorders. **Hairy-cell leukaemia**, for example, a lymphocytic and monocytic cancer, is an insidious cause of splenomegaly and pancytopenia. The peripheral blood mononuclear cells have piliform, cytoplasmic projections and contain rod-shaped inclusions.

The prognosis in both adults and children is influenced by aberrations in chromosomal structure (p. 92). Thus, in acute myeloid leukaemia, the identification of t(8;21) is good, the finding of t(6;9) poor. The outlook in many varieties of leukaemia, such as the acute lymphocytic leukaemia (ALL) of childhood, has been much improved by the use of cytotoxic and chemotherapeutic drugs.

LIPIDS

Lipids are an heterogeneous group of molecules that are insoluble in water. They can be extracted by certain solvents. In man, lipids are present in organ, tissue and cell compartments, as in adipocytes and their organelles; or as lipoproteins, for transport.

There are seven classes of lipid: triacylglycerol (formerly called triglyceride); fatty acids; phospholipids; glycolipids; sphingolipids; steroids; and vitamins A, D, E and K. Lipids are a major source of energy. A normal adult ingests ~60 to 150 g lipid/day. Ninety per cent is triacylglycerol. The remainder is cholesterol; cholesterol esters; phospholipids; and 'free' (unesterified) fatty acids. Some of the fatty acids are 'essential' in the sense that they are necessary components of a normal diet since they cannot be synthesised in the body

Digestion

Lipids undergo little digestion in the mouth or stomach and are borne virtually intact to the small intestine where they are degraded. Because of solubility problems, the enzymatic breakdown of lipids can only occur at the interface between a lipid droplet and adjacent water. It is therefore essential to emulsify lipids before they can be digested. Emulsification is brought about by mechanical mixing in the intestinal lumen, in the presence of bile salts.

Triacylglycerol, cholesterol and phospholipid are now degraded by pancreatic enzymes the secretion of which is regulated by the hormones cholecystokinin and secretin. Pancreatic lipase removes two of the three fatty acids of triacylglycerol. It is aided by a co-lipase. Cholesterol and phospholipid are broken down in a similar manner, yielding free cholesterol and other molecules that include glycerylphosphorylcholine. Rarely, they accumulate in the plasma in the course of the familial disorder, **type III hyperlipoproteinaemia**. Bile salts now enable the free fatty acids, free cholesterol and 2-monoacylglycerol to coalesce as a mixed micelle before they are absorbed through the intestinal mucosa.

The free fatty aids and free cholesterol are re-synthesised to yield activated triacylglycerol and cholesterol esters, respectively. These molecules are once again hydrophobic. They are therefore packaged as droplets called **chylomicrons** before they can pass into the intestinal lacteals, lymphatics that transport the lipid-rich material to the thoracic duct, and thence to the left subclavian vein.

Among many special forms of lipid are the fatty acids (prostanoic acids) termed **prostaglandins**. They are formed from the essential fatty acid (p. 180), linoleic acid, a process that takes place in almost every tissue. The immediate precursor of the predominant classes of prostaglandin is **arachidonic** Acid 180, released from membrane-bound phospholipids by the enzyme phospholipase A.

Utilisation

Conveyed as micelles in the blood, triacylglycerol is metabolised by adipose tissue, skeletal muscle, heart muscle, liver, kidney and lung. Free fatty acids gain direct entry to skeletal muscle cells or adipocytes or are carried in the blood bound to albumin. Glycerol, released from triacylglycerol, is either broken down or employed by hepatocytes to manufacture glyceryl-3-phosphate which then contributes to gluconeogenesis (p. 75). Any remaining chylomicrons are hydrolysed within the liver. A familial disorder, lipoprotein lipase deficiency, **type I hyperlipoproteinaemia**, is inherited as an autosomal dominant characteristic. It leads to chylomicronaemia.

Lipid malabsorption

Lipid malabsorption may be caused by defects in biliary or pancreatic secretions, or because of malfunction or disease of intestinal, epithelial cells. Malabsorption is common in any form of bile salt deficiency (p. 35). It is a feature of chronic liver disease and of obstructive jaundice, and is a consequence of resection of the distal part of the small bowel. Malabsorption is common in patients with inflammatory or neoplastic disease of the pancreas. Enteropathies such as coeliac disease severely limit the absorption of digested lipids.

LIVER

In addition to diseases centering on the liver itself, such as hepatitis, hepatocarcinoma and hydatid cyst, the organ is affected incidentally by many systemic disorders of surgical significance. They include shock (p. 290), malnutrition (p. 229) and cardiac failure (p. 149). Liver diseases and their treatment are strongly influenced by the high capacity of hepatocytes for rapid regeneration. The unusual arterial and portal venous blood supply, and the particular venous and biliary drainage of the liver, closely regulate the distribution of cellular damage (Fig. 37). Centrilobular disease and, in particular, fatty infiltration, are features of left ventricular failure; anaemia; hypoxia; and chronic venous congestion. Periportal disease is a feature of infection or of injury attributable to microorganisms or chemicals conveyed by the hepatic artery, via the portal vein, or within the bile ducts.

Now read Biliary tract (p. 35)

Biopsy diagnosis of liver disease

Percutaneous needle biopsy of the liver is often required for accurate diagnosis. The mortality of the procedure varies between 0.01 and 0.1% and is attributable either to bleeding or to biliary peritonitis caused by the inadvertent puncture of the gall

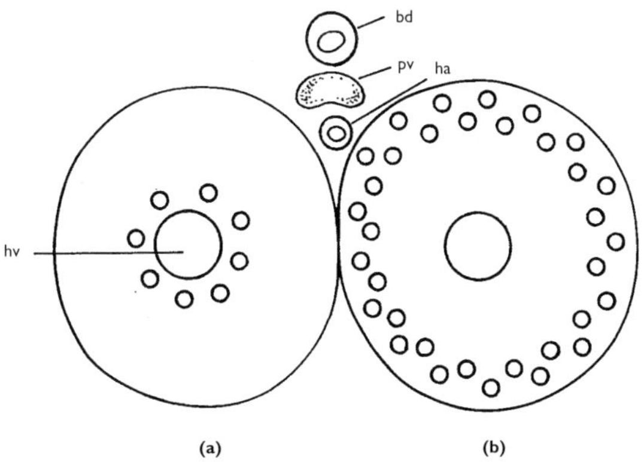

Figure 37 Cell injury in liver disease.
(a) Centrilobular. Centrilobular cells, remote from a hepatic arterial branch and a portal vein tributary, suffer in cardiac failure, shock and anaemia.
(b) Periportal. Periportal cells, adjacent to the vascular sources of oxygen and metabolites, suffer in intoxications, ethanol poisoning, infection, and cholangitis.
bd: bile duct; ha: hepatic arteriole; hv: hepatic venule; pv: portal venule.

bladder. Ultrasonographic guidance (p. 169) reduces the incidence of the latter but not of the former. Ultrasonography also enhances the precision of diagnosis of liver cancer. Laparoscopic guided-needle biopsy is now widely practiced. Transjugular biopsy is useful in patients with bleeding disorders or ascites. Although common conditions such as micronodular cirrhosis can be diagnosed by conventional needle biopsy, on rare occasions, a larger, wedge biopsy of the anterior border of the liver may be necessary to allow a disorder such as macronodular cirrhosis to be identified. In any report, the adequacy of the biopsy should be stated together with an opinion on the presence or absence of a defined liver disease and its severity.

DEVELOPMENTAL AND CONGENITAL DISORDERS

Alpha$_1$-anti-trypsin (α_1AT) deficiency

Alpha$_1$-anti-trypsin (α_1AT) is a protease inhibitor. In this rare, genetic disease, abnormal α_1AT accumulates in hepatocytes as cytoplasmic globules. Neonatal hepatitis is one result; it is usually followed by cirrhosis. There is a susceptibility to pulmonary emphysema (p. 215).

BILIARY ATRESIA

Atresia of bile ducts is described on p. 36.

Cystic disease

- **Single cyst**. Ultrasonography confirms that solitary, simple, developmental cysts are common. The cysts are usually small but may be sufficiently large to implicate a whole hepatic segment or lobe.
- **Polycystic disease**. This heritable disorder is determined by a mutant gene located on somatic chromosome 16. There is a strong association with polycystic renal disease (p. 197) and occasionally with intestinal malrotation and spina bifida. The cysts vary greatly in size, number and site. In many instances, cysts are asymptomatic but rupture or haemorrhage attract attention.

Now read Amoebic abscess (p. 9), Hydatid cyst (p. 113, 357)

LIVER FAILURE

In liver failure, there is a defective synthesis of protein and other macromolecules; impaired conjugation of metabolites and drugs; and defective intermediary metabolism. Hyperbilirubinaemia (p. 189) is common and jaundice may develop. The severity of disease can be graded from A (mild) to C (severe) (Table 44). The mortality of liver disease correlates with the grade. Additional, specific grading systems have been devised for individual diseases.

Table 44 The Child–Pugh classification of liver failure

Observation	A	B	C
Serum bilirubin (μmol/L)	<34	34–51	>51
Serum albumin (g/L)	>35	28–35	<28
Increase in prothrombin time (s)	<4	4–6	>6
Ascites	None	Mild	Moderate
Encephalopathy	None	Minimal	Advanced

Effects

The effects are widespread. Approximately half the glycogen reserve of the body is stored in the liver which is also the site for gluconeogenesis. Experimentally, total hepatectomy leads to death from hypoglycaemia. A similar sequence is likely in man. A plethora of protein deficiencies occurs. In particular, there is a fall in the serum albumin concentration. The subsequent decrease in oncotic pressure is one factor in the production of ascites. Most of the proteins required for blood coagulation (p. 95) are synthesised in the liver. Consequently, defective coagulation is an early feature of the disease. Many other compounds are detoxified by the liver. They are excreted in the bile after conjugation with amino acids, organic acids and other radicals such as glutamic acid, glucuronic acid and sulphate, respectively. Patients with liver failure consequently have a low tolerance of drugs such as the analgesic opiates.

Hepatic encephalopathy

The metabolic defects of liver failure often culminate in neurological changes that include coarse tremor; disorientation; deterioration in intellect; coma; and death.

In liver cell disease, increased quantities of insulin reach the systemic circulation. They induce the increased uptake by skeletal muscle of the branched-chain amino acids leucine, isoleucine and lysine. At the same time, the aromatic amino acids methionine, phenylalanine and tyrosine, normally metabolised in the liver, enter the circulation in excess. The change in the normal plasma ratio between these two forms of amino acid induces alterations in the concentrations of neurotransmitters in the central nervous system and an abnormal production of 'false neurotransmitters' such as octopamine and phenylethanolamine. The remedial, intravenous infusion of branched-chain amino acids can ameliorate hepatic coma. Serum ammonia concentration is elevated. Its incorporation into glutamine may deplete glutamate, an excitatory transmitter in the brain.

Causes

- **Acute failure** is a result of the destruction of hepatocytes by ischaemia; chemical reagents; drugs such as paracetamol; or viruses, particularly HBV and HCV (p. 152).
- **Chronic failure** is attributable to the replacement of hepatocyte lobules by fibrous tissue, for example in cirrhosis (p. 211).

CHEMICAL DISORDERS

Alcoholic intoxication and hepatitis

Acute

Acute alcoholic hepatitis is associated with episodes of very high ethanol intake. The chemical is metabolised by alcohol dehydrogenase the activity of which is lower in women than in men. Females are therefore more susceptible to the adverse effects of a sustained high intake of ethanol than males. Fever, hepatomegaly and jaundice are recognised. The first microscopic evidence of excessive intake is the asymptomatic and reversible accumulation of fat in hepatocytes. Vacuoles of fat displace the nucleus to one side. Some of the necrotic cells contain crescentic, hyaline perinuclear deposits called Mallory's bodies.

Chronic

The prolonged ingestion of large amounts of ethanol may culminate in cirrhosis. The response depends upon the quantity of ethanol consumed and the duration of its consumption. Some patients develop hepatic failure and encephalopathy. Post-operative complications are more common in alcoholics undergoing all forms of surgery. A prolonged period of abstinence before surgery reduces the post-operative morbidity.

INFECTION AND INFLAMMATION

Local infection and inflammation

The liver is frequently the site of local infection, occasionally caused by direct injury but frequently resulting from micro-organisms carried by arterial blood or by the systemic or portal venous circulations.

Liver abscess

Liver abscess results from biliary or abdominal sepsis and is a late consequence of purulent appendicitis, diverticular disease of the colon or other forms of peritonitis associated with portal pyaemia. Septic abortion may result in clostridial abscesses. Abscess is a common manifestation of amoebiasis (p. 8). It may also occur in hydatidosis (p. 357) and in fascioliasis (p. 357). In diabetics, the cause may be *Streptococcus intermedius* (*S. milleri*) but in many patients, the aetiology is not evident.

Tuberculosis

Solitary, tuberculous granulomas (p. 332) are rare. In miliary tuberculosis, a widespread scattering of pin-head-size lesions is characteristic.

Generalised infection and inflammation

Acute

Acute hepatitis is often the result of viral infection (p. 347) but may also be bacterial, protozoal or helminthic.

Now read Hepatitis (p. 152)

Chronic

Chronic hepatitis is the result of viral infection (p. 152); drugs; or auto-immune disease. The term indicates active but prolonged inflammation of the liver. There is hepatocyte necrosis that continues for at least 6 months. Mild forms progress little but severe forms advance to scarring and cirrhosis. The histopathological features are of value both in diagnosis and in prognosis, and biopsy is essential. With the exception of suspected cases of chronic hepatitis C, it is important to distinguish two forms, chronic persistent hepatitis and chronic active hepatitis

Chronic persistent/chronic lobular hepatitis

Patients have few symptoms or are asymptomatic. The progression to more severe disease is unlikely. There is no evidence of cirrhosis. Biopsy reveals:

- A mononuclear cell infiltrate restricted to the portal tracts, *without extension* of the inflammatory and destructive process into the liver lobules.
- An intact limiting plate of periportal hepatocytes.

In a lobular variant, foci of necrosis and inflammation extend into the liver lobules.

Chronic active hepatitis

Chronic active hepatitis is a progressive disorder liable to lead to cirrhosis, liver failure and death. The majority of patients are asymptomatic although laboratory tests of liver function may be abnormal. Biopsy reveals:

- A dense mononuclear cell infiltrate of the portal tracts *extending into* the liver lobule;
- The destruction of hepatocytes at the periphery of the liver lobule and of those that form the limiting plate (**piecemeal necrosis**). In severe cases, **bridging necrosis** extends between individual lobules.
- The extension of collagenous connective tissue into the liver lobules, isolating groups of liver cells.
- Active hepatocyte regeneration.

Chronic hepatitis C

In many cases, the microscopical features of this increasingly common disorder (p. 155) are intermediate between chronic persistent and chronic active hepatitis. In spite of little evidence of inflammation, the disease may advance to cirrhosis. This progression is more likely in older, alcohol-consuming, male patients with longstanding disease than in younger, abstemious females. High inflammatory activity and iron retention are also adverse features.

Cirrhosis

Cirrhosis describes a small, irregularly scarred, yellow-brown liver. There are three components:

- Liver-cell necrosis.
- Nodular hepatocyte regeneration.
- Fibrosis with obstruction to portal blood flow.

Fibrous tissue separates new islands of liver cells. Depending upon the distribution of the collagen, the appearances are micro- or macronodular.

In Western countries, the most frequent cause of cirrhosis is the sustained, excessive intake of alcohol. In Third World countries, viral hepatitis is the commonest agent. Other worldwide causes are metabolic, inherited and drug-related diseases; schistosomiasis; primary biliary cirrhosis; and cardiac cirrhosis.

Alcoholic cirrhosis

In this common condition, there is diffuse, fine scarring of the liver and many small, micronodular foci of regeneration. The cirrhotic lesion is periportal.

Continued alcohol intake leads to hepatocyte destruction. The ingrowth of myofibroblasts results in excess collagen formation. Fascicles of this fibrous protein extend between adjacent portal tracts, dividing the parenchyma of the liver into ill-defined and irregularly shaped territories. Residual liver cells multiply and regenerate but the rate of destruction exceeds that of regeneration. The liver becomes progressively smaller and firmer. Liver failure, with hepatic encephalopathy, may develop. Portal hypertension (below) is a result of the disordered hepatic blood flow. Cirrhosis is the consequence of a direct, toxic effect of ethanol upon hepatocytes. There is a high mortality rate but complete recovery is possible with abstinence.

It has been suggested that the daily consumption of smaller quantities of ethanol can protect against vascular diseases such as atheroma, extending life expectancy. However, not all alcoholic beverages are beneficial.

Biliary cirrhosis

Primary biliary cirrhosis

Primary biliary cirrhosis is a slowly progressive, auto-immune disorder (p. 28) that is much more frequent in females than males. Many patients have co-existent arthritis, scleroderma and hypothyroidism. Serum anti-mitochondrial antibodies are identified. The disease is an indication for hepatic transplantation.

Secondary biliary cirrhosis

There are many causes. In the West, it is an infrequent consequence of cholangitis associated with biliary obstruction. The end stages are characterised by fine (micronodular) or coarse (macronodular) scarring. Secondary biliary cirrhosis is commonplace in countries where portal vein obstruction is caused by *Schistosoma mansoni* (p. 356). The eggs of the adult worm produce an inflammatory reaction in the portal venules with massive fibrosis encircling the portal tracts, forming fibrotic sheaths of up to 20 mm in diameter. The appearances are described as 'pipe-stem' cirrhosis.

Now read Schistosomiasis (p. 356)

Portal hypertension

In this condition, the normal portal venous pressure of 5–7 mmHg is raised because of intra-hepatic or extra-hepatic obstruction. Relative to the hepatic sinusoids, obstruction to portal venous return may be pre-sinusoidal, sinusoidal, or post-sinusoidal. Relative to the anatomy of the portal veins, the obstruction may be within or external to the liver.

- **Intra-hepatic** obstruction is a late consequence of cirrhosis.
- **Extra-hepatic** obstruction in the neonate may follow umbilical infection or umbilical vein catheterisation. In adults, the obstruction is the result of pancreatic disease, particularly carcinoma; operative trauma; or, in certain countries, schistosomiasis.

Varices (p. 345) occur in the distal oesophagus and the upper third of the stomach, in the distribution of the left gastric vein. That variceal bleeding occurs in these sites is a consequence of the superficial situation of the veins. There is no increase in the incidence of haemorrhoids or variceal dilatation in other territories draining into the portal system. *Caput medusae*, with a cluster of dilated veins around the umbilicus, is very rare. Bleeding oesophageal varices represent only 5% of patients with haematemesis and melaena in the West but are the most frequent sources of gastro-intestinal haemorrhage in the Middle East.

Because the portal vein lacks valves, resistance to venous return at any level between the right side of the heart and the splanchnic vessels may lead to portal hypertension. One example of such a cause is constrictive pericarditis.

Budd–Chiari syndrome

In this rare condition, there is occlusion or thrombosis of the main hepatic veins. The aetiology is often uncertain. It may be due to a vascular web that forms at the junction of the hepatic veins and the inferior vena cava. Simple compression of the hepatic veins may accompany polycystic liver disease or hepatocellular carcinoma. Thrombosis of the hepatic veins may occur in patients taking oral contraceptive pills, in those suffering from myeloproliferative diseases or in paroxysmal nocturnal haemoglobinuria. The radicals of the hepatic vein undergo progressive intimal fibrosis.

TUMOURS

Metastatic cancer is very frequent. The majority of the cells from cancers of the gastro-intestinal tract metastasise via the portal vein but cells from tumours of the lung and breast may reach the liver via the hepatic artery.

Benign

Abdominal ultrasonography or CT scanning confirms that benign, often asymptomatic tumours are very common.

Haemangioma

Haemangioma is the most frequent benign tumour. Haemangioma may enlarge during pregnancy and under the influence of prophylactic or therapeutic oestrogens. Spontaneous rupture is rare and many haemangiomas are recognised only at operation or autopsy.

Adenoma

Unencapsulated islands of hepatocytes often arise in the livers of women during their reproductive years. There is a much higher frequency of these adenomas in patients taking oral contraceptives than in the general population. The cells are arranged in plates, two or three cells thick. There are no portal tracts within them. Blood may escape into the centre of a necrotic nodule. Spontaneous rupture results in haemoperitoneum.

Malignant

Hepatocellular carcinoma

The majority of primary malignant tumours are hepatocellular carcinomas although cholangiocarcinoma (p. 39) also occurs. Worldwide, this common cancer displays a male:female preponderance of 4:1. Hepatocellular carcinoma is found in only $30/10^6$ Western people. In South-East Asia, the prevalence is 30 times greater.

Causes

The majority of patients have been infected with HBV or HCV. Where mycotoxicosis is endemic, aflatoxins (p. 136) and HBV act synergistically as carcinogens. Irrespective of geographical location, there is an intimate association with liver cirrhosis. However, hepatocellular carcinoma is conspicuously uncommon in primary biliary cirrhosis and in Wilson's disease. There is a slightly increased incidence in patients taking oral contraceptive pills.

Structure

The tumour occurs in massive, nodular or diffuse forms.

- The **massive variety** is a solitary tumour of younger patients who do not suffer from cirrhosis. An important variant is the fibro-lamellar hepatoma that has a better prognosis. The cells are large, eosinophilic and polygonal. There is an abundant stroma.
- The **nodular form** is multifocal in origin and arises in cirrhotic livers.
- The **diffuse tumour** is a variety of the nodular form. Individual tumour cells are recognisable as hepatocytes but there is hyperchromasia and nuclear pleomorphism. The lobular architecture of the normal liver is lost and replaced by a trabecular pattern.

Diagnosis by aspiration biopsy, using a fine needle guided by ultrasound, is of high specificity and sensitivity. HBsAg (p. 152) is often demonstrable within liver cells surrounding the tumour.

Behaviour and prognosis

Metastatic spread is via the hepatic veins. Venous obstruction results and the Budd–Chiari syndrome (p. 212) is an occasional consequence. The majority of tumours are unsuitable for resection because of their extent or the co-existence of cirrhosis. In the absence of cirrhosis, depending upon cell type, the 5-year survival of resectable tumours is ~20–50%.

Hepatoblastoma

Hepatoblastoma is a rare tumour of young children usually under the age of two years. Like Wilms' tumour of the kidney (p. 200), it may be associated with congenital anomalies such as cardiac malformation. Serum levels of α_1-fetoprotein (p. 247) are elevated. The secretion of ectopic gonadotrophin by tumour cells may induce precocious puberty. The tumours occasionally rupture, leading to haemoperitoneum.

Haemangiosarcoma

Haemangiosarcoma, Kupffer cell sarcoma, is rare. It is multicentric and rapidly fatal. The tumour is recognised from time-to-time in individuals taking contraceptive pills or androgens. It is an occupational hazard of those exposed to arsenic in preparations such as insecticides, or to vinyl chloride monomer used in the manufacture of polyvinyl chloride. It was also detected in patients injected with thorotrast, a colloidal solution of thorium dioxide employed in early forms of angiography.

VASCULAR DISEASE

Hepatic artery obstruction

The hepatic artery is frequently surrounded by tumour cells but this rarely impedes blood flow. Iatrogenic obstruction may be accidental or produced deliberately during radiological embolisation or surgical ligation. Since 75% of the afferent hepatic blood flow comes from the portal vein, ligation of the common hepatic artery is rarely followed by infarction. However, embolisation or ligation, to control traumatic haemorrhage or in the treatment of hepatic tumours, should be confined to either the right or left branches of the hepatic artery or even to segmental branches. Embolisation or ligation must be attempted distal to the origin of the cystic artery. Unless this precaution is observed, gangrenous cholecystitis may develop. Local or zonal infarction may occur in systemic diseases such as polyarteritis nodosa and acute bacterial endocarditis.

TRANSPLANTATION

The first European liver transplant was performed by Calne (p. 370). An insufficient number of normal, cadaveric livers is now available to meet the demand for grafting. However, livers with insignificant disease can be used instead of normal organs. Moreover, the regeneration of liver tissue is so effective that donor organs can be subdivided into lobes or segments and the portions transplanted into multiple recipients. Liver allografting modulates the immune mechanism so that the success rate of simultaneous liver and intestinal transplantation is high.

LUNG

The lungs are susceptible to almost all forms of genetic or acquired, local or systemic disease. They can be investigated by a wide variety of imaging and functional procedures (p. 169) but biopsy is often a mainstay of diagnosis.

Biopsy diagnosis of lung and bronchial disease

A wide variety of techniques is available. The microscopical examination of sputum, pleural fluid, or fluid aspirated at bronchial lavage, enables the identification of cells from bronchial carcinoma. Culture reveals micro-organisms including bacteria, protozoa and fungi. Fibre-optic bronchoscopy with transbronchial biopsy is of value in the investigation of diffuse lung lesions and allows the rapid identification of parabronchial masses such as bronchial adenoma. Open biopsy at thoracotomy enables larger, representative parts of a lesion to be selected. This method, preferred by pathologists, establishes the diagnosis in more than 90% of cases of diffuse lung disease but in only 50% of cases of lung disease overall. Thoracoscopic biopsy may prove as accurate as open biopsy, without the need for thoracotomy. Percutaneous needle biopsy of the pleura is less rewarding than lung biopsy.

DEVELOPMENTAL AND CONGENITAL DISORDERS

Accessory lobes, sequestrated lung tissue (p. 123) and cysts are anomalous developments.
There are two varieties of cyst:

- **Bronchogenic cysts** lie near the trachea or hilum. The mural connective tissue contains cartilage.
- **Pulmonary cysts** form within the lung substance, in continuity with the air passages. The walls are devoid of cartilage.

IMMUNOLOGICAL DISORDERS

Asthma

Bronchial asthma is recognised with increasing frequency in surgical subjects. In young persons, asthma is the result of type I hypersensitivity (p. 160) to extrinsic materials such as the house mite. There may be an inherited predisposition. In adults, there is often no history of familial disease. Nevertheless, the development of hypersensitivity reactions to drugs such as aspirin and penicillin may provoke fatal attacks of bronchial spasm and obstruction.

Other immunological disorders

The lung is particularly prone to infections in immunodeficient patients such as those with AIDS (p. 2).

Transplantation

Lung transplantation has become practicable with the introduction of effective immunosuppression and with improvements in surgical techniques. Some uncommon or rare pulmonary diseases, such as the diffuse fibrosis that occasionally complicates the intake of anti-obesity drugs; paraquat poisoning; and amyloidosis, can be treated effectively by no other means.

Now read Transplantation (p. 329)

- **Unilateral transplantation** may be appropriate in individuals with emphysema or with primary pulmonary hypertension, depending upon the extent of damage to the right ventricle.
- **Bilateral lung transplantation** has proved especially effective in the treatment of end-stage pulmonary fibrosis.
- **Simultaneous heart–lung transplantation**. Patients with chronic lung infection, including those with cystic fibrosis; those suffering from the late effects of anti-obesity drugs; and others with particular forms of congenital heart disease, require both heart and lung transplants. Cardiac transplantation alone cannot correct the long-standing, associated abnormalities of the pulmonary vasculature. Technically, the operation is easier to perform than transplanting either organ individually. Occasionally, in patients receiving combined heart–lung transplants for primary respiratory disease, the heart removed from the recipient is used for further cardiac transplantation to another individual, a technique called 'domino' transplantation. Donor lungs are frequently sites of oedema and infection so that immunosuppressed recipients are prone to postoperative infection.

EMPHYSEMA

Interstitial (surgical) emphysema

Laceration of lung tissue by a perforating wound; rib fracture; and alveolar rupture are among conditions that allow air to escape into tissue planes. Sometimes the air is confined to the interlobular septa or to the pleural surface of the lung. When the collection is extensive, it may produce subcutaneous emphysema over the chest and in the neck. The air is detectable by palpable crepitus.

Pulmonary emphysema

Pulmonary emphysema is a **permanent** increase in the size of the alveoli and the air spaces distal to the terminal bronchioles, with destruction of their walls (Fig. 38). The changes are in contrast to the **transient** changes of bronchial asthma. There are two forms of pulmonary emphysema:

- **Centrilobular emphysema** is common in smokers and is associated with chronic bronchitis. It represents an enlargement of the terminal bronchioles.
- **Panacinar emphysema** is a feature of α_1-antitrypsin deficiency (p. 209). It begins with enlargement of the alveolar ducts and alveoli but progresses to involve the respiratory bronchioles and hence the whole acinus.

When part of one lung collapses or is occupied by a mass such as carcinoma, the remaining lung tissue expands to occupy the intrapleural space. The mediastinum shifts towards the side of the lesion. The changes in the non-collapsed lung are described as **compensatory emphysema**.

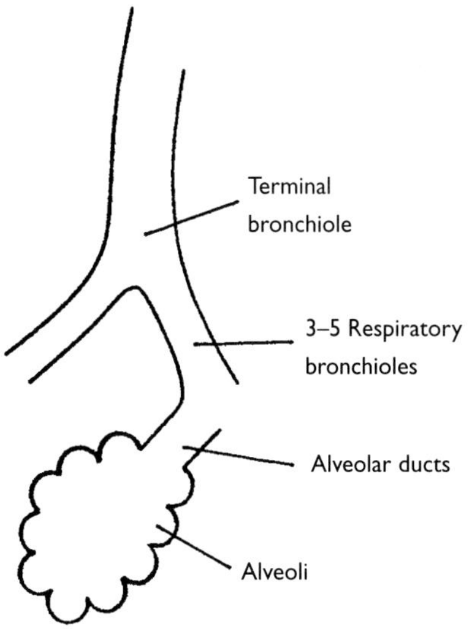

Figure 38 Defective gas exchange in lung periphery. Figure shows normal relationship between terminal bronchioles and alveoli. Diameter of terminal and respiratory bronchioles, and alveolar ducts, is closely similar. Active air flow ceases as respiratory bronchioles ends and air passes to alveoli by diffusion. Defective diffusion is result of:
(a) reduced, functional alveolar surface, as in pneumonia;
(b) increased distance for air to diffuse, as in emphysema;
(c) increased thickness of alveolar membrane as in the adult respiratory distress syndrome (ARDS).

Behaviour and prognosis
Abscesses may respond to conservative, antibiotic treatment. However, bronchoscopy or surgical intervention is often necessary when the cause is a foreign body, when the tissue destruction is extensive, or there is associated bronchiectasis. Bronchopneumonia is a frequent complication.

Tuberculosis

In pulmonary tuberculosis, infection of lung tissue is by *Mycobacterium tuberculosis* hominis (p. 237). The organisms are inhaled. They multiply within pulmonary macrophages and establish foci of infection that extend within the lung and destroy lung tissue.

- In **childhood type disease**, a peripheral focus of lung infection, the **Ghon focus** together with enlarged regional lymph nodes, constitute a **primary complex**. Healing, fibrosis and calcification are usual but lymphatic or vascular dissemination may occur. Miliary tuberculosis is one possible result.
- In **adult type disease**, the infection is superimposed on a state of partial immunity determined by the prior occurrence of a primary infection. The existence of cell-mediated, delayed hypersensitivity is indicated by a positive response in a Mantoux test (p. 229). Slowly progressive lung destruction, with cavitation, blood vessel erosion, pulmonary collapse and pleural fibrosis, are characteristic. However, a more rapidly advancing tuberculous bronchopneumonia is occasionally encountered. Among the complications is empyema.

Fibrosis

Pneumoconiosis

Pneumoconiosis is pulmonary dust disease. The inhaled particles may be inorganic or organic. Some are inert, others irritant or antigenic. The response they provoke is related to the size of the particles. Larger particles are retained by the respiratory epithelium; smaller particles are exhaled. Those between 1 and 10 μm in diameter are capable of inhalation into the alveoli. Some dusts, such as those derived from mining coal, iron, gold or copper or from quarrying, contain silicates. These materials cause lung fibrosis and increase the susceptibility of the individual to tuberculosis.

In **coal-workers' silicosis**, focal islands of fibrous tissue, impregnated with coal dust, are scattered throughout both lungs. Secondary emphysema is usual. There is impaired respiratory function and a predisposition to chronic bronchitis and to infection. The changes of **asbestosis** are described on p. 27.

MECHANICAL AND PHYSICAL CHANGES

Trauma

Lung tissue may be lacerated directly, for example in road-traffic accidents, or indirectly, for example by explosion. Pneumothorax and haemothorax are frequent results of direct injury. Hot gases or flame may reach the lungs via the bronchi. If the individual survives, the adult respiratory distress syndrome (ARDS – p. 219) is likely to develop.

Collapse

The persistent collapse of pulmonary segments, lobules or lobes predisposes to bronchiectasis.

Absorption collapse

The partial or complete collapse of lung lobules, segments or lobes, or, occasionally, of a whole lung results in the absorption of air from the lung tissue. It is one consequence of sudden and complete obstruction of a bronchus and may occur post-operatively, due to the accumulation of mucus. If untreated, a collapsed lung ultimately becomes fibrotic.

Pressure collapse

Pressure exerted on lung tissue by blood, pus or other fluids in the pleural cavity leads to collapse of the underlying tissue to an extent determined by the size of the haemothorax, empyema or effusion. The change is reversible unless the pleural lining becomes fibrotic.

Atelectasis

Atelectasis is incomplete expansion of the lung. It is common in premature infants in whom it is attributable to hyaline membrane disease. In elderly patients, it may follow airway obstruction after general anaesthesia.

Oedema

Oedema develops when the rate of accumulation of fluid in the lung exceeds the capacity of the lymphatics to remove it. Fluid collects first in the peribronchial, loose connective tissues, then in the alveolar walls, and finally in the alveoli themselves. The fluid collections exert profound effects upon gaseous exchange. Under normal conditions there is a net inward force of ~5 mmHg (Fig. 39). Pulmonary oedema therefore results from:

- **Increased vascular hydrodynamic pressure**. Examples are: excessive intravenous infusion or left ventricular cardiac failure.
- **Increased capillary permeability**. Examples are: inflammatory disease; the inhalation of noxious gases such as sulphur dioxide and chlorine; raised intracranial pressure; exposure to high altitudes by unaclimatised individuals; and renal failure with uraemia.

Now read Oedema (p. 251)

ADULT RESPIRATORY DISTRESS SYNDROME (ARDS)

The adult respiratory distress syndrome is the sudden onset of diffuse lung injury and respiratory embarrassment in critically ill patients. Some severely injured patients with shock respond initially to haemodynamic resuscitation but die ultimately from pulmonary failure. The syndrome has also been called 'shock lung' or 'post-traumatic pulmonary insufficiency'.

In earlier years, mechanical ventilation, the result of poor techniques, could seriously damage normal and injured lungs by regional overdistension. This is no longer likely.

Now read SIRS (p. 293)

Causes

ARDS is characterised by inflammation, oedema and atelectasis. The disorder may progress rapidly to fibrosis. The common cause is sepsis, particularly when combined with inadequate tissue perfusion. Other aetiological factors include:

- Massive blood transfusion, especially if the blood has not been filtered to remove micro-aggregates.
- Micro-embolism.
- Excessive infusion of saline.
- Prolonged ventilation, particularly with high oxygen partial pressures.
- Direct or indirect pulmonary damage attributable to inhalation of gases under high pressure.
- Shock waves or blows to the chest.

The role of circulating endotoxin is important. The syndrome is analogous to the generalised Shwartzman reaction. All the causal factors are thought to act through a final common pathway affecting the pulmonary surfactant lining the alveoli. A reduction in the quantity of surfactant or a change in the nature of the component lipoprotein are therefore possible common denominators.

Structure

The lungs display petechial haemorrhages together with engorgement of the capillaries and small veins. Alveolar congestion and zonal collapse are more evident in the lower and middle lobes than in the upper. The surface tension of surfactant increases. Within 24 hours, intra-alveolar haemorrhages appear and a hyaline membrane lines the alveolar walls. Thrombo-emboli are observed in small, pulmonary arteries and

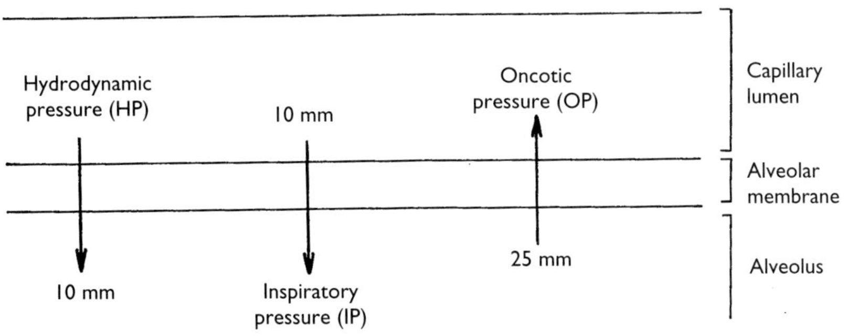

Figure 39 Fluid movement within normal lung tissue.
Several forces influence movement of fluid from pulmonary alveolus, into pulmonary capillaries, across alveolar membrane. Net force = (OP – (HP + IP)) = (25 – (10 + 10)) = 5 mm Hg. In pulmonary oedema, pneumonia and shock, balance is greatly disturbed.

arterioles. Interstitial and alveolar oedema develop and increase progressively. Oedema is accompanied by haemorrhagic pulmonary consolidation.

Behaviour and prognosis
By the fifth day, infection is the predominant feature and bronchopneumonia becomes confluent. The mortality is ~40%. In survivors, pulmonary fibrosis is a common sequel.

TUMOURS

Metastases to the lungs from distant sites are very frequent. The majority derive from gastro-intestinal, breast, renal, ovarian, thyroid and pancreatic carcinomas. Occasionally, the co-existence of two independent primary tumours results in two concurrent but entirely different forms of metastasis. Relative to their frequency, the metastasis to lung of osteosarcoma (p. 59) and other malignant mesenchymal tumours (p. 298) is very common and is due to the intimate relationship between the cells of the primary tumour and its small blood vessels.

Benign

Chondroma

Benign tumours, other than those arising in the bronchi, are rare. Chondroma is a developmental lesion, a hamartoma. The presence of a very slowly growing island of cartilaginous tissue within the lung is generally detected fortuitously, during radiological surveys. The mass of mature cartilage is incompletely divided by clefts of respiratory epithelium.

Malignant

The greatest number of primary malignant tumours are carcinomas originating in the bronchi. They are described on p. 70.

Now read Bronchus (p. 69)

VASCULAR DISEASE

Thrombo-embolism

Now read Embolism (p. 124), Thrombus (p. 320)

Vasculitis

Inflammation of the pulmonary arteries or arterioles may result from the lodgement of infected emboli, for example during narcotic abuse. It is also a feature of unusual forms of systemic connective tissue disease such as Wegener's granulomatosis (p. 25).

LYMPHOID DISEASE

LYMPHOID TISSUE

Lymphocytes and their precursors are assembled as primary and secondary organs.

Primary organs

Lymphocytes originate from bone marrow stem cells. Subsequently, B lymphocytes proliferate in the marrow, T lymphocytes in the thymus.

Bone marrow

In the adult haemopoietic marrow of the skull, ribs, vertebrae, proximal ends of femur and humerus, a large blood supply ensures the integrity of the stem cells and of the reticular fibre microskeleton that supports them. In the normal individual, the number of marrow lymphoid foci is very small; the majority of lymphocytes are arranged randomly.

Thymus

Lymphocytes within the thymus (p. 321) are thymocytes.

Secondary organs

Lymphocytes engaged in the immune response, in inflammatory reactions, and in foreign body and other episodes are concentrated in lymph nodes, in the spleen and in the mucosa-associated lymphoid tissues.

Lymph nodes

Lymph nodes (Fig. 40) are encapsulated masses of lymphoid tissue into which lymphatic vessels drain. Diseases of lymph nodes are intimately related to the immune response (p. 171). Normal lymph nodes are oval or bean-shaped. Their size is highly variable,

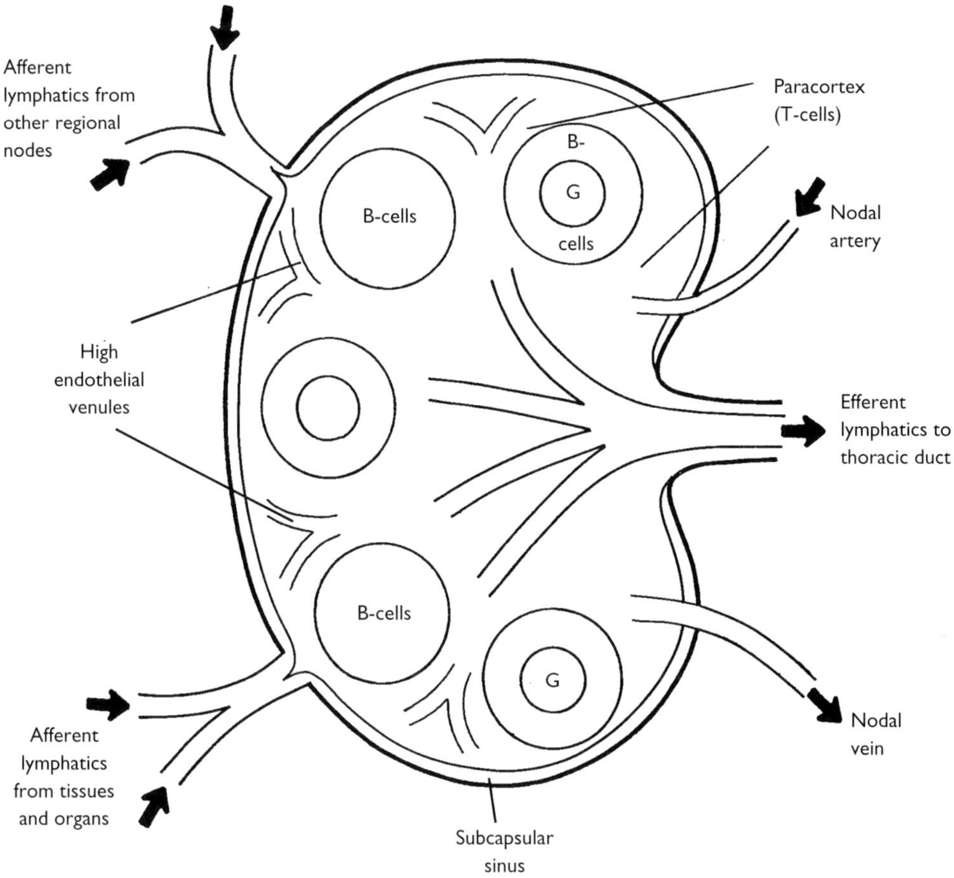

Figure 40 Lymph node structure.
Lymph reaches node from tissues or from another, more peripheral node. Lymph passes by afferent lymphatics to subcapsular sinus, thence into cortex, through the follicles, into paracortical zones, then to medulla. From here, lymph from medullary sinuses enters efferent lymphatics, then passes to larger lymphatic channels, thence to thoraric duct and blood.

Lymphocytes reaching node from tissues or from another, peripheral node, travel by afferent lymphatics to nodes and enter by high endothelial venules. Lymphoid follicles are rich in B-cells. Presence of germinal centres (G) mirrors activity of plasma cells in antibody synthesis. Paracortical zones, monitored by thymus, are replete with T-cells.

ranging from 2–5 mm to as much as 20 mm in diameter. There is an outer cortex and an inner medulla. Afferent lymphatic channels enter the periphery of the node. Efferent lymphatic vessels emerge from the hilus where blood vessels enter and leave. Viscera such as the respiratory and urinary tracts are further protected by widely dispersed, non-encapsulated lymphoid tissues. The pharyngeal tonsils are one example.

Lymph from the viscera and from territories drained by regional nodes, passes via the thoracic duct to the superior vena cava. Arteries convey this small circulating population of lymphocytes to the nodes where they enter a system of high endothelial venules, to the lining cells of which they adhere and from which they subsequently migrate. Simultaneously, the afferent lymphatic vessels transport lymph to the nodes from the organs and viscera. Through these dual mechanisms, antigen presenting cells (APC) and re-circulating lymphocytes are enabled to reach the cortical and paracortical tissue of the nodes.

The **cortex** of each node comprises follicles together with parafollicular zones. Inactive islands of B lymphocytes are 'primary' follicles. When active, the follicles acquire germinal centres and are 'secondary'.

The cortical lymphoid tissue around the follicles, the paracortex, is composed of T lymphocytes and dendritic cells. It is parafollicular.

The **medulla** of each node, the site of entry of the nodal artery and of the exit of the efferent vein, is populated by plasma cells (p. 172) and immunoblasts.

Now read Immunity (p. 171)

Spleen

The spleen (p. 301) acts as a filter for the blood stream. It is devoid of afferent and efferent lymphatics.

Mucosa-associated lymphoid tissues (MALT)

Much of the specialised lymphoid tissue of the intestine (p. 168) is arranged as Peyer's patches. It is extra-nodal. The overlying epithelium is permeable and permits the sampling of antigenic material from the gut lumen. There is a particular association with IgA and IgE synthesis and the term mucosa-associated lymphoid tissue (MALT) is used.

Biopsy diagnosis of lymph node disease

Needle aspirates of lymph nodes can be examined by the techniques of cytopathology although this approach is often inadequate for the precise diagnosis of lymphoreticular disease. Alternatively, the cut surface of a node may be smeared across the surface of a glass slide to give a similar preparation. When a whole node is excised, care should be taken that it is from a region draining the site of any suspected primary cancer. The groin nodes should be avoided. They are frequently sites for chronic inflammatory disease, even in normal individuals.

INFECTION AND INFLAMMATION

The lymph nodes are commonly involved in local infections of the skin and connective tissues and may be sites for viral disease such as infectious mononucleosis (glandular fever) and AIDS, for bacterial infection and for protozoal, worm and mycotic infestations. **Lymphadenopathy** is a general term signifying any disease of the lymph nodes. **Lymphangitis** is inflammation of lymphatic channels. In the skin, streptococcal lymphangitis, for example, can be recognised when red lines define the course of the affected lymphatics.

Lymphadenitis

Inflammation of a lymph node is **lymphadenitis**. It is commonly due to infection but may be caused by physical and chemical agents as varied as X-rays and silicates. Lymphadenitis may be diffuse in systemic infection or localised to specific anatomical regions.

Acute

Acute lymphadenitis often follows infection within an epithelium. If the lymphadenitis is due to pyogenic organisms such as Streptococcus spp., suppuration may occur. An affected node may become very large.

Chronic

Granulomatous inflammation of lymph nodes was often due to tuberculosis and this infection remains a common challenge among immigrants to Western Europe and in the Third World. Tuberculous lymphadenitis is a problem among the destitute and immunocompromised. Sarcoidosis, brucellosis, lymphogranuloma venereum and, occasionally, catscratch disease are other disorders recognised in the general population.

Lymphadenitis caused by worm infestations, such as filariasis, is recognised in immigrants from the Far East. Within the affected nodes, there is hyperplasia of the reticulo-endothelial cells with many altered macrophages. The phagocytes are frequently clustered and the term **granulomatous lymphadenitis** is used. In chronic inflammatory lymphadenitis, the lymph nodes are frequently matted together by perilymphadenitis. An abscess may develop and discharge spontaneously to the nearest epithelial surface, forming a sinus.

TUMOURS

Lymph nodes are the most frequent targets for carcinomatous metastases. Cancer cells readily invade lymphatic vessels and may grow by continuous extension (permeation) or be conveyed as tumour emboli to the peripheral sinuses of regional nodes. There they multiply, producing nodal enlargement. When they reach the efferent channel, tumour emboli may be disseminated again to more proximal nodes.

Lymphatic dissemination by this mechanism is usually sequential and is an important principal in the surgical treatment of malignant disease. This orderly spread may become disrupted due to blockage of lymphatic vessels by tumour so that the direction of normal flow becomes diverted or reversed. Nodal deposits may then occur in an unusual site and in an irregular manner. Occasionally malignant cells may reach the blood stream via the thoracic duct but venous dissemination is more commonly due to direct invasion of venules by a primary tumour.

Now read Dukes classification (p. 244), Sentinal lymph node biopsy (p. 40) Stomach carcinoma (p. 309)

Lymphoma

Lymphomas are malignant tumours occurring most commonly in nodal lymphoid tissue and, less often, in the spleen, bone marrow, liver and gut. They are closely allied to the leukaemias, from which they are distinguished immunologically by characteristic cell surface markers and, in most cases, by the absence of excess neoplastic cells from the circulating blood. Lymphomas vary greatly in their cellular nature, their natural course and their response to treatment. There are two major categories, Hodgkin's disease (HD) and the more frequent non-Hodgkin's lymphoma (NHL). Within these categories, there are numerous sub-divisions, particularly of NHL. These sub-divisions are not of major importance to the surgeon in a disease where the predominant treatment is chemotherapy. The surgeon is often required to obtain lymph nodes for histological and immunological examination and occasionally to excise extra-nodal, lymphoid disease, particularly from the gastro-intestinal tract or salivary and thyroid glands.

Hodgkin's disease

Hodgkin's lymphoma (HL) is much less common than non-Hodgkin's lymphoma (NHL) and occurs in two distinct age groups: young adults and middle-aged and older persons. Four microscopic types are defined. In increasing order of malignancy, they are: lymphocyte-predominant (15%), nodular sclerosing (70%), mixed cellularity (10%) and lymphocyte-depleted (5%). With advances in modern forms of chemotherapy, the significance of this differentiation has declined.

The annual incidence of HL in the UK is 20 and $30/10^6$ for males and females respectively. A geographic clustering of cases has been identified. In the USA, Epstein–Barr virus DNA has been detected in many cases of the mixed-cellularity or lymphocyte-depleted varieties. Cell-mediated immunity is depressed. The disease is confirmed at biopsy when the characteristic large Reed–Sternberg cell with its paired, 'mirror image', ovoid or bean-shaped nuclei, is found.

The behaviour and prognosis of HL is related both to the cell type and to the clinical stage. The Ann-Arbor classification comprises four stages:

I When a single lymph node or group of nodes is affected.

II When two or more groups of nodes are involved but the disease is confined to parts on one side of the diaphragm.

III When the disease is confined to lymph nodes but affects groups of nodes on both sides of the diaphragm.

IV When extra-nodal tissues such as the bone marrow and liver are also involved.

The absence (A) or presence (B) of systemic symptoms are features of staging. They influence prognosis.

Non-Hodgkin's lymphoma

Non-Hodgkin's lymphoma (NHL) accounts for 75% of all lymphomas. The peak incidence is in the seventh decade and there is an increased frequency in immunocompromised individuals. Identification of the cellular origin of NHL involves a combination of histology, immunophenotyping and chromosomal analysis. Immunological examination of biopsy tissue by polyclonal and monoclonal antibodies is undertaken.

Now read Histology (p. 157)

The classification of NHL is continually evolving. Old classifications (Rappaport, Lukes–Collins and Kiel) have been superceded by a Revised European–American Classification of Lymphoid Neoplasms (REAL). Assessment has shown improved inter-observer reproducibility and a more accurate prediction of prognosis and the necessary treatment. Further changes are predicted in order to establish a WHO classification.

The majority of NHL tumours are derived from B lymphocytes although a few, such as the Sézary syndrome, are of T-cell origin. Occasionally, NHL arises from histiocytes. The prognosis of NHL is regeneration, eradicating apoptotic cells. Antigenic material is processed and passed to lymphocytes, initiating immune reactions. Complement component C3 bound to macrophages assists the phagocytosis of bacteria that have been opsonised (p. 270).

Now read Phagocytosis (p. 270)

Activation

As a preliminary to killing intracellular micro-organisms, macrophages are activated by cytokines such as interferon gamma (IFNγ). Bacterial lipopolysaccharide (p. 30) and opsonised bacteria contribute to this process, during which some macrophages may themselves die. Prior to the process of phagocytosis, the cells increase in size and demonstrate raised lysosomal acid hydrolase and neutral proteinase activities.

Killing

The capacity to kill intracellular **micro-organisms** comes only after activation. Activated macrophages are effective in eliminating ingested Brucella, Mycobacteria and Salmonella spp. Ingested bacteria are destroyed by means of reactive oxygen and by NO (p. 133). The destruction of **tumour cells** is brought about by a specific antibody-associated mechanism (p. 247). Macrophages bear receptors for the Fc end of immunoglobulin molecules, enabling them to kill neoplastic cells non-specifically and by activating complement.

Antigen presentation and processing

Macrophages process antigens in an early phase of the immune response (p. 171) and this characteristic distinguishes them from the endothelial cells of the reticulo-endothelial system (p. 286), with which, however, they share the property of avid phagocytosis. Although resting macrophages do not express MHC class II molecules (p. 330), bacterial lipopolysaccharide and any nearby infective agent can prompt this expression. Nevertheless, macrophages do not prime native lymphocytes – this is a function of dendritic cells (Figure 30). Subsequently, antigen-pulsed macrophages can stimulate specific clones of B and T lymphocytes. Th-cells, primed to an antigen, recognise and bind to this combination with MHC class II molecules on macrophage surfaces, producing cytokines that include IL-2 (T-cell growth factor).

Now read Immunity (p. 171)

Granuloma, chronic inflammation and repair

Macrophages play a special part in initiating inflammation; in determining responses to tissue injury; in tissue re-organisation; and in granuloma formation. In tuberculosis, the organisms can remain alive within some macrophages for long periods. Macrophages ultimately aggregate together to destroy the organisms. Because of the resemblance of these macrophages to some forms of epithelium, they are known as **epithelioid cells**.

Amyloidosis

Macrophages take part in amyloid formation (p. 9).

MALFORMATION

A malformation is a primary structural defect that results from a localised error in the development of a tissue or organ. Among the most frequent are hypospadias; talipes; ventricular septal defect; hare lip and cleft palate; and congenital dislocation of the hip. The borderland between malformation and teratoma (p. 243) is narrow and ill-defined.

The causes of malformation are said to be **teratogenic**. They are genetic and environmental. Heritable causes constitute ~40% of the abnormalities. They are chromosomal defects (p. 93); faults in Mendelian inheritance (p. 183); and multifactorial genetic abnormalities (p. 184). A further 2% is due to infection; 7% to maternal diseases such as diabetes mellitus other than infection; and 1% to chemicals, hormones, drugs and alcohol. The remaining 50% are of unknown cause.

Injurious factors acting between the 4th and 5th week of intra-uterine development often result in embryonic death and abortion. Later, in the first trimester, agents such as rubella virus act to distort and disorganise the further growth of organs that have already been formed. A single teratogenic agent can induce different malformations when operative at different stages of embryonic and fetal development.

Now read Chromosomes (p. 90), Genes (p. 138), Inheritance (p. 182)

MALIGNANT MELANOMA

Malignant melanoma is a tumour derived from melanin-forming cells, melanocytes.

Biopsy diagnosis

With the exception of suspected subungual melanoma, biopsy is excisional. However, an incisional approach may be employed initially, to avoid the need for the skin graft that would be demanded after excisional biopsy. There is no place for frozen section since the appearances diagnostic of malignant melanoma cannot be identified reliably by this method. The value of sentinel node identification (p. 40) has not yet been tested adequately. However, lymphoscintigraphy with antimony bisulphide or technetium sulphur colloid can be used with benefit.

Origins

Malignant melanoma was recognised by Hunter. It is largely a disease of young and middle-aged individuals. The geographical prevalence differs widely. In Queensland, Australia, the incidence is $400/10^6$ persons. In black races the incidence is only $6/10^6$ but in the UK, it is $70/10^6$. Here, the frequency is rising by 5% annually and is commoner in females than males. In other countries, the sex ratio is the converse. The principal increase has been in the most common forms of neoplasm, that is, in superficial spreading malignant melanoma of the leg in females and malignant melanoma of the trunk in males.

Malignant melanoma occurs principally in the skin. However, a smaller proportion of tumours arises in the eye and in the mucous membranes of the oropharynx, nasopharynx, oesophagus, anorectal region (p. 14) and vulva (p. 354). Some malignant melanomas originate from a pre-existing junctional naevus.

Causes

With the exception of very small groups of island populations in Polynesia, where an heritable element has been shown, the principal known causes of malignant melanoma are the presence of pre-existing naevus and prolonged exposure to ultraviolet irradiation.

Malignant melanoma is a particular threat to white races living near the equator. Fair-skinned, red haired individuals carry the greatest risk. Although the presence of benign naevi, moles, can be identified in one in five patients with malignant melanomas, only those naevi that show junctional activity or are of a compound character are likely to undergo malignant transformation (p. 76). Intradermal naevi never become malignant. By contrast, the familial dysplastic naevus syndrome (p. 240) carries a high risk for the development of malignant melanoma, and there is a significantly heightened risk in those with xeroderma pigmentosum (p. 362).

Structure

Within the naevus cells are numerous mitotic figures, with hyperchromatism. The cytoplasm contains granules of melanin. The amount of pigment formed may be very large or extremely small. Malignant melanomas express S100 protein but this is a feature shared with the cells of naevi. At first, the tumour cells may show widespread, radial invasion of the epidermis. Later, the entire vertical thickness of the epidermis may be implicated.

The principal features that distinguish malignant melanoma from benign, pigmented naevus are:

- An irregular border.
- Asymmetry.
- A variegated colour.
- A diameter of more than 6 mm.

Four clinicopathological types are recognised:

Superficial spreading melanoma is the most common form of invasive tumour, representing 65% of cases. It appears as a small, brown-grey, flat or raised island of tissue, recognised on a skin surface or in the eye. The incidence is increasing worldwide, probably as a consequence of increased exposure to UV light. However, the prognosis is usually good.

Nodular melanoma is an ulcerating, pigmented mass that enlarges vertically. It accounts for ~ 25% of all malignant melanomas. It invades the dermis rapidly and has the worst prognosis of the four types.

Acral melanoma originates in the thick epidermis of palms and soles. It is the most frequent type in black races, the least common in white races. The prognosis is poor.

Lentigo maligna, a lesion of the atrophic, suntanned skin of the head, neck and hand of the elderly, is a flat lesion confined to the epidermis. It accounts for only 5% of cases of malignant melanoma. Ultimately, the basal epidermal melanocytes extend into the dermis to become **lentigo maligna melanoma**. In this variety of tumour, there is a 5-year survival rate of at least 90%, a prognosis attributable to the conspicuous location and early treatment of these lesions.

Behaviour and prognosis

The prognosis of melanoma varies considerably. Many surgeons are unjustifiably gloomy. In treatment, a combination of IL-2 and INF-α (pp. 23, 115) has proved of value.

Naevi of the skin of the palms, soles and genitalia are especially liable to undergo malignant change as are subungual naevi. This transformation is suggested clinically by a gradual increase in size and an alteration in colour, together with exudation, ulceration or bleeding. An altered irregular outline, nodularity and thickening, and a loss of normal skin markings are also suggestive signs. Satellite nodules may be identified in nearby skin.

For unknown reasons, the outlook is much better in women than in men. The future for peripheral lesions is more positive than for central lesions: treatment is more effective. The outcome is worse with nodular disease. The prognosis is optimal when a tumour has not extended into the subcutaneous tissues. The form and rate of growth of malignant melanoma is significant in prognosis; a tumour extends both radially and vertically. The Breslow index is an estimate of the invasion of the tumour into the dermis as measured from the corneal layer of the epidermis (Fig. 41). It is the single most important prognostic indicator in staging (Table 45). Favourable lesions are less than 0.75 mm thick, unfavourable more than 4 mm.

Metastases appear after 10 years in fewer than 6% of patients. The common targets for metastasis are skin 51%; lung 27%; liver 17%; brain 16%; bone 14%; and gastro-intestinal tract 4% where malignant melanoma is the most common secondary cancer.

Now read Melanin (p. 230), Naevus (p. 238)

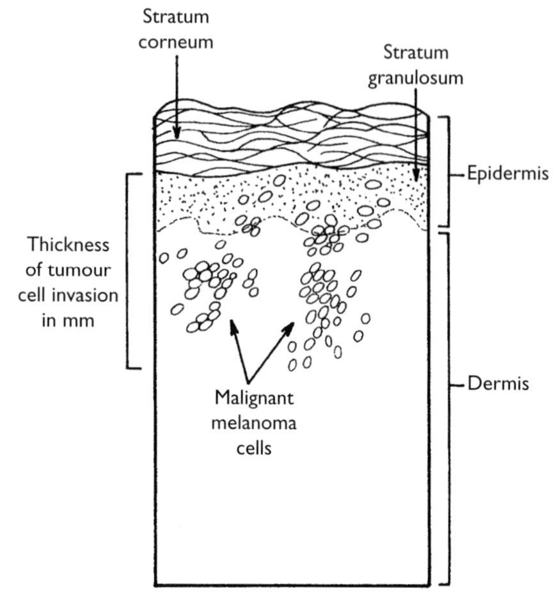

Figure 41 Prognosis of malignant melanoma – the Breslow index.
Diagram shows vertical section through skin containing malignant melanoma arising from junctional naevus. Extent of invasion of dermis by tumour cells offers valuable guide to tumour behaviour and prognosis. Infiltration is measured from superficial margin of stratum granulosum to deepest tumour cells.

Table 45 Four stages of malignant melanoma recognised by the American Joint Committee on Cancer Staging

Stage	5-year survival (%)
Stage I tumour confined to skin and less than 1.5 mm thick	
Stage IA: less than 0.75 mm thick and not invading papillary-reticular dermis interface	>90
Stage 1B: 0.75 to 1.5 mm thick and invading the papillary-reticular dermis interface	85
Stage II	<75
Stage III	<25
Stage IV	<25

MALNUTRITION

Malnutrition implies imperfect nourishment. It is a common challenge in hospital patients. The deficiency may be highly specific. Malnutrition is very frequent in impoverished, underdeveloped countries, particularly among children. In the West, malnutrition is most frequently seen in patients with diseases of the gastro-intestinal tract. The lack may be of a single substance, for example of vitamin B_{12}, or there may be a general deficiency of all the ingredients contained in a normal diet, 'protein-energy malnutrition'.

A common method of assessing gross nutritional state is to calculate the body mass index (BMI). This Index is the body weight/square of the height. It is expressed as kg/m^2. An ideal BMI is 20 to 25 kg/m^2 (Table 48, p. 251). A recent survey of patients in an UK teaching hospital showed that 40% of individuals had a BMI less than 20.

Kwashiorkor

Kwashiorkor is infantile protein malnutrition. It is a disease of young children and is characterised by a low concentration of plasma albumin, with oedema and ascites, normocytic anaemia (p. 10) and an enlarged, fatty liver. Ultimately, cirrhosis develops. Kwashiorkor is common in regions where infants and young children exist solely on maize. It is common in regions of Africa, Asia and South America where infants survive on this cereal alone. Because the diet is so unbalanced, kwashiorkor is frequently accompanied by other forms of deficiency such as rickets (p. 52).

Now read Cachexia (p. 73), Ketosis (p. 195), Starvation (p. 230)

MANTOUX TEST

The Mantoux test is the intradermal injection of the purified protein derivative (PPD) of *Mycobacterium tuberculosis*. PPD is the concentrate of a culture of *M. tuberculosis* that has been grown on a synthetic medium, purified by ultrafiltration. Although less frequently employed in the UK, the test is still used in many countries to identify children who may require BCG vaccination. BCG is of value in the prevention of tuberculosis.

Now read BCG (p. 333), Type IV Hypersensitivity (p. 161), Tuberculosis (p. 332)

In a person sensitised to mycobacteria by infection or prior vaccination, the injection of PPD is followed after 5–8 hours by a slowly developing focus of inflammation. A zone of oedema is surrounded by a wider area of erythema. Inflammation becomes maximal after 24–48 hours. The indurated zone is measured after 3 days. If a biopsy is made of this focus, the microscopical reaction is found to be dominated by mononuclear phagocytes ('epithelioid' cells, p. 143). A granuloma forms that has features in common with the tubercle (p. 332).

A positive reaction in the Mantoux test identifies individuals who have, at some time, been infected with *M. tuberculosis* or who have been inoculated with BCG. Non-reactors are still at risk of developing tuberculosis. In the face of massive active tuberculous infection, a positive test may become negative spuriously, as it may in the severely malnourished. In some countries, infections with 'atypical' mycobacteria are relatively frequent. In these circumstances, the Mantoux test is usually negative or weakly positive.

MAST CELLS

Mast cells are large, mononuclear cells with basophilic, cytoplasmic granules that are easily broken down and lost. They closely resemble circulating basophil polymorphs (p. 206). Mast cells are widely dispersed near blood vessels, in loose connective tissue and in the lung. The basophilic granules stain with metachromatic dyes because of their heparin content. In man, the granules also contain and release histamine; platelet-activating factor; leukotrienes; and a substance chemotactic for eosinophilic polymorphs.

One mechanism for the release of chemical mediators from mast cells is the binding of IgE antibody to the cell surfaces in individuals sensitised to antigens such as the house mite and pollen. Degranulation results and the chemical mediators liberated from the granules cause symptoms such as those of hay fever and allergic asthma (p. 161). Another role for mast cells is attributable to the small C3a and C5a fragments liberated during complement activation (p. 232). The complex which they form, together with mast cell mediators, aids the recruitment of polymorphs to sites of inflammation. The C3a and C5a fragments are **anaphylatoxins**.

Now read Anaphylaxis (p. 161)

MELANIN

Melanin is a brown–black pigment containing sulphur synthesised by melanocytes from the amino acid tyrosine. Melanocytes are clear, round cells within the basal layer of the epidermis. There is disagreement as to whether precursor cells, melanoblasts, are modified basal epidermal cells or migrate to the epidermis from the neuro-ectoderm. The latter view is more popular. Many consider melanoblasts to be part of the diffuse endocrine system (p. 127). The production of melanin is controlled in some species by a melanin-stimulating hormone (MSH) released from the pars intermedia of the pituitary gland. White and black races have the same proportion of melanocytes, but black races produce more melanin from each melanocyte. Melanophores are phagocytes that take up the pigment.

Now read Malignant melanoma (p. 227), Naevus (p. 238)

Melanosis

Melanosis is the excessive pigmentation of body surfaces by melanin. It is a consequence of prolonged solar ultraviolet – or of ionising radiation. An excess of melanin is synthesised in the skin in haemochromatosis (p. 117). The pigment also accumulates in Addison's disease, a result of the secretions of the closely related hormones adrenocorticotrophin (ACTH) and melanocyte stimulating hormone (MSH). Melanotic pigmentation of the lips occurs in the Peutz–Jegher syndrome (p. 256).

Melanosis coli

Melanosis coli is the presence of macrophages laden with melanin-like pigment in the lamina propria of the large intestine. Many believe that the pigment comes from purgatives containing anthracene, but it may be derived from the degradation of dietary phenylalanine or tyrosine in constipated individuals.

METABOLIC RESPONSE TO TRAUMA

After injury or operation, there are widespread alterations in intermediary metabolism. This sequence is the metabolic response to trauma or injury. The changes are governed by alterations in the secretions of the catabolic hormones adrenaline, noradrenaline, cortisol and glucagon, and by the anabolic hormones insulin and somatotrophin.

Now read Trauma (p. 332)

Catabolic phase

Following surgery, metabolic expenditure exceeds that observed before injury, leading to the '**catabolic response to surgery**'. The result of excess catabolism is weight loss and a reduction in body carbohydrate, fat and protein. The net catabolic effect is a consequence both of decreased molecular synthesis and of increased breakdown. Protein is mobilised for repair and for gluconeogenesis. All body proteins, whether skeletal, visceral or circulating, are functional or structural; they are not stored. Any reduction in protein levels implies disordered function or abnormal structure. The duration of the catabolic phase varies according to the severity of injury. After elective operations, it is usually not more than 5 days. Following severe injury, particularly after burns or sepsis, catabolism exceeds anabolism for a period of weeks.

Unlike starvation (p. 229), the simple restoration of nutritional intake does not reverse the changes in intermediary metabolism driven by catabolic hormones.

Anabolic phase

The recovering surgical patient enters an anabolic phase when the tissue lost during the catabolic phase is replaced. Most of this loss is made good within one month of an elective operation. However, a year may elapse before the body is entirely restored to its normal state.

Consequences

If the stimulus of injury is sufficiently severe or prolonged, a patient may die as a consequence of continuing, excess catabolism. The pattern of response to injury is inherited and may have survival value. Injured animals cannot hunt for food. They therefore mobilise fat and carbohydrate for energy, and protein for repair. This highly conserved and innate evolutionary response is inappropriate in hospital. The provision of nutrients, if necessary intravenously, may be life-saving.

REGULATION OF ACID/BASE BALANCE

Acidaemia/acidosis

Acidaemia is a decrease in the blood pH below 7.36, that is, an increase in the hydrogen ion concentration above the normal value. Acidosis is an accumulation of hydrogen ions (H^+) or a loss of base (protons) that will produce acidaemia in the absence of compensatory mechanisms. Examples of conditions in which acidosis occurs are renal (p. 201) and pulmonary (p. 214) failure; diabetic keto-acidosis (p. 117); and duodenal fistula. Acidaemia provoked by metabolic acidosis may be prevented by compensatory respiratory alkalaemia.

Alkalaemia/alkalosis

Alkalaemia is an increase in the pH of the blood above 7.44. Alkalosis is a loss of H^+ ions or an accumulation of base (protons) that will produce alkalaemia in the absence of compensatory mechanisms. Examples of conditions in which alkalosis occurs are hyperventilation due to anxiety or thyrotoxicosis; overventilation with a mechanical ventilator; and loss of gastric acid through persistent vomiting; or therapeutic aspiration.

MICROBIAL DEFENCE

The success and safety of surgery rests upon the principles of hygiene, asepsis and immunity. Immunity is inborn (innate) and non-specific. It may also be acquired and specific.

Now read Immunity (p. 171)

NON-SPECIFIC DEFENCE MECHANISMS

Micro-organisms are prevented from gaining access to the tissues by a variety of physical and chemical mechanisms. Skin surfaces, for example, are protected by the secretions of sweat and sebaceous glands; the lining of the stomach by acid secretions and proteolytic enzymes; the intestinal tract by mucus. In addition to these natural defences, many micro-organisms, in particular the staphylococci, can be denied access to human tissues by the artificial means of simple hygiene, disinfection (p. 118), antisepsis and asepsis (p. 23).

Inborn, non-specific defence against microbial agents is cellular and molecular. Cellular mechanisms are those of phagocytosis, particularly by neutrophil and eosinophil polymorphs (p. 206); macrophages; mast cells (p. 229); and natural killer (NK) cells. Molecular mechanisms are exemplified by the actions of complement. The role of the interferons in defence against viral infection is significant; it is considered on pp. 24 and 115.

Cells coated with low concentrations of IgG antibody can be killed by non-sensitised leucocytes, including polymorphs, macrophages and lymphocytes. The process is **antibody-dependent cell-mediated cytotoxicity** (ADCC). Contact with a target cell is essential. The lymphocytes are NK cells. They are large granular lymphocytes. When virus infects a cell, glycoproteins expressed at the plasma membrane surface distinguish the cell from normal, and activate NK cells. They release a cytolysin like the C9 complex of complement (p. 232). The cells are destroyed by lysis.

Now read Macrophages (p. 225), Phagocytosis (p. 270)

Acute phase proteins

When trauma or infection provokes macrophages to release interleukin-1 (IL-1), there is a sudden rise in the plasma concentration of molecules termed acute phase proteins. Together, these proteins act to minimise tissue damage, accelerate repair and resolution and, in the case of infection, enhance host resistance.

The most abundant of the acute phase proteins are C-reactive protein; mannose-binding protein; and serum amyloid P component. C-reactive protein can activate complement, opsonising micro-organisms prior to phagocytosis.

MOLECULAR AND CHEMICAL AGENTS

Complement

An important part of the non-specific defences against micro-organisms is provided by 'complement', a complex of 21 plasma proteins, some enzymes, constitutively present in normal and immune serum (Fig. 42). For historical reasons, the molecules called 'complement' have confusing, alphanumeric titles such as C5a.

There are two complement pathways. They are designated 'alternative' and 'classical'. The alternative pathway does not depend upon the presence of antibody whereas the classical pathway is activated in the presence of antibody.

Now read Antigens and antibodies (p. 19)

Alternative pathway

The first ('Alternative') pathway is **non-specific**. It is activated **directly** by micro-organisms. In surgery, it is particularly important because some Gram-negative bacteria and viruses can be neutralised by this mechanism.

Central to the alternative pathway for generating complement activity is the aim of splitting a protein named C3. There are three results:

- **Phagocytosis is facilitated.** An enzyme, C3 convertase, is stabilised on bacterial walls and leads to the formation of two subunits of C3 called C3a and C3b. The phagocytes have receptors that bind to C3b. It adheres to the walls of micro-organisms. Another component named C5a forms. It is chemotactic (p. 179) to polymorphs and macrophages, facilitating phagocytosis (p. 270).
- **Acute inflammation is promoted**. C3a and C5a are chemotactic. They increase capillary permeability and through their actions on mast cells, promote the molecular cascades of acute inflammation (p. 179). C3a, C4a and C5a are anaphylatoxins (p. 161). C3a and C5a together stimulate the respiratory burst (p. 133) that destroys bacteria.
- **Bacterial cell lysis and destruction are facilitated.** Changes in a series of molecules termed C5b, C6, C7 and C8 culminate in the formation of a membrane attack complex (MAC) (C5b-9) that can be inserted into the lipid bilayer of cell and microbial surfaces. A channel is created which pierces the cell membrane, allowing water to enter by osmosis and the contents of the disrupted cell to escape.

Classical pathway

The second ('Classical') pathway enhances the **specific** antimicrobial properties of antibodies. It is contrasted with the alternative pathway in Fig. 42.

Now read Immunity (p. 171)

Oxygen (O_2)-independent mechanisms

The **oxygen-independent** mechanisms of cells such as polymorphs are lysosomal (p. 225).

Oxygen-dependent mechanisms

After phagocytosis, bacterial destruction is brought about by oxygen-dependent mechanisms. There is a sudden burst of oxygen consumption, the respiratory burst, and the formation of free radicals (p. 133). A plasma membrane cytochrome oxidase reduces molecular O_2 to the superoxide anion ($O_2^{\bullet}$). $O_2^{\bullet}$ is converted to hydroxyl ($HO^{\bullet}$). Both $O_2^{\bullet}$ and $HO^{\bullet}$ are highly reactive chemically. They are potent microbicidal agents.

Nitric oxide

Nitric oxide (NO, p. 134) assists in the killing of micro-organisms like viruses that gain entrance both to phagocytic and to non-phagocytic cells.

Now read Free radicals (p. 133)

PHAGOCYTOSIS

The principle phagocytic cells are the blood and tissue macrophages; the other cells of the reticulo-endothelial system (p. 286); and the neutrophil polymorphonuclear leucocytes (polymorphs – p. 205) of the blood. Phagocytosis is enhanced when micro-organisms or other particles are opsonised by collectins and by the lipopolysaccharide endotoxins of Gram-negative bacteria.

Now read Macrophages (p. 225), Phagocytosis (p. 270)

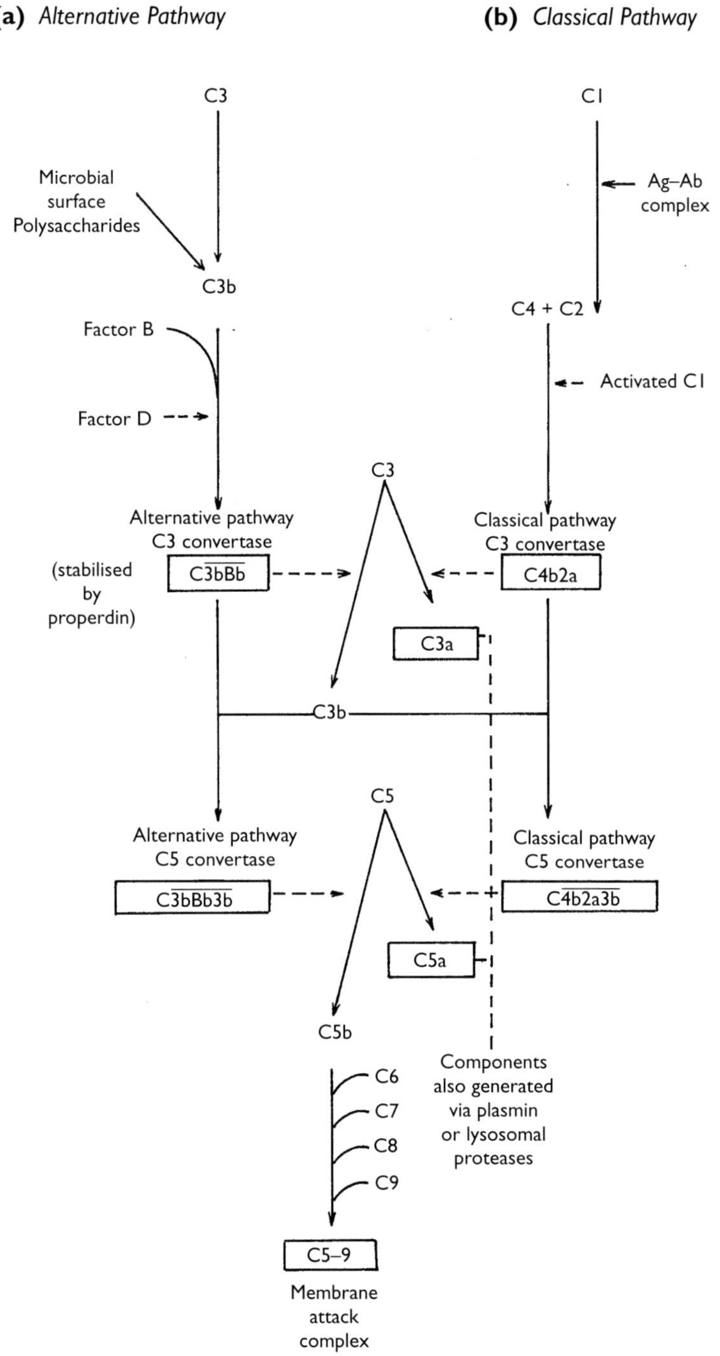

Figure 42 Microbial defence – complement pathways.

(a) Alternative pathway is very quickly activated by C3b during innate immune response. C3b binds to microbial cell surfaces. Bar over complex = enzyme activity. When a protein like B is cleaved, smaller products are designated 'a', larger products 'b'.

(b) Classical pathway is activated by binding of C1 to Ag–Ab complexes, formation of which takes 4–5 days after microbial infection.

In either case, pathways converge on C3a and C5a, resulting in production of membrane attack complex, C5–9. (Redrawn from Mitchell RN and Cotran RS: In *Basic Pathology*, 6th edition, Kumar V, Cotran RS, Robbins SL (eds). Philadelphia, London:

MICROSCOPY

The microscope is an indispensable tool in surgical laboratory diagnosis.

Light microscopy

In the binocular, compound microscope used in surgical, histopathological laboratories, white light is transmitted through stained sections or smears. There are many other forms of microscope; some do not employ visible light so that direct observation by the histopathologist is not required.

It is advantageous if a surgical pathologist becomes familiar with the principles of microscopy and of photography since the images must often be recorded, to provide permanent records and for education. The cameras now used are conventional or digital; video recording is frequent.

- **Fluorescence microscopy** enables the localisation, in cells and tissues, of antigens, antibodies and other reactants. Inverted fluorescence microscopes offer the possibility of viewing cells from below, at the bottom of a monolayer culture.
- **Telemicrosopy** is employed increasingly to transmit microscopic images by cable or by satellite. The technique allows pathologists in geographically separate centres to view and manipulate a single section or smear while active telephone discussion of a difficult case is in progress. The procedure is bidirectional.
- **Scanned laser light microscopes** allow optical sections to be 'cut' through blocks of wet or dry tissue without the need to prepare stained sections by the methods described on pp. 157, 158. They also facilitate immunohistochemical studies (p. 158) and chromosome analyses (p. 90). One or more lasers is used, permitting the use of multiple labelling. Dual photon confocal scanning microscopy, the focussing within a tissue of two beams of laser light, enhances the precision of 3-D localisation of fluorescence.

Electron microscopy

Transmission electron microscopy (TEM) remains an exotic diagnostic tool that is invaluable in the classification of tumours. It is useful in the identification of ultrastructural objects such as melanosomes and neurosecretory granules and for the recognition of some micro-organisms, particularly viruses. TEM is not applicable in routine, diagnostic histopathology but access to this technique is a desirable facility for regional surgical services.

- Electron probe X-ray analysis (EPXMA) allows elements of atomic weight above 4 to be located in tissues and measured.
- Many forms of EM can be undertaken with unfixed tissue, at low temperature.
- Scanning electron microscopy (SEM) permits the examination of surface and sub-surface structures. Biological SEM enables fully hydrated, living cells to be observed.

Now read Histology (p. 157)

MONOCLONAL ANTIBODIES

A monoclonal antibody (MAb) has single antibody specificity. MAbs are synthesised by a clone of B-cells. MAbs can be made commercially to order or are available 'off-the-shelf'.

MAbs are manufactured in bulk, cell cultures but can be produced in animals. Antibody-producing cells from the lymphoid tissues of an animal sensitised to a particular antigen are fused with myeloma cells to make 'hybrid myeloma' cells. These cells are grown in culture as a so-called **hybridoma**. The hybridoma cells combine the permanent growth potential and high rate of immunoglobulin protein synthesis of the myeloma with the specificity of the original animal antibody.

The ready availability of monoclonal antibodies against an almost limitless range of antigens has revolutionised laboratory diagnosis in those countries where the high cost of these reagents can be met (Table 46). Among the antigens that can be detected are hormones such as ACTH and parathormone; markers for individual cancer cells and macrophages; transplantation

Table 46 Some uses for monoclonal antibodies

Analysing embryological relationships	Blood grouping
	Cancer treatment
Cancer diagnosis	Cell isolation
Cell depletion	Counting immune cell populations
Clinical imaging	
Immunosuppression	Passive immunisation

antigens; bacterial serotypes; cell proteins such as actin and myosin; and drugs such as digoxin.

Monoclonal antibodies are valuable in radioimmunoassays and in establishing the histological identity and classification of tumours such as lymphomas; tumours of the diffuse endocrine system; and angiosarcomas. Radiolabelled Abs are used in staging and in tumour identification, for example:

- In cases of colorectal cancer in which carcinoembryonic antigen concentrations rise after CT scans have proved negative.
- To search for additional metastases that might not be resectable in cases of liver cancer with resectable hepatic lesions.
- During the re-staging of cancers, for the recognition of metastases.
- To identify somatostatin and other receptors overexpressed: by many neuro-endocrine tumours; by neuroblastoma; by some medullary carcinomas of the thyroid gland; by phaeochromocytomas; and by small cell carcinoma of the lung.

It is also possible to use monoclonal antibodies to select and destroy cancer cells *in vivo*. If anticancer-cell antibodies are 'labelled' with an appropriate radioactive isotope such as ^{14}C, ^{3}H or ^{32}P, the beta-particles emitted by the isotope irradiate and selectively destroy target cells.

Now read Antigens and Antibodies (p. 19)

MOUTH

See Oral cavity (p. 256), Pharynx (p. 270).

MUCUS

Mucus is the viscid, watery secretion of epithelial cells and some glands. The principal component is mucin, a glycoprotein. The majority of cells that secrete mucus are distended in the shape of a **goblet**. If there is inflammation of the epithelia lining the respiratory, gastro-intestinal or genito-urinary tracts, mucus secretion is increased and there is a rise in the number of goblet cells. In cystic fibrosis (mucoviscidosis), the mucus-secreting cells of the sweat glands, bronchi, intestines and bile ducts, as well as the pancreas, secrete an abnormally viscous mucin that ultimately obstructs the ducts of the glands. They atrophy. If the duct or orifice of any organ containing mucus-secreting cells is obstructed, a mucocoele may be produced as it is in the lip, appendix or gall bladder.

Some tumours of the breast, ovary, stomach and large intestine are composed largely of cells secreting mucin. They are mucinous adenomas or adenocarcinomas. Pseudomucinous cystadenomas of the ovary may rupture causing pseudomyxoma peritonei (p. 247).

MUSCLE, INVOLUNTARY

Involuntary muscle forms the contractile walls of the intestine, air passages, ureter and many other internal structures and ducts. Contractility of involuntary, 'smooth' muscle is regulated by the transmembrane flow of calcium (Ca^{2+}) ions. The movement of these ions takes place via L-type channels that are voltage-gated; that is, their responses are electrophysiological. Drugs termed Ca^{2+} channel blockers obstruct the passage of calcium through the L-type channels, decreasing vascular and non-vascular smooth muscle contractility. The channels also influence the growth of vascular smooth muscle cells and fibroblasts.

TUMOURS

Benign

Leiomyoma

Leiomyoma is a relatively frequent form of benign tumour originating in the involuntary muscle of the small intestine and myometrium. Within the skin of the legs of middle-aged women, leiomyoma occasionally forms single or multiple painful nodules. Less often, leiomyoma is encountered as a solitary lesion in the dartos muscle.

Angioleiomyoma is a recognised variant of leiomyoma and displays similar properties.

Now read Ileum and jejunum (p. 164)

Malignant

Leiomyosarcoma

By contrast with leiomyoma, this uncommon malignant soft tissue tumour is found most often within the deep tissues of the retroperitoneum in older women or in the limbs or skin. It is also a rare tumour of the intestinal tract (p. 168).

The tumour mass is not distinguishable macroscopically from other soft tissue sarcomas. Microscopical diagnosis is made difficult by appearances that offer no sharp transition between leiomyoma and leiomyosarcoma. A proportion of the tumour cells is pleomorphic and giant forms are usually present. Myofibrils may be identified by the use of stains such as phosphotungstic acid/haematoxylin. The application to tumour sections of MAbs against the muscle and connective tissue proteins actin and desmin, assists recognition.

Prognosis is adversely affected by site. A feature of leiomyosarcoma is invasion of the inferior vena cava. Leg oedema is one consequence, the Budd–Chiari syndrome (p. 212) another. The deep-seated retroperitoneal tumours offer a 5-year survival rate that rarely exceeds 30% whereas those of the skin, identified and diagnosed much earlier, are significantly better.

MUSCLE, VOLUNTARY

Biopsy diagnosis

The diagnosis of skeletal muscle lesions by biopsy alone remains an uncertain procedure. A sample of tissue may be taken from the quadriceps or other convenient muscle site. The tissue is gently fastened to a supporting surface of card or cork before fixation. The localisation of enzyme activities is crucial to the diagnosis of many conditions. The techniques are completed on fresh; fresh-frozen; or snap-frozen specimens.

TRAUMA

Crush syndrome

Crush syndrome, traumatic rhabdomyolysis, is encountered in earthquake victims, trapped miners and persons incarcerated after the collapse of masonry. There is an analogy with the compartment syndrome (p. 188). When long-continued forces compress the lower limbs, skeletal muscle cells break down. As a result, nuclear purines and cytoplasmic potassium and myoglobin are released into the bloodstream when the circulation is restored, causing myoglobinaemia and hyperkalaemia. Acute renal failure follows, caused partly by the accumulation of muscle-cell pigment in renal glomeruli, partly on account of the associated hypovolaemic shock. Some of the consequences of crush syndrome can be attributed to reperfusion injury (p. 134) and this sequence may be a partial explanation of the renal failure that is a frequent result of this form of trauma.

Now read Shock (p. 290)

TUMOURS

Benign

Rhabdomyoma

Rhabdomyoma is a rare benign tumour of voluntary muscle. It arises in the head or neck but is much less common than its malignant counterpart, rhabdomyosarcoma. Rhabdomyoma is not known to undergo malignant transformation.

Malignant

Rhabdomyosarcoma

This uncommon malignant tumour is encountered in three main categories: embryonal, alveolar and pleomorphic. It is also seen as a component of other tumours including malignant, mixed mesodermal tumour of the uterus or ovary.

Causes

Little is known of the causes. The tumour originates from a precursor population of primitive mesenchymal cells.

Structure

The three categories are distinctive:

- **Embryonal rhabdomyosarcoma** is a tumour of children, principally between the ages of 3 and 12 years. The most common location is in tissues of the head and neck, especially in the orbit and nasopharynx. However, the tumour is also encountered in the retroperitoneal tissues; bile duct; and urogenital tract. In certain locations, for example the nose, bladder and vagina, the tumour may grow as a large, polypoid mass, accounting for the name botryoid sarcoma (**sarcoma botryoides**), signifying a cluster of grapes.

- **Alveolar rhabdomyosarcoma** differs from the embyronal tumour in a variety of ways. The tumour occurs in an older age group, usually in the age range 10–25 years. The neoplasm is found most frequently in the extremities, especially in the arms, but also in the perirectal and perineal tissues. There is often a chromosomal abnormality, commonly t(2;13)(q35;q13).
- **Pleomorphic rhabdomyosarcoma** is a tumour of adults. It was originally believed to be the most common type. However, the advent of electron microscopy, the use of immunohistochemical techniques, and stricter criteria for classification, have combined to show that it is the least frequent.

The various tumours are composed of a population of rhabdomyoblasts interspersed with many small, densely staining cells. Rhabdomyoblasts are distinguished by their eosinophilic cytoplasm, cross-striations and strap-like form. Diagnosis is assisted by the application of MAbs against the muscle proteins actin and myoglobin and against the connective tissue cell protein desmin.

Behaviour and prognosis

Rhabdomyosarcoma extends locally, destroying calcified and non-calcified connective tissues. Distant spread is by lymphatic dissemination and via the bloodstream to the lungs, liver and bone. Prognosis has improved since the introduction of combined surgical, radiotherapeutic and chemotherapeutic treatment. The prognosis of alveolar rhabdomyosarcoma is significantly worse than for the embryonal type. Other adverse prognostic features include incomplete excision and lymph node involvement.

MYCOBACTERIA

Mycobacteria are rod-shaped bacilli closely related to the Actinomycetes (p. 5) and Nocardia. They are acid–alcohol fast organisms (p. 32). Mycobacteria divide infrequently and grow very slowly. They are identified by the use of selective media (p. 33). The distinction between strains is made by assessing antibiotic sensitivity, by growth characteristics, and biochemically.

Mycobacteria causing human and animal disease include *Mycobacterium tuberculosis* (tuberculosis – p. 332) and *Myco. leprae* (leprosy – p. 204); animal pathogens such as the vole bacillus; and *Myco. avium intracellulare*, the avian bacillus complex. There are also many less pathogenic mycobacteria such as *Myco. smegmatis*, the smegma bacillus; and numerous 'atypical' organisms such as *Myco. kansasii*, *Myco. marinum* and *Myco. fortuitum*. These organisms are normally not pathogenic but are able to cause disease under special circumstances, such as those of local injury; immunosuppression; or AIDS (p. 2). They are agents of opportunistic infection.

Mycobacterium tuberculosis hominis causes human tuberculosis (p. 332) and *Myco. tuberculosis bovis* also infects man and animals as well as cattle. Other mycobacteria such as *Myco. ulcerans* cause skin ulceration. Atypical, opportunistic mycobacteria, such as *Myco. kansasii* and *Myco. avium* intracellulare, are only occasionally pathogenic but the former can cause arthritis and the latter lymph node disease; pulmonary disease; or disseminated infection in immunocompromised patients.

Classically, infection by *Myco. tuberculosis* is air- or milk-borne. Occasionally, increased bacterial virulence rather than patient susceptibility or environmental circumstances may lead to extensive transmission within a community. Two to four hours exposure to virulent organisms in the course of a single air journey may be sufficient to cause infection to which steroid therapy predisposes. Resistance to antituberculous drugs is a global challange.

Now read Tuberculosis (p. 332)

MYELOMA

A myeloma is a unique malignant tumour derived from a single clone of plasma cells (p. 172). Although uncommon, myeloma is the most frequent primary tumour of bone and bone marrow in elderly persons (p. 59). Cells transform and multiply simultaneously in many sites so that the name multiple myeloma is used.

The proliferating cells destroy bone and cause hypercalcaemia. The skull, ribs and vertebrae are most susceptible but pathological fracture of a limb bone may be the first sign of disease. All the cells of a myeloma synthesise and secrete a single, identical immunoglobulin, usually IgG or IgA; or a single, identical immunoglobulin light chain (p. 19), which may be kappa or lambda (light-chain myeloma). The immunoglobulins and light chains are differentiated by immuno-electrophoresis. The light chains from myeloma proteins are secreted in large amounts in the urine as so-called Bence–Jones protein, a material which comes out of solution on gentle heating, redissolving with further heat. In 10% of cases, amyloidosis develops. The amyloid protein in myeloma, AL protein, is more frequently derived from kappa than from lambda light chains. Myeloma protein accumulates in the renal tubules and death may occur from renal failure.

Now read Antigens and antibodies (p. 19)

MYOSITIS OSSIFICANS

Myositis ossificans is metaplasia of mesenchymal tissue with bone formation. The process of myositis ossificans is analogous to the cell changes that occur at sites of fracture healing (p. 55). In the callus formed around a fracture, fibroblasts and osteoblasts are indistinguishable and are differentiated by the nature of the nearby extracellular matrix that they synthesise. The fibroblasts and osteoblasts have separate identities but come from the same stem cell. Their varied behaviour explains the complex cellular response seen in myositis ossificans.

Traumatic myositis ossificans

Localised myositis ossificans, **myositis ossificans circumscripta**, may follow repeated trauma to a muscle. One example is the development of rider's bone in the tendinous origin of the adductor longus muscle. Myositis ossificans may also arise after a single episode of trauma, for example in the tendinous insertion of the brachialis anterior muscle after supracondylar fracture of the humerus. The ossification is within an organised haematoma but there is argument as to whether the osteoblasts arise from the periosteum or from totipotent mesenchymal cells of the organising haematoma.

Progressive myositis ossificans

Myositis ossificans progressiva is a rare hereditary disorder in which ossification occurs in fascia, aponeuroses, tendons and muscles. The disease begins in childhood with painful swellings that ossify subsequently. There is an intermittent course. Ultimately, the body becomes rigid. Immobility leads to death from bronchopneumonia. Other congenital skeletal abnormalities, such as microdactyly and the absence of digits, are associated conditions.

N

NAEVUS

A naevus is a tumour of melanocytes (p. 230). It is often but not always pigmented. The term 'mole' is given to any congenital spot or blemish of the skin.

Biopsy diagnosis of pigmented skin lesions

The recommendations for biopsy of malignant melanoma (p. 227) should be followed. If malignancy is suspected, the pigmented lesion should be excised in totality. If a lesion is so extensive that excision would produce severe disfigurement then incisional biopsy is permissible. Full thickness biopsy is essential for accurate diagnosis and for determining treatment and prognosis. There is no place for frozen section.

Benign, melanocytic naevi

There are six main categories of benign, pigmented naevi (Fig. 43):

- **Simple naevus**. Simple naevi occur in infancy and early childhood. There is a uniform proliferation of melanocytes at the epidermo-dermal interface.
- **Junctional naevus**. Junctional activity describes the focal multiplication of melanocytes at the epidermo-dermal interface. Junctional activity (junctional 'change') is common in older children, before puberty.
- **Intradermal naevus**. Intradermal naevus, the common 'mole', is noticeable at puberty and conspicuous in middle age. Some are pigmented and bear hairs. The naevus may be flat or elevated, nodular or pedunculated. There is no junctional activity. Pre-existing intradermal naevi are found in 20% of patients with malignant melanoma.
- **Compound naevus**. Compound naevus describes the coincidence of junctional and intradermal naevus.
- **Halo naevus**. Halo naevus describes the brown, pigmented appearance of the skin around a lesion. It is a form of intradermal or compound naevus that has excited an extensive lymphocytic infiltrate.
- **Juvenile spindle-cell naevus**. This misnomer describes a naevus that may occur in adults. The naevus is usually raised, reddish brown and often

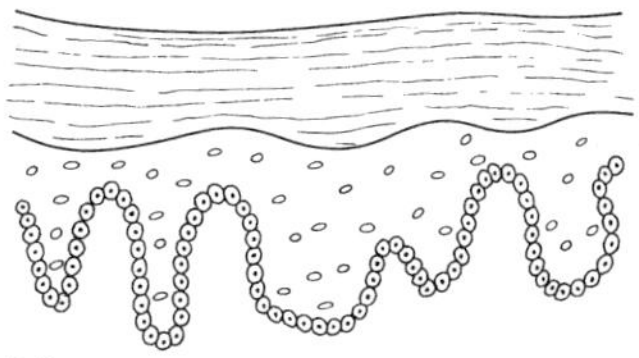

(a)

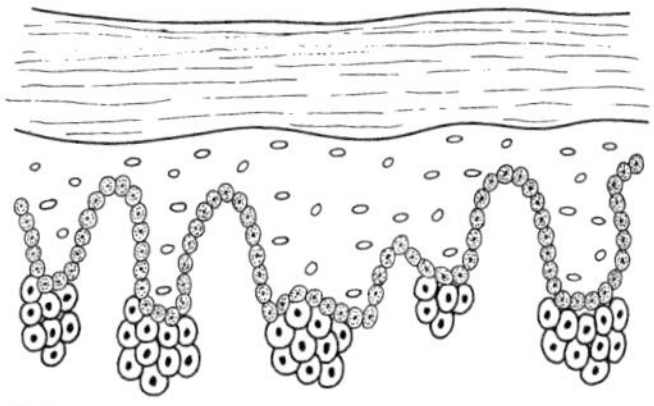

(b)

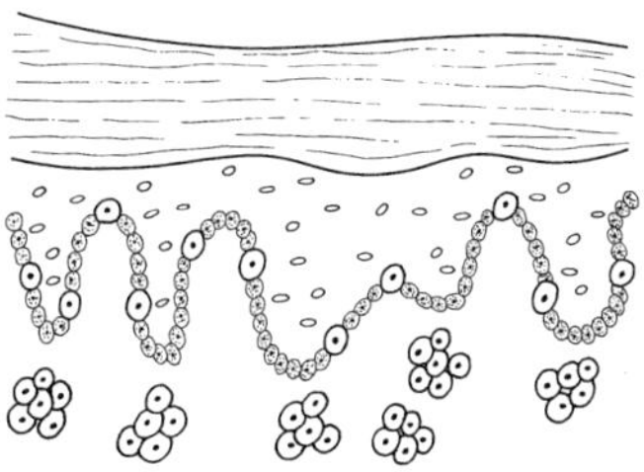

(c)

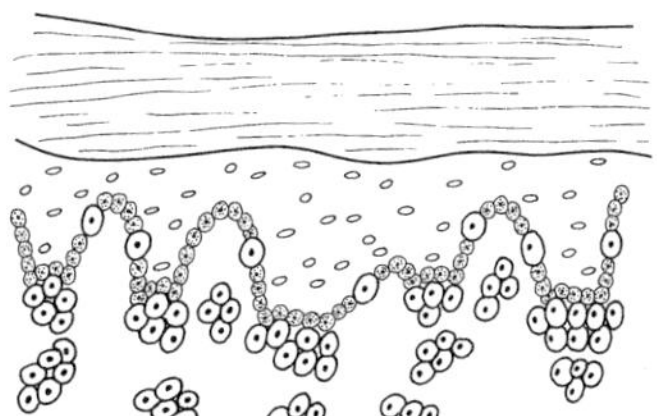

(d)

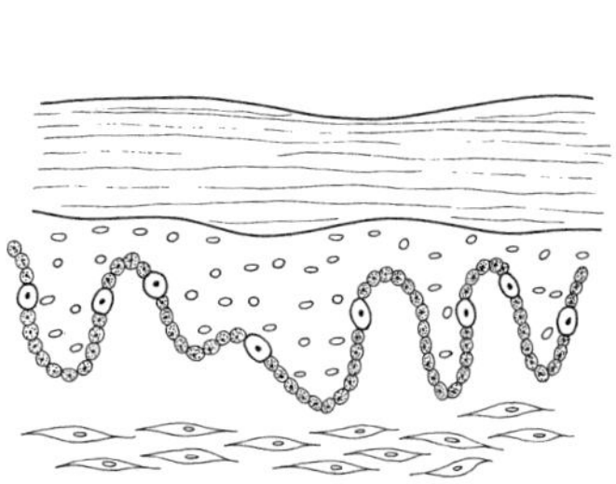

(e)

Figure 43 Naevus.

(a) Simple naevus. Basal layer of epidermis replaced by proliferation of melanocytes.

(b) Junctional naevus. Processes formed of proliferating melanocytes project like peninsulas into underlying dermis.

(c) Intradermal naevus. Small islands of naevus cells lie discretely within dermis. Junctional activity has ceased.

(d) Compound naevus. Features combine those of junctional and intradermal naevi. Clusters of naevus cells, detached from epidermal margin, mature as naevus cells, in dermis.

(e) Blue naevus. In a process entirely distinct from those described in (a) to (d), melanocytes originating in embryonic neural crest become isolated and lodge in dermis.

found on the face. It is compound and contains spindle shaped melanocytes, and single and multinucleated giant cells. There is no malignant predisposition. Involution is accompanied by replacement fibrosis.

Dysplastic naevus

Dysplastic naevi are large and irregular. They occur on the trunk and occasionally on the scalp and breast. Pigmentation is not uniform. The edge of the lesion is indistinct. Melanocytes proliferate within the epithelium, beyond the boundary of the dermal lesion. Some of these lesions are familial and predispose to malignant melanoma (p. 227). In families inheriting the predisposition, nearly every family member eventually develops this cancer.

Blue naevus

This naevus is found on the head, neck or upper limbs. The circumscribed lesion is slate blue and comprises heavily pigmented cells situated deep within the dermis. The cells contain DOPA, dihydroxyphenylalanine, a precursor of tyrosine and of melanin. The histological features are identical with those of the Mongolian spot occasionally found in the mid-sacral skin, and the naevus of Ota identified in the eye and facial skin. Malignant change is extremely rare.

NASOPHARYNX AND NOSE

INFECTION AND INFLAMMATION

The nasal passages are susceptible to acute infective rhinitis, sinusitis and nasopharyngitis. The causes of infection include adenovirus but *Streptococcus pyogenes*, *Haemophilus influenzae*, *Strep. pneumoniae* and *Staphylococcus aureus* are frequent agents. One in three asymptomatic, normal persons carries *Staph. aureus* in the anterior nares. The nasal passages are also frequent sites for hypersensitivity reactions (p. 160) provoked by allergens that include house dust and pollens.

The nasopharyngeal tonsils are common targets for bacterial and viral infection. The formation of nasal polyps is one result of a persistent chronic inflammatory reaction.

TUMOURS

Benign

Benign tumours of the nasopharynx include **squamous papilloma** and **haemangioma**. Less often, the soft tissues and bone of the nose are the sites of **juvenile angiofibroma**, a lesion of young males. Angiofibroma causes local bleeding and may erode bone as it enlarges. Tumour growth ceases as adolescence ends.

Malignant

The nose and nasal passages are susceptible to **transitional cell carcinoma** (p. 200) and to **squamous carcinoma** (p. 303).

Lympho-epithelioma

Nasopharyngeal lympho-epithelioma, a squamous carcinoma with an extensive lymphocytic infiltrate, is a common tumour of populations in Malaysia, southern China, Indonesia and East Africa. There is an association with Epstein–Barr virus (p. 351). The tumour is often poorly differentiated and anaplastic. Local spread takes place through retropharyngeal tissues to the base of the skull. Blood-borne metastasis occurs and implicates lung, liver, bone and brain.

Malignant midline granuloma of the nose

This locally destructive and ulcerating lesion erodes soft tissues and bone. It is a T-cell lymphoma (p. 223).

VASCULAR DISEASE

Vasculitis

Wegener's granulomatosis is a form of systemic vasculitis in which the pulmonary arterial branches and other, systemic blood vessels are implicated. The necrotising lesions centre on the small arteries and arterioles of the nasal sinuses, destroying bone and causing ulceration.

Now read Artery (p. 24), Blood vessels (p. 48)

NECK

The region of the neck is prone to a wide variety of lesions.

DEVELOPMENTAL AND CONGENITAL DISORDERS

Cystic hygroma

A cystic hygroma is a fluid-filled, multiloculated structure, usually found in the neck. It may also occur around the shoulder, upper arm and chest wall and occasionally within the mediastinum. Cystic hygroma is recognisable at birth but may not be apparent until infancy. The defect is a failure of embryonic lymphatics to unite with veins.

Branchial cyst

A branchial cyst is a fluctuant swelling at the anterior border of the sternomastoid muscle in the upper part of the neck of young adults. It may be a developmental remnant of a branchial cleft but usually contains lymphoid tissue and, like cystic hygroma, may be derived from embryonal lymphatics. Branchial cyst is more common in males than females. The cyst contains opaque, straw-coloured fluid but small amounts of blood may escape into this fluid, accounting for the presence of cholesterol crystals. Branchial cysts are lined by respiratory columnar or pseudocolumnar epithelium that slowly becomes flattened and squamous. A cyst may become infected. Rarely, carcinoma supervenes.

Branchial sinus and fistula

Exceptionally, branchial cyst communicates with the pharynx via a sinus that has an internal opening located on the anterior aspect of the posterior pillar of the fauces. Branchial cyst and sinus occasionally communicate with an external orifice anterior to the lower part of the sternomastoid muscle so that a fistula (p. 132) results.

Now read Cyst (p. 113)

TUMOURS

Carcinomas of the tongue; nasopharynx; oesophagus; larynx; stomach; and bronchus are among the tumours that metastasise to cervical lymph nodes.

Carotid body

The carotid bodies, like the jugulotympanic body, vagal body and analogous structures in the wall of the aorta and pulmonary artery, are chemoreceptors. They may lie:

- At the bifurcation of the carotid artery.
- Adjoining the jugular vein.
- Beside the inferior ganglion of the vagus nerve.
- In the walls of the aorta and pulmonary artery.

Carotid body tumour

The cells of chemoreceptors originate from paraganglionic cells and the uncommon carotid body tumour is often termed a chemodectoma. It develops with equal frequency in males and females. There is a large incidence in individuals living at high altitude, as in Peru, suggesting that prolonged hypoxia may be important aetiologically. The tumours are almost always benign. Malignancy may only be recognised after excision and histological examination. Like the majority of neuro-endocrine tumours and chemodectomas, there is a false capsule of compressed, nearby connective tissue.

Microscopically, there are uniformly ovoid or polygonal cells, the small nuclei of which are seen within an eosinophilic cytoplasm. The cells retain an acinar arrangement, separated by vascular, extracellular connective tissue. Malignancy is confirmed by the identification of:

- Large numbers of mitotic figures.
- The extension of tumour into vascular channels.
- Zones of necrosis.

Carotid body tumours are excised for cosmetic reasons in younger adults. They are also removed on account of compression of the carotid vessel nerves; because of speech impediment; on account of difficulty in swallowing; or when cancer is suspected.

NECROSIS

Necrosis is the death of part or the whole of a tissue. The physical form of the dead material varies both according to the cause and to the composition of the tissue.

- **Aseptic necrosis** is a term applied to necrosis of part of a bone resulting from ischaemia. A common example is aseptic necrosis of the head of the femur after fracture; in caisson disease; or in the courses of renal dialysis.
- **Caseous necrosis** describes the breakdown of tissue under the influence of *Mycobacterium tuberculosis*, with a conversion to a cheese-like material that forms a 'cold' abscess, an abscess with little surrounding inflammation (p. 1).
- **Coagulative necrosis** is a term that explains the conversion of dead tissue to a firm mass, as in ischaemic infarction of a kidney or of the myocardium. Structural proteins are retained but DNA and RNA are lost.
- **Colliquative necrosis** is the conversion of necrotic tissue to a fluid by autolysis, as in a cerebral infarct.
- **Fat necrosis** describes the breakdown of fatty tissue, with subsequent acute inflammation and sometimes haemorrhage. Known causes are trauma to breast or synovial tissue; the release of activated pancreatic enzymes; and bacterial infection.
- **Fibrinoid necrosis** is a term for the acellular zones, seen, for example, in the intima and media of arterioles in accelerated hypertension. Fibrinoid displays staining properties identical to those of fibrin. In the affected zones, other plasma proteins are also found.
- **Hyaline necrosis** (Zenker's degeneration) is a term applied to the segmental, skeletal muscle necrosis caused by *Salmonella typhi*.
- **Ischaemic necrosis** is the death of tissue by the deprivation of the blood supply. Aseptic necrosis is one variety.
- **Mummification** (p. 136) is erroneously called 'dry gangrene'.
- **Pressure necrosis** is tissue death due to local vascular stasis or ischaemia. This variety of tissue death is encountered in bedsores.
- **Radiation necrosis** is tissue death caused by the local action of ionising radiation (p. 186).

Now read Cell death (p. 89), Gangrene (p. 136), Ischaemia (p. 187)

NEOPLASIA/TUMOUR

Neoplasia means 'new growth'. A neoplasm is an abnormal mass of tissue the growth of which exceeds and is uncoordinated with that of the normal body tissues, persisting in the same excessive manner after cessation of the stimuli which evoked the change.

Neoplasms are usually called **tumours**, a word that in a literal sense means a swelling. Although many swellings are not tumours and the majority of tumours never appear as external swellings, the term is in universal use. Tumours are encountered in every form of multicellular animal and plant. They are apparently an inevitable consequence of life on earth. There are two categories: benign and malignant.

BENIGN TUMOURS

Benign tumours are well differentiated: their cell structure and arrangement closely resemble those of the parent tissue. They are classified by histogenesis, that is, by the cell and tissue of origin. There is often a true collagenous capsule. Growth is slow. It may cease. Mitotic activity is slight and nuclear pleomorphism rare. Metastasis does not occur but local recurrence after excision is not exceptional. Occasionally, patients may die from the anatomical consequences of benign tumours. Compression, displacement and torsion are among the mechanical effects. The brain (p. 60), encased within the rigid skull, is vulnerable and a rise in intracranial pressure (p. 61) may prove fatal. In addition, benign tumours may be a source of slight or catastrophic bleeding.

Some benign tumours secrete hormones and other humoral substances such as catecholamines and 5-hydroxytryptamine. The endocrine or chemical secretion may lead to a characteristic clinical syndrome and the tumour is said to be 'functional'. Thus, adenoma (p. 272) of the anterior pituitary may cause gigantism or acromegaly; a beta-cell adenoma, insulinoma (p. 266) of the pancreas may provoke hyperinsulinism; and adenoma (p. 267) of a parathyroid gland may culminate in osteitis fibrosa cystica (p. 267).

MALIGNANT TUMOURS

A malignant tumour is a **cancer**. The terms 'malignant' and 'malignancy' refer to invasive neoplasms and distinguish them from benign tumours. The critical characteristics of malignant tumours are uncontrolled growth and distant spread by metastasis. Malignant tumours characteristically invade and destroy host tissue locally and extend to a wide variety of anatomical sites. Tumours that show little spread clinically may have been identified early or may be growing relatively slowly. A good prognosis may be a consequence of either phenomenon.

Malignant tumours are composed of cells that have lost some or most of their resemblance to the structure and function of the parent tissue. Growth is often rapid. Mitotic figures are frequent: many are abnormal and there is aneuploidy. In the absence of effective treatment, the outcome is death, the result of destruction or disorganisation of essential structures such as brain, liver or lung, or of secondary haemorrhage, ulceration or infection. The abnormalities of cell behaviour that determine the pattern of growth are:

- Loss of the regulation of cell growth and synthesis.
- Loss of the regulation of cell motility.
- Loss of normal cell contact inhibition.

Malignant tumours often, but not always, retain structural, antigenic or functional characteristics that allow them to be classified according to the tissue or organ of origin. However, tumours are not homogeneous and may not even arise from a single cell. They are genetically unstable and display an over- or under-expression of normal gene products (p. 138). Metastatic behaviour may also be affected by gene amplification or mutation and by epigenetic factors. New characteristics develop as a tumour grows.

Now read Carcinogenesis (p. 76)

CLASSIFICATION

The categories of tumour are:

- **Epithelial.** Examples of benign tumours are adenoma and papilloma. Malignant tumours are carcinomas. Their predominant structure is indicated by a qualifying adjective such as squamous (scaly) or a prefix such as adeno- (glandular).

  Squamous carcinomas are epithelial tumours in which the cells have differentiated towards stratified squamous epithelium, with or without keratinisation.

  Adenocarcinomas are epithelial tumours in which the cancer cells have differentiated towards the formation of exocrine, glandular acini.
- **Mesenchymal.** Examples of benign tumours include fibroma and lipoma. Most malignant mesenchymal tumours are sarcomas (p. 298). Their predominant structure is indicated by a prefix such as osteo- (bone matrix-forming) or chondro- (cartilage matrix-forming).
- **Haemopoietic and lymphoreticular tissue.** This category includes the leukaemias and lymphomas (p. 223).
- **Undifferentiated.** Many malignant tumours display so few of the features of any normal tissue that they can only be described as undifferentiated and anaplastic.
- **Embryonic.** Embryonic tumours arise during embryonic, fetal or postnatal development; they derive from organ rudiments that retain immature growth characteristics and may result from genetic causes. Many are malignant. Examples include neuroblastoma of the adrenal medulla (p. 8); medulloblastoma of the cerebellum (p. 65); and retinoblastoma (p. 286). Some embryonic tumours also display divergent differentiation, forming tissues not normally present in the part or organ. Rhabdomyoblasts comprise an important element of the embryonic tumour of the kidney, Wilms' tumour (p. 200).
- **Mixed.** A mixed tumour is composed of cells of two or more kinds of neoplastic tissue. In behaviour, it may be benign or malignant. In the malignant mixed mesodermal tumour of the uterus, for example, striated muscle, cartilage and epithelial components are present. The metastases may be carcinomatous or sarcomatous. Occasionally, as in the oesophagus, a malignant tumour may be designated as a carcinosarcoma.
- **Teratomas.** Teratomas arise from stem cells. There are many differentiation options. Teratomas are tumours formed of two or more tissues foreign to those in which the tumour arises. Teratomas are distinct from, but may superficially resemble, non-neoplastic aberrations of development such as heterotopia (p. 123).

Now read Malformations (p. 226)

Diagnosis

There are few absolute criteria that allow the diagnosis of cancer except genetic and chromosomal changes (p. 93). On a balance of incomplete evidence derived from his/her knowledge and experience, a pathologist must decide:

- Whether the structure of a tumour permits a diagnosis of cancer to be made.
- The probable cell of origin and the extent of spread.

When a tumour is undifferentiated and anaplastic, a pathologist can offer only limited guidance. The use of labelled antibodies to identify neoplastic antigens and markers means that the proportion of tumours categorised as 'undifferentiated' is diminishing. Increasing assistance in precise diagnosis can be obtained by genetic analysis (p. 138). Tumour cell structural and functional proteins can occasionally be identified by electron microscopy.

Carcinoma *in-situ* describes the appearance of a malignant tumour in which an island of epithelial cells has assumed the cytological features of carcinoma but in which the basement membrane has not been breached and invasion has not begun. The individual, desquamated cells of carcinoma *in-situ* can be identified in smears. Precancerous states are differentiated from carcinoma *in-situ*.

A distinction is drawn between atypical hyperplasia, dysplasia and carcinoma *in-situ*, but this differentiation demands skill, experience and judgement in microscopy. Applied to the skin (p. 295); the uterine cervix (p. 340); the bronchus (p. 70); the oesophagus; and the stomach (p. 309), the diagnosis of carcinoma *in-situ* indicates an excellent prognosis by contrast with invasive carcinoma.

Now read Biopsy (p. 40), Cytodiagnosis (p. 114)

STAGING

The extent to which an invasive tumour has spread from its site of origin is described as the stage. Staging can be undertaken on a simple, clinical basis but becomes much more precise when joined with the results of scanning (p. 169) and microscopy (pp. 40, 234). The staging of some tumours before operation may correlate poorly with pathological staging after operation.

Staging is of surgical and oncological importance and enables the merits of different forms of treatment to be compared. It is one guide to prognosis. The choice of staging method depends on the apparent nature and site of a tumour and upon understanding of its probable metastatic behaviour.

Clinical staging – the TNM system

A method of general, clinical applicability, the TNM system, proposed by De Noix, was modified and applied to many tumours by the *Union Internationale Contre le Cancer*. Within this system, a tumour is staged according to three criteria. They are: T – the extent of the primary tumour; N – the involvement of regional and more distant lymph nodes; and M – the existence of distant metastases (Fig. 54). Sophisticated subdivisions are created within each category. Thus, a carcinoma of the colon with a colovesical fistula and spread to the para-aortic lymph nodes but no distant metastases is designated T3a/N4/M0.

Staging by imaging

With the help of modern imaging techniques, staging is often attempted pre-operatively. In addition to conventional imaging by CT and MRI, a variety of new methods now facilitates this approach.

Now read Imaging (p. 169)

Operative staging

Some cancers can be staged before surgery although many can only be assessed adequately after excision, by microscopic examination. During an operation, staging can be undertaken by frozen section and confirmed post-operatively by the microscopic survey of paraffin sections. One system, devised by Dukes for carcinoma of the rectum, adopted three stages: A, B and C (Fig. 44). Staging remains essential to the oncologist and radiotherapist for the planning of combined forms of treatment.

Now read Carcinoma of colon (p. 106)

The value of sentinel node biopsy in tumour staging is outlined on p. 40.

GRADING

The grading of tumours is a microscopic procedure. It attempts to define the degree to which a cancer is differentiated and may be of value in predicting the response to treatment by irradiation or chemotherapy. In Broder's classification (Table 47), malignant epithelial tumours can be divided into four grades. Such a precise numerical system is now rarely used; it is time-

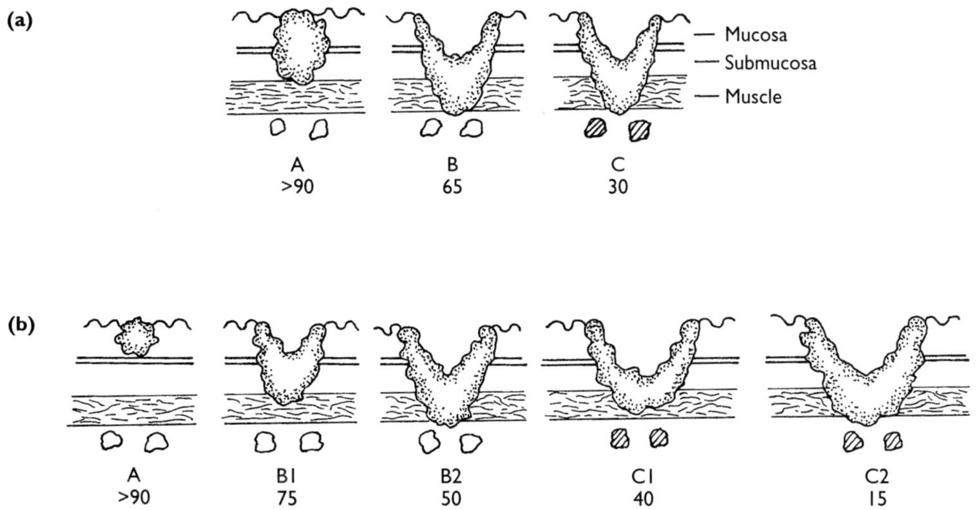

Figure 44 Staging of carcinoma of rectum.
(a) According to Duke's classification.
(b) According to Astler/Coller classification.
5-year survival is shown as per cent. Open islands represent lymph nodes devoid of metastases. Cross-hatched islands contain metastases.

consuming and histopathologists usually report a tumour as being well-differentiated, poorly-differentiated or undifferentiated.

In assessing the degree of differentiation, the histopathologist takes account of many factors. They include:

- The size and shape of the cells.
- The number of small blood vessels.
- The ratio between cell and nuclear size.
- The number of mitotic figures.
- The extent to which the tumour has reproduced a glandular structure (in tumours of glandular epithelium).
- The amount of cornification (in squamous carcinoma).

Attempts may be made to grade sarcomas but this is difficult and the degree of correlation between prognosis and grading is less than with carcinomas.

Table 47 Broder's classification of malignant tumours

Grade	**I**	**II**	**III**	**IV**
Proportion of differentiated cells (%)	>75	75–50	50–25	<25

GROWTH

Tumours arise when there has been an irreversible alteration in the genetic material of somatic or germ cells, leading to uncontrolled, purposeless, clonal multiplication. A tumour often appears in the host tissue as a swelling but diffuse growth or ulceration may occur. It is of interest that the growth of the most malignant tumours is rapid but no more rapid than that of normal embryonic or regenerating adult tissue. The ultimate outcome rests on a balance between host inhibiting factors and the stimulus for neoplasia.

Now read Carcinogenesis (p. 76)

Rate of tumour growth

Initially, growth of a neoplasm is a function of the frequency of cell division. A Mitotic Index (MI) describes the proportion of cells undergoing mitosis (p. 84). During this early period, the pattern of growth resembles the behaviour of multiplying bacteria (Fig. 7). After 10^9 cells have formed, a tumour may achieve a size of ~10 mm^3 and is recognisable clinically, for example by MRI. Even by this time, however, the further growth of a tumour is restricted by ischaemia (p. 187); by cell loss through inadequate nutrition; by necrosis and apoptosis; and by the impact of defence mechanisms such as cell mediated immunity. There is also a loss of cells by migration and metastasis.

Measures of tumour cell division and of tumour growth have value in assessing the urgency and variety of treatment. A tumour doubling time (Td) measures the time taken for a twofold increase in volume. Thus, the Td for Burkitt's lymphoma is ~14 days, for breast cancer ~80 days and for colorectal cancer ~500 days.

SPREAD

Metastasis

Metastasis is the distant extension of the cells of malignant tumours (p. 242). It is a dynamic, multi-step process involving, in sequence:

- Release from a tissue of single cells or of cell clusters.
- The penetration by such cells through the endothelial lining of blood vessels or lymphatics.
- Survival of the tumour cells in the blood or lymphatic circulation.
- Arrest of the transported cells in end-vessels.
- Invasion of the target tissue by infiltrating tumour cells.
- Local multiplication of the metastatic cells.

Some locally invasive tumours such as basal cell carcinoma do not metastasise.

Metastasis may be **direct**, by natural channels or ducts, or **remote**, via the blood, lymph or other body fluids. Blood-borne metastases are arterial or venous and may be within the systemic, pulmonary or portal circulations. It is not clear whether metastasis is a random process or whether certain cells only can behave in this way. Most cells released from a primary tumour die. The reasons for their death include destruction by turbulence; cell aggregation; and phagocytosis. In addition, immunity (p. 247) can exert a profound effect on the metastatic process.

Metastasis is often widespread before a tumour is apparent clinically. This behaviour is characteristic, for example, of malignant melanoma and carcinomas of the kidney and breast. Diffuse, occult, microscopic spread is frequently present in the liver in patients undergoing the resection of gastro-intestinal cancer. The metastatic tumour cells may be dormant. Reactivation can result from altered local endocrine secretion; from chemical, physical or mechanical factors; or from a change in the immune status of the host.

Influence of hydrodynamics

A simple, mechanistic concept supposes that all cancer cells are capable of being carried from the extracellular tissue spaces, via lymphatics, to the thoracic duct and venous system. Not all cancer cells transported in this way, or via the arterial tree, survive and grow.

Metastasis may be **retrograde** when, because of altered hydrodynamics, the normal direction of flow is reversed. **Paradoxical** metastatic spread is possible when there is an abnormal communication, such as a patent interatrial septum, between the venous and arterial circulations, and altered haemodynamics.

Influence of territory

Some tissues are clearly more supportive of metastatic tumour cells than others. The thyroid gland, for example, readily supports the growth of cells metastatic from renal cell carcinoma. Autocrine/paracrine control mechanisms; angiogenesis (p. 16); and adhesion molecules are among the agencies that play a part in selective cancer cell survival.

Influence of adhesion molecules

At the sites where cancer cells lodge, active attachment is influenced by adhesion molecules (p. 88). Tumour cells are usually less adhesive than normal. There is a paradoxical down-regulation of molecules such as E-cadherin (p. 88) and mutations in cadherin ligand-binding sites.

Lymphatic permeation

Lymphatic permeation is distinguished from the metastasis of cancer cells carried singly or as clusters, in the lymph. Permeation is the direct extension of cancer cells as continuous columns into and along lymphatic channels. It is a process characteristic of carcinomas such as those of the breast (p. 67) and stomach (p. 309).

Transcoelomic spread

Transcoelomic spread is the extension of the cells of a primary or metastatic malignant tumour across a body cavity. Upon reaching the serosal layer of a viscus, a tumour often provokes an effusion, allowing malignant cells to pass to other organs. The most frequent instances of transcoelomic spread are recognised within the abdomen, particularly from tumours of the stomach, pancreas, colon and ovaries. **Krukenberg tumour** describes bilateral ovarian metastasis from a mucin-secreting, gastro-intestinal carcinoma (pp. 260, 373). **Pseudomyxoma peritonei**, an occasional complication of coelomic spread, is described on p. 347.

Spread can occur throughout the pleural and pericardial cavities from tumours of the breast, lung and other organs.

MARKERS

As neoplastic cells grow, they manufacture proteins, polypeptides and other compounds not normally synthesised by the parent tissue. Some of these products are intracellular enzymes; others are hormones or embryonic, oncofetal proteins. The identification of these altered enzymes, or of increased levels of plasma hormones and oncofetal antigens, is often made by radio-immunoassay or, in tissue sections, by immunohistochemical techniques (p. 158). Identifying these markers can be of high diagnostic and prognostic importance but their main practical value is in assessing the response to treatment and in detecting tumour recurrence.

Some examples of neoplastic markers are:

- **Enzymes.** The cells of prostatic carcinoma form an acid phosphatase (PAP – p. 279) that escapes into the blood. Many hepatocellular and bronchial carcinomas liberate an alkaline phosphatase formed normally by the placenta. The enzyme is the carcinoplacental acid phosphatase or Regan iso-enzyme.
- **Hormones**. Functioning tumours of endocrine tissues secrete hormones appropriate to the parent tissue. For example, adrenal cortical adenomas may secrete aldosterone or cortisol. Many other non-endocrine tumours, including common carcinomas, such as those of the lung, kidney and liver, secrete inappropriate, ectopic hormones (p. 126). Thus, the cells of small cell bronchial carcinoma often release ACTH, gonadotrophin or ADH.
- **Cell proteins**. Other proteins formed by particular cancer cells include the cytokeratins; epithelial membrane antigen; leucocyte common antigen; and S100 protein. Prostate specific antigen (PSA) is described on p. 279.
- **Embryonic (fetal) proteins (oncofetal antigens).** Many malignant tumours form and secrete proteins that are normally synthesised only by embryonic or fetal tissue. These oncofetal antigens can elicit an immune response. They are expressed by many tumours, can have value in diagnosis and are recognised by radio-immunoassay.

  Oncofetal antigens behave as tumour-specific antigens (TSA). Carcino-embryonic antigen (CEA) is one example. It can be detected in the blood of patients with a variety of malignant tumours, including carcinoma of the colon and hepatocarcinoma. A changing titre of CEA may be an aid to monitoring the response of a tumour to treatment. Regression of the cancer leads to a fall in plasma levels of CEA and a rise in titre is often apparent before recurrence of the tumour is evident clinically. Alpha-fetoprotein (AFP) is another TSA. It is present in the serum of patients with hepatocarcinoma and the testicular teratomas. However, it may also be identified in patients with non-neoplastic diseases such as viral hepatitis.

TUMOUR IMMUNITY

Many but not all neoplastic cells bear antigens distinct from those of the host. In some ways a tumour behaves like a parasite, in others like an embryo, extending at the expense of the host or mother. The tendency is towards host destruction.

Those antigens that predispose towards tumour cell death are located at the neoplastic cell surface. They are the tumour-specific transplantation antigens (TSTA) and are distinct from histocompatibility (HLA) antigens (p. 330). TSTA cause the rejection of discrete cancer cells. Cells in larger masses are unaffected. In experimental chemical cancers (p. 80), the TSTA are unique to the individual tumour. In virus cancers (p. 80), these surface antigens may be shared.

It is convenient to classify tumour immunity as:

- **Non-specific.** Mononuclear macrophages play a part and can phagocytose cancer cells. NK cells (p. 231) may also be important.
- **Specific, cell-mediated.** The lack of co-stimulatory expression (p. 173) can enable tumour cells to evade an immune reaction. The influence of T-cells may be two-edged because lymphocytes can induce angiogenesis, aggregate with circulating tumour cells and assist in their lodgement. Cancer cells may also avoid a T lymphocyte immune response by selective, deficient expression of MHC class I molecules (p. 330).

- **Specific, humoral**. Humoral immunity may be protective so that the presence of antibodies to tumour cells may correlate with the absence of metastases, as in malignant melanoma. Antibodies to CD40 (p. 205) can stimulate CD40 and provoke tumour immunity. CD40 is an activator of B-cell proliferation. It is a transmembrane protein of the family of TNF receptors.

The use of immunisation in tumour therapy has been tested. The value of non-specific adjuvants is limited but there are many other specific approaches. They can be used to:

- Enhance innate (natural), non-specific immunity (p. 231) by the injection of non-specific adjuvants such as BCG (p. 333).
- Identify the causal virus, if there is one, and manufacture an anti-virus vaccine.
- Select tumour specific antigens, as in malignant melanoma, and prepare antisera against them.
- Promote clonal expansion and activation of tumour lymphocytes by the use of IL-2 (p. 172).
- Use monoclonal antibodies (p. 234) attached to toxins to target tumour cells.

NERVE, PERIPHERAL

TRAUMA

The nature of the response to nerve damage depends upon the type of trauma. Injury may be caused by contusion, compression, stretching, laceration or ischaemia. Motor nerves are more sensitive to compression than sensory nerves.

Degrees of injury

There are three degrees of neuronal injury: neuropraxia, axonotmesis and neurotmesis.

- In **neuropraxia**, (Gk *praxia*, action) there is physiological disturbance of nerve function without anatomical disruption. Following the injury, there is a period in which axons are unable to re-establish normal membrane potentials but complete recovery of function can be expected within 50–100 days. To the naked eye the nerve appears normal but there may be segmental demyelination. Examples include carpal tunnel syndrome and compression from tourniquets.
- In **axonotmesis**, (Gk *tmesis*, cutting, separation), the axons, but not the supporting tissue and cells, are completely divided or disrupted. The endoneuronal and perineuronal microskeletons of the neurone remain intact. Microscopically, the Schwann cells and myelin sheath are disrupted but the axon remains intact (Fig. 45). Degeneration occurs distal to the site of injury and there is a loss of both motor and sensory function. In the segment distal to the injury, these changes are known as **Wallerian degeneration** (Fig. 46). In myelinated fibres, degeneration extends proximally to the first node of Ranvier. During neurolysis, the Nissl granules disappear (**chromatolysis**), a change shown by electron microscopy to be a loss of endoplasmic reticulum. Functional restoration may be anticipated since the course of the axons is virtually intact. Several days after injury, neurofibrils emerge from the proximal end of the injured axon and grow into the regenerated distal sheath. The rate of neurofibril growth is ~1 mm/day. Many or all of the fibrils fail to reach their appropriate end-organ. Recovery is better in purely motor or purely sensory nerves than in nerves that comprise a mixture of both forms of fibril since it is likely that each proliferating fibril will reach an appropriate end-organ. Recovery in a mixed nerve is often poor since motor nerve neurofibrils may grow down sensory sheaths and *vice versa*. If the severed ends of the injured nerve are widely separated, fibrous tissue proliferates and forms a **traumatic neuroma**.
- In **neurotmesis**, the whole neurone is divided completely or partially. Any gap between the divided parts of the nerve is occupied by a fibrinous coagulum. If the division is complete, the proximal segment may develop a **stump neuroma** formed of convoluted and disorganised axons mixed with collagenous connective tissue and neurilemmal cells. Careful apposition of the nerve endings by means of an operating microscope restores continuity effectively. Grafting may be as beneficial as resuture if only small segments are replaced in either purely motor or purely sensory nerves.

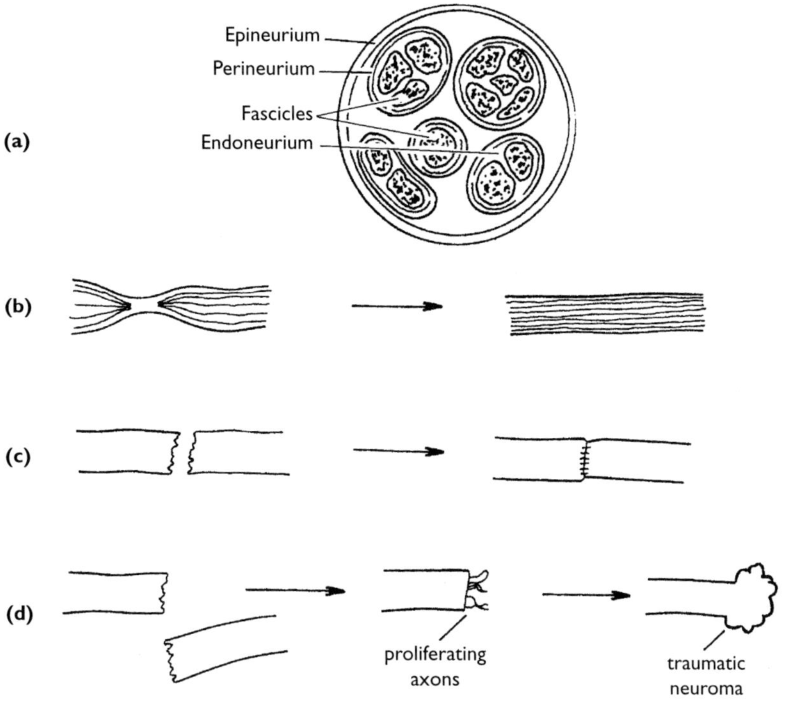

Figure 45 Nerve injury and regeneration.
(a) Cross-section of peripheral nerve showing microskeleton which has vital role in determining outcome of neuronal regeneration.
(b) Regeneration following **axonotmesis** due to crushing injury. Wallerian degeneration is usually followed by complete functional restoration. Motor and sensory axons regenerate within intact endoneural and perineural skeletons.
(c) Regeneration following surgical repair after **neurotmesis**. Functional result in mixed motor and sensory nerve depends greatly upon precise apposition of individual fascicles.
(d) Development of traumatic neuroma following **neurotmesis**. Axons that sprout from proximal end of divided nerve fail to reach and grow into microskeleton of peripheral end of divided nerve.

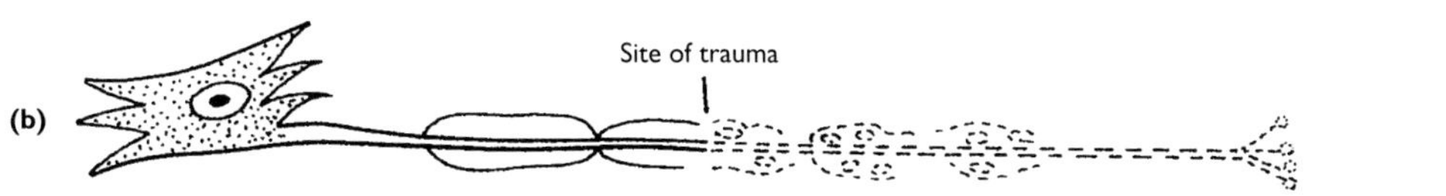

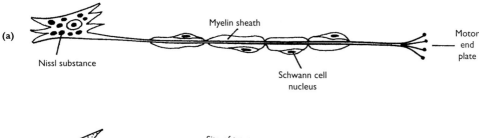

Figure 46 Peripheral nerve following trauma.
Following injury, there is Wallerian degeneration of the distal portion of the injured, peripheral nerve. There is also loss of Nissl substance (chromatolysis) in spinal neurone. Beyond injured site, fatty myelin sheath disintegrates as does the axon (axonolysis) but neurilemmal (Schwann) cells survive, a crucial factor in permitting axonal regeneration.
a. Normal structure of nerve. b. Wallerian degeneration.

TUMOURS

Benign

Neurilemmoma (schwannoma – p. 376)

Neurilemmoma is the most frequent nerve tumour. It is found on a peripheral nerve. Much less often, the neoplasm is recognised on the vestibular part of the eighth cranial nerve where it is designated '**acoustic neuroma**'. The fibres of the affected nerve are displaced and it is usually possible to enucluate the tumour. Malignant change is very rare.

Neurofibroma

Isolated neurofibroma is a fusiform swelling in which the nerve fibres of a peripheral nerve extend through a neoplastic mass formed of Schwann cells, perineural cells and fibroblasts. As a consequence, attempted surgical excision may have devastating consequences. In most instances, intervention is restricted to biopsy undertaken to establish diagnosis. When a group of nerves is affected, the condition is called **plexiform neurofibroma**. Malignant transformation is rare.

Neurofibromatosis

Peripheral neurofibromatosis (von Recklinghausen's disease – p. 377) is a rare genetic disorder inherited as an autosomal dominant characteristic. Approximately half the recognised cases are attributable to spontaneous mutation. The responsible gene, located on somatic chromosome 17, displays variable penetrance and occurs in 330 in every 10^6 births. It regulates the *ras* oncogene. The manifestations of the defect are widespread. Numerous neurofibromas develop on autonomic, sensory and motor nerves. A single, large nerve may be the site of plexiform neurofibroma. Other associated abnormalities are skeletal defects, *café-au-lait* skin spots and hamartoma of the iris.

In **central neurofibromatosis**, few peripheral nerve changes are recognised and the multiple lesions include astrocytoma, optic glioma, bilateral acoustic neuroma and spinal nerve root tumours.

Granular cell tumour

Granular cell tumour may occur in the larynx and other sites.

Malignant

Neurofibrosarcoma

Neurofibrosarcoma is a rare tumour of a peripheral nerve. It develops sporadically and in fewer than 10% of patients with peripheral neurofibromatosis.

O

OBESITY

Now read Fat (p. 128), Lipids (p. 207)

Obesity (adiposity – fatness) is an excess of body lipid in a solid or semisolid state. The most frequent cause of death worldwide is malnutrition but 21% of UK females and 17% of males were classed as obese in 1998 (Table 48). The implications for surgery are serious.

Obesity is defined by relating body weight to height. The ratio is expressed in kg/m^2 and provides a body mass index (BMI). Differences in the index between individuals are largely due to variations in the quantity of depot lipid (Table 48). Calculations of the BMI provide a reliable clinical index of obesity.

Table 48 Internationally accepted definitions of nutritional status based upon the body mass index (BMI) (kg/m^2)

Malnutrition	<18
Normal	20–25
Obesity	30–40
Morbid obesity	>40

Causes

Genetic

Comparisons of the BMI of similar twins, dissimilar twins and adoptees suggest that inheritance of obesity is polygenic. However, single gene mutations may also be significant. One inherited factor regulating weight change is the signalling protein leptin. It is coded by the *LEP* gene. The protein is derived principally from adipocytes. The amount of leptin secreted is proportional to the adipose tissue mass. Leptin interacts with specific receptors in the hypothalamus to regulate the balance between hunger and satiety. Feeding results in the release of leptin from gastric fundus cells into the blood plasma, a possible explanation for repletion. The molecule acts upon peripheral fatty tissues, inhibiting intracellular lipid concentrations by reducing fatty acid and triacylglycerol (triglyceride) synthesis, increasing lipid oxidation and improving glucose homeostasis.

Environmental

The prevalence of obesity is rising rapidly in the Western world. The rise is related to increased energy intake and decreased energy expenditure. These factors are strongly influenced by endocrine glandular activity and by psychological states.

Behaviour and prognosis

Obesity has a major influence upon life expectancy. The morbidly obese have a mortality twice that of those of normal weight. There is an increased risk of diabetes mellitus; osteoarthritis; hypercholesterolaemia; cholelithiasis; hypertension; atherosclerosis; and colorectal cancer. Obesity may be a major deterrent to surgery: obese patients are more likely to suffer post-operative chest infection; deep venous thrombosis; pulmonary embolism; wound infection; wound dehiscence; and incisional hernia, regardless of genetic or hormonal influences. The body is an energy store governed by the laws of thermodynamics. Even the morbidly obese can therefore attain a normal weight by prolonged dieting. Nevertheless, unsupervised dieting itself may be associated with enhanced morbidity and mortality, and drugs taken to diminish appetite may induce pulmonary disease sufficiently severe to require heart/lung transplantation (p. 149).

OEDEMA

Oedema is the presence of excess water in the interstitial tissue spaces. It may be localised or generalised. As much as 4 L of excess total body fluid may accumulate without obvious oedema.

Starling clearly defined the three principal factors that regulate the flow of water across capillary endothelium (Fig. 47), thus influencing the relative distribution of fluid between the intravascular and extracellular compartments. The factors are:

- The difference between intracapillary and interstitial hydrodynamic pressures.
- The difference between intracapillary and interstitial osmotic pressures.
- The permeability of the capillary wall.

There are two varieties of oedema, transudate and exudate (Table 49). They may co-exist. Osmotically active substances that cannot pass through semi-permeable membranes comprise a group of factors affecting the movement of fluid across the membrane. Within the intravascular compartment these substances determine **colloid osmotic pressure (oncotic pressure)**.

Now read Water (p. 355)

TRANSUDATE

In a transudate, the permeability of the vessel walls is unchanged. The increased escape of water is due either to an increased difference between intracapillary and interstitial hydrodynamic pressures or to a decrease in the difference between their osmotic pressures. The accumulated fluid has a low protein content. The oedema of cardiac failure (a result of obstruction to venous return and impaired capillary endothelial cell metabolism) and nutritional oedema (a result of decreased plasma oncotic pressure), are examples.

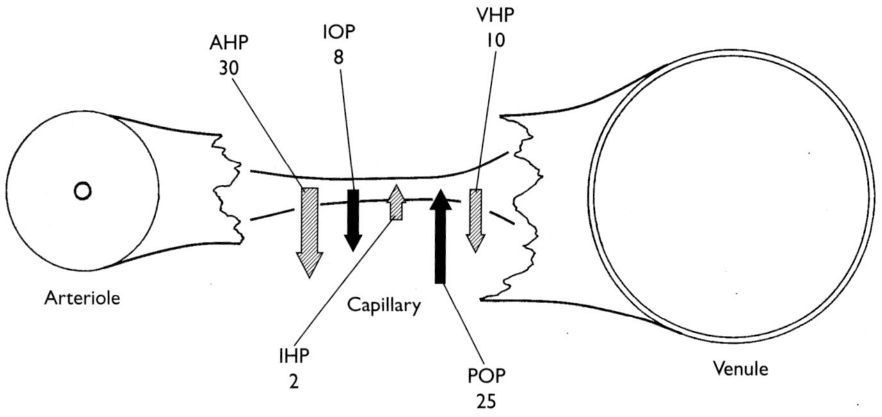

Figure 47 Transport of water across capillary wall.
Diagram shows high arteriolar, low venular and negligible interstitial hydrodynamic pressures. As Starling demonstrated, there is very small net gain of water external to capillary endothelium, accounting for daily flow of lymph.

Interstitial fluid pressure varies continually. It is sum of interstitial oncotic and hydrodynamic pressures. In subcutaneous tissue, interstitial fluid pressure is −2 mmHg; in brain it is +6 mmHg. In example shown, net outward force at arteriolar end of capillary is 11 mmHg ([30 + 8] − [25 + 2]). At venular end, there is net inward force of 9 mm Hg ([25 + 2] − [10 + 8]).

Oedema may be due to an increased hydrodynamic pressure or a diminished plasma oncotic pressure and causes large net accumulation of water within extravascular space. This is oedema. Correction of this imbalance, by enhanced removal of extravascular water through lymphatic drainage, returns water to circulation. Oedema persists if (a) arteriolar pressure remains excessive; (b) venular flow is obstructed; (c) oncotic pressure is lowered, for example by protein deficiency; (d) metabolism of capillary endothelial cells is impaired; or (e). there is obstruction to the flow of lymph.

AHP: arteriolar hydrodynamic pressure; IHP: interstitial hydrodynamic pressure; IOP: interstitial oncotic pressure; POP: plasma oncotic pressure; VHP: venular hydrodynamic pressure.

Table 49 Some common causes of oedema

Variety	Cause	Mechanism
Exudate	Increased capillary permeability to protein	Acute inflammation
Transudate	Increased venous capillary hydrostatic pressure	Cardiac failure (generalised) Venous thrombosis of a limb (localised)
	Lymphatic obstruction	Tissue permeation by cancer cells Surgical transection Worm infestation e.g. filariasis
	Hypoproteinaemia	Chronic malnutrition Nephrotic syndrome
	Increased pulmonary venous pressure	Left ventricular cardiac failure Vasoconstricting agents Neurogenic factors

EXUDATE

An exudate is fluid rich in protein, derived from the plasma during acute inflammation, injury or metabolic disorder. The exuded proteins include albumin, fibrinogen and the immunoglobulins. Leucocytes and some red blood cells are often present. The loss of protein has a slight effect on plasma osmotic (oncotic) pressure but a large effect on interstitial osmotic pressure. The selective filtration system of the post-capillary venules is impaired.

Ascites

Ascites is the accumulation of excess fluid within the peritoneal cavity as the result of exudation or transudation. Hepatic cirrhosis is a common cause in the treatment of which large volume paracentesis; transjugular intra-hepatic portocaval shunt, and liver transplantation have been used.

Pericardial effusion and hydrothorax describe the accumulation of excess fluid in the pericardial sac and in the pleural cavity, respectively.

OESOPHAGUS

Biopsy diagnosis of oesophageal disease

Suspicious lesions are examined at endoscopy. Cells are obtained with a brush. Biopsies are also taken with forceps. The identification of disease is enhanced if both techniques are used. The brush sample should be obtained before the biopsy and should be examined for hyphae when candidiasis is suspected. Oesophagitis may be due to infestation with Helicobacter (p. 151). An antral biopsy is taken if the presence of this organism is suspected. In the investigation of Barrett's syndrome, multiple biopsies are excised circumferentially. They should be obtained at recorded distances from the teeth, enabling a map to be drawn of the extent of the disease and of any dysplasia.

DEVELOPMENTAL AND CONGENITAL DISORDERS

Atresia

Atresia, with or without tracheo-oesophageal fistula, is recognised in $330/10^6$ neonates (1/3000). It is frequently associated with cardiac and other congenital abnormalities.

Further forms of developmental anomalies include:

- **The VATER syndrome** of **V**ertebral defects, **A**nal atresia, **T**racheo-o**E**sophageal fistula and **R**enal dysplasia. Oesophageal webs or stenoses may be found in the upper oesophagus.
- **Schatzki's ring**, a web of mucosa in the lower oesophagus, the upper surface bearing squamous epithelium, the lower columnar epithelium. The defect becomes apparent in later life because of defective oesophageal motility.
- **Duplication of the oesophagus**, leading to cyst formation. One part is obstructed. Because the epithelial glands lining this part continue to secrete, a cyst is formed that compresses the other component.

Achalasia

Achalasia is a 'failure to relax'. It describes the defective opening of sphincters. In surgical practice, the term is confined to abnormal function of the lower oesophageal sphincter.

Causes

The aetiology remains uncertain. The condition has an equal sex distribution and is diagnosed most frequently in the fourth decade of life. Achalasia is an uncommon cause of dysphagia and affects no more than 1 in every 10^6 persons in the UK.

Structure

There is loss of argyrophil ganglion cells from Auerbach's myenteric plexus. The defect is similar to that of Hirschprung's disease (p. 105). Degenerative changes in the vagal nuclei and trunks are described. Later, the lumen above the lower sphincter is much dilated, giving rise to mega-oesophagus (p. 254). At the lower end, the oesophagus tapers uniformly, producing a smooth, so-called 'bird-beak' deformity. The mucosa is frequently inflamed. Initially, the muscle layer is hypertrophied; later, it becomes attenuated.

Behaviour and prognosis

At first, there are vigorous, painful contractions of the oesophageal musculature. Peristalsis is disordered. The main defect is incomplete relaxation of the lower oesophageal sphincter resulting in a raised, resting intraluminal pressure. Among the complications are aspiration bronchopneumonia and lung abscess. These pulmonary complications are due to an overspill of oesophageal contents into the bronchi. It is claimed but not proven that oesophageal cancer is six times more probable in those with achalasia than in a normal population.

Mega-oesophagus

Mega-oesophagus is very common in Brazil and the Argentine, countries in which Chagas' disease (South American trypanosomiasis – p. 282) is endemic. The parasites destroy the ganglion cells of Auerbach's plexus. The resulting dilated, oesophageal segment is comparable to that recognised in achalasia. The demand for remedial surgery is very high.

MECHANICAL DISORDERS

Hiatus hernia

Sliding

This is relatively more common in the obese than in those of normal build and can be found in ~30% of the population. As a consequence of the displacement of part of the stomach into the chest, ~30% of these individuals have symptoms of oesophageal reflux.

Rolling

Rolling hiatus hernia (para-oesophageal hiatus hernia) develops when the fundus of the stomach passes into the chest beside the oesophagus. The lower oesophageal sphincter is within the abdomen. Oesophageal reflux is uncommon but the hernia often produces obstructive symptoms and may become incarcerated.

Now read Hernia (p. 156)

Perforation

Oesophageal perforation is usually iatrogenic. It is caused by manoeuvres to dilate strictures or by the insertion of endoprostheses. Perforation by ingested fish bones and other foreign bodies is uncommon. Spontaneous perforation of the oesophagus, **Boerhaave's syndrome** (p. 370), is an unusual complication of severe vomiting. Whatever the cause, interstitial emphysema, mediastinitis and empyema are secondary consequences.

Stricture

Stricture develops in 10% of patients with severe, untreated reflux oesophagitis. It is the result of excess collagen deposition in the oesophageal wall. Stricture may also be due to the action of swallowed caustic chemicals; of ionising radiation; or of trauma or carcinoma (p. 255). It is a feature of the uncommon disease, systemic sclerosis (scleroderma – p. 74).

INFECTION AND INFLAMMATION

The stratified squamous epithelium of the normal oesophagus resists bacterial, mycotic and viral invasion effectively. The most frequent infections are with *Candida albicans*, herpes simplex virus and cytomegalovirus, disorders often encountered in immunocompromised patients; following radiotherapy or chemotherapy; and in those suffering from AIDS (p. 2).

Barrett's oesophagus

The normal oesophagus is lined by non-keratinising, stratified squamous epithelium. Barrett (p. 369) described patients in whom the distal part of the oesophagus was lined by columnar epithelium. The defect was thought to be congenital, a short oesophagus causing the stomach to be drawn into the thorax. It is now viewed as an acquired metaplasia encountered in 10–15% of patients with acid reflux. The extent of the abnormality corresponds to the frequency, duration and severity of acid exposure. It has been suggested, however, that bile, not acid, provokes metaplasia. Endoscopy reveals reddened, columnar epithelium, confined to a few small islands of mucosa or extending circumferentially. In severe cases, ulceration and stricture develop. In ~25% of patients, microscopy reveals low-grade epithelial dysplasia that may regress. If high-grade dysplasia occurs, the risk of developing adenocarcinoma is ~40 times greater than in the general population. Malignant change is much more frequent in men than in women with this condition.

In the absence of dysplasia, there is disagreement concerning the incidence of adenocarcinoma and, consequently, debate regarding the merits of subjecting affected patients to annual screening. Routine endoscopic surveillance may be justified in those with epithelial dysplasia and is obligatory in patients with high grade dysplasia.

Candidiasis

Painful dysphagia in malnourished or immunocompromised patients is often due to this fungal infection which is called 'thrush'. The friable mucosa bleeds easily. Small, white islands of mycelia are recognised on endoscopy.

Now read Mycoses (p. 135)

Reflux oesophagitis

The prevalence of this condition is difficult to determine. Many otherwise healthy persons experience heartburn and spasm intermittently throughout their lives. Reflux oesophagitis is significantly more frequent in obese, middle-aged women than in the remainder of the adult population. Individuals with the disorder often have a co-existent, sliding hiatus hernia. In those with histological evidence of oesophagitis, functional abnormalities of the lower oesophageal sphincter may be demonstrable and the intra-abdominal part of the oesophagus is short. The incidence of adenocarcinoma of the oesophagus is eight times greater than among unaffected persons.

Ulcer

Gastric mucosa may exist within the tissue of the lower, cardiac end of the oesophagus. Peptic ulceration may occur. In most instances, it follows recurrent reflux. In the upper oesophagus, gastric-type epithelium is ectopic. Ulcers found within the wall of the oesophagus may be malignant.

Haemorrhage

Bleeding from oesophageal varices is responsible for ~5% of admissions to UK hospitals for gastro-intestinal haemorrhage. Microscopic haemorrhage and anaemia may occur in patients with reflux oesophagitis or malignant neoplasia. Occasionally, frank haemorrhage may originate from these causes. Mucosal tears at the cardia can be caused by violent retching or vomiting. The resultant bleeding is not usually severe but surgery may be necessary if the blood loss becomes excessive.

TUMOURS

Benign

The most frequent benign tumour is the rare leiomyoma, an occasional cause of gastro-intestinal bleeding. Polyps may also be encountered.

Malignant

Carcinoma

In all countries, the frequency of carcinoma of the oesophagus is increasing. Carcinoma of the oesophagus is particularly prevalent near the Caspian Sea, in the Transkei and in northern China and in these regions the incidence is greater than $350/10^6$ individuals. In England and Wales, the annual incidence is $\sim 110/10^6$ population. The mortality in men has doubled since 1960 and has increased by 50% in women. However, the disease accounts for only 2% of cancer deaths in the UK.

Causes

- **Heredity**. In spite of irrefutable evidence implicating race, the significance of heredity remains uncertain. One genetic factor is **tylosis**. This rare condition is inherited as an autosomal dominant trait. Hyperkeratosis of the palms and soles accompanies abnormal maturation of oesophageal mucosal squamous cells.
- **Environment**. The role of environmental factors is well established. In northern Europe, there has been a change in the prevalence of oesophageal carcinoma within the different social classes: the tumour is now as common in the affluent as in the poor. Nicotine, alcohol, opium and nitroso-compounds are implicated. Cigarette smoking and ethanol excess act synergistically. There is a high risk of cancer many years after chemical injury due to the ingestion of sclerosants such as lye. The increased incidence in those with achalasia and strictures of all types suggests that stagnation may be important. Other possible contributory, local factors are discussed (above).

Structure

Dysplasia of varying severity inevitably precedes malignant change. In countries with a high prevalence of oesophageal carcinoma, this change may be identified by exfoliative cytology. Oesophageal mucus is obtained ingeniously by traction upon a balloon inflated in the stomach and pulled back through the mouth. The apparatus resembles a Foley urinary catheter.

- **Squamous carcinoma**. The most frequent primary malignant tumour worldwide is squamous carcinoma (p. 303).

- **Adenocarcinoma**. In the UK, however, adenocarcinoma is equally common although it is unusual to find this variety of carcinoma in the proximal two-thirds of the oesophagus. Imaging appearances are those of a 'shouldered' and irregular deformity. Endoscopically, the tumour may appear as a plaque, as an ulcer or as a circumferential zone of stenosis: it is usually exfoliative. Both squamous carcinomas and adenocarcinomas display varying degrees of differentiation.
- **Small cell carcinoma** is very uncommon.

Behaviour and prognosis

Because of the extensive lymphatic system of the oesophageal submucosa, tumour cell permeation and distant lymphatic metastasis are early features of this cancer. Fewer than 10% of patients in the UK have tumours confined to the mucosa or submucosa (stage 1). Metastasis is both prograde and retrograde. Satellite nodules may form. Local extension within the mediastinum establishes a tracheo-oesophageal fistula. Rarely, invasion of the aorta leads to fatal haemorrhage. Haematogenous spread to the liver and lungs is the most frequent cause of death and is responsible for the poor prognosis that is closely related to TNM staging.

OPERATING THEATRES

The design of modern operating theatres is complex and involves special forms of lighting, heating and ventilation.

A smooth, constant, laminar flow of air is impelled into the operating theatre. A downward displacement of air is more effective than lateral displacement in reducing the dispersion of bacteria and dust. The air is heated or cooled, saturated with water vapour or dehumidified to maintain an environment of 20°C and 40–60% humidity. The entire volume is replaced at ~5–10 minute intervals. This arrangement is necessary for the welfare of anaesthetised patients in whom thermoregulation is paralysed and in whom heat and fluid are lost uncontrollably to the environment. However, the atmosphere is uncomfortable for gowned staff.

The air entering an operating theatre is filtered to remove bacteria, fungi and spores. Sampling of the air is frequent. If more than 30 bacterial colony-forming units (cfu)/m^3 are detected in a sample, the theatre is shut and cleaned. Because of the dangers posed by *Staphylococcus aureus* (p. 303), the finding of a single colony of this organism is sufficient reason for closure.

To minimise microbial contamination from outside, staff change into clean clothes and wear clean caps to cover their hair. Patients are transferred across a physical barrier from the trolley used to transport them from the ward, to another, clean trolley that does not leave the theatre suite. Dirty instruments, gowns, drapes and pathological specimens are taken from the theatre complex by a different route from that used for clean materials.

When operating on patients in whom wound infection is likely to prove devastating, as it is in hip replacements, particular precautions are necessary. Specially designed, ultra-clean air enclosures or transparent plastic envelopes are used to isolate the wound. All personnel except the surgeons and operating personnel are excluded from this enclosure. Those within the enclosure wear 'space-suits' that allow gaseous exchange through flexible pipes. Operating theatres are cleaned early each morning. 'Clean' operations are therefore performed first each day, potentially infective cases, particularly those on HIV-1 or HBV-positive patients, last.

ORAL CAVITY

Biopsy diagnosis of oral disease

The recognition of dental disease is not described in this account. The diagnosis of non-dental, oral diseases is undertaken by methods closely similar to those used for other mucosal surfaces.

DEVELOPMENTAL AND CONGENITAL DISORDERS

Pigmentation

Patches of brown–black melanin pigmentation are a feature of the oral mucosa in the Peutz–Jegher syndrome (p. 106) and in Addison's disease (p. 7).

Hare lip and cleft palate

Defective formation of the lip and palate constitutes a relatively frequent congenital malformation.

Congenital epulis

In newborn female children, this soft pedunculated or sessile mass is recognised on the anterior aspect of the maxilla.

MECHANICAL AND TRAUMATIC DISORDERS

Ulcer

Ulcers of the lip result from trauma, malnutrition and herpetic infection. Ulcers of the oral epithelium are often the result of poorly fitting dentures; impact with sharp teeth during sporting activities; excessive brushing; and dental, surgical procedures.

Fibrous hyperplasia

Sustained mechanical irritation, caused, for example, by dental irregularities, results in the formation of small fibrous tags covered by non-keratinising, stratified squamous epithelium. Prolonged or repetitive local trauma may result in a **fibrous epulis**, an island of vascular, collagenous connective tissue originating in the gum. When the lesion assumes a polypoidal form, perhaps due to malaligned biting, it becomes a **fibro-epithelial polyp**.

INFECTION AND INFLAMMATION

Viral infection

From time-to-time, clusters of vesicles outlined by an inflamed red margin appear on the oral mucosa in young persons. The lesions follow exposure to ultraviolet light; cold; heat; infection by a common cold virus; or systemic disease. They are attributable to HSV-1 or HSV-2 (p. 351). Virus survives indefinitely in the tissues of the dorsal root ganglia of the trigeminal nerve. Herpetic vesicles may re-appear when there is a precipitating disorder such as a concurrent bacterial infection. All body tissues are prone to direct injury by HIV. The lips and oral cavity are no exception. In AIDS, hairy cell leukoplakia (p. 207) can be caused by the Epstein–Barr (EB) virus. The oral cavity is also the site for infections by agents such as *Candida albicans* and the herpes and cytomegaloviruses.

Bacterial infection

Acute necrotising ulcerative gingivitis, Vincent's angina, is a disorder of malnourished, immunocompromised or cachectic individuals. As a result of impaired immunity, there is synchronous infection of the oral tissues by two or more commensal organisms that exist in symbiosis. The most frequent agents are an anaerobic, Gram-negative, fusiform bacillus, *Fusiformis fusiformis;* and a spirochaete, *Borrelia vincenti*. Untreated, tissue destruction spreads locally and may culminate in **cancrum oris** (noma) (p. 137).

Mycotic infection

Candidiasis

Candidiasis (p. 135), infection by *Candida albicans*, is one consequence of impaired immunity, malnutrition or debility. The infection, in which white patches and aphthous ulcers form on the oral mucosa, is commonplace in AIDS; in immunosuppressed individuals; and as an indirect consequence of antibiotic therapy.

Other inflammatory disorders

Pyogenic granuloma

Pyogenic granulomas originate on the gingiva near inflamed or infected teeth. Clinically, they resemble capillary haemangioma and are compact, raised, hyperaemic islands of vascular fibrous tissue.

Oral leucoplakia

Leucoplakia (p. 207) and erythroplakia are descriptive terms, signifying adherent white or red patches on the oral mucosa, respectively. The patches may be of uniform appearance or have a speckled structure due to a mixture of the white and red areas. Microscopically, there is hyperkeratosis and acanthosis. In a minority of cases, epithelial cell abnormalities are recognised. They range from dysplasia and carcinoma *in-situ* to overt squamous carcinoma, a change seen in one case in 20. Leucoplakia is particularly likely to represent a premalignant state in female patients with iron-deficiency anaemia, a condition recalling that of the Plummer–Vinson (pp. 10, 375) syndrome of atrophic glossitis, oesophageal web and dysphagia.

Now read Leucoplakia (p. 207)

Crohn's disease

The appearance of a chronic ulcer of the lip or mouth may precede the recognition of intestinal disease. The ulcer is punctuated by islands of proliferating epithelium. The appearances recall those of the cobblestone structure of the chronic intestinal lesions. Biopsy confirms the presence of non-caseating granulomas encircled by clusters of lymphocytes.

Now read Crohn's disease (pp. 104, 165)

TUMOURS

The lips and mouth are susceptible to several classes of carcinogens including chemical and physical agents and viruses.

Benign

Squamous papilloma

Oral squamous papillomas closely resemble the warty lesions encountered in other sites and a papilloma virus (pp. 80, 340) aetiology is suspected. A central pedicle of vascular connective tissue is surmounted by well-differentiated stratified squamous epithelium.

Haemangioma

Haemangioma of the lip or mouth does not differ significantly in structure or behaviour from capillary haemangioma in other sites (p. 49).

Lymphangioma

Lymphangioma is occasionally recognised as a small, superficial, circumscribed, cyst-like focus.

Giant-cell epulis

Giant-cell epulis is a local proliferation of gingival fibrous tissue.

Giant-cell tumour

Giant-cell tumour of bone (Table 12, p. 58) may extend into the soft oral tissues and mimic fibrous epulis. Rarely, a localised lesion of osteitis fibrosa cystica can cause identical changes.

Malignant

Carcinoma

Carcinoma of the oral cavity and oropharynx accounts for 3 to 5% of all cancers. The annual incidence in England and Wales of mouth, lip and pharynx cancer together is ~$70/10^6$ persons. The prevalence has declined steeply since 1945. Ninety five per cent of oropharyngeal tumours are squamous carcinomas. The part played by HPV-16 is outlined on p. 340. There are a small number of lymphomas and sarcomas, while malignant melanoma (p. 227) is a rare but rapidly invasive tumour of the hard palate. In decreasing order of frequency, squamous carcinoma is found in the tongue (30%); lower lip (25%), floor of the mouth (15%) and the gingiva, cheek and palate (each 10%).

Causes

Epithelial dysplasia may be a precursor of oral and of pharyngeal cancer but progression from dysplasia to carcinoma *in-situ* and invasive cancer is not invariable. Particularly in the tongue and the floor of the mouth, both high risk sites, the early changes may regress.

- **Heredity**. The role of heredity is not established but a high prevalence in some Asian countries suggests a racial predisposition.
- **Environment**. Cancers of the tongue and lower lip are disorders of the elderly. Many more men than women are affected. Pipe and cigar smoking; tobacco and betel nut chewing; and the exposure (of the lower lip) to prolonged, strong sunlight; are among the known agents. There is an increased frequency of oral as well as pharyngeal cancer in the Plummer–Vinson syndrome (pp. 10, 257, 375). Contrary to earlier views, poor oral hygiene is not now believed to be a predisposing factor.

Structure

The appearances of carcinoma of the tongue and of the lip are similar but not identical.

- **Carcinoma of the tongue** originates most frequently in the middle third of the lateral border but other parts, including the posterior and upper surfaces, are occasionally implicated. The earliest recognisable changes are those of erythroplakia and induration; they progress to ulceration. The ulcer is characteristically bounded by raised, firm margins. On palpation, the extent of the tumour is usually found to be greater than the appearances suggest. Much the most frequent tumour is well-differentiated squamous carcinoma (p. 303). The tumour cells aggregate as epithelial pearls and there is active keratinisation. Poorly differentiated, anaplastic and small cell tumours are very uncommon.

- **Carcinoma of the lip** evolves in a similar manner, through epithelial dysplasia, to invasive carcinoma. The tumours form small, exophytic, localised masses which quickly ulcerate, retaining indurated margins and a firm base. The lower lip is affected much more often than the upper.

Behaviour and prognosis

Biopsy is a prerequisite for diagnosis and planned treatment. Tissue is excised from the edge of a lesion under general anaesthesia.

- **Carcinoma of the tongue** extends locally by penetrating the lingual basement membrane. Tumour cells pass directly to the adjacent soft tissues of the mouth and neck. Lymphatic permeation is early. In the case of the common, anterior tumours, unilateral lymph node metastasis takes place to the submental and submandibular nodes and thence to those of the lower neck. In the case of the rarer, posterior tumours, bilateral spread occurs to the upper cervical nodes. Blood-borne metastasis is commonplace and the deposits are recognised in bone, liver and other sites. The prognosis is poor. Tumours are staged by the TNM system. Those that are unilateral, of small size and without metastasis have a much better outlook than large, posterior tumours with bilateral lymph node involvement. There is a mean 5-year survival rate of no more than 25%. Treatment is by radical excision followed by irradiation.
- **Carcinoma of the lip** behaves in an analogous manner but its superficial position and easy recognition benefit prognosis. Early complaint enables swift biopsy and prompt diagnosis. In the absence of regional lymph node metastasis affecting the submental, submandibular or deep cervical nodes, the 5-year survival rate is at least 80–85%.

OVARY

Biopsy diagnosis of ovarian disease

When a general surgeon encounters an ovarian disease at laparoscopy or laparotomy, he/she should seek the assistance of a gynaecologist. In the absence of such expertise, difficult decisions may be required. The usual concern is the possibility of malignant change. The great majority of ovarian tumours are epithelial in origin. Diagnostically, any fluid that can be aspirated from the pouch of Douglas is highly likely to contain malignant cells. If the lesion is cystic, fluid may be aspirated from the cyst but the surgeon must then be prepared to control any bleeding that may occur. If the disease can be identified at laparotomy, a wedge biopsy should be taken. The results of treatment for ovarian cancer differ widely. Inexperienced surgeons should not undertake 'occasional' oophorectomy.

DEVELOPMENTAL AND CONGENITAL DISORDERS

Cysts

Functional, non-neoplastic cysts (p. 113) are frequent, proliferative, neoplastic cysts less so. Both types can rupture, twist or infarct.

Luteal cyst

Luteal cysts are lined by granulosal and thecal cells and contain yellow fluid or altered blood. They are usually single and asymptomatic but may rupture into the peritoneal cavity. There is slight haemorrhage.

Follicular cyst

Follicular cysts are frequently multiple and contain clear fluid. They are lined by granulosal cells and may secrete enough oestrogen to inhibit FSH secretion, with the subsequent production of anovulatory cycles and endometrial hyperplasia.

The **Stein–Leventhal syndrome** is a triad of infertility, obesity and hirsutism, in which polycystic ovaries secrete an excess of androstenedione.

Chocolate cyst

Chocolate cysts are a feature of endometriosis (p. 341).

Theca lutein cyst

Theca lutein cysts develop in the luteinised granulosa cells of atretic, ovarian follicles. The change occurs in women subject to the effects of excess gonadotrophic hormone secreted by hydatidiform moles or during gonadotrophin treatment.

TUMOURS

Ovarian **metastases** (p. 246) are often from gastric or colonic cancers. The deposits are frequently formed of signet-ring cells containing much mucin. When bilateral, the lesions are Krukenberg tumours (p. 373). There is debate as to whether the mode of spread is vascular or transcoelomic. The surface of the ovaries is often free of deposits and similar metastases have been found in patients with mucin-secreting carcinoma of the breast. Consequently, retrograde lymphatic or haematogenous spread may explain this mode of extension.

Primary tumours

In England and Wales, the annual incidence of primary malignant ovarian tumours is ~110/10^6 females. Primary tumours are often mixed cystic and solid masses that reach a very large size. The greater the extent of the solid component of the tumour, the more likely it is to be malignant.

The three main categories of primary, ovarian tumour that arise from specialised tissue, originate in the surface epithelium, the sex cords and the germ cells. Other uncommon tumours may originate in non-specialised stromal cells.

Surface epithelial tumours

The majority of ovarian tumours are epithelial. They arise from the coelomic surface. Benign and malignant categories are recognised but many of these tumours occupy an intermediate position and are described as tumours of low malignant potential. They have a limited capacity for invasion and a better prognosis than overt cancer.

Serous tumours

Serous tumours are the most frequent of all ovarian neoplasms. They are encountered between the ages of 30 and 40 years.

Sixty per cent of serous tumours are benign **cystadenomas** composed of thin walled cysts. Of these, one quarter is bilateral. Smaller tumours have a single cavity but larger tumours may be multiloculated. A single cell layer lines the cavity.

Serous **cystadenocarcinomas** have solid, papillary components that project into the cyst lumen. There is epithelial ingrowth and invasion of the stroma. The prognosis is poor and ultimately, almost all those with this form of ovarian cancer die from the effects of the tumour. Confined to the ovary, there is a 70–75% 5-year survival rate. When the capsule has been penetrated, the survival rate is ~13%. The tumour extends in contiguity through the cyst wall, thence throughout the peritoneal cavity so that the cancer may provoke intestinal obtruction or urinary bladder dysfunction. Regional lymph node involvement is frequent, distant metastasis less so.

Mucinous tumours

A total of 80% of mucinous **cystadenomas** is benign. They form abdominal cysts, sometimes of extraordinarily large size. The abdominal distension that they cause can be mistaken for ascites or even for pregnancy. Few cystadenomas are bilateral. On the peritoneal surface, the cells may continue to secrete mucin, resulting in pseudomyxoma peritonei (p. 347).

Mucinous **cystadenocarcinomas** are less likely to display invasive characteristics than serous cystadenocarcinoma. Many are multiloculated. The appearance and growth of solid islands of cells within the cyst is an index of malignancy. Extension of the tumour through the stroma and the cyst wall culminates in peritoneal seeding and pseudomyxoma peritonei. The prognosis is significantly better than for serous carcinomas and the 10-year survival rate is ~35%.

Other epithelial tumours

Further forms of epithelial ovarian tumour include endometrioid tumour, cystadenofibroma and Brenner tumour. Endometrioid tumours are solid or cystic. They are usually malignant.

Sex cord tumours

An important category of ovarian tumour is derived from the sex (germinal) cords.

Granulosa cell tumour

Granulosa cell tumour is the most frequent sex cord tumour. It is of low-grade malignancy, secreting large quantities of oestrogen. The consequences include precocious puberty in young girls and postmenopausal bleeding in elderly women.

Androblastoma

Androblastoma is composed of Sertoli cells or Leydig cells or, more commonly, an admixture of the two. Most are benign. They secrete an excess of androgens. These hormones lead to virilisation with breast atrophy; amenorrhoea; facial hirsutism; and clitoral enlargement.

Germ cell tumours

Dysgerminoma

Dysgerminomas are undifferentiated tumours, microscopically analogous to testicular seminoma (p. 318). The tumours soon metastasise to para-aortic lymph nodes.

Benign cystic teratoma

In this common tumour, a large cyst is filled with a viscous and gelatinous fluid. The cells of the solid cyst wall exhibit varying degrees of differentiation into organised embryonic tissues. The cysts are lined by squamous epithelial cells and contain hair follicles and hair. However, other tissues, particularly teeth, bone, cartilage and thyroid, are frequently present. Some cystic teratomas include only a single tissue and those in which only thyroid is represented are described as **struma ovarii**. Malignant transformation is rare.

Other tumours

Fibroma

Fibromas are common. They are occasionally associated with Meigs' syndrome (p. 374), a condition in which pleural and peritoneal effusions accompany the growth of fibroma. The cause of the effusions is not understood.

Stromal tumours

The cells comprising tumours of stromal origin retain a diverse potential for differentiation. One form of stromal tumour, **theca cell tumour**, secretes oestrogen. Unlike granulosa cell tumour, its behaviour is generally benign.

OXYGEN

Oxygen excess and oxygen deficiency may both lead to disease.

OXYGEN EXCESS

High concentrations of oxygen, or prolonged exposure to moderately increased concentrations of this gas, result in a state of oxygen toxicity. The local effects of oxygen excess include **retrolental fibroplasia**, a condition provoked by exposure of the premature infant to prolonged, high oxygen concentrations. In this infantile cause of blindness, retinal blood vessels dilate and retinal swelling is followed by detachment.

OXYGEN DEFICIENCY

Acute deprivation of oxygen, resulting, for example, from a loss of pressurisation in an aircraft, is rapidly fatal. Prolonged, partial oxygen deprivation leads to impaired tissue metabolism or to infarction, depending upon the degree and rapidity of the loss and the sensitivity of the tissues.

Cells and tissues are vulnerable to a reduction in the partial pressure of oxygen in their immediate micro-environment. They suffer damage to essential structures and, in particular, to cell membranes. The degree of sensitivity of different parts to reduced oxygen concentrations is identical to their sensitivity to ischaemia (p. 187), the effects of which are attributable to a diminished availability of oxygen. Thus, if a tourniquet is applied for ~2 hours, a patient experiences parasthesiae when the constriction is released. However, neurological recovery is the norm. Irreversible muscle damage occurs by 6 hours. Plastic surgical operations on limbs may take up to 8 hours and tourniquets are released every 2 hours during these procedures.

Now read Ischaemia (p. 187), Oxygen free radicals (p. 133)

P

PANCREAS

The exocrine and endocrine components of the pancreas are each subject to a distinct pattern of disease.

Biopsy diagnosis of pancreatic disease

The appearances of tissues viewed by endoscopic retrograde cholangiopancreatography (ERCP), computed tomography (CT), and magnetic resonance imaging (MRI), can yield more valuable information than aspiration cytology or biopsy.

The prime aim of biopsy and of aspiration cytology is to differentiate chronic pancreatitis from pancreatic cancer. Attempts at biopsy may be made both before and during laparotomy. In addition, bile and pancreatic juice and brushings from the biliary and pancreatic ducts can be obtained for cytological examination during ERCP.

Percutaneous fine-needle aspiration cytology is performed with ultrasound or computed tomographic guidance although many pancreatic lesions are small: even in expert hands, representative samples can be obtained in no more than 70% of patients.

At laparotomy, transduodenal needle biopsy and wedge biopsy may be performed to obtain a frozen tissue diagnosis.

DEVELOPMENTAL AND CONGENITAL DISORDERS

The pancreas develops from the foregut as ventral and dorsal buds. Each bud has an axial duct system (Fig. 48). After 2 months, the ventral part rotates and comes to lie next to the dorsal moiety, on the left side of the duodenum. The two channels fuse and form a main duct of Wirsung, which drains into the duodenum through the major pancreatic papilla. The residual portion of the dorsal duct becomes the accessory, Santorini's duct. The corresponding accessory or minor papilla is prone to partial or complete obliteration. When it remains patent, the risk of gallstone pancreatitis (p. 263) is reduced since the orifice acts as a valve, diminishing the pressure changes that occur when a gallstone impacts in the ampulla, blocking the main pancreatic duct.

Pancreas divisum

The dorsal and ventral duct systems fail to fuse in 4% of embryos. In the majority of individuals, pancreas divisum is of no consequence as the drainage of the dominant dorsal duct is sufficient. In some individuals, drainage through the minor papilla is inadequate. These patients are more likely than normal persons to develop acute or chronic pancreatitis.

Annular pancreas

In this uncommon anomaly, a portion or all of the dorsal duct and its associated parenchyma fails to rotate to the left and remains encircling the second part of the duodenum. The defect is more common in patients with trisomy 21 (p. 92) than in normal persons. In a few children, annular pancreas may cause neonatal duodenal obstruction but this condition does not predispose to acute or to chronic pancreatitis.

Heterotopic and ectopic pancreas

Heterotopic pancreatic tissue is occasionally present in the duodenum and less often in the stomach. Ectopic pancreatic tissue is infrequent but may be discovered at endoscopy or necropsy when it is found in the colon; vermiform appendix; Meckel's diverticulum; mesentery; and omentum. Ectopic pancreatic tissue results from metaplasia of the embryonic foregut endoderm.

Developmental cyst

Congenital cysts are rare. They are multiple, asymptomatic and associated with inherited polycystic disease of the kidney and liver. Enterogenous cysts that are

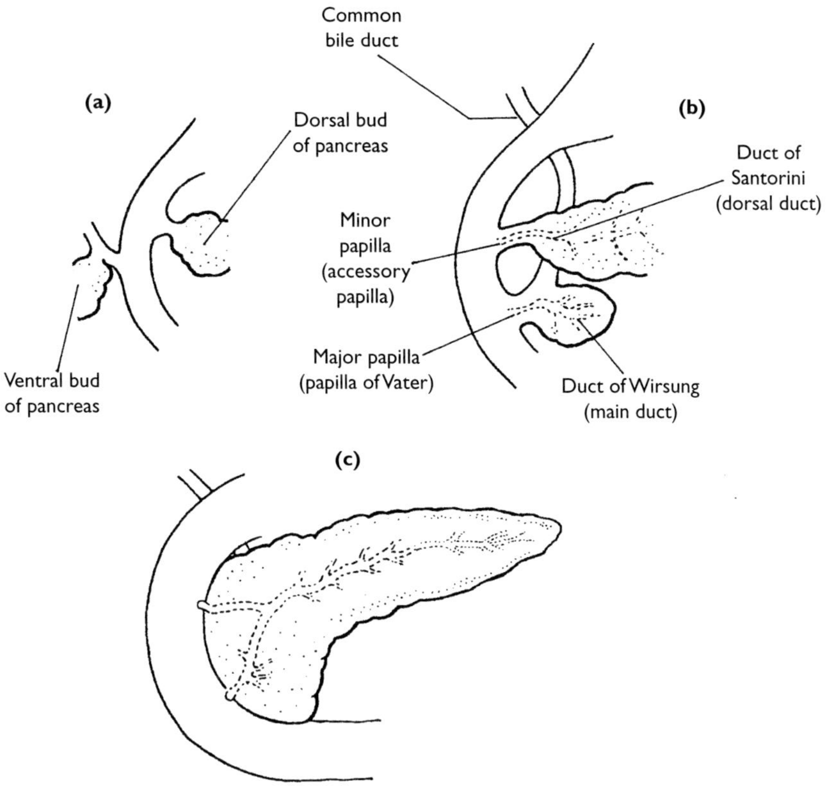

Figure 48 Pancreatic duct anomalies.
(a) Dorsal bud lies proximal and medial to ventral bud which is associated with bile duct.
(b) Ventral bud and bile duct rotate. They come to be immediately beyond dorsal bud.
(c) Ventral and dorsal buds fuse and form duct of Wirsung. Duct of Santorini does not always remain patent.

congenital duplications of the duodenum may be present in the head of the pancreas.

CALCULUS

Calculi containing calcium phosphate and carbonate are found occasionally in the major pancreatic ducts in patients with chronic pancreatitis.

INFECTION AND INFLAMMATION

Acute pancreatitis

In all countries, acute pancreatitis is becoming increasingly common. There are large geographical differences in prevalence. In the UK, the annual incidence is $150/10^6$ persons. In Finland, the incidence is $900/10^6$.

Causes

The increased frequency of acute pancreatitis reflects a rise in the incidence of cholelithiasis and alcoholism, particularly the latter (Table 50).

The initial mechanism is not understood nor is it known whether the provocative agent first takes effect within the pancreatic ducts, the interstitium or the glandular acini. It is, however, agreed that autodigestion begins within the pancreas. In the presence of cholelithiasis, obstruction to the outflow of pancreatic secretions is believed to be caused by a gallstone impacted in the ampulla of Vater. Reflux of bile into the pancreatic duct renders the mucosa permeable to

Table 50 Aetiological factors in acute pancreatitis. More than 90% of the cases are attributable to alcoholism or cholelithiasis

Alcoholism	Cholelithiasis
Abdominal cardiac and renal operations, including transplantation	ERCP
Direct trauma	Connective tissue disorders
Addictive drugs	Hypercalcaemia
Hyperlipidaemia	Hypothermia
Pancreas divisum	Viral infections, particularly mumps

macromolecules that activate pancreatic enzymes. Ethanol exerts a similar effect upon mucosal permeability.

Structure

There is oedema of the interstitial tissue and proteolytic destruction of the parenchyma, the process of autodigestion. Blood vessels are disrupted and zones of free haemorrhage appear, giving the gland a blue-black appearance. Fat necrosis occurs and may extend throughout the adipose tissue of the abdominal cavity. Saponification of tissue lipids takes place. Calcium combines with the fatty acids liberated by the action of pancreatic lipase on triacylglycerols, creating chalky, white deposits.

Islands of necrotic tissue become segregated from the duct system, forming cysts with no discernible epithelial lining. The contents of these pseudocysts are usually sterile, reflecting the activity of digestive and lysosomal enzymes; they may compress and obstruct the duodenum or the common bile duct. Larger cysts rupture into the peritoneal cavity, leading to peritonitis. Bacterial infection may involve all or part of the gland, leading to abscess. However, there may be complete resolution of the inflammatory process.

It was customary to divide the pathological features of acute pancreatitis into oedematous; haemorrhagic; and necrotising varieties, on the basis of increasing severity. However, these categories are difficult to correlate with the clinical features of the disorder.

Behaviour and prognosis

Acute pancreatitis produces severe physiological derangements throughout the body. They cannot be ascribed to simple translocation of fluid, the result of peritonitis. Adult respiratory distress syndrome (p. 219); acute renal tubular necrosis (p. 201); cardiogenic shock (p. 291); and disseminated intravascular coagulation (p. 119), can occur individually or as part of a multisystem, organ failure (p. 292). The mediators of this damage have not been identified but do not appear to originate within the pancreas. They may be derived from leucocytes.

When treatment has proved adequate in Western countries, death from acute tubular necrosis or cardiogenic shock is uncommon. The overall mortality rate, now 5–10%, is proportional to the extent of the disturbances measured by an injury scoring system such as APACHE (p. 264). The majority of patients who die succumb to pulmonary failure. A few patients have recurrent attacks. Occasionally, these repeated attacks progress to chronic disease.

Chronic pancreatitis

Chronic pancreatitis is a progressive inflammatory disorder with irreversible morphological changes often associated with permanent exocrine and endocrine insufficiency.

Causes

Alcoholism is responsible for ~85% of European cases of chronic pancreatitis. In a further ~15%, no cause can be found. They are 'idiopathic'.

The persistent, excessive consumption of ethanol is associated with pancreatic calcification. Gallstones are an uncommon cause of chronic disease but long-standing bile duct obstruction by a gallstone may lead to fibrous stenosis of the sphincter of Oddi. Hypercalcaemia due to hyperparathyroidism, or other causes, may be responsible for the formation of protein plugs within the pancreatic duct system. Similarly, calcification of mucus plugs appears to be a factor in the development of tropical pancreatitis. Other infrequent causes include pancreas divisum; cystic fibrosis; haemochromatosis; hypertriglyceridaemia; and hyperlipoproteinaemia.

Structure

The surface of the gland is irregular and hard. As fibrosis progresses, the gland becomes white and small. Calculi form in the ducts. There is atrophy of the exocrine glandular acini with inflammatory cell infiltration and fibrosis. The islets and ducts survive. The ducts are often dilated, containing inspissated mucus that may become calcified. The main duct is frequently much enlarged but there are many constrictions that can be recognised as a 'chain of lakes' on pancreatography. True cysts with an epithelial lining are common and arise behind a focus of duct obstruction.

Behaviour and prognosis

Exocrine insufficiency is not recognised until 95% of the parenchyma of the pancreas has been destroyed. Many patients with chronic pancreatitis develop insulin-dependent diabetes mellitus. In fewer than 5% of patients, obstruction of the distal part of the common bile duct by the inflammatory process culminates in obstructive jaundice. The integrity of the splenic vein may be prejudiced so that thrombosis occurs. As a result, hypersplenism develops, occasionally complicated by haemorrhage from gastric varices. There is a small increase in the frequency of pancreatic cancer.

TRANSPLANTATION

Transplantation of the body and tail of the pancreas has been made possible by the development of effective immunosuppressive drugs. The one-year graft survival is ~80%. Because of the high frequency of arteriolar and glomerular disease in diabetes mellitus, the operation is now usually combined with renal transplantation. Transplantation of the pancreatic islets is an alternative but largely unsuccessful procedure (p. 117).

TUMOURS

Tumours originate in the endocrine and in the exocrine pancreas. The sources of the exocrine tumours are the acinar or ductal cells. Ninety per cent of primary tumours of the pancreas are ductal adenocarcinomas. All the epithelial elements of the pancreas are derived from endodermal stem cells and, consequently, pancreatic tumours are often composite. They include acinar, ductal and endocrine components. Because of differences in prognosis, it is essential that the clinician and pathologist distinguish between malignant tumours arising from the distal common bile duct; from the pancreatic duct in the head of the pancreas; from the ductal cells of the papilla of Vater; and from the duodenum.

EXOCRINE

Benign

Papillary adenoma

This is a rare tumour occurring late in life and causing obstruction of the pancreatic duct.

Cystadenoma

Cystadenoma comprises only 1% of pancreatic tumours.

- **Serous cystadenoma** occur in elderly women. Those in the head of the pancreas lead to biliary and pancreatic obstruction; those in the body and tail are asymptomatic.
- **Mucinous cystic tumours** occur in middle-aged women. They are located in the tail of the pancreas and form abdominal masses.

Malignant

Carcinoma

The prevalence of this tumour in Western countries has doubled in the past 40 years. There is an annual incidence of ~$100/10^6$ population. It is frequent in the elderly and is more common in males than in females.

Causes

Race, cigarette smoking, alcohol and coffee may be aetiological factors. The associations are not strong.

Structure

More than 80% of the tumours occur in the head of the gland or uncinate process, resulting in obstructive jaundice. Concurrent obstruction to the pancreatic duct occasionally provokes acute pancreatitis. The tumour comprises a hard, ill-defined, pale, yellow–white mass distinguished with difficulty from the surrounding normal pancreatic tissue. Well-differentiated tumours predominate. They are formed of glandular acini in which the cells have large, deeply-staining nuclei displaying loss of nuclear polarity, an excess of mitotic figures and nuclear pleomorphism. Poorly differentiated tumours merge as groups or attenuated columns of cells within the collagenous connective tissue that gives the carcinoma its firm, 'scirrhous' character. Variants of pancreatic carcinoma include serous and mucinous cystadenocarcinoma.

- **Serous cystadenocarcinoma** displays a characteristic honeycomb or spongy appearance due to the presence of numerous small, fluid-containing cavities. The cysts are lined by cuboidal or columnar epithelium with papillary projections. The cytoplasm is clear and contains glycogen. The lesion may be mistaken for a pseudocyst.

- **Mucinous cystadenocarcinoma** forms a large and well-circumscribed mass with multilocular cysts containing mucin. Calcification is common. There is a desmoplastic reaction and the fibrous tissue contains duct-like structures with various degrees of differentiation. The tumour acini are lined by columnar epithelium including goblet and argentaffin cells.

Behaviour and prognosis

Tumours in the head of the gland spread directly to involve the uncinate process, the duodenum and the superior mesenteric and portal veins. Spread to regional lymph nodes has already occurred in the majority of patients coming to surgery. Carcinomas of the body and tail of the pancreas do not cause jaundice and are not recognised easily: by the time of diagnosis, the disease is extensive and resection rarely possible.

The 5-year survival of those undergoing resection is ~5%. Tumour cells are conveyed to the liver in the venous circulation and death is the result of hepatic metastasis. This sequence also accounts for the mode of death in ~60% of patients with stage I disease who have undergone 'curative' resection.

ENDOCRINE

Endocrine tumours of the pancreas have a circumscribed margin, a faint red colour and a firm consistence. These characteristics reflect their generally benign, encapsulated structure; their high vascularity; and the presence of a fibrous microskeleton. The majority do not secrete hormones actively although their hormone precursors can frequently be demonstrated by immunohistochemical techniques.

Insulinoma

Insulinomas constitute 75% of the endocrine tumours. They are small, solitary and benign and are more common in the body and tail than in the head of the gland. Immunoassays demonstrate inappropriately elevated plasma insulin concentrations accompanied by low concentrations of glucose.

Gastrinoma

Gastrinomas arise from pancreatic G-cells. They account for 20% of pancreatic endocrine tumours. The excess secretion of gastrin leads to the Zollinger–Ellison syndrome (pp. 121, 363). Nine of 10 gastrinomas arise in the head of the pancreas, the duodenum or the porta hepatis. By the time of diagnosis, most have metastasised to the liver. When part of a MEN syndrome (p. 126), gastrinoma is often multiple.

Glucagonoma

Glucagonomas are large, solitary tumours. Many are malignant. They are more common in adult females than in males. The hyposecretion of glucagon results in abnormal glucose tolerance.

VIPoma

Named after **V**aso-active **I**ntestinal **P**olypeptide, so-called VIPomas account for 3% of pancreatic endocrine tumours. They lead to the Verner–Morrison syndrome of **W**atery **D**iarrhoea, **H**ypokalaemia and **A**chlorhydria, alternatively designated the WDHA syndrome. More than half are malignant.

Other endocrine tumours

Tumours secreting somatostatin and pancreatic polypeptide are rare.

Now read Hormones; Multiple endocrine neoplasia (p. 126)

PAPILLOMA

A papilloma is a nipple-shaped or stalked, benign neoplasm of epithelium. Papillomas may be villous or seaweed-like, as in the urinary bladder, or sessile and less prominent, as on weight-bearing skin.

The term **'papillary'** is applied to other structures, including carcinomas, to describe their shape and histological pattern. Examples include papillary cystadenocarcinoma of the ovary (p. 260) and papillary carcinoma of the thyroid (p. 325).

PARATHYROID GLANDS

Biopsy diagnosis of parathyroid disease

Convention dictates that there are four parathyroid glands but there may be as many as eight. They can be difficult to identify. Occasionally, one or more is located within the mediastinum. Pre-operative MRI has revolutionised the localisation of those glands that are in the neck. ^{99m}Tc-MIBI (p. 170) may aid the identification of glands elsewhere.

Repetitive biopsy samples are examined at once, by intra-operative frozen section, enabling the distinction of parathyroid glands from foci of lymphoid, thyroid and other tissue. Expert histopathologists can differentiate between hyperplasia or adenoma on the one hand, and carcinoma on the other. The differentiation of adenoma from hyperplasia may be difficult. If an adenoma is not found and the diagnosis is of hyperplasia, the surgeon must identify all the glands and remove what is judged to be an appropriate proportion of functioning parathyroid tissue.

HYPERPARATHYROIDISM

Primary hyperparathyroidism

Causes

In 85% of instances, the cause of primary hyperparathyroidism is the presence of a single or, occasionally, two functioning adenomas. In a further 12%, the disease results from unexplained hyperplasia. Functioning carcinoma accounts for only 3% of cases. Primary hyperparathyroidism may also be caused by the inappropriate secretion of excess parathormone from functioning, non-parathyroid tumours. It is a feature of MEN 1 and MEN 2 (p. 126).

Structure

Parathyroid adenoma resembles other endocrine tumours. On average, it is 100–120 mg in weight, red–brown, highly vascular and bounded by a capsule of compressed normal glandular tissue. Parathyroid carcinoma is distinguished from adenoma by a firm consistence, adhesion to nearby structures and recognisable infiltration at the tumour margin. Microscopically, there is a predominance of chief cells and varying proportions of oxyphil and transitional cells.

Behaviour and prognosis

The effects of hyperparathyroidism are first recognised by the insidious onset of systemic symptoms such as fatigue and nausea. Diagnosis is confirmed by raised plasma levels of parathormone or by elevated calcium and lowered phosphate concentrations, changes that are particularly pronounced in cases of parathyroid carcinoma. Untreated disease results in the ectopic calcification of renal tubules and blood vessel walls. Renal calculi, peptic ulceration and pancreatitis are frequent. Eventually, skeletal changes are detected. They include osteoporosis and osteitis fibrosa cystica (p. 51).

Secondary hyperparathyroidism

Secondary hyperparathyroidism is the result of persistent hypocalcaemia. It is caused by chronic renal disease with impaired phosphate excretion and hyperphosphataemia. There is a low concentration of plasma calcium and hyperplasia of the parathyroid glands. The four or more parathyroid glands enlarge, not necessarily uniformly. Enlargement is due to chief cell hyperplasia or, less often, to clear cell change. Ultimately, one or more adenomas develop within the enlarged glands in a process of **tertiary hyperparathyroidism**. The skeletal changes of the primary, secondary and tertiary forms of hyperparathyroidism are identical.

Now read Osteitis fibrosa cystica (p. 51)

HYPOPARATHYROIDISM

Parathyroid atrophy and hypoplasia are rare. The parathyroid glands may, however, be excised accidentally at thyroidectomy. Tetany (p. 319) due to hypocalcaemia is one result.

PENIS

Biopsy diagnosis

The principles of diagnosis do not differ from those followed in diseases of the skin or of the urinary tract.

DEVELOPMENTAL AND CONGENITAL DISORDERS

Rarely, the organ may be absent or of excessive or diminished size. The urethra may be duplicated or open upon the upper (**epispadias**) or lower (**hypospadias**) surface. Other defects, recognised in infancy, include stricture; meatal stenosis; phimosis; the presence of urethral valves; or diverticulum.

INFECTION AND INFLAMMATION

The penis is susceptible to infections by *Candida albicans*, Streptococcus spp., *Chlamydia trachomatis*, *Trichomonas vaginalis* and *Neisseria gonorrhoeae* (the gonococcus), as well as to skin pathogens that include *Staphylococcus aureus*. Primary chancre attributable to *Treponema pallidum* is now seldom seen in Western countries. HHV infection is occasionally identified.

Fibromatosis

Peyronie's disease is analogous to other forms of fibromatosis (p. 130).

Paget's disease

The appearances closely resemble those of Paget's disease described at other sites (p. 68).

TUMOURS

Primary tumours of the penis are very uncommon. The only tumour of significant frequency is squamous carcinoma.

Squamous carcinoma

Causes

Squamous carcinoma, is a rare tumour in Western countries where it accounts for <2% of all male cancers. It is relatively frequent in some African and Central American communities. Dysplasia, presenting as **Queyrat's erythroplasia** (p. 207), is a predisposing factor. The recognition of carcinoma-*in-situ* may warn of the development of invasive carcinoma.

Structure

The tumour is a firm or hard, fixed nodular and ulcerating mass, seen on the glans. Biopsy reveals a well-differentiated squamous carcinoma (p. 303).

Behaviour and prognosis

The tumour extends first to the corpora cavernosa, subsequently to the corpus spongiosum and urethra. Enlarged regional lymph nodes may, however, be due not to metastasis but to persistent and coincidental, chronic inflammation. Subsequently, blood-borne metastasis is via the periprostatic venous plexus and pelvic veins to the paravertebral plexus and thence to the systemic circulation. Treatment is by amputation. The prognosis depends greatly upon the TNM stage. The 5-year survival is >50%.

VASCULAR DISEASE

Thrombosis of the corpora cavernosa is one cause of priapism, a disorder that may occur spontaneously, or as a result of neurological disease, or in thrombotic or occlusive vascular states including leukaemia; systemic neoplasia; sickle-cell disease; and local forms of inflammation.

The penis may be implicated in Fournier's gangrene (pp. 136, 374).

PERITONEUM

The peritoneal cavity is a serous sac the lining of which is a thin, mesothelial lamina together with a very small quantity of subserosal, connective tissue. The surfaces are separated by a liquid film. The sac therefore constitutes a complex, potential space that becomes engorged with fluid in ascites (p. 251). The peritoneum is closely attached to the surfaces of the underlying viscera, enveloping the abdominal organs and covering their parietal surfaces and those of the abdominal cavity. For reasons of practical convenience, the peritoneal space is subdivided into several compartments such as the greater and lesser sacs, and the left and right subphrenic spaces.

Biopsy diagnosis of peritoneal disease

Cytological examination of ascitic fluid may reveal evidence of suspected peritoneal disease. Biopsy of lesions under laparoscopic vision is more accurate than the analysis of aspirated fluid and often reveals unsuspected minute metastases in patients with neoplastic disease of the pancreas and ovary.

DEVELOPMENTAL AND CONGENITAL DISORDERS

Cysts

Mesenteric and other cysts are encountered in the peritoneum and peritoneal recesses.

INFECTION AND INFLAMMATION

The responses of the peritoneum mirror the inflammatory, infective and neoplastic disorders that occur within the superficial parts of the organs and tissues that it covers. Localised infection within the compartments of the peritoneum often results in abscess formation.

Peritonitis

Peritonitis is generalised or localised inflammation of the vascular tissues covered by the peritoneum.

Causes

Diffuse peritonitis, with or without abscess formation, is usually attributable to acute appendicitis; cholecystitis; colonic diverticultitis; salpingitis; or perforation of a viscus. However, in 20% of instances, the site of origin of the infection is not known. The three most frequent causes of diffuse, bacterial peritonitis are *Escherichia coli*, *Bacteroides fragilis* and the enterococci. *Streptococcus milleri* may also be implicated. *E. coli* plays a crucial part in the acute ('septic') phase of many examples of intra-abdominal infection while *B. fragilis* promotes the late complications of abscess formation. The acute peritonitis that accompanies salpingitis is attributable to *Neisseria gonorrhoeae* while chronic salpingitis may be due to *Mycobacterium tuberculosis*.

Structure

The changes are those of acute, exudative inflammation, with an outpouring of a fibrin-rich exudate; hyperaemia of peritoneal tissues; pus formation; and abscess.

Behaviour and prognosis

Acute peritonitis leads to paralytic ileus with hypovolaemic shock. There is a severe loss of water. Electrolyte disturbances result from vomiting. In addition, there are local changes in gut absorption and a loss of fluid into the intestines. The inevitable escape of fluid into the peritoneal cavity itself constitutes a so-called 'third-space' loss. The gut mucosa becomes permeable to bacterial toxins so that endotoxic shock and multiple organ systemic failure (p. 292) may supervene.

Acute peritonitis may respond to antibiotics and to the correction of fluid and electrolyte imbalance. Nevertheless, there is often an overriding demand for adequate surgical treatment of the underlying cause. In community-acquired peritonitis, most of the organisms isolated are susceptible to a combination of co-amoxiclavulonate and gentamicin or to cephalosporin and metronidazole. In nosocomial infections, resistant organisms are common among patients undergoing multiple operations. The most frequent of these organisms are methicillin-resistant *Staphylococcus aureus* (MRSA), *Pseudomonas aeruginosa*, multiresistant Klebsiella, *E. coli*, Serratia and Acinetobacter. The mortality rate for those with susceptible organisms is 16% compared to a rate of 45% in those with resistant organisms.

Foci of inflammation and abscesses are bounded by fibrous tissue and localised to the pelvic or subphrenic regions. Eventually, the fibrous adhesions arising in this way bind loops of bowel and viscera together. The possible consequences include kinking of the bowel; mechanical obstruction; hernia; and volvulus. The mortality rate reflects the nature of the underlying cause.

Pelvic abscess

This is the most frequent form of intra-abdominal abscess. It is occasionally due to infected fluid tracking from upper abdominal conditions such as perforated peptic ulcer. However, most pelvic abscesses are attributable to lower abdominal infections. They include appendicitis; sigmoid diverticulitis; regional enteritis; and salpingitis. Many pelvic abscesses drain spontaneously into the rectum. Occasionally, pus escapes into the vagina. The formation of adhesions involving loops of terminal ileum is a common consequence of pelvic abscess.

Subphrenic abscess

When peritoneal infection and abscess arise in or near the diaphragm, there is a tendency for pus to accumulate beneath the right or left dome, provoking subphrenic abscess. Among the causes are undiagnosed acute appendicitis; perforated peptic ulcer; liver abscess; and leaking anastomoses following operations within the upper abdomen.

Now read Abscess (p. 1)

TUMOURS

The peritoneum is frequently the site for:

- The direct spread of malignant tumours from nearby viscera.
- The indirect, transcoelomic spread of tumours across opposed peritoneal surfaces.
- Distant metastasis of which Krukenberg tumour is one example (pp. 260, 373). Pseudomyxoma peritonei is described on p. 247.

Retroperitoneal tumours

A number of soft tissue sarcomas originate in the connective tissue of the retroperitoneal spaces. They include liposarcoma (p. 299) and rhabdomyosarcoma (p. 236).

PHAGOCYTOSIS

Phagocytosis is the ingestion by a cell of foreign solids or of altered, autologous solids. It is characteristic of mononuclear macrophages, histiocytes and neutrophil polymorphs but may be displayed by B lymphocytes, Kupffer cells, endothelial cells and many other cell forms. Phagocytosis is an important end stage of apoptosis (p. 89).

The response may be local or systemic. When there is a systemic response, the splenic sinus cells, continually vigorous as scavengers for circulating cell debris, and in the removal of effete and aged cells, are among those activated. The most common materials ingested by phagocytosis are old red blood cells; injured or anoxic body cells; bacteria; immune complexes; and foreign bodies ranging from insoluble fibres, polymers and metals, to crystals.

The cell membrane of a phagocyte throws out a pseudopod-like process that closes around an object such as a bacterium, to form a vacuole, the phagosome. The phagocytic vacuole unites with a lysosome. Lysosomal enzymes at once begin to degrade the vacuolar contents.

Lysosomes (p. 225) are storehouses of inactive, degradative enzymes that are activated when exposed to an appropriate substrate at acid pH. The enzymes include a nuclease; cathepsin B; glucuronidase; a collagenase; and plasminogen. The enzymes are activated during phagocytosis. **Endocytosis** of a small foreign object such as a bacterium results in the formation of a phagosome, with which the lysosomal membrane fuses to form a phagolysosome. The lysosomal enzymes are activated within the phagolysosome. Digestion of the foreign solid follows.

Within the cell, micro-organisms are killed or inactivated by free radicals (p. 133); by nitric oxide (p. 134); by defensins; by proteolytic enzymes; and by other, oxygen-independent mechanisms. Digestion of the killed micro-organisms or of engulfed solids takes place within the phagosome and is brought about by acid hydrolases. The products of digestion are excreted from the cell by **exocytosis**, a process of 'reverse phagocytosis'. If digestion is incomplete, residual living or inert objects may remain within the phagocyte indefinitely. The tubercle bacillus is an example of the former, haemosiderin of the latter. The carbon that accumulates in pulmonary and splenic lymphoid tissue originates in this way, rendering the pulmonary and lymphoid tissues of city dwellers permanently grey–black.

Defects of phagocytosis, and thus of bacterial destruction, arise when cytotoxic drugs or ionising radiations deplete the bone marrow of leucocyte precursors. Rarely, defective phagocytosis is encountered in inherited oxidase deficiencies, for example in chronic granulomatous disease.

Now read Inflammation (p. 179), Macrophages (p. 225)

PHARYNX

Biopsy diagnosis of pharyngeal disease

Lesions of the oropharynx and hypopharynx may be apparent both upon indirect mirror examination and with flexible or rigid endoscopy. Reliance upon a single method may result in a failure to identify a lesion but the likelihood of error varies with the site. Accurate localisation is recorded upon printed diagrams. Cells or tissue may then be obtained with a spatula, a scalpel or biopsy forceps.

DIVERTICULUM

The pharynx is the site of diverticula caused either by compressive forces acting on a zone of weakness within the pharyngeal wall, or by tensile forces drawing the wall outwards. There are three anatomical categories.

- **Pulsion**. Pharyngeal pulsion diverticulum, or **pharyngeal pouch**, is a protrusion of the mucosa and submucosa between the oblique fibres of the inferior constrictor muscle and the transverse fibres of the cricopharyngeus. Undigested food collects within a pouch and causes dysphagia. Pulmonary aspiration (p. 217) and chest infections may culminate in lung abscess.
- **Lateral pharyngeal**. A variant of pharyngeal pouch, this is a much less common abnormality that may be congenital or acquired. In the former case, the defect is recognised in the tonsillar fossa or pyriform recess. It arises at the site of the first, second and third branchial clefts. In the latter, injury or infection promote a defect in the pyriform recess.
- **Traction**. As infected and inflamed lymph nodes undergo fibrosis, the collagenous tissue contracts and draws the pharyngeal wall outwards. Tuberculous lymphadenitis is one well-recognised cause.

PIGMENTATION

Pigmentation is the coloration or discoloration of tissues by the formation or deposition of a coloured substance.

Pigmentation may be generalised or localised. The physiological pigments are organic compounds. They often contain metals such as iron or copper.

- **Generalised**, physiological, yellow, brown or black skin pigmentation is usually racial; there is much melanin in the basal layer of the epidermis. It is exaggerated in Caucasian races by chronic exposure to ultraviolet light and is common in pregnancy when it is termed **chloasma**. The prolonged, excessive ingestion of foods such as carrots can result in a temporary, yellow skin coloration due to the accumulation of large quantities of carotene.
- **Localised** melanin pigmentation is recognised in the axillary and perineal skin and in the facial skin of white persons exposed to excess sunlight.

PIGMENTATION DISEASES

Abnormal pigmentation may be genetic or environmental in origin, generalised or localised in distribution.

Haemoglobin derivatives

- **Carboxyhaemoglobinaemia and methaemoglobinaemia**. Smoking one cigarette leads to a measurable increase in the concentration of carboxyhaemoglobin (HbCO) in the blood. The presence of larger amounts of this haemoglobin derivative is sufficient to change the colour of the blood to a persistent, bright pink. In methaemoglobinaemia, the blood appears a dull blue. The tissues are correspondingly discoloured, simulating cyanosis.
- **Haemosiderosis**. Excess iron is stored as the brown pigment haemosiderin. Generalised haemosiderosis can follow parenteral iron therapy; multiple transfusions of blood (p. 47); and haemolysis (p. 145). In haemochromatosis (p. 117), some of the pigment is haemosiderin, some lipofuscin and some melanin. Localised aggregates occur in haematomas (contusions).
- **Jaundice**. Jaundice is described on p. 189.
- **Porphyria**. Porphyrins are tetrapyrroles, natural components of haemoglobin. Small quantities of iron-free porphyrins are present normally in the plasma and the urine. In hereditary porphyria, abnormal quantities are formed. The skin becomes photosensitive and neurological disorder with mania may develop, as in the case of King George III. If the urine is left standing, it turns a deep red colour. Porphyria may be acquired as a consequence of the ingestion of some metals, organic agents or drugs.

Foreign substances

- **Inorganic pigments.** The prolonged ingestion of silver compounds is one example of the effects of inorganic substances and metals. It results in a permanent, grey–blue discoloration of the tissues, argyria.
- **Tattooing.** This is a Tahitian word. It implies the production of indelible markings in the skin. Deliberate tattooing is usually decorative. It is brought about by puncturing the skin and inserting pigments such as carbon (black) and mercuric sulphide (red). The process introduces the hazard of HBV infection (p. 2) since the needles are rarely sterilised adequately.

  Accidental tattooing occurs around entry wounds caused by gunshots (p. 358) at close range.
- **Organic pigments.** The consequences of prolonged exposure to organic substances are shown by the pigmentation of the skin that resulted from the occupational exposure to trinitrotoluene (TNT) during the manufacture of this explosive.

DEPIGMENTATION

Generalised lack of pigment is characteristic of **albinism**. There is a genetic deficiency of tyrosinase. Localised depigmentation, **vitiligo**, is the focal absence of melanocytes.

PITUITARY GLAND, ANTERIOR

The anterior pituitary gland (adenohypophysis) develops from the upward growth of the embryonic oral cavity. The endocrine cells of the anterior pituitary are:

- Growth hormone (somatostatin) (GH) – secreting somatotrophs.
- Prolactin (PRL) – secreting lactotrophs.
- Adrenocorticotrophic hormone (ACTH) – secreting corticotrophs.
- Follicle-stimulating hormone (FSH) – secreting gonadotrophs.
- Luteinising hormone (LH) – secreting gonadotrophs.
- Thyroid-stimulating hormone (TSH) – secreting thyrotrophs.

VASCULAR DISEASE

Because of a tenuous arterial blood supply, the anterior pituitary gland is prone to the effects of ischaemia. Infarction is one result of large, prolonged falls in arterial blood supply. **Sheehan's syndrome** of hypopituitarism may be a consequence of anterior pituitary gland ischaemia after postpartum haemorrhage. It may also follow cardiogenic and other forms of shock.

TUMOURS

Adenoma is the most frequent disorder of the anterior pituitary gland. There are two distinct results: anatomical and functional.

- **Structure.** The lesion is space-occupying. It slowly destroys nearby bone and compresses the optic chiasma, restricting the temporal parts of the visual fields and culminating in blindness.
- **Function.** There is an overproduction of hormones that may precipitate characteristic endocrine syndromes. Functioning tumours usually secrete excess growth hormone (GH). Excess GH may also be released by the action of growth hormone releasing factor (GRF) secreted, for example, by an islet cell tumour of the pancreas. Occasionally, functioning pituitary adenomas secrete other hormones such as TSH. Hyperprolactinaemia, the result of excess PRL secretion from a functioning adenoma, causes amenorrhoea and infertility in women. In men, the signs are those of a local, space-occupying lesion of the pituitary gland together with gynaecomastia.

ENDOCRINE CONSEQUENCES

Acromegaly

Acromegaly (Gk '*akron*': extremity, '*megas*': great) describes the large hands, feet, jaw and face that are consequences of the secretion of excess growth hormone (GH) in those whose skeletons have reached maturity. The viscera are also enlarged. When such a neoplasm liberates excess GH before the growth of the long bones has ceased, the condition of **gigantism** follows.

The term **local gigantism** describes the excessive growth of an appendage, for example a finger or a limb. However, the congenital presence of an enlarged limb or part, or an increase in size, is occasionally attributable to other disorders such as neurofibromatosis (p. 250) (von Recklinghausen's disease) or a large arteriovenous fistula.

Cushing's disease

Cushing's disease is a specific disorder of the anterior pituitary gland. It is a consequence of excess ACTH release, usually from an ACTH-secreting corticotrophic cell pituitary adenoma but sometimes from hyperplasia of these cells. The result is hyperstimulation of the adrenal cortices. There is diffuse or nodular cortical hyperplasia and the release of excess glucocorticoid (p. 6). The clinical signs closely resemble those of Cushing's syndrome (p. 6).

Now read Adrenal cortex (p. 5)

PITUITARY GLAND, POSTERIOR

The posterior pituitary gland or neurohypophysis, structurally and functionally distinct from the anterior pituitary gland, develops from a downward growth of cells from the floor of the third ventricle. The gland secretes two polypeptide hormones, oxytocin and vasopressin, synthesised in the supra-optic and paraventricular nuclei, respectively. The hormones are attached to carrier proteins, the **neurophysins,** and conveyed to the posterior pituitary gland within the nerve fibres of the hypophysopituitary tract.

Destruction of, or injury to, the posterior pituitary gland by head injury; infection; granulomatous disease; tumour; or haemorrhagic shock is likely to result in **diabetes insipidus**.

PLATELETS

Platelets are convex, anucleate cells, 2–5 μm in diameter. They are formed by the disintegration of megakaryocytes, giant cells (p. 142) with 184 chromosomes. Each megakaryocyte has a single, multilobed nucleus and gives rise to more than 3000 platelets. Normally, there are 150 to 350 × 10^9 platelets/L in blood. They are vigorously contractile, 15 to 20% of their protein being actomyosin. Platelets are phagocytic, have granules that are lysosomal, and dense bodies containing calcium, ADP and 5-HT.

The platelet membrane has an associated phospholipid, platelet factor 3, part of the blood clotting mechanism (p. 95). The platelet adhesion receptor $\alpha_{IIIb}\beta_3$ is one of 20 integrins (p. 88). Platelet activation ensues as cells engage these adhesive ligands or encounter soluble agonists such as thrombin, ADP or noradrenaline. The hallmark of platelet activation is the metamorphosis of $\alpha_{IIIb}\beta_3$ to its active state when it serves as a receptor for the soluble proteins, fibrinogen and vWF (p. 100).

Platelets have two distinct haemostatic functions:

- The prevention of leakage of red cells from sites of minor endothelial damage.
- The formation of thrombus.

To correct a deficiency of platelets, the fresh cells are given in concentrated suspension, by transfusion (p. 45). However, stored platelets survive less than 24 hours.

Now read Coagulation (p. 95), Platelet disease (p. 99)

PLEURA

Biopsy diagnosis of pleural disease

Pleural disease can be identified by examination of fluid aspirated from the thoracic cavities. The cytological changes call for expert opinion since macrophages, for example, may readily be mistaken for tumour cells. Fine-needle aspiration biopsy enables lung tissue to be sampled. Thoracoscopy and thoracotomy provide an opportunity for overt lesions to be examined. Bronchial and lung biopsy are described on pp. 69 and 214.

TUMOURS

Benign

Fibroma

Pleural fibroma is a very uncommon, benign tumour with a capacity for intrathoracic but not systemic spread. The tumour, pedunculated and either parietal or visceral, may be as much as 60 mm in diameter by the time of diagnosis. The development of hypertrophic pulmonary osteo-arthropathy or episodes of hypoglycaemia, evidence of ectopic hormone secretion, may constitute the first evidence of tumour growth. The fibroma is formed of spindle cells growing in a collagen-rich stroma within which are abnormally thick-walled blood vessels. The prognosis is good.

Malignant

Mesothelioma

Malignant mesothelioma is a malignant tumour of the mesothelial cells of the pleura and peritoneum. It is a disease of modern, industrial society.

Causes

There are fewer than 500 cases each year in the UK (~$9/10^6$ persons) yet the tumour has attracted interest out of proportion to its global importance. This is because of the proven association between the development of the tumour and exposure to a family of inorganic fibrous minerals, collectively called asbestos (p. 27). Signs of the tumour may first emerge as long as 30 or more years after the last exposure to this carcinogen. Males are affected much more often than females. There is a clustering of cases near manufacturing plants and examples have been recognised in nearby populations. Cigarette smoking enhances the hazard.

Structure

Malignant mesothelioma arises at the pleural surface of the lung at sites to which asbestos fibres have been conveyed. The lung is encased in broad, deep sheets of dense fibrous tissue. The tumour is rich in collagen and the material covering the surfaces of the lungs may be as much as 20 mm in thickness. Much less often, an analogous mesothelial response is elicited in the peritoneum. Similar, but smaller, localised plaques are found on the peritoneal surface of organs including the spleen.

Four categories of tumour are recognised: epithelial; sarcomatous; mixed; and undifferentiated. The spindle, or epithelial-like cells of malignant mesothelioma have distinctive appearances and react positively for vimentin and cytokeratin but negatively for carcino-embryonic antigen (CEA – p. 247).

Behaviour and prognosis

Tumour spread is via the bloodstream to distant sites and only a minority of cases display regional lymph node involvement. Treatment of pleural mesothelioma is by pneumonectomy. There is little response to chemotherapy or radiotherapy although combination treatment may offer alleviation. The prognosis of pleural and peritoneal mesothelioma is poor. Malignant mesothelioma is an aggressive tumour and there are few 5-year survivors.

Now read Asbestos (p. 27)

Askin tumour

Askin tumour is a rare disorder, principally affecting young females. It is of peripheral neuro-ectodermal origin. There are analogies with Ewing's sarcoma, with which Askin tumour shares a common chromosomal translocation, and with other small cell tumours.

The tumour forms a soft tissue mass within the chest wall or in peripheral lung tissue. Closely similar tumours may be found, however, in the head and neck; the arms or legs; the retroperitoneum; or the pelvis. Askin tumour comprises small, round or ovoid, undifferentiated cells. The distinction from neuroblastoma; Ewing's tumour; embryonal rhabdomyosarcoma, and lymphoma can be made by immunohistochemical tests and electron microscopy. The prognosis is less good than with Ewing's tumour and the 5-year survival rate in response to surgical excision, combined chemotherapy and radiotherapy, is no more than 50%.

MECHANICAL AND TRAUMATIC DISORDERS

Hydrothorax

Excess fluid in a pleural cavity, hydrothorax, results from:

- Increased capillary pressure, a change encountered in left- or right-sided cardiac failure.
- Enhanced capillary permeability as in acute inflammation.
- A decreased concentration of circulating plasma proteins (Appendix Table).
- Defective lymphatic drainage.

Thus, the collection of fluid may be an exudate or a transudate (p. 251). In the presence of tumour, the fluid is often haemorrhagic.

Empyema thoracis is pus in a pleural cavity (p. 1).

Chylothorax

Chylothorax is the accumulation of lymphatic, chylous fluid within a pleural cavity.

Chylothorax is a result of obstruction to, or transection of the thoracic duct or right bronchomediastinal lymphatic trunk. The causes of this rare condition are usually trauma, infection or metastatic tumour. The duct may be injured surgically, but abrupt hyperextension of the spine may have the same effect and obstruction by tuberculous lymph nodes is a further cause. Untreated, specific nutritional deficiencies may evolve. Protein malnutrition is one consequence and there is a possibility that lymphocyte depletion may result.

Haemothorax

Haemothorax is a collection of blood in a pleural cavity. The principal causes are direct injury by sharp objects, such as fractured ribs; and metastatic or primary lung carcinoma. Disruption of the coagulation mechanism (p. 95) underlies some cases so that haemothorax may develop during treatment with anticoagulant drugs or as a result of thrombocytopenia, leukaemia and other bone marrow disorders.

Pneumothorax

Pneumothorax is air in a pleural cavity. The many causes include:

- Trauma, particularly rib fracture.
- Rupture of small blebs or bullae on the surface of the lung in otherwise normal, young individuals.
- Rupture of emphysematous bullae.
- Over-inflation of a lung, either during anaesthesia or during assisted ventilation in an intensive care unit.

Pneumothorax also follows the escape of air into a pleural cavity via **bronchopleural fistulae** created by staphylococcal, tuberculous or other infection or by the erosion of bronchogenic carcinoma. It is an occasional result of the rupture of a bronchus. When air is present above an empyema, the disorder is **pyopneumothorax**. It is usually a result of rupture of lung abscess or carcinoma into the pleural cavity. The same effect may follow the breakdown of a bronchial stump after pneumonectomy.

Now read Bronchus (p. 69), Lung (p. 214)

POLYCYTHAEMIA

Polycythaemia is an increase in the number of circulating red blood cells in excess of 7×10^9/L. There is a rise in both total blood volume and in the packed cell volume (PCV) which may be as high as 60%. There is consequently an increase in haemoglobin concentration to a level of more than 18 g/dL. Because of the increased proportion of red blood cells, blood viscosity is high. Sludging (p. 330) occurs and there is an abnormal tendency to thrombosis.

- **Primary polycythaemia**, polycythaemia vera, arises without demonstrable cause. In the UK, the annual incidence is $15/10^6$ people.
- **Secondary polycythaemia** occurs when there is a persistent stimulus to new red blood cell formation. The response can be caused by life at high altitude; chronic heart failure; chronic respiratory disease; the persistent binding of carbon monoxide to haemoglobin in heavy smokers; or excess secretion of erythropoietin by a renal neoplasm.

The imprecise term 'relative polycythaemia' is occasionally used to describe the increased proportion of red blood cells that is a transient result of fluid loss due to burns or fulminating gastro-enteritis. Total blood volume is usually decreased and the disorder is better described as **haemoconcentration**.

POLYP

A polyp is a pedunculated cell mass arising from an epithelial surface as a result of neoplasia, metaplasia or inflammation (Fig. 49). Some polyps are hamartomas. Most polyps are gastro-intestinal and neoplastic. When the surface of a polyp forms finger-like processes, the polyp is said to be villous. The majority are benign.

It is important that surgeon and pathologist agree on the criteria used to define malignant change in a polyp. Under these circumstances, there is an initial zone of cellular atypia. Later, epithelial cells are judged to be neoplastic because they have extended through the muscularis mucosae and invaded the connective tissue stalk of the polyp. There is evidence that many, if not all, carcinomas of the large intestine arise in benign polyps.

Now read Carcinoma of colon (p. 106), Polyposis (p. 105)

PSEUDOPOLYP

Pseudopolyps are polyp-like masses of vascular granulation tissue and glandular crypts, partly or

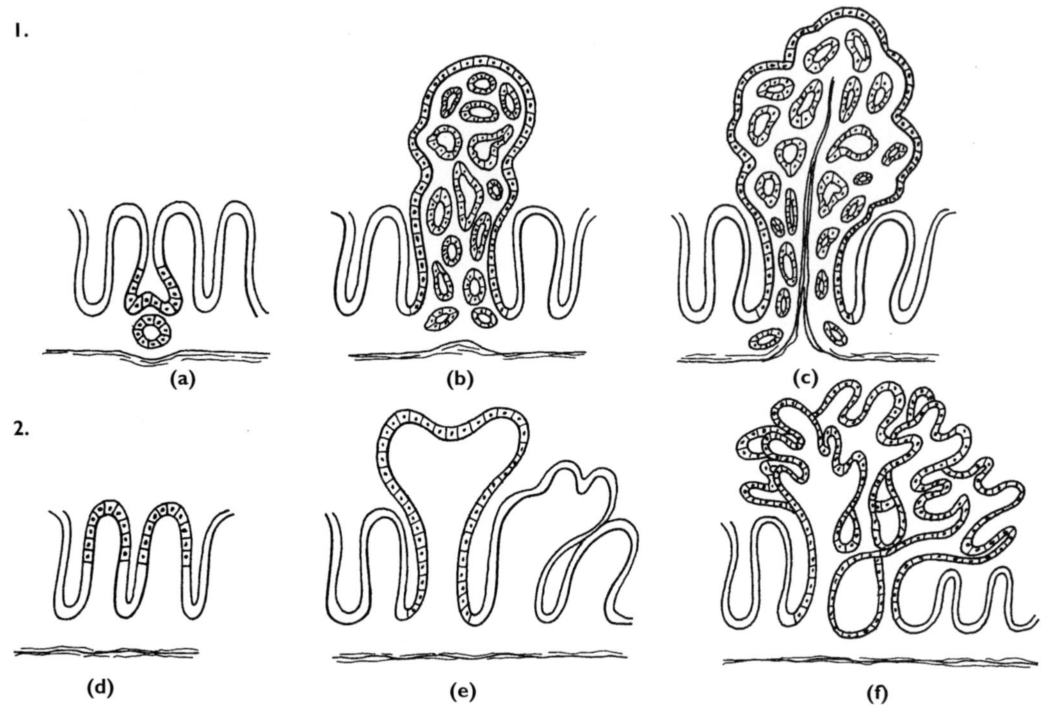

Figure 49 Intestinal polyps.
1. **Tubular adenoma**
(a) Origin of polyp is from epithelial cells at base of intestinal crypt.
(b) Islands of multiplying cells form small mass.
(c) Physical constriction of base of mass, by intestinal peristalsis, results in pedicle formation.
2. **Villous adenoma**
(d) Origin of polyp is from epithelial cells at surface of intestinal villus.
(e) Multiplying cells result in papilliform structure.
(f) Tumour mass is exophytic but sessile.

wholly covered by hyperplastic colonic epithelium. The pseudopolyps, long and pendulous or shorter and broad, are often conspicuous. Their presence characterises ulcerative colitis (p. 103). Unlike the true adenomatous polyp, there is no distinction between the structure of the body of the pseudopolyp and the stalk. Both lesions may occur together.

POTASSIUM

POTASSIUM DEPLETION

Extra-cellular and later, intra-cellular potassium (K^+) depletion is characteristic of vomiting, aspiration and severe diarrhoea. It develops after surgical operations or other injury, and in starvation. Much potassium may be lost from a villous papilloma of the large intestine. The body of a healthy 70 kg male contains ~3000 mmol of potassium (K^+) within cells but only 60 mmol outside cells. Measurements of the plasma concentration of K^+, estimated by assays, therefore provide no guide to total body K^+ content. Whole-body monitoring of potassium is used in research but is of little value in clinical practice.

Potassium concentrations have a profound effect upon neuromuscular conductivity. Muscular weakness develops when the serum K^+ level falls to ~2.5 mmol/L – the condition of hypokalaemia. Because of its low concentration in the extracellular fluid, the rapid loss of moderate amounts of potassium soon causes symptoms of K^+ depletion. Patients suffering from villous papilloma of the large bowel, for example, may lose up to three litres of mucus per day, containing 120 mmol/L of K^+. Following operation or injury (p. 230) the urinary excretion increases from 50 mmol/day to 100 mmol or more. The potassium/nitrogen ratio in muscle is 3 mmol K^+/gN. After a surgical operation, the urinary excretion is approximately 5–15 mmol K^+/gN. During starvation, the urinary K^+/N ratio is similar to that in muscle.

POTASSIUM EXCESS

The most frequent cause of **hyperkalaemia** is renal failure (p. 201). The ingestion of normal quantities of K^+ may produce hyperkalaemia when renal output falls below 500mL/d. Acidosis increases the serum K^+ concentration: K^+ is released from cells containing an increased concentration of H^+ in order to maintain electrical neutrality on either side of the cell membrane. Acidosis is also common in patients with renal failure. Iatrogenic hyperkalaemia due to intravenous infusion of excessive quantities of potassium salts is sometimes fatal. Massive transfusion, particularly of old blood, is now a rare cause of hyperkalaemia. There is both *in vitro* and *in vivo* haemolysis of effete red blood cells.

The initial signs of hyperkalaemia are not dramatic. Muscle weakness may not be obvious until flaccid paralysis develops; it is usually observed first in the lower limbs. The serum K^+ is already dangerously high as may be apparent from the ECG. The initial feature is the appearance of tall, peaked T waves. The P waves then disappear. Ultimately abnormalities of the QRS complex indicate that the development of ventricular fibrillation and death are imminent.

PROSTATE GLAND

Biopsy diagnosis of prostatic disease

Needle aspiration enables cell preparations to be made. Multiple samples should be taken. Their interpretation calls for histopathological expertise (p. 40). Conventional needle biopsy, with the retrieval of a fine core of tissue for fixation and paraffin section, may be by perineal or transrectal routes and is facilitated by ultrasonography or MRI. Bleeding and bacteraemic shock are recognised complications and the procedure is undertaken under antibiotic cover.

During transurethral resection, the gland is removed piecemeal in the form of numerous fragments ('chips'). In effect, they provide multiple biopsies. It is essential that a representative proportion of all the tissue removed be examined microscopically since the chances of detecting a small carcinoma varies directly with the number of fields surveyed. By consensus therefore, not less than two-thirds of the gland should be processed for histopathological analysis. The surgeon may select fragments from the centre and from the periphery of the gland to allow the location of suspicious zones to be differentiated spatially.

DISORDERS OF GROWTH

Benign prostatic hyperplasia

Benign prostatic hyperplasia (BPH) describes a common disorder of prostatic growth that increases in frequency with advancing age. Autopsy surveys suggest that at least 50% of males aged 50 years display the pathological signs of BPH and the condition is present in four-fifths of men in the seventh and subsequent decades. BPH is the most frequent of all diseases of middle-aged and older men. It is the second most common reason for any form of surgery.

Causes

Like comparable disorders of the thyroid gland and female breast, BPH is closely related to alterations in tissue hormonal responsiveness. Although plasma levels of testosterone tend to rise with advancing age while levels of oestrogen diminish, neither agent acts directly upon prostatic tissue. Rather, the causes of BPH centre on the effects of testosterone metabolites on the behaviour of both glandular and smooth muscular tissue. Testosterone is metabolised to the active agent 5-alpha-dihydrotestosterone (5-αDHT) by a 5-alpha-reductase. Although plasma levels of this metabolite do not change as BPH develops, the tissue content is increased, perhaps due to the decreased activity of enzymes catalysing the conjugation and degradation of the compound. The raised tissue concentration of 5-αDHT may be a direct stimulus to glandular hyperplasia. At the same time, the expression of androgen receptors within the prostate gland may be enhanced because of changes in the circulating levels of oestrogens.

Structure

BPH evolves gradually and gland enlargement precedes the onset of clinical signs and symptoms. However, the severity of the clinical features is not directly related to the size of the prostate gland. There is enlargement of all lobes. The enlargement evokes the formation of a false, thickened, periprostatic connective tissue capsule. Cross-sections of the hyperplastic prostate reveal the presence of many small nodular zones which assume a microcystic appearance if the abnormality is mainly one of glandular change, a firm, fibrous structure if the changes are principally smooth muscular.

Microscopically, the double layer, epithelial lining of the prostatic glands is thrown into excessive folds and the glandular spaces are enlarged and cystic. The smooth muscular and stromal fibrous tissue is proportionately increased. The prostatic ducts may undergo squamous metaplasia but this change is inconstant. Foci of infarction are recognised and there is often an infiltrate of inflammatory cells.

Enlargement of the median lobe, in particular, results in progressive obstruction to urinary outflow. It culminates in distension of the urinary bladder; increased trabeculation of the bladder wall; and diverticula formation. With obstruction come stasis, infection and calculus formation. The final consequences in untreated cases are hydro-ureter; hydronephrosis; and renal excretory failure with uraemia.

Behaviour and prognosis

BPH is not a precancerous lesion although small, coincidental carcinomas often co-exist. Attempts have been made to delay or prevent glandular enlargement by anti-androgen drugs and by the administration of inhibitors of 5-alpha-reductase. The hydrodynamic disturbances to urinary outflow can be alleviated by the insertion of a stent and by balloon dilatation of the prostatic urethra; they are corrected by transurethral resection. The genito-urinary symptoms can now be lessened by finasteride, a drug that slows the conversion of testosterone to dihydrotestosterone. The need for prostatectomy can be significantly reduced although impotence is one complication of treatment.

MECHANICAL DISORDERS

Calculus

Calculi composed of calcium phosphate and carbonate, form in the ducts of elderly patients with benign prostatic hyperplasia. They are multiple. Prostatic secretions become inspissated to form corpora amylacea which act as niduses for calculus formation (p. 75).

INFECTION AND INFLAMMATION

Prostatitis

Acute prostatitis

Gonorrhoea is one cause. Particularly in the presence of urinary obstruction, *Escherichia coli*, *Klebsiella pneumoniae*, Enterobacter spp., *Pseudomonas aeruginosa* and *Proteus vulgaris* are micro-organisms likely to initiate ascending infections. Abscesses may form.

Chronic prostatitis

Chronic prostatitis is a consequence of persistent or recurrent acute bacterial infection. Very occasionally, it is tuberculous. Alkalinity of the urine and the presence of calculi promote and exacerbate chronic infection. Prostatitis can be caused by micro-organisms other than bacteria. *Chlamydia trachomatis* is one such agent. *Schistosoma haematobium* can lodge in the prostate. The ova of this worm are conveyed to the periprostatic venous plexus.

Granulomatous prostatitis

There are at least two forms: the first resulting from tuberculous infection of the epididymis or kidney; the second a hypersensitivity response in which rheumatoid nodule-like granulomas are formed.

TUMOURS

Malignant

Carcinoma

Carcinoma of the prostate is one of the most common malignant tumours. It is the second most

PSEUDARTHROSIS

A pseudarthrosis is a false joint formed in living bone and connective tissue because of heritable or acquired disease.

INHERITED PSEUDARTHROSIS

This is a rare connective tissue disease.

ACQUIRED PSEUDARTHROSES

False joints may form at sites where the healing of fracture of a long bone is delayed or prevented (p. 56). The predisposing factors include inadequate immobilisation after fracture; impaired local blood supply; and the presence of necrotic or foreign tissue.

Now read Bone (p. 50), Joints (p. 190)

PUTREFACTION

Putrefaction is the decomposition of dead animal and vegetable matter by saprophytic bacteria and other organisms. Enzymatic degradation of proteins produces cadaverine; putrescine; trimethyl amine; ammonia; hydrogen sulphide; and mercaptans. There are consequently nauseating odours. Absorbed, these products are toxic.

Now read Gangrene (p. 136)

PYAEMIA

Pyaemia is an obsolete term. It was defined as the presence and multiplication of pyogenic bacteria in the blood and their carriage by micro-emboli to other organs. The distinction between pyaemia and septicaemia has little therapeutic significance. The effect of pyaemia/septicaemia is to produce micro-abscesses distal to the source of the emboli. Thus, 'systemic pyaemia' results in abscesses in viscera such as the kidney, whereas 'portal pyaemia' leads to abscesses in the liver.

Now read Bacteraemia, Septicaemia (p. 34)

PYROGENS

Pyrogens are substances that provoke fever. Some are formed by bacteria. Among the most important are those produced by water-borne bacteria. They are filterable and thermostable. Others include foreign proteins and an endogenous substance produced by polymorphs.

Endogenous pyrogen is a lipoprotein. It causes the fever that develops during severe, acute inflammation. Endogenous lipoprotein, like other pyrogens, acts on the temperature-regulating centres of the brain.

Q

QUEYRAT'S ERYTHROPLASIA

Queyrat's erythroplasia is described on p. 268.

QUINSY

The term 'quinsy' is applied to the presence of large, unilateral or bilateral tonsillar abscesses attributable to group A streptococci (*Streptococcus pyogenes)*, or to *Staphylococcus aureus*. Oedema may lead to pharyngeal obstruction. Antibiotic treatment is required and surgical incision may be necessary.

R

RAYNAUD'S PHENOMENON

Raynaud's phenomenon (p. 188) is digital ischaemia due to vascular spasm. When severe and prolonged, infarction of the tips of the fingers or toes may occur. Raynaud's phenomenon is often initiated by minor degrees of environmental cold but the phenomenon can occur at a relatively high ambient temperature. Systemic connective tissue disease (p. 111); macroglobulinaemia; and prolonged occupational exposure to vibration are underlying causes. A comparable form of vascular occlusion may occur if cryoglobulins are formed in excess by multiple myeloma.

An occasional response, analogous to Raynaud's phenomenon, is the activation of antibodies, haemagglutinins and haemolysins, that are normally inactive at 37°C. Red blood cells agglutinate in small, peripheral vessels. Haemolysis may then lead to 'cold' haemoglobinuria.

RECTUM

The rectum is a component of the large bowel and consequently may be involved in the congenital and acquired conditions described under Colon (p. 101). There are differences in the structural and functional consequences of disease in the two parts of the intestine because the external, longitudinal muscle coat of the colon is in the form of taeniae whereas the longitudinal muscle layer of the rectum is an entire, encircling layer.

Now read Colon and Rectum (p. 101)

Biopsy diagnosis of rectal disease

Mucosal biopsies can be obtained at proctoscopy or sigmoidoscopy using biopsy forceps. Polyps of various types can be removed in their entirety by diathermy snare. Incisional, whole-thickness biopsies obtained by scalpel are required to diagnose Hirschprung's disease (p. 105).

INFECTION AND INFLAMMATION

In patients with ulcerative colitis, the rectum is the most severely affected portion of the large intestine. In Crohn's colitis, the rectum is often spared.

Now read Crohn's disease (p. 104, 165)

MECHANICAL DISORDERS

Prolapse

Rectal prolapse may be complete, involving the full thickness of the wall, or partial, involving only the mucosa.

- **Complete**. The majority of patients with complete rectal prolapse are females. In some, damage to the pudendal nerves at childbirth causes lax anal sphincters and perineal descent on straining. However, many patients are nulliparous with a healthy pelvic floor and normal anal sphincter tone. In these patients, the origin of rectal prolapse may lie partly in heritable factors, partly in occupational - and other forms of mechanical stress.
- **Partial**. Partial prolapse is the most frequent form in children. It is attributed to repeated attacks of diarrhoea or to prolonged straining as a result of constipation. In adults, slight mucosal prolapse inevitably accompanies third-degree haemorrhoids.

Diverticular disease

Diverticular disease of the large bowel (p. 102), so common in the colon, spares the rectum. The explanation lies in the structure and behaviour of the taeniae coli where the vascular cores constitute foci of relative weakness in the intestinal wall that are not present in the rectum.

Haemorrhoids

Haemorrhoids are described on p. 12.

Solitary ulcer

The term 'solitary ulcer' is applied loosely to a disorder of the rectum in which one or more zones of smooth muscle hyperplasia, with or without ulceration, are accompanied by fibrosis. Affected individuals are usually under the age of 40 years. There is rectal bleeding and the passage of mucus, although these phenomena may occur in the absence of ulceration. The aetiology of solitary ulcer remains uncertain. One explanation is incomplete, recurrent mucosal prolapse. Another is self-digitation or other trauma.

Ulceration when present, is of a chronic character. It is found on the anterior wall of the rectum, 70 to 100 mm from the anal verge. Characteristically, smooth muscle hypertrophy implicates both muscularis mucosae and the circular muscle of the rectum. In the absence of ulceration, a zone of mucosal erythema or mucosal nodularity is often recognised.

TUMOURS

The rectum is the most frequent site for carcinoma of the large intestine. In England and Wales, there is an annual incidence of $220/10^6$ persons. Tumours of the rectum are considered with those of the colon (p. 105) and anal canal (p. 13).

REGENERATION

Regeneration is the repair of an injured but viable part, tissue or cell by the formation of an identical structure. It is accomplished by the new formation of cells and tissues that have the same structure and function as those that have been lost.

Although animals as complex as the newt can regenerate whole limbs, in man the scale upon which regeneration can take place is severely restricted. It is most active in highly vascular tissues. Regeneration is vigorous in facial skin; liver; renal tubules; bone; gut; stomach; and haemopoietic bone marrow but of limited degree in skeletal muscle; arterial medial muscle; and pretibial skin. The process is rapid in skin; liver; renal tubules; bone; and adrenal cortex but may not occur at all in the neurones of the central nervous system. The cornea and hyaline articular cartilage are avascular and do not regenerate.

In some cases, for example the adrenal cortex, destruction or removal of one of the two paired organs rapidly provokes mitotic activity in the remaining organ. The combined mass is restored within 4 weeks provided the secretion of growth hormone continues. Removal of one kidney evokes a similar response in the tubules of the remaining organ. Excision of part of the liver is quickly followed by cellular multiplication within the remaining hepatocytes. Where regeneration is not possible in a living part, repair takes place by the formation of a substitute collagenous, fibrous tissue.

Now read Cell growth (p. 84), Fibrosis (p. 131), Scar (p. 290), Transplantation (p. 329)

RESPIRATORY FAILURE

Two forms of respiratory failure can be recognised. The signs may overlap. The forms are distinguished by the absence or presence of carbon dioxide retention.

- **Type I failure** is present when the arterial oxygen tension is less than 60 mmHg (8.0 kPa) as a result of lung disease in an individual breathing air at sea level. There is no associated retention of carbon dioxide. The causes of type I failure include pulmonary oedema or collapse; pneumonia; thromboembolism; bronchial asthma and interstitial lung disease.
- **Type II failure** exists when the same criteria are evident but, in addition, there is carbon dioxide retention. The causes of type II failure include narcotic overdosage in head injury; traumatic, crushing injuries of the chest; severe thoracic deformity, for example with kyphoscoliosis; and chronic bronchitis and emphysema.

RETICULO-ENDOTHELIAL SYSTEM

The concept of a reticulo-endothelial system (RES) was advanced by Aschoff (p. 369) to describe a family of cells, widely distributed throughout the body but sharing the properties of phagocytosis and intravital staining.

The cells of the RES derive from stem cells that differentiate in the bone marrow to become the precursors of the red (p. 10) and white (p. 204) blood cells and platelet series (p. 273). RES cells are grouped in organs such as the spleen but they are also dispersed in vascular and stromal tissues; they are therefore intravascular or extravascular. The intravascular cells include the blood monocytes and the endothelial cells of the liver capillaries, the Kupffer cells, together with those of the lymph node sinuses, splenic sinuses and the adrenal and hypophyseal capillaries. The extravascular cells are the macrophages of the connective tissues. These cells may be 'fixed' in location or may 'wander' freely as they enter the tissues from the blood. Unlike the dendritic macrophages of the lymphoid tissues, they cannot 'present' antigens to initiate an immune response.

Now read Immunity (p. 171), Macrophage (p. 225), Phagocytosis (p. 270)

RETINOBLASTOMA

Retinoblastoma is a rare form of malignant tumour which develops in 1 in 23 000 ($43/10^6$) live infants. It is more common in males than females. In 40% of cases, other relatives within the family are affected. The tumour may arise spontaneously or on a genetic basis.

- **Spontaneous**. In the spontaneous form, the tumour is unilateral and develops at a later age. It originates when two acquired somatic mutations occur within the same area of the retina. The prognosis is good since enucleation of the eye allows the prolonged survival of 90% of cases.
- **Familial**. In the familial cases, the disorder is inherited as an autosomal dominant characteristic (p. 183). The tumour may be bilateral and sometimes multiple in an affected eye. There is an additional hazard of a further malignant tumour, usually a soft tissue sarcoma. The prognosis is guarded.

Tumorigenesis is initiated when the first 'hit', in the form of the inherited, mutant allelic gene, is succeeded by a second 'hit', a somatic mutation at the same site. The 'retinoblastoma gene', *RB1* is located on the long arm of somatic chromosome 13, at 13q14. It has proved of importance in understanding the regulation of cell growth and carcinogenesis (p. 286). It is a universal 'brake'.

Now read Carcinogenesis (p. 76)

RETROPERITONEUM

Acute retroperitoneal disease is uncommon but often of extreme gravity. Prolonged or chronic disorders affecting the retroperitoneal tissues share certain characteristics. There is insidious weight loss; diminished health; and progressive ureteric obstruction.

INFECTION AND INFLAMMATION

From time-to-time, acute bacterial infections spread through the retroperitoneal tissues from the pancreas; kidneys; large intestine; liver; adrenals; and vertebrae. One example is anaerobic streptococcal infection of muscle; another is tuberculosis. Originating in vertebral bone, infection extends within the retroperitoneal sheath of the psoas muscle.

Periodically, renal pyaemic abscess implicates retroperitoneal tissues and a comparable disorder may occur in amoebiasis.

Now read Retroperitoneal fibrosis (p. 131).

TUMOURS

Metastatic tumours of the retroperitoneal tissues include those arising in the kidney; adrenal glands; ovary; stomach; pancreas; and large intestine.

Primary tumours originating in the retroperitoneal tissues are largely those of the soft tissues (p. 298). They include liposarcoma, leiomyosarcoma and fibrosarcoma.

ROBOTIC SURGERY

The design of robots and the application of voice-operated computers, have allowed the introduction of surgical techniques in which a surgeon is assisted by a robot, not by a live individual.

S

SALIVARY GLANDS

The paired parotid, submandibular and sublingual salivary glands, together with the many small glands scattered throughout the oral cavity, are frequent sites for inflammatory and neoplastic disease but are rarely affected by developmental abnormalities or vascular disorders.

Biopsy diagnosis of salivary gland disease

The majority of biopsies are undertaken to establish the diagnosis of salivary gland swellings. In the case of cancers, incisional and Trucut needle procedures are likely to cause tumour seeding and should not be performed. Fine needle aspiration cytopathology with magnetic resonance imaging is now used in specialist centres to assess tumour malignancy.

INFECTION AND INFLAMMATION

Acute

- Viral sialadenitis is often due to mumps, epidemic parotitis. The infection is a systemic disorder that periodically provokes encephalitis, orchitis and pancreatitis and is a possible cause of thyroiditis.
- Bacterial sialadenitis may develop in elderly, dehydrated and debilitated patients when the flow of salivary secretions is low. The causative organisms are usually streptococci or anaerobes. The presence of a calculus in a main parotid duct predisposes to infection.

Chronic

Persistent or recurrent bacterial infection, often in the presence of calculus, culminates in glandular atrophy and fibrosis. Granulomatous inflammation of the principal salivary glands is a feature of sarcoidosis and may be encountered in Crohn's disease. Mycobacterial and mycotic infections are rare.

Sjögren's syndrome

In this auto-immune disorder, a condition that may arise spontaneously or as one part of generalised diseases such as rheumatoid arthritis and systemic lupus erythematosus, there is low-grade, persistent sialadenitis with a widespread lymphocytic infiltrate and a diagnostic pattern of circulating auto-antibodies (p. 28). Glandular acini atrophy.

MECHANICAL AND TRAUMATIC LESIONS

Mucocoele

Within one of the main glands; in a small intra-oral gland; or on the lip, there arise isolated, thin-walled, blue swellings. They are cysts formed by the extravasation of mucin or by local injury to a gland or duct, perhaps during dental surgery. A **ranula** is a larger variant of the same condition, usually affecting the submandibular gland. It has a tendency to increase in size within the nearby submucosal connective tissues.

Now read Cyst (p. 113)

Calculus

Salivary calculi contain calcium phosphate and carbonate. They form around a central nidus of desquamated epithelial cells and bacteria following infection and are most frequent in the submandibular duct. Subsequent obstruction of the duct is partial, producing a painful distension of the salivary gland from which the duct originates. When there is obstruction and subsequent stasis, infection occurs within the duct, predisposing to the development of secondary calculi. A vicious circle is established. Acute sialadenitis with suppuration may follow.

Now read Calculus (p. 75)

TUMOURS

Salivary gland tumours are infrequent. The majority arise in one of the parotid glands and are benign. Tumours of the submandibular, sublingual and minor glands comprise no more than 20% of salivary gland neoplasms but a higher proportion is malignant.

Benign

Pleomorphic adenoma

This is the most common salivary gland tumour. Three-quarters originate in the parotid gland, a smaller proportion in the submandibular gland. Pleomorphic adenoma of the minor salivary glands is unusual.

Pleomorphic adenoma of the parotid gland is a slowly growing, painless, unilateral swelling near, and in front of the ear, close to the facial nerve. The cut surface of the tumour displays a variegated structure in which glandular and solid zones are interspersed with islands resembling cartilage. There are many myo-epithelial cells thought to be the source of the loose connective tissue and cartilaginous tissues that are invariably present. There is a false capsule formed of compressed glandular and connective tissues. Formerly, the designation 'mixed' tumour was used on the assumption that the adenoma derived from more than one embryonic germ layer. Now it is believed to be entirely epithelial.

Pleomorphic adenoma extends finger-like processes insidiously within adjoining salivary glandular and other tissues but does not metastasise. These processes may be incompletely excised by a surgeon intent on protecting the facial nerve. Rarely, carcinoma arises within the adenoma.

Adenolymphoma

Adenolymphoma is an infrequent form of papillary adenoma usually recognised in elderly males. It forms an insidious swelling within a major salivary gland. It is occasionally bilateral and multifocal. The diagnosis may not be made until histological examination is undertaken. There is a characteristic double layer of eosinophilic epithelial cells interspersed among conspicuous islands of lymphoid tissue.

Malignant

Malignant tumours are very uncommon. They affect ~20/10^6 persons each year in the UK and are more common in women aged >40 years than men.

Adenoid cystic carcinoma

Adenocystic carcinoma is the most frequent of the malignant salivary gland tumours. Aggregates of small, darkly staining cells are arranged in a sieve-like pattern. The description 'cribriform' is applied to this structure. Adenoid cystic carcinoma is a slowly growing lesion that spreads locally along the paths of nerves. The tumour is not easy to eradicate but metastasis is late.

Muco-epidermoid carcinoma

As the name indicates, muco-epidermoid carcinoma comprises a blend of mucin-secreting, glandular cells together with islands of squamous cells. Although the degree of differentiation of this rare tumour is a guide to its behaviour and thus to prognosis, it is unpredictable. Tumours that appear well-differentiated may recur. Metastasis to regional lymph nodes precedes spread via the bloodstream. Alternatively, muco-epidermoid carcinoma may follow a less aggressive pattern.

Acinic cell carcinoma

This rare tumour forms a circumscribed, slowly-growing mass composed of acinar cells. Its behaviour is difficult to predict and prognosis remains uncertain.

Other malignant tumours

Even less common malignant tumours of the salivary gland include adenocarcinoma; squamous carcinoma; and lymphoma. The latter is a recognised complication of Sjögren's syndrome (p. 288).

Now read Oral cavity (p. 256)

SARCOIDOSIS

Sarcoidosis is a local or widespread, multisystem, chronic granulomatous, inflammatory disease of unknown aetiology. Any part of the body may be affected but lung lesions are the most frequent. Pulmonary infiltrates are accompanied by the presence of firm, grey–pink and rubbery, enlarged mediastinal lymph nodes. The eye, skin and other lymphoid tissue are commonly implicated.

The characteristic lesion is a sterile epithelioid cell granuloma in which the mononuclear cells are arranged in follicles without the caseous necrotic centres of tuberculosis. The granulomas include large, multinucleate giant cells containing cytoplasmic inclusions, Schaumann bodies (p. 376). They are rich in calcium.

The causes of sarcoidosis are not known. Hypersensitivity to mycobacteria; to mineral dusts; and to pine pollen, are among the agents proposed. Th lymphocyte activity is enhanced. A diagnostic procedure, the Kveim test, could be performed by injecting sterile material from known sarcoid lesions intradermally. Now seldom performed, it was often positive. Another diagnostic sign is hypercalcaemia: sarcoidosis stimulates vitamin D activity.

SARCOMA

A sarcoma is a malignant tumour of mesenchymal tissue. Suffixes such as fibro-, chondro-, lipo-, angio- and myxo- are added to indicate the differentiation shown by the neoplastic cells and demonstrated by the nature and amount of the extracellular matrix that is formed. When more than one extracellular matrix material is present, the tumour is designated by the most mature material seen. Thus, even minute islands of osteoid are sufficient to categorise a collagenous tumour as osteosarcoma.

Sarcomas have a solid, flesh-like structure with many small, thin-walled blood vessels. The neoplastic cells lie close to the basement membrane of these vessels and gain ready access to the circulation. Consequently, blood-borne metastasis to the lungs is common. Rarely, the microscopic features of carcinoma and sarcoma co-exist. The term **carcinosarcoma** can then be applied.

Now read Bone (p. 59), Cartilage (p. 83), Soft tissue tumours (p. 298)

SCAR

The replacement of injured or dead tissue is by repair or by regeneration. A scar is a focus or island of fibrous connective tissue that forms when healing (p. 147) occurs by repair. The quantity of tissue is large if healing is delayed and complicated by infection, or by the presence of foreign bodies. Scar tissue, initially pale pink, abundant and soft, becomes dense, hard and white and contracts with time. These changes are accompanied by an increase in strength and are closely related to the formation and maturation of fibrous collagens.

The creation of a scar is dependent on the availability of essential nutritional factors such as ascorbic acid. However, scar formation is not impaired in old age. Abnormal scars form in rare inherited diseases of collagen, such as the Ehlers–Danlos syndrome. In occasional patients, the growth of a scar is progressive and excessive, resulting in hypertrophic scar or keloid.

Now read Fibrosis (p. 131), Keloid (p. 195), Regeneration (p. 285), Wound (p. 357)

SCROTUM

Hydrocoele

Hydrocoele is a collection of serous fluid within the tunica vaginalis.

The cause of congenital hydrocoele is a failure of obliteration of the processus vaginalis. The result of this defect is the persistence of a communication with the peritoneal cavity. **Infantile hydrocoele** develops when the processus closes proximally but persists distally. Closure takes place at the deep inguinal ring. A segment of the processus may persists within the inguinal canal producing an **encysted hydrocoele** of the cord.

The cause(s) of most hydrocoeles is debatable. They are therefore said to be primary (idiopathic). Hydrocoeles that form as a consequence of inflammatory or malignant disease of the testis are secondary. Their nature is determined by ultrasound and/or biopsy.

Epididymal cyst

Epididymal cysts develop in middle age. They are often multiple and bilateral. The cysts contain clear fluid. They are the result of degeneration of the paradidymis or epididymis.

Spermatocoele

Spermatocoeles are cysts arising in the vasa efferentia. They lie above and behind the testis. Their fluid content is rich in sperm.

INFECTION AND INFLAMMATION

Sebaceous cysts are common in scrotal skin and may become infected. Fournier's gangrene is described on p. 136. In the East, filariasis (p. 357) may result in elephantiasis.

TUMOURS

Malignant

Carcinoma

Squamous carcinoma of the scrotum is rare under the age of 60. The tumour was first recognised in chimney sweeps (Pott, p. 375); its growth was associated with the persistent adherence of soot to the scrotal skin. The paraffin oil used to lubricate spinning machines in cotton and woollen mills was another responsible carcinogen.

The cancer spreads locally to inguinal lymph nodes. The 5-year survival rate is ~70%.

SHOCK

Shock is a state of disturbed body functions due to inadequate perfusion of tissues. It may be caused by any large-scale interference with cell metabolism, including sepsis. In clinical terms, inadequate perfusion is the persistence of a systolic blood pressure of <90 mmHg or a fall of 40 mmHg below the individual's normal systolic pressure. The varieties of shock are:

- Hypovolaemic.
- Normovolaemic.

HYPOVOLAEMIC (OLIGAEMIC) SHOCK

Hypovolaemic shock is attributable to the loss of blood, plasma or water. Ultimately, there is a reduction in circulating blood volume; tachycardia; and impaired cardiac output.

Haemorrhagic

Common causes of haemorrhagic shock include simple fracture of a large bone, and blood loss from the alimentary tract. In the former, bleeding takes place into the soft tissues around the broken bone. In the latter, oesophageal varices, carcinoma and peptic ulcer are frequent sources of bleeding. Other causes of haemorrhagic shock include bleeding from diverticular disease of the colon; from ruptured abdominal aortic aneurysm; from placenta praevia; and from ruptured ectopic pregnancy. Early vasoconstriction and reduced blood volume are followed by the diffusion of interstitial fluid into the intravascular compartment, with haemodilution and a consequential restoration of blood volume.

Now read Blood loss (p. 42)

Plasma loss

The rapid loss of plasma is a characteristic feature of extensive burns or scalds. Plasma collects in blisters under the epithelium and exudes from the exposed, subepithelial tissues. However, the greatest loss is into the interstitial tissue spaces. Other causes are severe crushing injuries to the limbs, and the peritonitis associated with acute pancreatitis.

Now read Burns (p. 71)

Water and electrolyte loss

Shock may follow the inadequate intake or excessive loss of water and electrolytes. In the UK, the most frequent cause is so-called 'third space loss' due to peritonitis and intestinal obstruction. Elsewhere, the most common explanation is severe diarrhoea due to dysenteric organisms. An extreme form is encountered in cholera (p. 165).

Now read Peritonitis (p. 269)

NORMOVOLAEMIC SHOCK

Neurocardiogenic (vasovagal) syncope

A subject may faint because of emotion or pain. Loss of consciousness is due to bradycardia and hypotension induced by vagal stimulation. Bradycardia distinguishes the condition from the tachycardia of hypovolaemic shock. The same vagal response may occur when general anaesthesia, for example of a dental patient, is induced in an upright, seated position. Unless blood flow is quickly restored, cerebral infarction may occur.

Cardiogenic shock

Cardiac output is severely reduced following myocardial infarction; myocarditis; cardiac tamponade; dissecting aortic aneurysm; or the onset of cardiac arrhythmias. There is metabolic acidosis (p. 231) due to underperfusion of the tissues.

Pulmonary shock

Patients with severe pulmonary lesions such as embolism; atelectasis; pneumothorax; and haemothorax exhibit the classical features of shock.

Septic shock

Septic shock is the multi-system result of severe local or systemic infection. Unlike other forms of shock, the condition does not respond to the correction of fluid imbalance or underperfusion. There is a mortality of 40–70%.

Many micro-organisms form exotoxins or endotoxins (p. 327) that are potent causes of normovolaemic shock. Clostridia spp. and Staphylococci spp. exemplify the former, coliforms the latter. In the initiation of septic shock, a role for innate (natural) immunity (p. 231) is suspected.

Endotoxic shock

Endotoxic shock (p. 327) results from the liberation of cell wall lipopolysaccharide from dead Gram-negative bacteria (Fig.50). All tissues may be damaged by bacterial endotoxins but the lungs are particularly susceptible. To promote shock, it is not necessary for the bacteria to reach the bloodstream; shock may result from the actions of the toxins alone. The term 'bacteraemic' shock is therefore often inappropriate.

Anaphylactic shock

Type I antigen–antibody interactions in the body liberate vaso-active substances such as histamine. This form of hypersensitivity (p. 161) is more common in atopic than in normal individuals. The blood pools in the capillaries and there may be laryngeal oedema. Circulatory stagnation may produce severe tissue hypoxia.

MULTIPLE ORGAN SYSTEMIC FAILURE

The widespread nature of the tissues affected in septic shock has led to the terms **multiple organ systemic failure** (MOSF) or **multiple organ dysfunction syndrome** (MODS).

Scoring systems have been devised to measure the severity of MOSF or MODS. A cytokine cascade (p. 114) mediates the tissue injuries. MOSF and adult respiratory distress syndrome (ARDS) are very often due to the release of bacterial lipopolysaccharides (LPS). In Gram-negative bacteraemia (p. 34), endotoxic shock is initiated when these macromolecules interact first, with LPS-binding protein, second, with the CD14 receptor on monocytes and macrophages. Many intracellular signalling pathways are then activated with the release of cytokines such as TGF-β. IL-10 is secreted. Positive and negative feedback loops operate within the system. If the regulation of cytokine secretion is abnormal, an exaggerated, harmful inflammatory response may ensue.

Now read ARDS (p. 219)

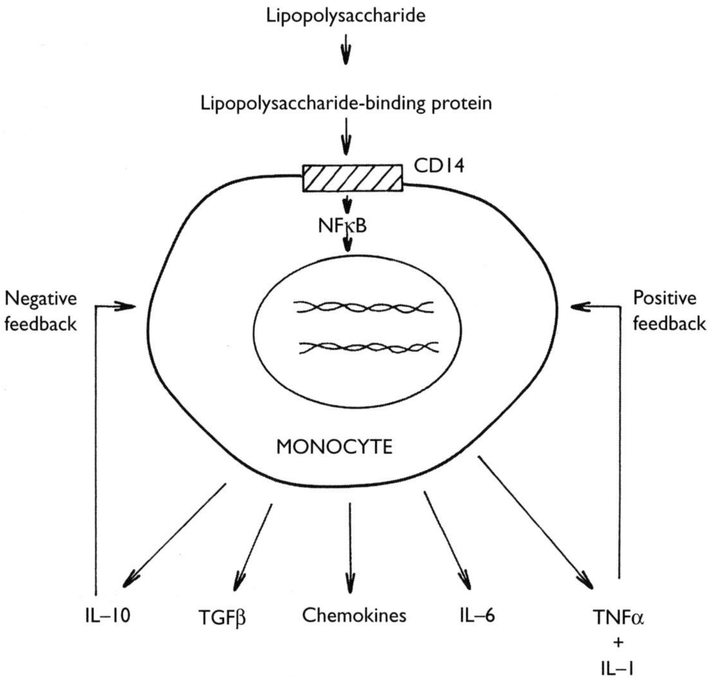

Figure 50 Gram-negative endotoxic shock.
Diagram emphasises role of bacterial cell membrane lipopolysaccharide (LPS) in bacteraemic shock. Molecular patterns of LPS (at top) are shared among all Gram-negative bacteria: they are highly conserved in an evolutionary sense. Innate immune system receptors, encoded in germ line, respond rapidly to presence of bacteria. Receptors activate NFκB and cytokine genes. Cytokines (at bottom) are formed, generating both beneficial and adverse effects regulated by positive and negative feedback control. One example of a damaging result is disseminated intravascular coagulation (DIC, p. 119).

Systemic inflammatory response syndrome

During the last two decades it has become apparent that identical pathological changes to those seen in individuals dying from septic shock can be identified in patients with MOSF who display no evidence of infection. The term **systemic inflammatory response syndrome** (SIRS) has been introduced to describe their condition. Many consider septic shock to be a variant of SIRS. The syndrome may also be induced by trauma, burns and pancreatitis. The American College of Chest Physicians defines the syndrome by specific criteria (Table 51).

Table 51 The systemic inflammatory response syndrome (SIRS). bpm = beats/minute; rpm = respiratory movements/minute

Temperature:	<36° C or >38° C
Tachycardia:	>90 bpm
Tachypnoea:	>20 rpm
Or	
Hyperventilation:	pCO_2 <4.25 kPa
Leucocytosis:	>12 × 10^9/L

The presence of a condition producing endothelial damage and two or more of the criteria shown in Table 51 are required for the diagnosis of SIRS. In overwhelming sepsis, there may be leucopenia because of bone marrow depression.

Septic shock (p. 291) and SIRS share several cytokine mediators including TNF±, IL-1, IL-6 and IL-8 but there may be differences in the extent of the release of individual cytokines according to the pathological stimulus. Cytokines are also liberated following elective surgical operations, during the acute phase response of the metabolic response to trauma (p. 230). Following elective operations and moderate injury, the concentrations of these cytokines falls and the acute systemic inflammatory response resolves. In severely injured patients, particulary those with overt sepsis, TNFα, interleukins, PGE_2, leukotrienes and thromboxane (p. 180) contine to be released. Ultimately many patients die from MOSF, not because of infection but due to excessive inflammatory response.

SICKLE-CELL PHENOMENON

Sickle cells are red blood cells, the shape of which is altered because of the heritable presence of an abnormal sickle-cell haemoglobin, HbS (Fig. 35). Normal adult haemoglobin (HbA) and HbS possess the same solubility when oxygenated. On de-oxygenation, HbS becomes poorly soluble and forms a semi-fluid gel. The affected cells change shape, and become sinusoidal and curved. The altered shape and changed physical properties of these sickled cells determines that blood flow through capillaries is obstructed and blood viscosity increased. The sickled cells are avidly phagocytosed by the reticulo-endothelial cells of the spleen (p. 270). The decreased life-span of sickled cells is the reason for the development of sickle-cell anaemia.

INHERITANCE

The presence of HbS is the result of an inherited mutation in the gene coding for glutamic acid which is replaced by the gene coding for valine (p. 183). Because of shifts in populations, the sickle-cell trait and the fully expressed disease are now recognised with increased frequency in Europe.

When an individual is heterozygous for this defect, both HbA and HbS are formed. The individual is then said to have the **sickle-cell trait**. The red blood cells do not deform *in vivo*, but sickling can be induced by exposing them in the laboratory to an atmosphere containing less oxygen than normal.

When the sufferer is homozygous, normal HbA is not formed. The red blood cells readily deform *in vivo* and **sickle-cell anaemia** develops.

Now read Genes (p. 138)

PATHOLOGICAL EFFECTS

Sickle-cell disease may create great difficulties for the surgeon. Patients may develop signs that can mimic intra-abdominal catastrophes. There is often fibrosis and calcification of the spleen and an increased formation of pigmented biliary calculi. The anaemic individual responds poorly to infection and trivial bacterial infection can precipitate widespread sickling with massive tissue infarction, for example, of an entire kidney. Septicaemia may develop. Osteomyelitis, sometimes attributable to Salmonella spp., is a further complication.

SINUS

Anatomically, the term sinus implies a wide venous channel; a pouch or recess; or an air-containing cavity lined by mucosa. Pathologically, a sinus is a narrow, infected tract lined by granulation tissue and leading from an abscess to the skin, or to a body cavity. It is a consequence of incomplete resolution of an inflammatory process. Sinuses are often due to the presence of a retained foreign body such as a non-absorbable suture, hair or dead bone; to constant re-infection; or to the persistence of indolent, chronic infections such as tuberculosis or actinomycosis. Untreated, sinuses become chronic. They are then lined by squamous epithelium.

SKIN

Biopsy diagnosis of skin disease

Biopsy may be incisional but is more often excisional. Biopsy of all skin lesions suspected of malignancy is mandatory. If an excisional biopsy has been performed, the pathologist must confirm that the margin of normal tissue includes the entire circumference of the lesion.

Now read Biopsy (p. 40), Histology (p. 157), Malignant melanoma (p. 227)

DEVELOPMENTAL AND CONGENITAL DISORDERS

Many heritable diseases affect skin structure and function. Examples include connective tissue disorders such as the Ehlers–Danlos syndrome; disorders of pigmentation such as albinism; xeroderma pigmentosum (pp. 78, 362); and dysplastic naevus (p. 240).

INFLAMMATION AND INFECTION

The skin is susceptible to viral; bacterial; protozoal; and helminthic infections and infestations, as well as to fungal disease. Skin infections are one complication of AIDS. The existence of overt bacterial skin infection is of clear relevance to attempts to prevent wound sepsis. Common skin disorders in this category include impetigo; folliculitis; and a variety of staphylococcal infections, such as furuncles and carbuncles. In indigent populations, scabies and maggots contribute to the persistence of skin infections. Viral infections include verruca vulgaris; verruca plana; condyloma acuminata; and molluscum contagiosum.

Now read Wound infection p. 361

Furuncle

A furuncle or boil is a localised infection of the skin that results in the formation of a small abscess. The causative organism is usually *Staphylococcus aureus*. The lesion originates in an obstructed hair follicle.

Carbuncle

A carbuncle is a large zone of infected skin and subcutaneous tissue. It is caused by pathogenic staphylococci, particularly *Staphylococcus aureus*. Carbuncles are prone to occur in individuals and especially in diabetics, in whom resistance to infection is low. The affected site is covered by hair-bearing skin and a hair follicle may be the portal of entry of bacteria. Characteristically, the site is one where the skin is relatively thick and firmly attached to the subcutaneous tissue. The occipital area and the back are particularly susceptible. There is widespread, diffuse subcutaneous tissue necrosis, contrasting with the localised focus of necrotic, subcutaneous tissue in a boil. There are multiple sinuses through which staphylococcal pus (p. 1) is often discharged.

Condyloma acuminata

These multiple, papillary, viral warts are the result of sexually transmitted infection by human papilloma virus (HPV). The abnormal epithelium is sharply demarcated from nearby normal tissue. The virus particles are recognisable by electron microscopy.

So-called **giant condyloma acuminata** is verrucous carcinoma.

TUMOURS

A very considerable variety of tumour-like lesions require excision. They include tags of skin that form at sites of chronic irritation or repair, and cutaneous horns. Epidermoid cysts are non-neoplastic, unilocular inclusion lesions of the dermis that contain inspissated sebum and keratin.

Benign

Basal cell papilloma – seborrhoeic keratosis

This common lesion of the elderly takes the form of prominent, circumscribed, grey–black, raised plaques on the limbs or trunk. Microscopically, zones of hyperplastic basal cells are interrupted by varying numbers of small, keratin-containing cystic spaces. By contrast with malignant melanoma (p. 227) to which it bears a superficial resemblance because of its colour, the deep margin of the tumour is level with the basal layer of the adjacent epidermis.

Kerato-acanthoma

Kerato-acanthoma, **molluscum sebaceum**, is a small swelling that appears on the face of middle-aged individuals. The lesion grows rapidly for 6–8 weeks and soon assumes the appearance of an elevated, pale mass. The centre of the lesion is a keratinous 'plug' that may be extruded. Growth is followed by an equally short phase of regression and resolution. It is important to distinguish this benign condition from squamous carcinoma (p. 303).

Granular cell tumour (granular cell myoblastoma)

'Granular cell' describes the large cells of which this benign tumour is formed. The cells are thought to be of Schwann cell derivation. They contain many large, secondary lysosomes, accounting for their appearance. Granular cell tumour is encountered in the skin but also, characteristically, in the tongue and larynx. The tumour extends locally by direct infiltration but does not metastasise. The growth of granular cell tumour excites the overlying epithelium causing pseudo-epitheliomatous hyperplasia. It is necessary to guard against a mistaken diagnosis of squamous carcinoma.

Premalignant lesions

Both the exposed and the covered surfaces of the skin are susceptible to a range of precancerous disorders. Some are heritable, others acquired.

Solar (senile) keratosis

With advancing age, the exposed skin surfaces of fair-haired individuals often develop flat, grey–brown foci in which zones of parakeratosis and hyperkeratosis alternate. In themselves, these changes are of little other than cosmetic consequence. However, the epithelium undergoes progressive atrophy and the cells begin to show the signs of dysplasia (p. 85). When these abnormalities become pronounced, carcinoma *in-situ* is diagnosed.

Bowen's disease

Elevated plaques of red, scaly epithelium form on the skin of exposed surfaces and, from time-to-time, on the penile and peri-anal skin. The term Bowen's (p. 13) disease is applied to the disorder. Nearby, hair follicular epithelium is affected. The lesions are foci of epidermal carcinoma *in-situ*. There is a loss of the normal structured layering of the epidermis, the cells of which are replaced by others that are large and pale-staining. Mitotic figures are numerous and often abnormal. Squamous carcinoma evolves at the affected site in 15–30% of afflicted individuals but only after a long latent interval.

Xeroderma pigmentosum

In this rare autosomal recessive disorder, enzymes necessary for the repair of epidermal cell DNA are deficient or absent. There is a greatly enhanced risk of developing squamous carcinoma on exposure to sunlight.

Now read Carcinogenesis and Cancer (p. 76), Irradiation (p. 185)

Chemical keratoses

Skin lesions closely resembling those of solar keratosis develop in persons habitually exposed to carcinogens such as tar or arsenical compounds.

Malignant

Basal cell carcinoma (rodent ulcer)

Basal cell carcinoma (BCC) is the most common malignant tumour of the skin of elderly people.

Causes

Basal cell carcinoma is a locally invasive tumour of older, white persons that arises in skin frequently exposed to sunlight. The mean age of onset declines as the duration of exposure lengthens. Predisposing factors are genetic and environmental. There is an increased likelihood of BCC in the autosomal recessive disorder, xeroderma pigmentosum. Multiple tumours may arise in the autosomal dominant, basal cell naevus syndrome.

Structure

BCC is first recognised as a slightly raised, painless skin nodule located on the skin of the face, eyelids, ear or forehead. The tumour may be multifocal. Occasionally, the tumours are pigmented or cystic. In others of sclerosing or cicatrising form, there is either a relative excess of collagen, or a red, scaly margin with a scar-like centre, respectively. A delicate skein of small blood vessels extends over the tumour. As growth continues, the central loss of necrotic tumour cells results in ulceration. This indolent 'rodent' ulcer displays a rounded, raised edge (Fig. 53b).

BCC arises from the basal cells of the epidermis. The deeply stained cells, with compact, orderly nuclei, assume a pallisaded format at the margins of the tumour processes. Islands of neoplastic cells are frequently separated by collagenous connective tissue. There are microscopic variants including differentiation towards a squamous or sebaceous pattern. Solid and microcystic forms are frequent. BCC is sometimes multifocal and tumour buds may be identified at scattered points along the epidermo-dermal junction.

Behaviour and prognosis

Spread takes place locally. BCC does not metastasise but local tissue destruction may be very extensive. If the tumour remains untreated, skin, soft connective tissue, cartilage and bone are destroyed progressively, leading, for example, to loss of an ear or the nose. Early, wide excision is curative. Radiotherapy is also effective and other forms of topical treatment such as cryotherapy are used. Given prompt diagnosis, the prognosis is excellent.

Squamous carcinoma

Less common than in earlier industrialised societies, squamous carcinoma (p. 303) of the skin remains of great importance because early removal almost guarantees cure.

Causes

With the exception of populations where occupational or social factors lead to prolonged solar exposure at an early age, squamous carcinoma is a disease of elderly Caucasians. It is rare among black races. The risk of developing squamous carcinoma in response to chronic exposure to sunlight is 1000 times greater in individuals with xeroderma pigmentosum than in a control population. Other provocative environmental agents include ionising radiation; chronic inflammation, as in varicose ulcer; prolonged contact with chemical carcinogens, of which tar is the classical example; and immunosuppression for renal and other transplantation. Solar keratosis and Bowen's disease (p. 295) are precancerous.

Structure

Squamous carcinoma is first evident as a focus of roughened, red, hyperkeratotic skin on sites such as the forearm and hand; the nose, ear and lip; and the forehead. An uncommon, poorly differentiated tumour may be mistaken for an infective or inflammatory lesion. Finger-like processes composed of cells with eosinophilic cytoplasm and relatively large, pale nuclei, insinuate themselves through the epidermal basement membrane into the underlying dermis. In the usual, well-differentiated tumour, spinous processes bridge intercellular gaps. Keratin secretion continues, leading to focal aggregates of this material in the form of 'pearls'. A number of different tumour forms are recognised. Poorly differentiated squamous carcinoma is of high cellularity with many mitotic figures and anaplastic cell forms. A variant of this tumour is a spindle cell category that may be mistaken for sarcoma.

Behaviour and prognosis

Squamous carcinoma extends locally, by lymphatic dissemination and via the bloodstream. Tumours arising at sites of varicose ulcers, like those originating on the basis of burns or ionising radiation, and those developing in the skin of the ear, penis (p. 268) and vulva (p. 353), behave aggressively and metastasise early. Following early treatment by excision or radiotherapy, the prognosis is very good, although there is still a low, residual mortality in those cases in which block dissection of regional lymph nodes has been necessary.

SKIN APPENDAGES

Sweat gland-bearing skin is frequently affected by hidradenitis suppurativa, a chronic, folliculitis of the axillary; breast; peri-anal and genital zones. The infection is usually caused by *Staphylococcus aureus*. If the patient is a hospital employee, the disease precludes active work with patients until bacterial cultures are negative. The infection results in abscess formation and scarring.

TUMOURS OF HAIR FOLLICLE ORIGIN

The hair follicles, with their sebaceous glands, the eccrine sweat glands and the less frequent apocrine glands, are frequent sites for benign and malignant tumours.

Benign

Sebaceous glands undergo hyperplasia. Benign tumours are rare.

Pilomatricoma

This common tumour arises on the face and scalp of young persons, where it may recur after incomplete excision. Microscopically, the lesion is a mass of deeply staining cells among which there is dystrophic calcification.

Tricho-epitheloma

Tricho-epithelioma forms an isolated facial nodule in adults. The component cells resemble those of basal cell carcinoma but among them are characteristic, keratin-filled horn cysts. If a cyst ruptures into adjacent dermal and subcutaneous tissue, the keratin excites a foreign body giant cell reaction.

Malignant

Sebaceous carcinoma

Sebaceous glandular carcinoma is located particularly near the eyelids. There is sebaceous glandular cell differentiation, with mitotic activity and local tissue infiltration. It is an aggressive tumour and metastasis culminates in death.

TUMOURS OF ECCRINE GLAND ORIGIN

Benign

Syringoma

Syringoma is a frequent, small tumour of sweat glands that appears as a yellow papule on the head and neck, chest or genitalia. Not infrequently, the tumour is multiple. The double cell layer of the tumour acini is distinctive. Cartilage-like change is common.

Eccrine poroma

Eccrine poroma is a tumour of the margin or flexor surface of the hand or foot. Whereas syringoma originates from the substance of a sweat gland, eccrine poroma arises from that part of the sweat gland duct that extends within the epidermis. The presence of intercellular bridges is identified. The tumour cell is small, uniform and deeply staining. There is no propensity to malignant transformation.

Malignant

Eccrine glandular carcinoma

This is a rare skin cancer that may originate on the basis of an existing benign tumour.

TUMOURS OF APOCRINE GLAND ORIGIN

Benign

Hidradenoma papilliferum

In regions such as the vulvar or peri-anal skin, where apocrine glands predominate, small, slowly growing, pale yellow tumours are found. Papillary glandular cell processes, comprising a double layer of epithelial and myo-epithelial cells, lie within a cyst-like structure.

Cylindroma

However rare, multiple cylindromas attract attention because, untreated, they grow in the skin of the scalp to assume an enormous size and striking appearance. They are 'turban' tumours. Their formation may be inherited as an autosomal dominant characteristic.

Malignant

Apocrine glandular carcinoma

Apocrine glandular carcinoma is a rare tumour of sites such as the axilla, nipple and vulva.

SOFT TISSUE TUMOURS

A wide range of benign and malignant tumours arise within the loose connective tissues (p. 110). For practical reasons of diagnosis and treatment, these neoplasms are described as 'soft tissue tumours'. It has been found valuable to divide them into three broad categories of benign, intermediate and malignant. Many display specific chromosomal translocations leading to the expression of chimaeric genes that encode transcription factors.

In practice, the soft tissue tumours are distinguished:

- First, from the **tumour-like**, infiltrating and recurrent but non-metastasising condition of fibromatosis (p. 130).
- Second, from a class of quickly growing but non-neoplastic, **reactive** lesions that includes nodular fasciitis and myositis ossificans (p. 238).

The cells of soft tissue tumours are of fibrous; histiocytic; adipose; vascular; smooth or striated muscular; neurilemmal; cartilaginous; or bony origin. The tumours are classified on the basis of these cell types. Some remain unclassified: they arise from undifferentiated, mesenchymal cells. Vascular and neurilemmal soft tissue tumours are discussed on pp. 48 and 250, respectively; tumours of muscle on pp. 235–236; and those affecting cartilage and bone on pp. 82 and 57, respectively.

Biopsy of soft tissue tumours

The management of malignant soft tissue tumours calls for referral to special centres and for close collaboration between surgeon, pathologist and oncologist. Fine-needle aspiration biopsy and cytology is neither a reliable nor a recommended technique. However, Trucut needle biopsy has been authenticated. Accurate diagnosis can be assured and the technique may replace initial, incisional biopsy. The interpretation of frozen sections of soft tissue tumours is difficult and uncertain. Definitive diagnosis rests upon the availability of conventional, paraffin-embedded sections.

Benign

Lipoma

Lipoma presents as a slowly growing, lobulated mass, most commonly within the soft connective tissues of the neck, shoulder or back of adults. Occasionally, lipoma occurs within a large synovial joint. It is much less common in the mediastinum or retroperitoneum where it is imperative to distinguish the mass from liposarcoma. Variants of lipoma include a pleomorphic form. Inter- and intramuscular lipoma is recognised when a lobulated mass forms in a skeletal muscle. A similar lesion occasionally grows within the confines of the median nerve at the wrist.

Dercum's disease, adiposa dolorosa, is an inherited condition in which the afflicted individual develops multiple, tender, subcutaneous lipomas, sometimes associated with a peripheral neuropathy.

Angiolipoma is a painful skin nodule of young adults.

Dermatofibroma

Dermatofibroma is a lesion of young and middle-aged adults. It forms a subcutaneous nodule in the skin of the leg or arm and has an ill-defined edge. The tumour comprises slowly proliferating, spindle-shaped cells of histiocytic origin but foamy, lipid-rich macrophages and a few multinucleated giant cells are seen and the presence of iron-containing, haemosiderin granules is characteristic. The cells of the tumour may be arranged in a cartwheel pattern.

Myxoma

Myxoma originates as a firm or gelatinous tumour of the mandible and other connective tissue sites. It is also encountered as a mass in the right atrium of the heart where it can function as a ball valve to occlude blood flow.

Now read Heart (p. 150)

Fibroma

Fibroma is a very frequent benign tumour of organs such as the kidney but is surprisingly rare in the soft connective tissues.

Malignant

The annual incidence of these rare but important tumours is ~$2.5/10^6$ population. The most frequent are rhabdomyosarcoma (p. 236), in children; and malignant fibrous histiocytoma, in adults. Some exhibit defined chromosomal translocations but the genotypes of many have not yet been determined. Synovial sarcoma (p. 194) is an exception. The prognosis of soft tissue sarcoma is closely related to histological grade assessed by mitotic counts and by ploidy. Adverse features are advanced age; a deep as opposed to a superficial site; and local recurrence. Venous metastasis is usual and lymphatic dissemination is not a feature.

Now read Angiosarcoma; Kaposi's sarcoma (p. 49)

Malignant fibrous histiocytoma

Many tumours previously classified as fibrosarcoma are regarded as malignant fibrous histiocytoma (MFH), now the commonest soft tissue sarcoma of the elderly but a relatively rare disorder of children and young adults. A frequent mutation is the result of a chromosomal translocation that represents t(12;16) (q13;p11).

The tumour forms a slowly growing, deep-seated mass within the muscular and connective tissues of the leg or in the retroperitoneal tissues. The predominant cell is fibroblast-like. Characteristically, these cells are often arranged in a cartwheel pattern. They are interspersed with groups of pleomorphic and anaplastic cells that display abnormal mitotic figures and which, in turn, lie among varying proportions of macrophages, lymphocytes and occasional multinucleated giant cells. Tests with monoclonal antibodies confirm that the fibroblasts express the fibrillar protein, vimentin.

Prognosis is adversely influenced by the size of the tumour; by a deep location; and by evidence that incomplete resection has been followed by recurrence, a feature of half of all cases. MFH extends locally within the connective tissue planes of the limb. Distant spread is by blood-borne metastasis to the lungs. The 5-year survival rate is ~30%.

Liposarcoma

Liposarcoma is a relatively frequent malignant soft tissue tumour of adults. It is rare in children. The tumour arises within the deep fascial, mesenchymal connective tissues as a slowly growing mass in the leg or retroperitoneal tissues. It forms an ill-defined, soft or gelatinous mass. The unique cellular component is a population of polygonal cells with heavily staining, indented nuclei and vacuolated cytoplasm. They are seen against a background of cells ranging from mature lipocytes to small, undifferentiated cells, the proportions of which vary with the tumour grade. There are occasional pleomorphic giant cells.

Prognosis is guarded. Adverse factors are large size; a proximal situation; failure to excise satellite tumour nodules that arise in nearby connective tissues; and a tendency for loss of differentiation among low-grade retroperitoneal tumours. Distant spread is to the lungs, pleura, liver and gastro-intestinal tract. The 5-year survival rate ranges from ~40% for the poorly differentiated tumours to ~60% for tumours of lower grade.

Fibrosarcoma

Fibrosarcoma is a malignant soft tissue tumour of middle-aged adults. The tumour may arise in any collagenous connective tissue but the most frequent locations are the lower limb adjacent to the knee; the trunk; the forearms; and the lower leg. Retroperitoneal tumours are not uncommon and, from time-to-time, fibrosarcoma is identified in the paranasal sinuses. The tumour forms a deep-seated mass defined by a false capsule of compressed, circumferential connective tissue and composed of islands of undifferentiated spindle-shaped cells extending locally into nearby muscle and fat. Bundles of cells may assume a herring-bone pattern. Local spread, often in the form of apparently independent nodules, precedes blood-borne metastasis to lung, liver and bone.

Prognosis is uncertain. Adverse factors include inadequate excision; high tumour grade; and a deep location. The 5-year survival rate is ~50%.

Synovial sarcoma

The name synovial sarcoma is still given to a very unusual neoplasm of young adults. Synovial sarcoma is not a tumour of synovial cells but, like liposarcoma and malignant fibrous histiocytoma, originates in mesenchymal cells. A chromosomal translocation, t(X;18)(p.11.2; q11.2), is demonstrable.

Synovial sarcoma is a slowly growing, sometimes painful and often cystic mass located near the knee but occasionally at other sites. There is a close association with tendons, ligaments and joint tissues but the tumour is not intra-articular. There are two varieties: monophasic and biphasic.

- **Biphasic**. Islands or columns of epithelial-like cells lie within broad zones of spindle cells. Epithelial-like cells often line a cleft or space.
- **Monophasic**. Only one of the two cell types is represented.

At first, it may be difficult to distinguish synovial sarcoma from malignant fibrous histiocytoma, fibrosarcoma and metastatic carcinoma. Focal calcification is frequent. The demonstration in both spindle cells and epithelial-like cells of a positive reaction with monoclonal antibodies against the cytokeratins and epithelial membrane antigen, assists diagnosis. The spindle-cell component reacts with antivimentin antibodies.

Prognosis is guarded. There is a 5-year survival rate of ~70% but many synovial sarcomas recur locally. Metastasis to lung and liver is a late result of blood-borne spread.

Now read Sarcoma (pp. 243, 289)

SPINE

The spine comprises 24 vertebral bodies together with the five fused bones of the sacrum. The vertebral bodies are separated by 23 intervertebral discs – there is no disc between C1 and C2. Whereas the main intervertebral joints are fibrocartilaginous and relatively fixed, the posterolateral, facet joints are synovial and freely moving. The spine is subject to virtually all of those heritable and acquired diseases that affect bone, articular cartilage, joints and associated tissues including the bone marrow. Diseases of the vascular, freely moving, spinal joints are distinguished from those affecting the avascular, fixed joints.

Now read Bone (p. 50), Cartilage (p. 82), Joints (p. 190)

DEVELOPMENTAL AND CONGENITAL DISORDERS

Spina bifida is discussed on p. 63.

Now read Brain (p. 60)

MECHANICAL DISORDERS AND TRAUMA

Intervertebral disc protrusion and prolapse

In response to physical exertion, generally in flexion, the nucleus pulposus of the lower thoracic and upper lumbar intervertebral discs may protrude through the posterolateral parts of the ligaments that bind the discs to each other and to the underlying vertebral bones. Systematic MRI surveys show that the protrusions are very often asymptomatic. However, when the displacement of disc tissue becomes more severe and prolapse occurs, it is commonplace for the nuclear tissue to compress the nerve roots as they emerge from the intervertebral canals, resulting in a segmental loss of sensation and selective motor nerve irritation. In the cervical region, the C3 and C4 segments are particularly susceptible to compression. In the lumbar region, the L5, S1 nerve roots are very often implicated.

Ankylosing hyperostosis

In this condition, common in male patients with diabetes mellitus, the vertebrae are joined by new bone formation that is of greater degree on the right than on the left side of the spine.

INFECTION AND INFLAMMATION

Spinal abscess is one result of vertebral osteomyelitis. In Western societies, the cause is usually infection with *Staphylococcus aureus* or Gram-negative bacilli but in less affluent, malnourished and immunocompromised populations, *Mycobacterium tuberculosis* infection is again becoming frequent. One consequence is Pott's disease (p. 54).

TUMOURS

Metastatic tumours of the spine are exceedingly frequent. There are two broad categories: osteolytic and osteosclerotic. The former is exemplified by metastatic carcinomas of the bronchus, breast and gastro-intestinal tract. The most characteristic osteosclerotic metastases are from carcinoma of the prostate gland (p. 278).

Primary benign tumours of the spine include haemangioma, osteochondroma and giant osteoid osteoma.

Primary malignant tumours are recognised very much less often than metastases. Multiple myeloma is the most common in the elderly. Saccrococcygeal chordoma (Table 13, p. 58) is rare.

VASCULAR DISEASE

The anterior aspects of the thoracic and lumbar spine are prone to compression by enlarging aortic aneurysms. There is bone atrophy but the intervertebral discs remain intact, resulting in a 'scalloped' appearance of the spinal outline.

SPONDYLITIS AND SPONDYLOARTHROPATHY

An important category of inflammatory diseases affecting the joints of the spine is associated with the inheritance of the antigen HLA-B27 and with the absence of rheumatoid factors (p. 29) from the blood. The conditions are termed seronegative **spondyloarthropathies**. They include ankylosing spondylitis (p. 192); psoriatic arthropathy; and the reactive, axial joint disorders associated with Crohn's disease, ulcerative colitis and *Yersinia enterocolitica* infection.

SPLEEN

In the fetus, the spleen is a site of haemopoiesis. This function may be retained after birth or resumed if much bone marrow is replaced or destroyed by disorders such as myelofibrosis or metastatic carcinomatosis. In the adult, the most important function of the spleen is to combat systemic, blood-borne infection. The white pulp, comprising 25% of the body's lymphoid tissues, has immunological functions important for defence against micro-organisms. Bacteria coated with opsonic antibody are phagocytosed by macrophages. The sinusoids of the red pulp, lined by vigorously phagocytic cells, engulf and destroy aged and abnormal red blood cells.

Now read Haemopoiesis (p. 10), Immunity (p. 171)

DEVELOPMENTAL AND CONGENITAL DISORDERS

Splenic agenesis is rare and often associated with cardiac abnormalities. Hypoplasia is also very unusual; there is an increased susceptibility to infection, particularly in infants. Splenunculi (accessory spleens) are found near the hilum in ~10% of individuals.

Cysts

- **Congenital cysts** have a lining of cuboidal cells and a serous content. The cysts are usually multiple and subcapsular. In some countries, hydatid cyst (pp. 113, 357) is frequent; it may rupture and cause haemorrhage. Dissemination of the contents of a hydatid cyst within the peritoneal cavity may initiate anaphylactic shock.
- **Pseudocysts** may form in the spleen as a consequence of infarction or haematoma.

SPLENOMEGALY

Enlargement of the spleen may be transient or permanent. The causes are hereditary and acquired.

- **Hereditary**. The rare hereditary lipid storage diseases, Gaucher's disease and Niemann–Pick disease, lead to massive splenomegaly.
- **Acquired**. Among the frequent environmental causes are malaria; enteric fever; infectious mononucleosis; infective endocarditis; tuberculosis; and schistosomiasis. Haematological disorders that commonly produce splenomegaly include lymphoma; leukaemia; polycythaemia; haemolytic anaemias; thrombocytopenic purpura; and myelofibrosis. Portal hypertension due to various causes is usually associated with moderate splenomegaly.

  In **Banti's syndrome**, splenomegaly and hypersplenism are secondary to portal hypertension (p. 212) due to cirrhosis or portal vein thrombosis.

  In **Felty's syndrome**, a variant of rheumatoid arthritis, there is hepatomegaly, splenomegaly and hypersplenism, leading to anaemia and leucopenia.

HYPERSPLENISM

Hypersplenism describes over-activity of the spleen, with trapping and destruction of all forms of blood cell. The result is pancytopenia. There is splenomegaly but the degree of hypersplenism is not related directly to the size of the spleen.

INFECTION AND INFLAMMATION

Pathogenic bacteria such as encapsulated type III *Streptococcus pneumoniae* are frequently associated with hyposplenism (below) as are *Haemophilus influenzae* and *Neisseria meningitidis*. The spleen also acts as a reservoir for viruses and other parasites. When the defensive mechanisms of the spleen are overcome by bacterial infection, one or more abscesses may form.

TUMOURS

Direct invasion of the spleen by the extension of intra-abdominal tumours is uncommon. Distant metastasis to the spleen is frequent. Microscopic examination of the spleen in patients with carcinomatosis reveals deposits in ~30% of cases. Melanoma, choriocarcinomas and carcinomas of the breast, ovary and lung frequently spread to the spleen.

Benign

Benign primary tumours are uncommon. Hamartomas comprising blood and lymphatic vessels are described.

Malignant

Lymphoma

The spleen is commonly implicated in lymphoma, regardless of the primary cell type. At laparotomy, the examination of the spleen and lymph nodes was part of a system for staging lymphoma. Now, CT provides an accurate assessment for decisions regarding treatment.

Now read Lymphoma (p. 223), Neoplasia/Tumour staging (p. 244)

Leukaemia

The spleen is involved in all forms of leukaemia. Gross splenic enlargement is particularly characteristic of the chronic disease. In chronic granulocytic leukaemia the organ may weigh as much as 10 kg. The red pulp is infiltrated with leukaemic cells that obscure the Malpighian bodies. As an indirect consequence of the replacement of haemopoietic bone marrow by leukaemic cells, there is frequent evidence of extramedullary haemopoiesis shown by the presence in the spleen of megakaryocytes and erythroid precursors.

Now read Leukaemia (p. 207)

VASCULAR DISORDERS

Infarction

Occlusion of a branch of the splenic artery by embolus leads to infarction of a wedge-shaped island of peripheral, splenic tissue. The infarct is pale since the splenic arteries are end-arteries. As organisation advances, the necrotic splenic tissue is converted to a shrunken, fibrotic scar. Splenic artery emboli often complicate endocarditis. Atheroma, aneurysm or thrombosis of the splenic artery lead to splenic ischaemia. Multiple zones of infarction also characterise sickle-cell disease (Figure 35).

SPLENECTOMY

Within hours of splenectomy, granulocytosis (p. 206) develops and persists for two weeks when it is accompanied by lymphocytosis and monocytosis. The blood granulocyte count may reach ~50 × 10^9/L (p. 205). There is a comparable thrombocytosis. The platelet count may rise to ~500 × 10^9/L. Episodes of thrombosis and embolism occur. The loss of splenic tissue reduces the capacity of the spleen to destroy immature or abnormal red cells: within a few days, target cells, reticulocytes and siderocytes appear in the circulating blood.

Small islands of splenic tissue may survive after excision of the spleen and are sometimes incorrectly termed splenunculi. Following splenectomy, this tissue hypertrophies. There may be total restoration of immune and other functions. The state of the revitalised tissue can be examined by radio-active isotope tests.

The intra-abdominal implantation of splenic tissue

may be beneficial after splenectomy for trauma. It often restores vascularity but not physiological activity and can be detrimental if splenectomy was performed for reasons such as the treatment of thrombocytopenia. Indeed, it may permit the re-emergence of diseases such as haemolytic anaemia for which the operation was originally performed.

Individuals from whom the spleen has been removed are unduly susceptible to infection. Encapsulated bacteria such as *Streptococcus pneumoniae*, *Haemophilus influenzae*, and *Neisseria meningitidis,* the meningococcus, are particular hazards and death from septicaemia may follow.

Overwhelming, post-splenectomy infection (OPSI) is uncommon but carries a high mortality. Patients should therefore be immunised against these micro-organisms at least 2 weeks before elective surgery. In addition, all patients from whom the spleen has been removed abruptly, after accident or injury, should be given the vaccine immediately before they leave hospital. It has been suggested that they should also receive daily oral penicillin prophylactically for the remainder of their lives.

SQUAMOUS CARCINOMA

Squamous carcinomas are epithelial tumours in which the cells have differentiated towards expressing the features of stratified squamous epithelium. Sometimes, but not always, there is keratinisation. The microscopic features of squamous carcinoma include intercellular ('prickle') process formation and neoplastic cells arranged as 'nests', often with central keratin. There are cytoplasmic filaments, keratohyaline granules, and intercellular junctions. There are no intracellular lumina but long, slender microvilli may exist within intercellular spaces.

Squamous carcinomas of the skin of the hand were the first occupational tumours attributed to the prolonged effects of ionising radiation (p. 185). Later, experimental squamous carcinomas were produced by painting the skin of mice with coal tar and, subsequently, with carcinogens such as dibenzanthracene. Squamous carcinomas often arise from metaplastic epithelium such as that of the bronchi (p. 70). Squamous carcinomas of the lung; oesophagus; uterine cervix; oral cavity; and skin are discussed on pp. 70, 255, 340, 258 and 296, respectively.

STAPHYLOCOCCUS

Staphylococci are Gram-positive cocci that form grape-like clusters. The organisms exist in the nose and on the skin of many healthy persons; they provoke opportunistic infection when skin or mucosae are damaged. Individuals with exfoliative skin diseases such as eczema are liable to carry *Staphylococcus aureus*. Pathogenic *S. aureus* invade and destroy tissue locally, causing suppuration. The virulence of *S. aureus* is due to a combination of numerous surface components, toxins and enzymes that enable the bacteria to resist phagocytosis, kill leucocytes and avoid opsonisation (Table 52).

Common suppurative infections caused by *S. aureus* include boils (furuncles); styes; carbuncles; wound infection; cellulitis; and arthritis. Septicaemia, osteomyelitis and bacterial endocarditis are other results. *S. aureus* often causes hospital infections, par-

Table 52 Some virulence factors and toxins of *Staphylococcus aureus*

Virulence factor/toxin	Actions and effects
Protein A	Cell-wall structural protein binding to Fc region of Ig
Coagulase	Inhibits opsonisation. Enzyme activating prothrombin, producing fibrin barrier that impairs movement of leucocytes towards micro-organisms. Production of coagulase is good index of pathogenicity
Leucocidin	Toxin that kills leucocytes
Alpha toxin	Toxin that kills leucocytes, causes vascular smooth-muscle contraction, lyses red blood cells
Enterotoxins	Five types recognised. Type C has three sub-types. Type F responsible for toxic shock syndrome. Enterotoxin is formed by bacterial multiplication in contaminated food kept at ambient temperatures where it may be identified. Resists destruction by heat. Food poisoning follows ingestion
Epidermolytic toxin	Toxin produced by *S. aureus*, usually of phage group II. Effects range from scattered blisters to 'scalded skin'. Most common in neonates

ticularly of the newborn; the old; the surgical patient; and the diabetic, and is responsible for some outbreaks of food poisoning.

The capacity of staphylococci to spread (**epidemicity**) does not always correlate with their **pathogenicity**, their capacity to cause disease. The source and spread of staphylococcal infection in a surgical ward is investigated by epidemiological analysis, a plot of antibiotic sensitivities and, perhaps, by phage typing (pp. 34, 35). Some phage types are more **virulent** than others, that is, they result in more severe disease. These types are especially likely to be responsible for surgical infections.

Most strains of *S. aureus* remain sensitive to flucloxacillin, erythromycin and gentamicin but at least 85% of hospital strains are resistant to benzyl penicillin. Strains resistant to flucloxacillin are a growing challenge. They are termed methicillin-resistant *Staphylococcus aureus* (MRSA). There are few therapeutic options apart from the selection of vancomycin for oral treatment. The parenteral antibiotics that can now be employed are glycopeptides (vancomycin and teicoplanin), streptogranin and oxazolidonone. However, vancomycin-resistant strains (VRSA) have emerged.

Now read Methicillin and vancomycin (p. 18)

TOXIC SHOCK SYNDROME

The toxic shock syndrome is infection with a type F toxin-producing strain of *Staphylococcus aureus*. Originally described in young women in association with the use of superabsorbent vaginal tampons, the toxic shock syndrome may occur in any person harbouring a focus of *S. aureus* infection. There is fever; vomiting; diarrhoea; rash; desquamation; and circulatory collapse.

STATISTICS

Many of the greatest advances in medicine and surgery owed nothing to statistical assessment. The recognition of the circulation of the blood; the mechanism of genetic inheritance; the existence of the endocrine system; and the isolation of penicillin, for example, were the consequences of a mixture of scientific forethought, careful observation, intuition and chance. However, the use of medical statistics has been responsible for major advances in determining the cause of human disease. The controlled studies that identified smoking as the cause of the rise in deaths from cancer of the lung after World War II offer a classical example. The comparison of different methods of surgical treatment has also required statistical evaluation. More than 70% of papers published in the world's leading medical journals contain some form of statistical analysis and it is not uncommon for this analysis to provoke more comment than the medical point at issue or the relevant data.

Two fundamentals must be taken into account when a surgeon assesses a published paper.

- **Biological variation**. A major feature of biological science is variability. The atomic weight of a specified element does not vary but measurements of human indices vary from minute to minute. A carefully designed study reduces the possibility of confounding variables.
- **Sample size and power**. Many published studies that include valid methods of statistical analysis fail to reach the desired conclusion because of the inadequate size of the study. In any statistical analysis, the number of observations required to identify changes of a certain magnitude with a specified probability, can be calculated. For example, a statistician can estimate the number of patients needed to test the efficacy of an antibiotic in preventing wound infection. He/she is told that the natural incidence of infection without antibiotics is 10%. The predicted response to prophylactic antibiotic might be a 20% reduction in the rate of infection. Such a study would demand the recruitment of hundreds of patients.

Statistics in audit and research

The advice of a medical statistician should be sought before analysing data for audit or research. The principles of frequency, normal distribution, range and means, standard deviation, standard error, confidence limits, Student's *t* test, the chi squared test, Fisher's exact test, Mann–Whitney U test, Wilcoxon signed-rank test, analysis of variance, and correlation and linear regression, require to be understood.

STERILISATION

Sterilisation is the entire destruction of micro-organisms, including their spores and cysts, by a solid, fluid or gas.

Most viruses survive at temperatures as low as −70°C or in a dry state after freeze-drying. The majority, including HIV, are killed by moderate heat. There are important exceptions. The viruses of serum hepatitis and poliomyelitis resist much higher temperatures. The agent of CJD (p. 351) resists boiling for 1 hour and is inactivated with difficulty. Viruses are not destroyed by pH changes from 5 to 9. Those with a lipid-containing envelope are sensitive to solvents such as ether. Hydrogen peroxide and other oxidising agents, such as hypochlorite, are good viral disinfectants. Phenols are seldom effective, although this depends on the concentration at which they are used. Viruses with envelopes are also sensitive to bile. Many viruses are inactivated by ultraviolet light (UVL). Dyes such as acridine orange that bind to nucleic acids increase this susceptibility.

CHEMICAL

Chemical agents are considered as disinfectants (p. 118).

PHYSICAL

Heat

Dry heat

Many objects do not withstand the high temperatures required for sterilisation by dry heat. Those that can be sterilised by this means include metal instruments, dishes and cloths. They are held in sealed containers from which they can be removed conveniently in an operating theatre or other room. Dry heat can be produced by infra-red irradiation as well as by conventional and microwave ovens.

Moist heat

Solids

Moist heat is more effective than dry heat in killing micro-organisms on or near solid objects. It penetrates porous materials well and denatures the proteins of microbial cell walls. Boiling at 100°C, at normal atmospheric pressure, is effective if continued for many hours although bacterial spores and hepatitis B virus withstand short periods under these conditions. Bacteria, fungi and their spores are destroyed in 10 minutes by steam at 126°C; in 15 minutes by steam at 121°C; but only after 1 hour by dry heat at 160°C. The transmissible agents of scrapie, Creutzfeld–Jacob disease (CJD) and bovine spongiform encephalopathy (BSE) are very difficult to destroy and material suspected of carrying these agents requires to be autoclaved three times, at 134°C, on each occasion for 30 minutes.

- **Autoclaves**. Sterilisation by steam under raised pressure is the most commonly used method in hospitals and in industry. The devices employed for this purpose are autoclaves. In the closed autoclave, steam is heated to a temperature of 121°C by increasing the pressure. The steam condenses upon the surfaces of cool instruments and containers placed within the autoclave, giving up the large amount of latent heat of vaporisation required for its production. It is essential that the steam be able to penetrate all these objects. The sterilising cycle must be sufficiently long to ensure that this happens. To confirm that sterilisation has been completed, a recording of temperature is made from the coolest, lower part of the autoclave. Browne's glass tubes, placed amongst the instruments, change from red to green on exposure to a temperature of 115°C for 25 minutes (type 1) or 15 minutes (type 2). Sterile packs can be identified by the colour of the heat-sensitive inks used in a Bowie–Dick test. A colour change develops after sufficient heating.
- **Pasteurisation** is described on p. 119.

Fluids

Many of the fluids employed in surgery require sterilisation.

Gases

Some gases used in surgery are sterilised before use.

Radiation

Non-ionising irradiation

Solar and artificial sources of ultraviolet light (UVL) of wavelength less than 330 nm can kill micro-organisms.

Ionising irradiation

High energy, gamma-rays penetrate materials for substantial distances. They are employed commercially to sterilise heat-labile articles; plastic syringes; and dressings.

Filtration

Bacteria and spores can be removed from heat-labile, biological and biochemical solutions and gases, by filtration through earthenware, sintered glass, or Seitz (asbestos) filters. Cellulose acetate (Millipore) membrane filters can be chosen with a pore size sufficiently small to remove mycoplasmas and viruses. The efficiency of sterilisation is determined by the pore size.

The air entering operating suites is filtered to remove dust particles that carry bacteria, but the glass fibre filters do not remove particles as small as individual bacteria or spores.

Now read Antisepsis/Asepsis (p. 23), Disinfection (p. 118)

STERILISATION OF VENTILATORS

Anaesthetic ventilators

The most effective method of avoiding infection is to use disposable components but these are expensive. Most ventilators are used for comparatively short periods in anaesthetised patients undergoing operations. In this type of ventilator, the expiratory circuit from the patient is the key component. Ideally, this circuit is changed for each patient. In practice, this procedure is not followed because the components are made of rubber, plastic and metal that offer limited support for bacterial growth. Under these circumstances, cleaning with disinfectants (p. 118) at regular intervals is sufficient. However, the expiratory circuit is changed and disinfected when it has been used in a patient with pulmonary tuberculosis or pulmonary sepsis and in those who are HIV or HBsAg-positive. After operations on patients with clostridial infections or MRSA, the entire contents of the operating theatre are disinfected.

Methods of sterilisation vary according to the type of ventilator. Modern ventilators are designed so that they can be dismantled to allow easy access to the contaminated units. Some components can be sterilised by autoclaving but this reduces the life of the part. Other components, particularly transducers and electronic devices, can be damaged by heat. Pasteurisation (p. 119) and the use of disinfectants is possible but less effective than costly techniques employing ethylene oxide and gamma-irradiation. Water in any ventilator system is likely to contain organisms such as antibiotic-resistant Pseudomonas spp. and the coliforms that are found commonly in a hospital environment.

ICU ventilators

Some ventilators are used for the prolonged ventilation of severely ill patients, usually in intensive care units (ICUs). Patients requiring prolonged ventilation often become infected with virulent, pathogenic bacteria that are resistant to antibiotics. Sterilisation of the inspiratory and expiratory circuits is essential before the ventilator is used for another patient. Most ICUs are now equipped with ventilators that incorporate disposable circuits.

STOMACH

Biopsy diagnosis of gastric disease

Suspicious lesions identified at endoscopy are examined cytologically. The cells are obtained with a brush. Biopsies are also taken with endoscopic forceps: numerous samples should be obtained from various parts of the lesion. The precision of diagnosis is enhanced if both techniques are employed. The brush sample should precede conventional biopsy. If there is an ulcer, tissue is excised from the edge rather than from the base which is likely to be necrotic.

The pathologist should seek the presence of *Helicobacter pylori*. If there is a possibility that the lesion is malignant, biopsies are taken from additional parts of the stomach, allowing the extent of a mucosal lesion to be demarcated pre-operatively. Severe dysplastic changes in other sites indicate the need for total – rather than for partial – gastrectomy. Pedunculated polyps are removed in their entirety by diathermy snare.

Accurate records must be kept concerning the precise site from which biopsies are removed. The record should include a diagram indicating and numbering the sites sampled.

DEVELOPMENTAL AND CONGENITAL DISORDERS

Congenital abnormalities of the stomach, other than pyloric stenosis, are uncommon.

- **Pyloric stenosis**. In this condition, more common in male than female infants, there is hypertrophy of the circular muscle of the pylorus. Severe, persistent vomiting develops two weeks after birth. In the absence of surgical treatment, death may occur.
- **Dieulafoy's anomaly** is a vascular abnormality located high in the fundus. A large, tortuous submucosal vessel is found in the base of a gastric erosion. The anomaly is more common in males. The condition has occurred in twins, suggesting a genetic predisposition. Life threatening haemorrhage may result.

INFECTION AND INFLAMMATION

Acute gastritis

Acute mucosal inflammation is frequent in those consuming aspirin and non-steroidal anti-inflammatory drugs (NSAIDs) that inhibit prostaglandin synthesis. Another cause of acute gastritis is infestation with *Helicobacter pylori* (p. 151): the organism exerts a direct, cytotoxic effect upon gastric epithelium.

Acute gastritis may progress to **acute erosion**. This is a mucosal defect without penetration of the muscularis mucosae. Acute erosions often develop in patients in intensive care units, a sequence that may be related to local ischaemia. Deficient blood flow may prevent the dispersal of H^+ ions that have penetrated epithelial cells. Acute erosions may produce haematemesis and melaena but in the majority of patients, acute gastritis resolves spontaneously. Those treated with NSAIDs are often subject to intractable anaemia.

Chronic gastritis

There are three principal varieties, superficial, atrophic and granulomatous. The characteristic feature of all is mucosal infiltration by plasma cells (p. 172) and lymphocytes (p. 206). Infestation with *Helicobacter pylori* is the commonest cause.

Chronic superficial gastritis

In chronic superficial gastritis (CSG), persistent inflammation is confined to the mucosa. The lamina propria is not implicated. The cellular infiltrate is plasmacytic and to a lesser extent, composed of lymphocytes and macrophages. When polymorphs are present, the chronic inflammation is regarded as active.

Chronic atrophic gastritis

Progression of CSG leads to the disappearance of much of the glandular tissue: the gastric glands atrophy and are replaced by collagenous connective tissue. The condition is then termed chronic atrophic gastritis (CAG). Where there are residual glands, intestinal metaplasia (IM) is often detected. In this condition, the gastric glands assume the appearance of those of the small intestine and the epithelium comprises enterocytes with a brush border. There are both goblet and Paneth cells.

Chronic atrophic gastritis and intestinal metaplasia are common. The structural changes are accompanied by the synthesis of antiparietal cell antibodies although these immunoglobulins are identifiable in 10% of normal individuals over the age of 50 years. Intestinal metaplasia is associated with an increased incidence of gastric carcinoma of intestinal type. Populations with a high prevalence of gastric cancer manifest a high frequency of IM. Relatives of patients with gastric cancer often have IM and this abnormality is a common histological feature of the mucosa adjacent to gastric cancer.

The significance of CAG and IM in the aetiology of gastric cancer remains uncertain: the varieties of chronic gastritis and IM display differing susceptibility to neoplastic change.

Chronic granulomatous gastritis

In chronic granulomatous gastritis (CGG), non-caseating, mucosal granulomas are found within the gastric mucosa. In some cases, the explanation for their presence is sarcoidosis, in others tuberculosis. CGG may be a variant of regional enteritis, Crohn's disease (p. 165).

Dysplasia

Gastric mucosal dysplasia is a common sequel to gastric IM but may occasionally be recognised in the normal epithelium. The epithelial cells are large with pleomorphic, hyperchromatic nuclei. There are abnormalities in the architecture of the gastric pits. The dysplastic epithelium may revert to normal and does not invariably undergo malignant transformation.

Now read Dysplasia (p. 85)

Ménétrier's disease

Ménétrier's disease is hypertrophic gastritis of unknown aetiology. Giant rugae are confined to the body and fundus of the stomach. These mucosal folds remain after inflation of the stomach at endoscopy. There is a loss of parietal cells resulting in hypochlorhydria and an increased risk of carcinoma.

Ulcer

Gastric ulcer is most frequent in the sixth decade but the prevalence has declined in recent years. It may be acute or chronic.

Acute

Acute gastric ulcers penetrate the muscularis mucosae whereas, in erosions, the muscularis remains intact. Acute ulcers may follow aspirin or NSAID ingestion and may be provoked by exposure to bile. Cushing (p. 371) described acute gastric ulceration after intracranial trauma or surgical operations. Curling (p. 371) reported comparable duodenal ulcers following severe burns, sepsis and shock. One factor linking these phenomena is mucosal ischaemia.

Chronic

Chronic gastric ulcer is slightly more common in males than females. The sex difference is not apparent in the elderly, probably because of the influence of NSAIDs. The peak incidence is some 10 years later than for duodenal ulcer (p. 121).

Causes

The aetiology of gastric ulcer is uncertain. Impaired mucosal protection is evidently more important than excess acid secretion. Indeed, acid secretion rates are often normal or reduced although achlorhydria is exceptional. Furthermore, infection with *Helicobacter pylori* can be demonstrated in 70% of patients. There is a higher prevalence among those who smoke cigarettes than in those who do not.

Structure

Simple, chronic ulcers occur on the lesser curve of the stomach or in the antrum. The majority lie at the incisura. The edges of the ulcer frequently overhang. Contraction produces radiating mucosal folds not found in malignant ulcers. Ulcers at other sites are likely to be cancerous. At endoscopy, the edges of an ulcer appear red with a pale slough at the base. Restoration of a normal gastric mucosal architecture cannot be achieved. When inflammation subsides, repair begins. The base of the ulcer comes to be formed of fibrous tissue. Here, the obliteration of small arteries by endarterial fibromuscular regeneration, endarteritis obliterans, confirms that inflammation has been long-standing. Cytological and histological examin-ation of tissue obtained with a brush and with biopsy forceps is necessary to exclude the presence of carcinoma.

Behaviour and prognosis

The complications of chronic gastric ulcer are bleeding; perforation; stenosis; and malignant transformation.

- **Bleeding**. Gastric ulceration is the cause of bleeding in 20% of patients admitted with haematemesis to hospitals in the UK.
- **Perforation** is nine times less frequent in gastric ulcer by comparison with duodenal ulcer. Perforation may take place into the lesser sac. A posterior gastric ulcer may penetrate into the pancreas.
- **Stenosis**. If an ulcer on the lesser curve heals with much fibrosis, contracture may produce the hourglass deformity of pyloric stenosis.
- **Cancer**. Malignant transformation of benign gastric ulcer is thought to occur in less than 1% of instances. The size of a chronic peptic ulcer is not a reliable sign that the lesion is malignant. In patients with chronic peptic ulceration, carcinoma may arise at sites remote from the ulcer. The origin of the neoplasm may be related to infection with *Helicobacter pylori* (p. 151).

MECHANICAL DISORDERS

Bezoar

Bezoar is an intragastric mass of insoluble, ingested material usually found in individuals of low intelligence. **Phytobezoar** is derived from plant material and **trichobezoar** from hair, the presence of which often leads to ulceration or perforation. Bezoars composed of inspissated bile may also develop after repetitive gastric operations. They are attributable to biliary reflux with gastric stasis.

Foreign bodies

Occasionally, foreign objects like coins; nails; marbles; pieces of glass and wood, are swallowed accidentally or deliberately. Whether they are removed surgically depends on their size: objects larger than 20 mm in diameter are unlikely to pass the pylorus spontaneously.

Dilatation

Acute gastric dilatation is a dynamic phenomenon akin to ileus (p. 166). It is an infrequent complication of simple laparotomy. Post-operative acute dilatation is more common in diabetics than in non-diabetics, and may occur spontaneously in diabetic coma. In most cases, however, acute dilatation is due to local conditions such as acute pancreatitis (p. 263) that cause peritonitis. Chronic dilatation may be caused by pyloric obstruction resulting from gastric or duodenal ulceration or from gastric carcinoma.

Volvulus

Volvulus (p. 167) twisting is likely to be orientated about the pylorocardiac axis. It is therefore **organo-axial** and may be associated with large para-oesophageal hiatus hernias. Much less commonly, the rotation is about the **mesenteric axis** of the stomach. Recurrent volvulus may result in episodes of transient vomiting and obstruction. If spontaneous resolution does not take place, obstruction; strangulation; haemorrhage; gangrene; or perforation, are potential consequences.

Haemorrhage

Haematemesis is a complication of oesophageal varices and gastric ulcers (p. 308) and may accompany diseases of the blood, bone marrow and coagulation systems. Microscopic blood loss is a common feature of gastric erosions; varices; neoplasms; severe acute gastritis; and Dieulafoy's lesion. The **Mallory–Weiss syndrome** (p. 254) is haemorrhage from a mucosal tear in the upper part of the stomach or the lower part of the oesophagus. It is a consequence of forceful retching and vomiting. Occasionally, such haemorrhage can be life threatening.

TUMOURS

Benign

Polyps

Hyperplastic or regenerative polyps are of a sessile form. Their development is associated with gastritis but they are not precancerous. **Adenomatous polyps** are villous and display varying degrees of metaplasia and dysplasia. They are precancerous but do not usually become malignant until they are at least 20 mm in diameter. Multiple adenomatous polyps may occur in patients with familial adenomatous polyposis (FAP – p. 105).

Leiomyoma

Leiomyomas are very uncommon. They arise from the muscularis mucosae, project into the lumen of the stomach, and can be recognised endoscopically. In small tumours the overlying mucosa is frequently normal so that endoscopic biopsy is unrewarding. However, large tumours have a typical endoscopic appearance with a central ulcer or pit from which profuse haemorrhage may occur.

Malignant

Carcinoma

Gastric carcinoma remains the second most frequent form of cancer worldwide and the fourth commonest in Europe. The prevalence of gastric cancer is high in Western countries but the overall incidence, now $200/10^6$ persons in England and Wales, has declined during the past three decades. This decrease has been confined to tumours of the distal part of the stomach. There has been an increase in the incidence of tumours of the cardia.

Causes

There are substantial geographical differences in frequency. Gastric carcinoma is particularly common in Japan, China and Brazil. It is more frequent in males than females and in those of blood group A than in the other ABO blood groups. Environmental factors are important. The consumption of diets rich in meat but poor in fruit and vegetables increases the risk. There is also a greater risk, not apparent for 15–20 years after surgery, among those who have had a prior operation on the stomach. The effect of diet and gastric operations may be attributed to an increase in nitrosamine formation (Table 19, p. 81). Bacterial proliferation induces enzymatic degradation of dietary nitrate to nitrites in patients with atrophic gastritis and a high mucosal pH. There is an increased incidence of gastric carcinoma in patients with chronic atrophic gastritis.

The role of *Helicobacter pylori* in the aetiology of gastric carcinoma is debatable. Although there is a relationship to gastric carcinogenesis, the prevalence of gastric cancer is low in some countries where infestation with the organism is high, perhaps reflecting the different pathogenicity of various strains.

Now read *Helicobacter pylori* (p. 151)

Structure

The majority of tumours are polypoidal or ulcerogenic; some show rudimentary gland formation and are 'intestinal'. **Polypoidal carcinoma** forms large, fungating, cauliflower-like masses that protrude into the lumen of the stomach. The surface is often ulcerated (Fig. 53). **Ulcerating carcinoma** is frequently sited on the greater curvature, near the pylorus. Since diagnosis is often late, the local and regional lymph nodes commonly contain metastatic cancer cells.

Five per cent of gastric cancers infiltrate only diffusely, creating an appearance called **linitis plastica**, leather bottle. This old-fashioned term referred to the non-distensibility of the affected organ that may be the only sign evident at endoscopy. Biopsy of the overlying mucosa may be normal as the neoplasm spreads through the submucosa. There is little gland formation. The cells are discrete and widely scattered. They are designated 'signet-ring' cells because they are distended with mucin and have eccentric nuclei.

Behaviour and prognosis

The term 'early' gastric cancer can be applied to malignant tumours confined to the mucosa or the submucosa. Intra-mucosal carcinoma without penetration of the muscularis mucosae is associated with a 5-year survival rate of over 90%.

At the time of diagnosis, 30% of tumours of the distal third of the stomach extend beyond the pylorus into the duodenum. Direct spread through the gastric wall is early and insidious and has prognostic significance. Lymphatic spread is prompt and follows a circumferential sequence recognised in other parts of the gastro-intestinal tract. Virchow's (p. 377) node describes a left supraclavicular lymph node enlarged because of its involvement by metastatic gastric or other intra-abdominal carcinoma. Blood-borne metastasis of gastric cancer cells to the liver, lungs and other viscera is frequent. Transperitoneal spread to the ovaries results in the appearance of Krukenberg tumours (p. 373).

To describe the sequence of nodal metastasis, the Japanese use concentric rings of tumour spread designated N1, N2 and N3 (Fig. 51). The N2 nodes are more than 30 mm distant from the tumour and lie around the coeliac axis and the three arteries of its trifurcation: the left gastric, the common hepatic and the splenic arteries. Surgical resections of increasing extent are now designated D1, D2 and D3 (D signifies dissection), to remove N1, N2 and N3 nodes respectively. Curative resection requires the excision of the next ring of uninvolved nodes. If N1 nodes only are positive, then a D2 dissection is required for a curative resection. A D3 dissection is required if N2 nodes are positive. It remains to be determined whether the increased morbidity and mortality of the D2 and D3 resections justifies the theoretical improvement in the chances of performing a curative operation.

Lymphoma

The stomach is the most frequent site for primary gastro-intestinal tract lymphoma but lymphomas account for less than 2% of gastric cancers. All gastric lymphomas are of non-Hodgkin's type (p. 223). They are a particular variant of extranodal lymphoma and are MALTomas since they arise from the **M**ucosa-**A**ssociated **L**ymphoid **T**issue (p. 224).

Helicobacter pylori is probably of pathogenic significance. In individuals with *H. pylori* infection, gastritis is associated with the formation of mucosal lymphoid follicles. A few cases have been treated successfully by antibiotics, eradicating the micro-organisms. If the lymphoma is confined to the stomach, the 5-year survival exceeds 75%. However, the majority display extragastric spread with direct involvement of retroperitoneal structures. The prognosis is related to the histological type.

Carcinoid tumour

Carcinoid tumours of the stomach are infrequent complications of megaloblastic, pernicious anaemia.

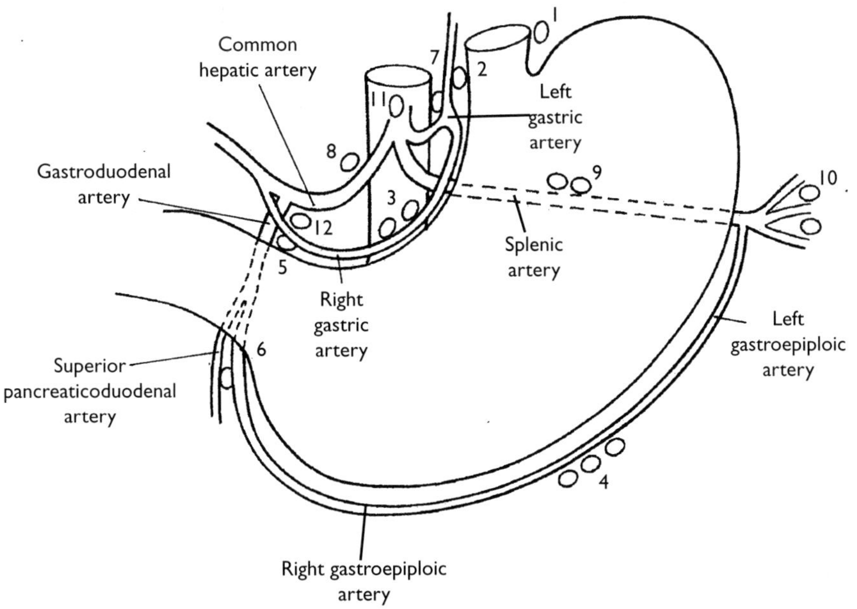

Figure 51 Carcinoma of stomach.
Identification of lymph node metastases is critical for assessment of surgical demands. Classification proposed by the Japanese Research Society for Gastric Cancer, now adopted internationally. Lymph node groups are:
1, Left cardiac; 2, right cardiac; 3, lesser curvature; 4, greater curvature; 5, suprapyloric; 6, subpyloric; 7, left gastric; 8, common hepatic; 9, splenic artery; 10, splenic hilum; 11, coeliac axis; 12, right gastric. Additional lymph nodes not shown are identified in the hepatoduodenal ligament, behind the head of the pancreas, in the root of the small bowel mesentery, along the middle colic artery, and beside the abdominal aorta.

They are commonly multiple. The tumour cells are often argyrophilic but not argentaffin. They rarely secrete 5-hydroxytryptamine (p. 82).

Leiomyosarcoma

Gastric leiomyosarcoma (p. 235) is very uncommon. It may be possible to identify the tumour endoscopically but it is usually covered by healthy, normal gastric mucosa. Mucosal biopsy may fail either to confirm the identity of the underlying lesion, or to differentiate between leiomyoma and leiomyosarcoma. A microscopic diagnosis of leiomyosarcoma rather than leiomyoma may be made if there are more than 10 mitotic figures in each high power field. The 5-year survival is ~50%.

STORAGE DISEASES

In the rare storage diseases, there is an inherited biochemical deficiency of the activity of one or more enzymes in a metabolic pathway. The majority of storage diseases are inherited as autosomal recessive characteristics (p. 182). Intermediary metabolites or metabolic products accumulate in excess, often in the viscera. In the many types of **glycogen storage disease**, for example, there is an enzyme deficiency affecting carbohydrate metabolism. Excess glycogen accumulates mainly in either the liver or heart. In the **mucopolysaccharidoses**, lack of a single lysosomal enzyme results in the accumulation of glycosaminoglycans in the brain, skeleton and skin. In the **mucolipidoses**, there is a comparable lysosomal deficiency affecting multiple enzymes, so that both glycosaminoglycans and lipids accumulate.

STREPTOCOCCUS

Streptococci are Gram-positive cocci seen as pairs or as short or long chains. Some streptococci exist as normal commensals; others are responsible for a wide range of infections of surgical importance. Many grow better anaerobically than aerobically. There is a correlation between the appearance of colonies on blood agar plates and the behaviour of the organisms as pathogens. On this basis, streptococci are divided into three categories:

- Those bacteria that produce clear zones of haemolysis around their colonies on blood agar plates are designated **beta-haemolytic**. They may be further divided on the basis of a system of grouping devised by Lancefield so that *Streptococcus pyogenes*, for example, is a Group A streptococcus.
- Those that cause green coloration around their colonies on a blood agar plate are **alpha-haemolytic** e.g. *S. pneumoniae*.
- Those causing neither plate response are said to be **non-haemolytic** e.g. faecal type streptococci.

The toxins and enzymes (Table 53) of the streptococci injure or break down cells and tissues and contribute to the spread of infection. However, some of these enzymes have a role in therapy, for example in the treatment of thrombosis.

Group A beta-haemolytic streptococci – *Streptococcus pyogenes*

The majority of beta-haemolytic streptococci causing human infections are of this group. They are designated *Streptococcus pyogenes*, the Group A streptococci. The organisms (Table 53) can be divided into more than 80 Griffith serotypes using a classification based on an M surface bacterial antigen. A further T-protein may be used as a marker in tracing the epidemiology of outbreaks of infection.

Table 53 Toxins and enzymes of *Streptococcus pyogenes*

Toxin or enzyme	Properties
Haemolytic exotoxins	Toxins that damage polymorphs and other cells
NADase and DPNase	Enzymes that kill leucocytes
DNAase	An enzyme able to degrade nuclear material in pus
Hyaluronidase	The 'spreading factor'
Erythrogenic exotoxin	Encountered in erysipelas (p. 112)
Fibrinolysin; streptokinase A and B	Have therapeutic uses e.g. in the therapy of myocardial infarction; catalyse the spread of infection

S. pyogenes is an occasional cause of a series of hazardous, surgical infections that include erysipelas; lymphadenitis; cellulitis; suppurative wound infection; necrotising fasciitis; and abscess formation. Infection often progresses rapidly and frequently demands an extended course of antibiotic therapy. *S. pyogenes* infection is a well-recognised threat to laboratory staff handling infected biopsy or autopsy material. Such infections may complicate open wounds and compound fractures and are a risk in domestic procedures such as gardening and following insect bites.

The micro-organism is a frequent cause of pharyngitis and tonsillitis and occasional strains of the organism have been associated with outbreaks of scarlet fever and acute glomerulonephritis. Rheumatic fever follows an episode of streptococcal upper respiratory tract infection. The reason for the onset of this disorder of immunity may be the possession of common antigens shared by a component of the bacteria and by macromolecules of the connective tissue of the host's heart; synovial joints; blood vessels; brain; lung; and skin.

Streptococcal infections spread readily from staff to patients and between patients with open wounds. Transmission is often by contact but may be airborne. The spread of infection can be traced by testing staff and patients for streptococcal Griffith serotypes or by searching exposed individuals for antistreptolysin D; anti-DNAase B; and anti-hyaluronidase.

From the earliest days of antibiotic and chemotherapy, it has been apparent that many strains of *S. pyogenes* are highly susceptible to these forms of treatment. Penicillins remain the drugs of first choice but erythromycin is an alternative. The optimal treatment of necrotising fasciitis is with high doses of parenteral penicillin combined with low dose gentamicin.

Now read Hospital Acquired infection (p. 159)

Group B beta-haemolytic streptococci – *Streptococcus agalactiae*

These beta-haemolytic organisms are normal inhabitants of the gut and vagina but their presence in vaginal blood or wounds should not be ignored if the patient is symptomatic. Babies are at risk of neonatal meningitis and septicaemia if a mother carries a pathogenic strain. Following apparently successful treatment, women with group B streptococcal vaginitis frequently recolonise from their sexual partner. The micro-organisms display cultural differences from *S. pyogenes* so that, for example, they grow on bile salt agar. Serious *S. agalactiae* infections can be treated by a combination of penicillin and gentamicin or netilmicin.

Groups C and G

Group C and G organisms are increasingly recognised as important pathogens; they behave very similarly to those in group A and are treated in the same manner. The streptococci of groups A, C and G interact synergistically with *Staphylococcus aureus* in wound infections and cellulitis; they are often found in the throat or vagina of patients with infections elsewhere.

Streptococcus intermedius (milleri) group

This category of micro-aerophilic streptococcus includes the bacteria formerly called *Streptococcus milleri*. The organisms have considerable surgical significance. They are particularly likely to be found in intra-abdominal abscesses and are often the organism responsible for the colonisation of intravenous catheters (p. 34). In diabetics, the *S. intermedius* group bacteria are prone to cause hepatic and cerebral abscesses (p. 63). Unlike the enterococci, they are susceptible to penicillin.

Alpha-haemolytic streptococci

Alpha-haemolytic streptococci such as *Streptococcus pneumoniae*, the pneumococcus, normally inhabit the upper parts of the respiratory tract. This organism is the commonest cause of community-acquired pneumonia but may also contribute to post-operative lung infections.

Oral streptococci

The majority of these 'viridans' bacteria are commensals found in the mouth and nasopharynx where they are distinguished from *Streptococcus pneumoniae*. One example is *S. mutans*, associated with the development of dental caries. Whereas *Staphylococcus epidermiditis* is the most frequent cause of endocarditis of prosthetic heart valves, viridans streptococci remain the common cause of bacterial endocarditis affecting non-prosthetic valves.

Enterococci

Group D streptococci include the faecal streptococci, Enterococci. They normally inhabit the intestinal tract. *Streptococcus bovis* is often associated with colon cancer and may lead to endocarditis. Enterococci can initiate alpha-, beta- or no haemolysis on blood agar culture and tolerate the presence of bile salts in the culture medium. They cause wound and central line infections; bacteraemia; and septicaemia after surgery, and are a common agent of urinary tract infection.

After the coliforms, enterococcus is the most frequent cause of biliary infection. The organism is readily and quickly identified by biochemical tests but does not respond to penicillin or cephalosporins; cephalosporins may, in fact, provoke bacterial proliferation. Enterococci are frequently resistant to amoxycillin. Combined treatment with aminoglycoside antibiotics and amoxycillin or piperacillin may be necessary for severe infection but some strains have become resistant to virtually all available antibiotics and are designated vancomycin resistant enterococci (VRE) (p. 18).

STRESS

Stress may be psychological or physical. Prolonged mental distress can reduce resistance to disease and increase the probability of a fatal outcome to infection and injury. There is an effect upon immunity, related to the regulatory mechanisms of the hypothalamo-pituitary-adrenal cortical axis. Physical stress increases the rate of the adrenal secretion of cortisol. There are changes in the appearance and behaviour of the cells of the zona fasiculata (p. 5), which becomes lipid-depleted. Under these conditions, relatively minor surgical and anaesthetic procedures, such as those used in dentistry, may cause serious effects including neurogenic shock and cerebral infarction.

SUTURE MATERIALS

Clean surgical wounds of epithelial and vascular tissue heal quickly but the restoration of even half the normal mechanical strength of tissues rich in collagen requires 3 or more months. The half-life of fibrous collagen is ~2 years.

An ideal suture material should:

- Retain sufficient tensile strength to ensure wound integrity until healing is complete.
- Resist damage during sterilisation.
- Be chemically and biologically inert.
- Undergo natural re-absorption.

These ideal properties are not found in a single material. A variety of sutures is therefore employed for different surgical purposes: their choice is often a compromise.

Absorbable sutures

Absorbable sutures are degraded by enzymatic dissolution.

- **Catgut**, a material obtained from the submucosa of the small intestine of the sheep, produces a profuse tissue reaction within 24 hours, with oedema and polymorph infiltration. It delays healing but is usually rapidly dissolved, with a corresponding reduction in tensile strength. After catgut has been tanned with chromic acid, its absorption is delayed and its capacity to cause inflammation reduced. It loses half its strength within ~14 days. The use of catgut has declined rapidly with the advent of synthetic, absorbable materials.
- **Collagen** sutures are obtained from the Achilles tendon of cattle and provoke less tissue reaction than catgut. They are now rarely used.
- **Polymers**. Synthetic polymers of glycolic acid (**dexon**), glactin (**vicryl**) and dioxanone (**PDS**) are less irritant than the catgut and collagen that they have replaced. However, their enzymatic dissolution is not as rapid as that of the older materials.

Non-absorbable sutures

Non-absorbable sutures resist enzymatic dissolution but may fragment and lose tensile strength over a period of months. They are made as a single strand (**monofilament**), or as a number of strands twisted or braided together (**multifilament**). There is a lesser tissue reaction to monofilament than to multifilament sutures. Bacteria may lodge in the interstices of the latter.

Sutures made of the **natural fibres**, silk, cotton and linen are multifilament and induce a tissue reaction almost as severe as that caused by catgut: they are being replaced by inert synthetic plastics such as polyamide (**nylon**) and polypropylene (**prolene**).

Metal sutures of stainless **steel** or **tantalum** are almost inert, as is **carbon fibre** (p. 281).

Now read Prostheses (p. 280)

SYPHILIS

Venereal infection by *Treponema pallidum* causes a prolonged, complex disease which, if untreated, may evolve through primary, secondary and tertiary stages. In Western countries, where effective, early treatment is available, the late gummatous, vascular, bone and nervous system sequelae are much less common than formerly. Infection may also be transplacental or by accidental or coincidental inoculation.

Congenital syphilis

Large numbers of bacteria are particularly likely to infect a fetus exposed during the maternal primary and secondary stages. Necrotic foci appear in the liver, lungs and pancreas and the long bones display a characteristic disorganisation of the growth plate. Exposure at a later stage of the disease exerts a less dramatic effect. Fetuses infected in subsequent pregnancies develop deformities of the incisor teeth; saddle nose; keratitis; and signs of central nervous system disease.

Adult syphilis

Following venereal infection, the organisms are disseminated very quickly but there is an incubation period of 3 weeks before a primary chancre appears. Anorectal lesions may be overlooked. After a further 6 weeks, the spirochaetes settle secondarily in many parts of the body. The skin lesion is an erythematous rash. There is also a rash on the palms of the hands and generalised lymphadenopathy. Mucosal ulcers develop on the pharynx and genitalia, while raised, papular lesions in sites such as the perineum and axilla constitute **condylomata lata**. There may also be concurrent low-grade meningitis, hepatitis, uveitis and an immune complex-mediated nephrotic syndrome.

The micro-organisms are demonstrable in the primary and secondary lesions but, after one or more relapses, the microscopic appearance of the secondary lesions is granulomatous rather than acute. The prototype lesion of tertiary syphilis is the **gumma**, a necrotic focus surrounded by macrophages and occasional compact, multinucleated giant cells. Without treatment, as many as a quarter of all cases formerly died from the tertiary manifestations of the disease. Although this is no longer the case, tertiary lesions of the aorta and brain are life-threatening, while those of the skin; liver; bones; testes; and other organs are destructive and deforming.

LABORATORY TESTS FOR SYPHILIS

Although *Treponema pallidum*, the cause of syphilis, can occasionally be identified in primary lesions by dark-ground microscopy, the bacterium cannot be grown in culture. The diagnosis of syphilis therefore rests on methods for the demonstration of anti-treponemal antibodies in serum.

There are now two tests, the first a screening procedure. It is the non-treponemal rapid plasma reaginic (RPR) test. If this test is positive, or to confirm positivity, a second investigation is performed comprising the *Treponema pallidum* haemagglutination assay (TPHA) and the indirect fluorescence treponemal antibody (FTA) test.

The Wasserman, complement fixation reaction (p. 232) is no longer employed. False-positive tests were given in recent respiratory infections; pregnancy; auto-immune diseases; yaws; and glandular fever.

T

TALC GRANULOMA

Early latex gloves (p. 142) worn by surgeons required lubrication. The powder chosen was insoluble talc. Talc is native, hydrous magnesium silicate. It is sometimes mixed with a small amount of aluminium silicate. Released from a glove inadvertently, talc could be retained within wounds and body cavities. The silicates provoked acute inflammation followed by giant cell granuloma formation (p. 143). Within the peritoneal cavity, adhesions formed. Their presence was liable to lead to intestinal obstruction. When talc gained access to the fallopian tubes, sterility was one consequence of the chronic inflammatory response.

Now read Gloves (p. 142)

TELEPATHOLOGY

Telepathology is the transmission of digitised histological, cytological and other images by telephone line or cable. It provides a means of remote consultation enabling problematical diagnoses to be reviewed by one or more experts. There is no geographical limit to the distance over which discussion can take place. The microscopic equipment necessary for this procedure is very expensive but the costs are decreasing as the practice extends. Telepathology is most useful when the signals can be sent in both directions simultaneously and has proved of great value in countries such as Norway where hospitals are geographically remote from a reference centre. In Asia, live consultation with experts in Europe and North America is now commonplace.

The histological images are viewed on a monitor on which a picture of the participating pathologist is also displayed. With modern communication technology, and software incorporating high-speed image transfer and video-conferencing, a pathologist at one site can take full control of a motorised microscope at any remote site to view diagnostic quality images while discussing a case with a colleague. Sets of images including scans of a whole slide can be annotated and stored along with case details for teaching, clinical meetings and quality assurance.

risk in those with Klinefelter's syndrome (p. 93). The incidence is highest in white males in the USA and Northern Europe. The frequency is increasing rapidly but still accounts for less than 1.5% of all male cancers. Patients who have been successfully treated for a neoplasm in one testis have a much greater chance of developing a second, primary tumour in the other testis than unaffected individuals. There is also a relationship with infertility. A single, common factor may depress fertility and, simultaneously, increase the likelihood of malignancy. There is a comparable risk in those who have undergone testicular biopsy, perhaps related to the development of anti-sperm antibodies. A similar mechanism has been suggested for any increased risk following vasectomy.

Malignant testicular tumours may be staged according to the Royal Marsden classification (Table 54).

Table 54 Royal Marsden classification for testicular tumours

Stage	Classification
I	Confined to the testis
II	Abdominal lymph node metastases
III	Supra-diaphragmatic lymph node metastases
IV	Extra-lymphatic metastases

Germ cell tumours

Seminoma

Seminoma is the most frequent testicular tumour, comprising 40% of all cancers in this location. It is uncommon before puberty. The peak incidence is ~30 to 40 years of age.

Structure

The cut surface of the testicular mass is uniformly grey–white. There are sheets of large cells with pale cytoplasm, recalling the appearances of spermatogonia. The stroma is densely infiltrated with lymphocytes.

Behaviour and prognosis

The tumour is confined to the testis in ~75% of patients. When metastasis occurs, it is initially by lymphatic channels to the iliac and para-aortic nodes. Blood-borne metastases to the lungs, liver and bone occur later. Plasma lactate dehydrogenase concentrations are raised in many patients with metastases. Seminoma is exceedingly radiosensitive. Patients with stage I or stage II disease are treated by orchidectomy and radiotherapy: 95% are cured.

Teratoma

Teratomas account for 30% of testicular cancers. The peak incidence is at 20–30 years of age.

Structure

The testis is nodular. The cut surface of the tumour displays areas of haemorrhage, necrosis and cyst formation. There are four categories. Varieties of gross structure and of microscopic differentiation parallel differences in behaviour:

- **Differentiated teratomas** comprise ~5% of testicular tumours in adults but are the most common testicular tumour in children. A variety of epithelia are present, resembling normal glandular structures. Usually benign, in rare instances the tumour is malignant and metastasis occurs.
- **Intermediate malignant teratoma** is the most common variety, comprising ~55% of cases. Like differentiated teratoma, there are zones in which normal epithelia reproduce glandular structures but others that are clearly malignant. Some tumour cells resemble those of the yolk sac and liberate abnormal amounts of α-fetoprotein. The prognosis depends upon the extent of the cancer.
- **Undifferentiated malignant teratoma** accounts for ~40% of cases. It comprises sheets of pleomorphic cells with numerous mitotic figures.
- **Malignant teratoma, trophoblastic** or **choriocarcinoma,** is rare. There are zones of haemorrhage and necrosis. The component cells are derived from both syncytio- and cytotrophoblast. The synthesis of human chorionic gonadotrophin (HCG) is demonstrable immunocytochemically within those cells that are derived from the syncytiotrophoblast. An elevated concentration of this hormone is found in the serum. The prognosis is very poor.

Behaviour and prognosis

Teratomas have also been staged according to the Royal Marsden Classification. By contrast with seminoma, only 40% present with stage 1 disease. Testicular teratomas spread to the epididymis and to the spermatic cord. Venous metastasis to the lungs and liver is common, as is lymphatic spread to the abdominal and mediastinal lymph nodes. Teratoma is not radiosensitive. Treatment is by orchidectomy and chemotherapy. Survival for stage III and stage IV disease is ~80%.

Combined seminoma and teratoma

Ten per cent of testicular tumours are formed of seminomatous and teratomatous elements. In some, the two components co-exist; more commonly, they occur in separate nodules. Prognosis rests upon the degree of differentiation of the teratomatous, not the seminomatous, zones.

Sex cord tumours

Sex cord or gonadal stromal tumours of the testis are relatively much less frequent than those of the ovary.

Androblastoma (Sertoli cell tumour)

Androblastoma is associated with gynaecomastia in ~30% of patients. It is encountered in patients under the age of 40 years. Ten per cent are malignant. There are varying numbers of Sertoli cells, often arranged in tubules, together with spindle-shaped, stromal cells.

Interstitial cell tumour (Leydig cell tumour)

Ten per cent of these rare tumours are malignant. There are two peaks of incidence, the first between the ages of 5 and 10 years, the second between the ages of 30 and 35 years. The tumours appear yellow–brown *naked-eye*. The eosinophilic cells of which they are formed contain a pigment resembling lipofuscin. The tumours secrete large quantities of androgens. Prepubertal, precocious virilisation is a consequence. After puberty, there is gynaecomastia and loss of body hair.

Yolk sac tumour (orchioblastoma)

This is a tumour of infancy. It is yellow–white. The component cells display tubular and papillary patterns. Alpha-fetoprotein can be shown by immuno-histochemistry; raised plasma concentrations of this marker are demonstrable.

Lymphoma

The testis is occasionally affected by primary diffuse, non-Hodgkin's lymphoma (p. 223).

MECHANICAL INJURIES AND TRAUMA

The testis is vulnerable to gunshot wounds; impacts sustained in sport and road traffic accidents; and other forms of injury. The complications include hydrocoele and haematocoele (p. 290).

Torsion

Testicular torsion is relatively common between 10 and 25 years of age. It is encountered in patients in whom the testis lies horizontally within a tunica vaginalis that extends to a high position on the spermatic cord. The location encourages abnormal mobility. Torsion is usually of both testis and epididymis. Either testis may be affected. Initially, the veins are obstructed, causing oedema. Later, there is arterial obstruction and testicular infarction. The result is scarring and permanent dysfunction.

TETANY

Tetany is the painful, tonic spasm of muscle. It is induced by changes in the concentrations of extracellular ions. Neuromuscular irritability can be increased by a reduction in the concentrations of Ca^{2+}, Mg^{2+} and H^+ ions, or by an increase in the concentrations of Na^+, K^+ and OH^- ions. Tetany is induced more often by respiratory alkalosis than by metabolic acidosis (p. 231).

The most frequent cause of tetany is hypocalcaemia but changes in the concentration of more than one ion frequently coincide. Paraesthesiae and muscular spasm develop. Spasm of forearm muscles produces the *main d'accoucheur*, Trousseau's sign. Latent tetany can be diagnosed by tapping a branch of the facial nerve, inducing twitching of the facial muscles, Chvostek's sign. It can also be recognised by inflating a sphygmomanometer on the upper arm, occluding blood flow.

Tetany is an uncommon complication of partial thyroidectomy when parathyroid gland tissue may be excised or injured. It is unusual for all parathyroid tissue to be removed, or for the arterial blood supply to every gland to be prejudiced. Tetany is also uncommon following operations on the parathyroid glands unless pre-operative hyperparathyroidism has been severe.

Now read Hyperparathyroidism (p. 267)

Biopsy diagnosis of thymic disease

Needle biopsy is unreliable. Endoscopic biopsies may be taken during mediastinoscopy. Open biopsy should be performed through a small incision in the second intercostal space, lateral to the sternum.

TUMOURS

Thymic infiltration by nearby mediastinal tumours is a regular occurrence and bronchial carcinoma is commonly responsible. The thymus is occasionally the target for carcinomatous metastases from distant primary sources. It is often implicated in lymphoma and leukaemia. Hodgkin's and non-Hodgkin's lymphoma may originate in the gland or it may be invaded by lymphoma arising at other sites.

Now read Lymphoma (p. 223)

Thymoma

Thymoma is a rare tumour of the epithelial elements of the thymus gland.

Causes

Thymoma is a tumour of older adults although, very occasionally, the neoplasm is identified in the young. It exerts pressure on the organs and vessels of the mediastinum. One-third of cases is detected when myasthenia gravis develops. In combination with medical treatment, this disease responds well to thymectomy. A smaller proportion of individuals has other associated diseases such as aplastic anaemia.

Structure

Thymomas are lobulated, anterior mediastinal masses. The majority are encapsulated. A cystic structure is often recognised. The neoplastic epithelial cells occupy varying proportions of the tumour mass and are intimately associated with the lymphocytic population of the gland.

Behaviour and prognosis

Based upon the degree of dedifferentiation of the thymic epithelial cells, the tumours are judged to be:

- **Benign**. Benign thymoma is a slowly growing tumour, formed of well-differentiated epithelial cells. The tumour does not infiltrate beyond the confines of the organ.
- **Malignant**. The cells of the second category, malignant thymoma, appear little different from those of the benign form but growth is unrestrained and the tumour infiltrates adjoining tissues.
- **Poorly differentiated**. The cells of the third category, **thymic carcinoma**, are poorly differentiated and the tumour extends by uncontrolled spread. Adverse prognostic features are high tumour grade and large size. There is also a close relationship between prognosis and the degree of local and remote metastasis.

Teratoma

Thymic teratoma, of developmental origin, is a benign dermoid cyst. Thymic tissue lies at the tumour margin but it is not certain whether this represents residual, compressed thymus or a part of the neoplasm.

THYROID GLAND

The thyroid gland develops within the first month of fetal life. It arises from the endoderm of the posterior third of the tongue. The thyroglossal duct descends anterior to the hyoid bone and fuses with components of the fourth branchial pouch to form two lobes united by an isthmus. Thyroid C cells develop from this pouch. The proximal end of the thyroglossal duct often remains as the foramen caecum of the tongue. The remainder of the duct atrophies but the pyramidal lobe of the thyroid is a normal, distal remnant.

Biopsy diagnosis of thyroid disease

Biopsy of the thyroid gland is usually undertaken for the diagnosis of tumour.

In the differential diagnosis of thyroid disease, the expert survey of fine-needle aspirates yields a false-positive diagnosis of malignancy in ~2% of cases, a false-negative in ~5%. The core of tissue provided by needle biopsy leads to fewer false-negative results but there is a higher risk of haematoma. The distinction between follicular adenoma and carcinoma depends on the identification of capsular invasion. This diagnosis cannot be determined by fine-needle aspiration and is difficult to make by frozen section. Some surgeons therefore prefer to perform lobectomy for all solitary thyroid nodules.

DEVELOPMENTAL AND CONGENITAL DISORDERS

- **Lingual thyroid**. Particularly in females, the embryonal thyroid gland may not descend but develops within the tongue, below the foramen caecum. It forms a small lingual thyroid that may constitute the entire thyroid tissue. Lingual thyroid does not contain residues of the fourth branchial pouch: the development of medullary carcinoma (p. 127) from thyroid C cells is not possible at this site. However, other malignant tumours are more frequent in lingual thyroid glands than in thyroid tissue located normally.
- **Ectopic thyroid**. Ectopic thyroid tissue may be identified in any location on the path leading from the foramen caecum to the normal site of the gland. Thyroid tissue may also be found within the mediastinum.
- **Accessory thyroid tissue**. Accessory glandular tissue can sometimes be recognised close to the normal thyroid lobes or above the isthmus. The tissue must be distinguished from metastatic papillary carcinoma, the usual explanation for an aberrant mass.
- **Thyroid aplasia and hypoplasia**. Aplasia and hypoplasia are rare. They lead to abnormalities of growth and development.
- **Thyroid cyst**. A remnant of the thyroglossal duct may persist into adult life, resulting in a midline cyst. The majority of such cysts lie at the level of the hyoid bone. The mucoid contents are secreted by the columnar lining cells but squamous epithelium may predominate. Occasionally, disruption or inadequate surgical extirpation of a cyst leads to the formation of a fistula. More often, an opening on the skin is the orifice of a thyroglossal sinus originating from a persistent thyroglossal duct. Within it, papillary carcinoma (p. 266) may arise.

GOITRE

A goitre is a swelling of the thyroid gland. All forms are more common in females than males.

Toxic goitre

Toxic goitre describes the association of glandular enlargement with hyperthyroidism. The swelling may be **diffuse** as in Graves' disease, or **nodular** and more evident in one lobe than the other.

Diffuse, toxic goitre

Diffuse thyroid hyperplasia (Graves' disease) occurs in $20/10^3$ women in the UK, usually between 20 and 40 years of age. There is a familial tendency. On the basis of this predisposition, circulating IgG auto-antibodies, designated long-acting thyroid stimulator (LATS) bind to and activate thyroid stimulating hormone (TSH) receptors. The thyroid epithelium responds by hyperplasia but there is a greatly reduced content of stored colloid. Vascularity increases. Epithelial cells hypertrophy, become columnar and form papillary ingrowths. The plasma levels of tri-iodothyronine (T3) and thyroxine (T4) rise. In many patients there is co-existent enlargement of the thymus gland. In these patients, there may be lymphocytic infiltration within the thyroid, indicating the existence of auto-immune thyroiditis. Proptosis may develop; exophthalmos is believed to be due to the binding of one of the IgG auto-antibodies to a retro-orbital antigen. Paradoxically, pretibial myxoedema, a sign of hypothyroidism, may be identified.

Toxic, nodular goitre

Toxic, nodular goitre is recognised much less frequently than diffuse, toxic goitre and is usually found in those aged 50 years or more. It is often a late sequel to the presence of long-standing, multinodular, non-toxic goitre. Exophthalmos is uncommon.

Non-toxic goitre

Non-toxic or simple goitre, is endemic or sporadic. Racial and familial factors have been implicated. Lack of iodine in the diet in mountainous regions such as the Andes and Himalayas, where much water flows from molten snow, may explain endemic goitre in these regions but this does not account for the preponderance of goitres in females. In some Western countries, iodine is added to commercial table salt to lessen the possibility of this hazard. Elsewhere, endemic goitre cannot be accounted for simply by an insufficiency of dietary iodine.

Lack of iodine produces a reduction in circulating T3 and T4, resulting in increased secretion of thyroid-stimulating hormone (TSH). TSH secretion continues until T3 and T4 return to normal plasma concentrations. Release of these hormones then ceases and the follicles become filled with colloid. The enlarged gland is a **colloid goitre**. Some of the follicles rupture, producing haemorrhage, cysts and fibrosis in a cycle of events that may be repeated many times.

Sporadic, non-toxic goitre may result from dyshormonogenesis, a consequence of uncommon inborn errors of metabolism. Other instances are attributable to unusual dietary habits or to the action of chemicals and drugs, such as paraminosalicylic acid, that interfere with the synthesis of T3 and T4.

Non-toxic goitre may be sufficiently large to compress the trachea and oesophagus. Enlargement into the mediastinum may cause obstruction of the superior vena cava. After many years there is a tendency for thyrotoxicosis to develop. Contrary to previous concern, there is only a small risk of malignant change. Cancer develops in less than 1% of patients.

HYPOTHYROIDISM

Myxoedema (hypothyroidism in adults) or cretinism (hypothyroidism in infants), results from:

- Developmental abnormalities of the thyroid.
- Iodine deficiency.
- The ingestion of goitrogens.
- Hashimoto's disease.
- Surgical or radioactive treatment for thyrotoxicosis.

The clinical effects are the converse of those attributable to thyrotoxicosis.

Cretinism

Cretinism (congenital hypothyroidism) is due to thyroid aplasia or hypoplasia. The defect leads to abnormal thyroid development. The disorder may be endemic or sporadic. The consequences are not immediately evident after birth since maternal thyroxine readily crosses the placenta. The signs that develop in the young child include mental defect, short limbs, coarse dry hair and skin; a protruding tongue; and a protuberant abdomen, with umbilical hernia. A definitive diagnosis is made after the estimation of thyroid hormone.

Myxoedema

The onset of adult hypothyroidism is dangerously insidious and culminates in the classical syndrome of myxoedema. There is dry skin; alopecia; bradycardia; low metabolic rate; weight gain; constipation; anaemia; and mental depression. They accompany a predisposition to osteoporosis and osteoarthritis.

HYPERTHYROIDISM

Hyperthyroidism is a feature of Graves' disease but transient hyperthyroidism may occur with thyroiditis. Thyrotoxicosis may also develop in toxic, multinodular goitre and toxic adenoma. The increased release of T3 and T4 stimulates the metabolism of all body cells.

INFECTION AND INFLAMMATION

Thyroiditis

The causes are infective or non-infective. The thyroid gland is rarely infected by bacteria and fungi but more often by viruses. The cause of De Quervain's **giant cell thyroiditis**, a febrile illness of adult females, is unknown. The patients develop a painful goitre and transient thyrotoxicosis. The gland is infiltrated with neutrophils, macrophages and multinucleate giant cells. Fibrosis follows. Serum antibodies to several viruses are recognisable but none has been identified as the causal agent. The condition resolves spontaneously, usually without the development of hypothyroidism.

Hashimoto's disease

Hashimoto's disease is an **auto-immune thyroiditis** of middle-aged women. The incidence is increasing. The disorder is often associated with other auto-immune abnormalities such as rheumatoid arthritis; pernicious anaemia; Addison's disease; and diabetes mellitus (p. 117). Circulating antibodies are demonstrable against thyroid antigens that include thyroglobulin. There is painless, symmetrical goitre and hypothyroidism. The excised gland is a conspicuous pale, yellow–white colour without evidence of haemorrhage, cysts or necrosis. It is widely infiltrated by lymphocytes and plasma cells. Later, discrete foci of lymphoid tissue appear with well-formed germinal centres. There is an increased risk of lymphoma but not of carcinoma.

Riedel's thyroiditis

Riedel's thyroiditis is an increasingly common inflammatory disorder of middle aged individuals. The aetiology is unknown. There is no evidence of auto-immune disease in the thyroid or elsewhere. The gland is replaced by dense fibrous tissue. Only one lobe or part of a lobe may be affected, with a clear distinction between the normal and the abnormal tissue. Characteristically, fibrosis extends to involve the thyroid capsule, promoting obstruction to the trachea or oesophagus. Many sufferers develop fibrosis in the orbit, mediastinum and abdomen, resulting in retroperitoneal fibrosis (p. 131) and sclerosing cholangitis (p. 38).

Now read Fibrosis (p. 131), Fibromatosis (p. 130)

TUMOURS

The incidence of primary malignant thyroid tumours in the UK is $50/10^6$ persons, although the frequency is less in England and Wales than in Scotland and the North of Ireland. Five per cent of the adult population has a palpable lump in the gland and many more are apparent upon ultrasonography. Much effort is required to identify which are malignant.

Benign

Adenoma

Thyroid adenomas are distinguished from nodules within a multinodular goitre. Follicular adenoma has a well-defined capsule. Within an adenoma, the follicles vary considerably in size compared with those of the surrounding, compressed, normal thyroid. Haemorrhage; cyst formation; and calcification occur in the adenomatous tissue.

Malignant

The thyroid gland is infiltrated directly by the cells of bronchial and oesophageal carcinoma. Blood-borne metastases from carcinoma of the kidney, bronchus and other sites, and from malignant melanoma, are unexpectedly frequent. They are almost always asymptomatic although metastatic renal carcinoma may provoke hyperthyroidism.

Carcinoma

Primary carcinoma of the thyroid may originate from either the follicular or the parafollicular C-cells. Follicular cell tumours are papillary, follicular or anaplastic, depending upon the degree of differentiation.

Causes

Thyroid tumours can be caused by exposure to endogenous or exogenous, ionising radiation. There is evidence that beta-particle radiation from the isotopes used in diagnosis can induce thyroid cancer although ^{131}I, used in the treatment of thyrotoxicosis, has not been shown to be carcinogenic. Following the Chernobyl atomic power station explosion in 1986, a raised incidence of thyroid tumours was recognised in children 100 miles distant. By 1995, the total number of individuals who had died as a consequence of assimilating radioactive iodine was estimated to be ~125 000. It is thought that 60% of the exposed local population may ultimately develop thyroid cancer.

Structure and behaviour

- **Papillary carcinoma** accounts for more than 50% of malignant thyroid tumours. The symptomless swelling arises in women aged 30–40 years. Cysts develop and arrays of cuboidal or columnar cells exhibit a characteristic papillary structure without a capsule. Psammoma bodies are often found. The tumours are small and multifocal. They affect both lobes and may invade other structures in the neck directly.

  The prognosis is good and is largely unrelated to the extent of the surgical procedure performed. The tumour is very sensitive to stimulation by TSH. If the secretion of this anterior pituitary hormone is suppressed by exogenous thyroxine, the majority of patients survive. Total thyroidectomy may be indicated in those with large (>20 mm diameter) tumours; in those with aneuploid tumours; and in those with cervical lymphadenopathy.

- **Follicular carcinoma**, a solitary tumour of middle-aged women, accounts for ~20% of thyroid cancers. At first the cancer is encapsulated. The absence of capsular and vascular invasion assists differentiation between follicular adenoma and carcinoma. However, the distinction is rarely possible by fine-needle aspiration biopsy. Consequently, lobectomy is preferred for solitary nodules that appear adenomatous when examined by this biopsy technique. Unlike papillary carcinoma, fewer than 10% of follicular carcinomas spread to the cervical lymph nodes but blood-borne metastases are conveyed to lungs and bones. Treatment is by lobectomy or total thyroidectomy followed by radiotherapy. Survival is not as long as with papillary carcinoma and is related to the degree of extracapsular spread.
- **Anaplastic carcinoma**, a rapidly growing tumour of women aged >60 years, comprises ~15% of thyroid cancers. It is composed of spindle and giant cells. Local infiltration leads to compression of the trachea and oesophagus. The majority of patients present with advanced disease and fewer than 10% survive 1 year.
- **Medullary carcinoma** arises from parafollicular C-cells. This unusual cancer constitutes only 5% of thyroid cancers. In sporadic cases, the patient is elderly and the tumour unilateral. However, one in five originates in young adults and is familial, part of a MEN 2 syndrome (p. 127). There are raised serum calcitonin levels and sometimes evidence of the secretion of 5-hydroxytryptamine, ACTH and the polypeptide, bombesin. In these familial cases, the neoplasm may be bilateral.

  The tumour appears as a grey mass. The component cells are arranged in groups and linear arrays but a variety of microscopic types has been described. Immunohistochemical tests for calcitonin demonstrate that this polypeptide is invariably present. In half the cases, calcitonin-derived amyloid (Table 1) accumulates within the interstitial tissues. The cancer spreads via lymphatic channels and the bloodstream. Prognosis is related to the presence or absence of metastasis to the cervical lymph nodes. Evidence of increased calcitonin secretion in clinically unaffected members of the family is an indication for prophylactic thyroidectomy.

Lymphoma

The thyroid gland is an occasional primary site for high grade, non-Hodgkin's lymphoma. The gland may also be implicated by the extension of secondary lymphoma. Primary lymphoma is found most commonly in middle-aged females. It comprises 2% of primary thyroid tumours one form of which is a mucosa-associated, lymphoid tissue tumour, MALToma (p. 224). Prognosis is related both to extrathyroid spread and to histological grade. The 5-year survival of low grade lymphoma is ~80%, of high grade tumours only ~20%.

TISSUE CULTURE

Under sterile conditions, cells can **grow** *in vitro* in a process of culture. Alternatively, small pieces of tissue can be **maintained**, without cell growth, in organ or tissue culture. Cell and tissue culture techniques are central to recent advances in carcinogenesis, cytogenetics, and molecular biology.

CELL CULTURE

Cells from many tissues and organs can be grown outside the body, without a supporting stroma or blood circulation. Initially, the cells are suspended in a fluid medium to encourage multiplication. They are then deposited in a flat chamber or on a slide where growth can be watched and measured. The media in which cells are grown are often entirely synthetic. Alternatively, a medium may be wholly or partly natural, in the sense that it includes serum together with a population of growth factors and cytokines.

The practical applications of cell culture include:

- The use of monkey kidney cells to allow viral growth and identification.
- The growth of cells in searches for carcinogens.
- The growth of macrophages in tests of immunity mediated by lymphocytes or lymphokines.
- The culture of bone marrow stem cells to replace those ablated by irradiation or immunosuppression.
- The culture of connective tissue cells to test and identify pharmacological agents.

ORGAN CULTURE

Organ culture implies the maintenance, without cell multiplication, of very thin slices or minute solid parts of tissue in special dishes or chambers. The explants are placed in a chamber containing an appropriate oxygen/carbon dioxide gas mixture and incubated at 37°C. Organ cultures are valuable for:

- The testing of drug actions *in vitro*.
- The bioassay of hormones such as ACTH.
- The organ culture of parts of tumours to study their characteristics.
- The development of implants.

Bone grafts, for example, can be prepared by encouraging cells such as osteoblasts to grow into and colonise honeycombs made from calcium hydroxyapatite.

TOXINS

A toxin is a poisonous substance manufactured during the growth of some micro-organisms, plants and animals. Among the toxins that have achieved notoriety are ricin (castor seeds: *Ricinus communis*) and cobra venom. In surgery, bacterial toxins are of special significance. They are liberated from the bacterial cell (exotoxins) or are an integral part of its structure (endotoxins).

EXOTOXINS

Exotoxins are synthesised by actively growing bacteria. They exert their pathogenic effects remotely from the organism that produces them. Most bacteria producing exotoxins are Gram-positive; a few, including *Vibrio cholerae* and *Shigella dysenteriae*, are Gram-negative. Many of the lesions produced by exotoxins are systemic although the site of bacterial infection remains localised.

Exotoxins exert specific effects on selected tissues where they behave as enzymes or enzyme inhibitors. For example, the alpha-toxin of *Clostridium perfringens* is a phospholipase and acts on the phospholipids of the cell membranes of red blood cells. The exotoxin of *C. tetani* potentiates neurotransmission at the synapse of the upper motor neurone with the anterior horn cells of the spinal cord, whereas the neurotoxin of *C. botulinum*, the most potent of all bacterial exotoxins, blocks transmission at cranial motor-nerve endings. The actions of the haemolytic, cytolytic and leucocidal toxins of the pathogenic staphylococci (p. 303) and streptococci (p. 311) are equally specific.

Toxoid

Exotoxins are proteins of high molecular weight and are therefore sensitive to heat. When changed in this way or by chemicals such as formaldehyde, pathogenicity is destroyed, antigenicity retained. An altered, non-pathogenic toxin is a toxoid. It can be used safely for active immunisation (p. 175).

ENDOTOXINS

Endotoxins are phospholipid–polysaccharide–protein complexes that form the outer layer of the cell wall of Gram-negative bacteria (Figs 5 and 6, p. 30 and p. 31). The endotoxin of *Neisseria meningitidis*, the meningococcus, is one of the most potent. Within hours of infection, it can lead to peripheral ischaemia and gangrene resulting in the need for amputation of one or more digits or parts of limbs.

When endotoxin is incorporated into the plasma membranes of host leucocytes, macrophages, endothelial cells or platelets, it disrupts cell function. The lipid component determines toxicity, the carbohydrate antigenic specificity. Endotoxins resist heat but are of low potency and specificity. They cannot be changed to toxoids. In the same way, combining endotoxin with antibody does not destroy toxicity. Complexed or modified endotoxins cannot be used in immunisation.

Endotoxin is an exogenous pyrogen (p. 283), provoking leucocytes and macrophages to release endogenous pyrogen that acts on the temperature-regulating centre of the hypothalamus. Repeated exposure to endotoxin results in some tolerance and the activity of mononuclear phagocytes may be enhanced. Pyrogenic endotoxin may come from environmental Gram-negative bacteria that have grown in fluids used for intravenous administration. The endotoxin is not destroyed by autoclaving (p. 305). Similar organisms may multiply in fluids that have been autoclaved but are contaminated during storage.

TRACE ELEMENTS

Minute (trace) quantities of certain dietary elements are essential for normal development, growth and function. Most of these substances are cofactors for enzymes. Iron; zinc; copper; cobalt; manganese; iodine; and fluorine are required by man. Chromium; selenium; molybdenum; nickel; silicon; tin; and vanadium are needed by other animals. The pathological effects of a trace element may result from deficiency or excess.

Deficiency

The lack of a trace element may be relative or absolute. Deficiency is very unusual in individuals who consume a normal, balanced diet. Prolonged partial or complete deficiency of a trace element tends to culminate in a pathognomonic syndrome. The conditions under which signs of deprivation appear are exemplified by those that follow gastroplasty, or those that result from the operation of intestinal by-pass performed for morbid obesity (p. 250). Trace element imbalance should not develop in patients being 'fed' intravenously: modern regimes of surgical treatment include appropriate supplements.

Excess

Substances present in excess, for example in the water used for renal dialysis, may cause adverse reactions. Among these compounds are: aluminium; calcium; chloramines; copper; fluoride; formaldehyde; hydrogen peroxide; sodium; sodium azide; sodium hypochlorite; and zinc.

Syndromes

- **Iron** is a crucial part of the haemoglobin and myoglobin molecules, and a component of the peroxidases and cytochromes. Iron absorption is controlled by intestinal epithelial cells, regulated by serum ferritin levels, and facilitated by vitamins A and C and by β-carotene. Persistently raised serum transferrin saturation leads to the deposition of iron throughout the body but particularly in the liver and pancreas. **Haemochromatosis** (bronzed diabetes) is a heritable disorder of iron metabolism. In this disease, pancreatic islet cell obliteration leads to insulin deficiency (p. 117). 0.5% of affected individuals are homozygous for a mutation in the *HFE* gene on somatic chromosome 6.
- **Zinc** is a component of enzymes such as carbonic anhydrase, lactate dehydrogenase and the carboxypeptidases. Zinc is necessary for the healing of wounds; in malnourished patients, the local application or systemic administration of zinc may accelerate wound healing. There is no effect upon wound healing in normal individuals.
- **Copper** is a component of cytochrome oxidase; mono-amine oxidase; and tyrosinase. Copper deficiency impairs the maturation of red and white blood cells and the mineralisation of bone. In the absence of copper, hair is depigmented, and cerebral function deteriorates.
- **Cobalt**, part of the vitamin B_{12} molecule, is required for the normal function of the nervous system, and for the development of red and white blood cells.
- **Manganese** is necessary for the activity of enzymes, such as pyruvic carboxylase, that catalyse oxidative phosphorylation. Manganese deficiency is rare.
- **Iodine** is required for the iodination of tyrosine in the formation of tri-iodothyronine (T3) and thyroxine (T4) (p. 323). Iodine deficiency may develop when there is a persistent intake of less than 50 μg iodine/day, a quantity ingested by most individuals in their table salt.
- **Fluorine** assists the development of healthy teeth and the formation of normal bone. Added to drinking water, calcium fluoride prevents dental caries although less than 10% of the UK population receives fluorinated water. Fluoride ingested for prolonged periods in great excess causes skeletal abnormalities, a problem encountered in Hyderabad-Deccan, India.

TRACHEA

The trachea extends from its origin at the cricoid cartilage to the bifurcation of the right and left main bronchi.

DEVELOPMENTAL AND CONGENITAL ABNORMALITIES

Tracheo-oesophageal fistula

This congenital abnormality may exist in isolation, when it is readily correctable surgically, or may accompany other defects, for example of the heart (p. 147).

INFECTION AND INFLAMMATION

Tracheobronchitis

Tracheobronchitis is a complication of endotracheal intubation, trauma and the inhalation of irritant gases and flames. It is often caused by adenoviruses and Respiratory syncitial virus (RSV), as well as by the viruses of influenza and measles.

TRANSPLANTATION (GRAFTING)

A transplant or graft is an organ or piece of tissue *deliberately* implanted in a different site in the same individual, or in the same or different site in another individual. Tissue is transplanted from a **donor** to a **recipient** or host. Occasionally, as a result of trauma, a portion of one tissue is *accidentally* implanted in an abnormal site.

Tissue for transplantation may be living and survive in its original form. It is then said to be **vital**. Alternatively, grafted tissue such as bone or tendon may be dead. It is a **static** graft, performing a passive, mechanical function and acting as a nidus for the new growth of cells derived not from itself but from those of the recipient.

A transplant from one site to another in the same individual is an **autograft**. When transplanted human tissue has a genetic structure identical with that of the recipient, for example if donor and recipient are identical twins, it is **syngeneic**. A transplant from one individual to another of the same species is an **allograft**. Under these circumstances, when the donor and recipient are of the same species but otherwise genetically dissimilar, the graft is **allogeneic**, as in dissimilar twins. Transplants between different species, **xenografts**, display species differences in antigenic structure and the genetic relationship is **xenogeneic**.

Other terms denote the anatomical site of grafts. When a graft is placed in the tissue from which it came, as in the case of corneal grafts, it is a **syngraft** (isograft). The tissue is, of course, syngeneic. If a graft is placed within the same type of tissue as its origin but in a different anatomical position, as for example skin grafted from the thigh to the arm, it is **orthotopic**. When a graft is inserted in a different type of tissue, it is **heterotopic**.

Different types of graft dictate the required procedure. Autografts, such as those used in head and neck surgery, may require a temporary vascular pedicle but many are now sustained by free vascular anastomosis, made by the use of an operating microscope. Large allografts, such as those of whole kidney, liver and heart, also require vascular anastomosis. Some grafted tissues including epidermis; articular cartilage; and cornea, can survive without a vascular pedicle: they are normally avascular (p. 188).

Now read Immunity (p. 171)

GRAFT REJECTION

Autograft rejection

The reasons for autograft rejection are vascular; mechanical; endocrine; and microbial. An autograft that has an adequate blood supply and receives appropriate mechanical, nervous or hormonal stimuli is not rejected provided that the transplanted tissue is healthy and sterile.

Allograft rejection

When a carefully sited graft from an individual to an unrelated person is rejected, the cause is usually immunological. Occasionally, the graft is rejected extremely rapidly because of the presence of preformed antibodies. More often, the response is less rapid. The recipient's circulating lymphocytes recognise foreign histocompatibility (MHC) antigens (p. 330) on the surface of the grafted cells and initiate rejection. A further reason for rejection is vascular insufficiency. After months or years of normal function, a graft may be rejected because of slowly progressive arterial obliteration.

Graft rejection patterns are classified according to their time scale.

Hyperacute

In hyperacute rejection, blood flow through a graft decreases within minutes of transplantation. Sludging of red cells and microthrombi cause blood vessels to be obstructed (p. 320). The adverse changes are due to preformed antibodies already present in the recipient's circulation. These immunoglobulins include anti-red and anti-white blood cell antibodies formed during pregnancy, and anti-class I MHC antibodies formed after previous blood transfusion or due to blood group incompatibility.

Acute

A human allograft may be vascularised and function well for an initial period but then undergo rejection. There are two mechanisms of which one predominates.

An **acute, early** parenchymal rejection occurs within 10 days of transplantation. It is attributable to a cell-mediated hypersensitivity reaction and results in infiltration by CD8 cytotoxic T lymphocytes. Vascular changes are minimal.

Now read Cell-mediated hypersensitivity (p. 161)

An **acute, late** rejection occurs within 42 days of transplantation. The response is mediated by antibodies and complement that bind to small blood vessels blocked by platelet aggregates and fibrin. Immunoglobulins can be identified in the vessel walls by immunofluorescence (pp. 158, 234). Injury may also be caused by antibody-dependent, cell-mediated cytotoxicity (ADCC – p. 231).

Chronic

Rejection due to progressive occlusion of the vessels may occur insidiously, months or years after transplantation. The endothelial deposition of fibrin and platelets is followed by arterial collagen and proteoglycan formation in the vascular intima. One explanation may be immune complex deposition. A second implicates the co-stimulatory signal needed for T lymphocyte activation when antigen is presented by class I MHC molecules (p. 173).

Second set phenomena

After graft rejection, a second graft implanted from the same donor is rejected at an increased rate. Accelerated rejection is a consequence of recipient sensitisation to donor cell histocompatibility antigens. Sensitised lymphocytes mediate the accelerated response.

HISTOCOMPATIBILITY ANTIGENS

Histocompatibility surface antigens are recognised by lymphocytes taking part in transplant rejection and are important in determining the outcome of grafting. The antigens are inherited and are coded by genes on somatic chromosome 6 in the major histocompatibility complex (MHC). The sequence that promotes the activation of high-affinity IL-2 receptors by IL-2, catalyses the clonal expansion of activated T-cells. In prophylaxis, this sequence can be blocked by a molecularly engineered human IgG1 monoclonal antibody that binds to but does not activate the high-affinity receptor.

Major histocompatibility complex

In man, the complex of antigenic determinants that comprises the major histocompatibility complex (MHC) is the human leucocyte antigen system (HLA) (Fig. 52). Maps of the MHC show three main sites (I, II and III) coded by HLA genes and others that code for components of complement (p. 232).

The outcome of allografting is best when the HLA antigens of donor and host are matched before transplantation. Advances in the design and use of immunosuppressive drugs such as cyclosporin mean that perfect donor–host matching is no longer an absolute requirement for success. Nevertheless, it is still true that the result of grafting is improved if blood group and minor histocompatibility antigens are matched as well as those of the major HLA antigens. To achieve this aim, lymphocytes or other cells from a prospective donor are tested against anti-HLA sera. The sera come from three sources:

- Multiparous women who have reacted to form antibodies against paternal antigens on fetal cells.
- Recipients of multiple blood transfusions.
- Individuals subject to planned immunisation schedules.

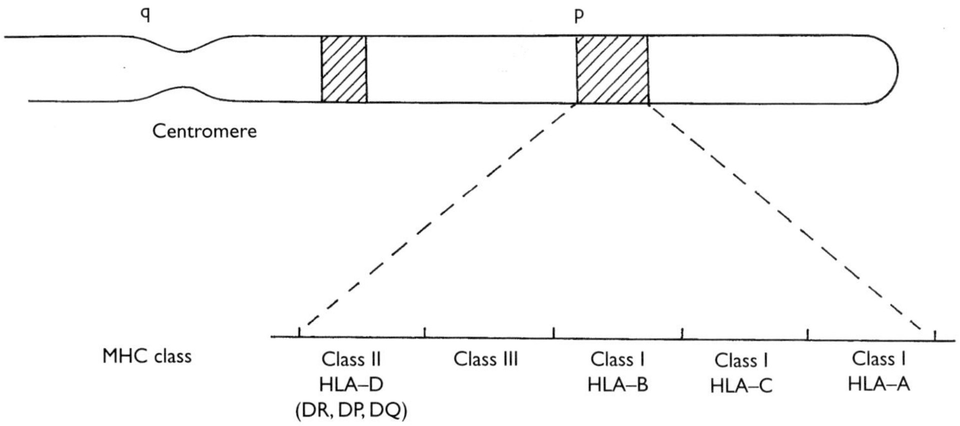

Figure 52 Organ transplant rejection.
Main cause of tissue transplant rejection are antigens, encoded by MHC locus located on somatic chromosome 6, and found on all nucleated cells. In man, MHC locus is termed HLA (human leucocyte antigen). Diagram shows location of HLA antigens. HLA antigens direct functions of T-cells. Genetic coding for HLA antigens is complex so that chances of all HLA antigens of donor and recipient being same is no more than ~$1/10^6$. Human blood incompatibility is mainly determined by ABO antigens of surfaces of erythrocytes.
q: long arm of chromosome; p: short arm of chromosome

GRAFT-VERSUS-HOST REACTION

When foreign cells were injected into embryonic or neonatal animals, some died from a wasting 'runt' disease. This graft-versus-host reaction takes place:

- When a host contains tissue antigens not present in the donor of the graft.
- When the grafted cells are immunologically competent.
- When the host is tolerant of the graft.

Foreign lymphocytes, included with the graft, attack the tissues of the host. The reaction is exemplified by the response that follows allogeneic transplantation of bone marrow to patients whose marrow has been destroyed during the treatment of leukaemia. In these patients, the iatrogenic disease is limited to exfoliative dermatitis; anorexia; diarrhoea; and opportunistic infection.

TRANSPLANT CANCERS

The development of cancer is a highly undesirable complication of immunosuppression in tissue and organ transplantation. A balance has to be struck between preserving graft function and invoking carcinogenesis. In heart, liver and lung transplants, there is no dilemma because there is no alternative way of sustaining life. In renal transplants, the difficulty is much greater. Dialysis offers a poorer quality of life than transplantation but the overall incidence of cancer is not increased. Indeed, the probability of squamous carcinoma may be reduced by comparison with healthy controls. There is a high frequency of cancers in patients given cyclosporin after transplantation. The effect is dose-related. However, the disadvantage of reducing dosage is an increased tendency to acute late rejection of the transplant.

The immune response plays a larger part in the natural history of some transplant cancers than others. The nature of the cancers is selective. The incidence of breast cancer is not increased. However, the response varies geographically. Lymphoma and cancers of the thyroid, kidney and uterus are more common in Japan, skin cancer in Australia and Kaposi's sarcoma in Saudi Arabia. In Australia, the prevalence of skin cancer increases from 20% at 5 years after transplantation to 75% at 20 years. The corresponding figures in Europe are 10% and 40%. However, any assessment of these frequencies must consider changes in the general population among whom basal cell carcinoma, for example, has increased in frequency by 240% during the past 15 years.

TRAUMA

Trauma is the third most frequent cause of death worldwide. In Western Societies, it is the most common cause of death in the first half of life although the UK mortality has fallen steadily during the last decade. This benefit may be related to better health and safety at work; to improved roads; to careful vehicle design; to the use of seat belts and helmets; and to a reduction in drink-driving. The reduced mortality is also, beyond doubt, due in part to the improved care of the injured.

Nevertheless, a challenge remains. The annual cost of treating all injuries occurring in the UK is still approximately £1.6 billion. It is a particular problem for the young and the old. Almost 75% of deaths after major trauma occur in patients who are >70 years of age or who have sustained severe head injury. Many patients have injuries to more than one organ or system. Falls account for 46% of patients with blunt trauma; road traffic accidents for 36%; and assaults for 5%. Penetrating injuries occur in <3% of patients. In assaults within the UK, knife wounds are more frequent than gunshot injuries. The converse is the case in Europe. Severe blunt abdominal trauma is relatively uncommon: fewer than 10% of severely injured patients require laparotomy.

The risk of dying from trauma in the UK is proportional to the extent of the injury. It is also influenced by age with a progressive increase in risk within each decade over the age of 55 years. Prior health may influence the outcome. The effect of previous disease upon the outcome of trauma is considered in the *Acute Physiology And Chronic Health Evaluation* (APACHE) system which assesses acute physiology, age and chronic health.

To audit treatment, objective scoring systems have evolved. They include the *Glasgow Coma Score* (CGS) for head injury and the *Ranson score* for acute pancreatitis. Other systems assess nutritional status and the severity of sepsis. In the UK, 97 hospitals, half of those that admit injured patients, contribute data to the UK Trauma Audit and Research Network (UK–TARN).

Now read Fracture (p. 54), Bleeding, Haemorrhage (p. 42), Shock (p. 290), Wound (p. 357)

TUBERCULOSIS

Tuberculosis is an infectious disease caused by *Mycobacterium tuberculosis hominis*. Man is also susceptible to *Myco. tuberculosis bovis* which infects cattle and other animals. Under particular circumstances, the *Myco. avium-intracellulare* complex is pathogenic. It is an agent that affects individuals with AIDS. Such opportunistic mycobacteria are often difficult to treat because of their resistance to many anti-biotics.

During the years between 1945 and 1960, tuberculosis was gradually eradicated from the UK by combining the X-ray screening of susceptible populations, with Mantoux testing (p. 229). Immunisation with BCG (p. 333) was adopted for those who were Mantoux negative. More recently, immigration, poverty, AIDS, the cessation of BCG vaccination, and resistance to anti-mycobacterial antibiotics, have combined to encourage a resurgence of infection. In Western countries, the threat posed by tuberculosis is now greater than it has been for 50 years.

Now read Mycobacteria (p. 237)

INFECTION

Mycobacterium tuberculosis reaches the tissues by the inhalation of droplets expectorated or expelled when patients with open disease speak, cough, or sing. Very small numbers of organisms are sufficient to provoke disease in susceptible individuals. Infection may be contracted during a single air journey. One index case can provoke widespread community infection. Large droplets are particularly hazardous and *Myco. tuberculosis* can survive in dust. Infection can also be spread directly to the small intestine when infected milk is drunk after contamination with *Myco. tuberculosis bovis*. In nosocomial outbreaks of multidrug resistant (MDR) tuberculosis, virulent disease may be associated with the immunosuppressive actions of HIV (p. 2). Genetic factors are also important in determining susceptibility to tuberculosis (p. 182).

At sites of infection, mycobacteria are phagocytosed by macrophages and can remain alive within these cells for long periods. Many macrophages and tissue cells die and a focus of ischaemic, caseous necrosis results. The focus is surrounded by residual, living macrophages, and by lymphocytes responding to mycobacterial antigen in the processes of delayed hypersensitivity and cell-mediated immunity (p. 172). Some macrophages fuse to form Langhans (p. 373) giant cells. The focal lesion originating in this way is a granuloma; it is a **tubercle**. The skin reactions in a positive Mantoux test (p. 229) and the response at sites of BCG vaccination are indistinguishable from those of tuberculosis microscopically.

Now read Mycobacteria (p. 237)

Primary disease

Infection of an individual who has not previously been in contact with pathogenic mycobacteria leads to a primary disease; there is neither acquired immunity nor hypersensitivity. The lung is a common site. Bacteria lodge in the lung periphery where a focus of infection, a **Ghon focus**, together with the associated regional lymph-node disease, constitute a **primary complex**. The organisms may gain entry to the bloodstream from necrotic lymph nodes adjoining the pulmonary vein. Blood-borne, miliary spread is then a complication. In cases where the intestine is infected, the bacteria multiply in the lymphoid tissues and cause circumferential ulcers of the adjacent mucosa. Ileocaecal tuberculosis may provoke intestinal obstruction. When mesenteric lymph nodes are, in turn, infected, the old description **'tabes mesenterica'** is sometimes used.

Post-primary disease

Pulmonary disease

If there has been previous, healed or localised infection, or vaccination with BCG, the post-primary response to infection is much modified by cell-mediated, delayed hypersensitivity. There is little humoral immunity. The organisms elicit a vigorous inflammatory reaction, Koch's phenomenon, generally in the apex of a lung lobe. Infection, localised to this site, becomes chronic, with slowly progressive, caseous, tissue destruction and fibrosis. Healing is accelerated by antibiotics such as rifampicin, streptomycin, isoniazid, pyrazinamide and ethambutol. Surgical removal of lung segments or lobules is now rarely necessary to control advancing disease.

BACILLE CALMETTE ET GUÉRIN (BCG)

Vaccination with BCG can give protection against the hazards of primary tuberculous infection. BCG is an attenuated strain of *Mycobacterium tuberculosis bovis* that has been grown for long periods on artificial media in a laboratory. The organism loses its virulence but retains its antigenic structure so that it can induce cell-mediated immunity when injected into a non-immune individual. BCG vaccination protects efficiently against the hazards of primary tuberculous infection. It was therefore given to all children in the UK who had been shown, by the demonstration of a negative Mantoux test, not to have had contact with *Myco. tuberculosis* by the age of 13. This policy has now ceased.

BCG has been used in the attempted immunosuppression of tumour growth (p. 247).

TUMOUR

Readers are referred to Carcinogenesis, Cancer (p. 76) and Neoplasia, Tumour (p. 242)

U

ULCER

Ulcers are interruptions in the continuity of an epithelial or endothelial surface. They can be caused by any mechanism that initiates tissue destruction. Trauma, ischaemia, bacterial infection and cancer are the most common agencies but ionising radiation; parasitic infestation; the action of chemicals; and occupational factors, are of importance. There are early signs of acute inflammation. Healing takes place by the regeneration of the epithelial or endothelial surface.

Acute

Acute ulcers penetrate through skin or mucosal surfaces into subjacent tissue. A slough of dead tissue and inflammatory exudate forms the ulcer floor. An acute ulcer is distinguished from an acute erosion by the extent of the tissue loss. Acute gastric erosion, for example, causes the transitory destruction of an area of mucosa whereas acute peptic ulcer results in the loss not only of mucosal but also of submucosal tissue.

Chronic

The causes of ulceration often persist so that many forms of ulcer become indolent or chronic (Fig. 53). Alternatively, chronic ulceration results from infection of a previously uninfected lesion; from secondary vascular disease; or from failed attempts at treatment.

In chronic ulceration, scar tissue formation is almost inevitable. In some sites, the contraction induced by fibrous repair may lead to stenosis. Pyloric

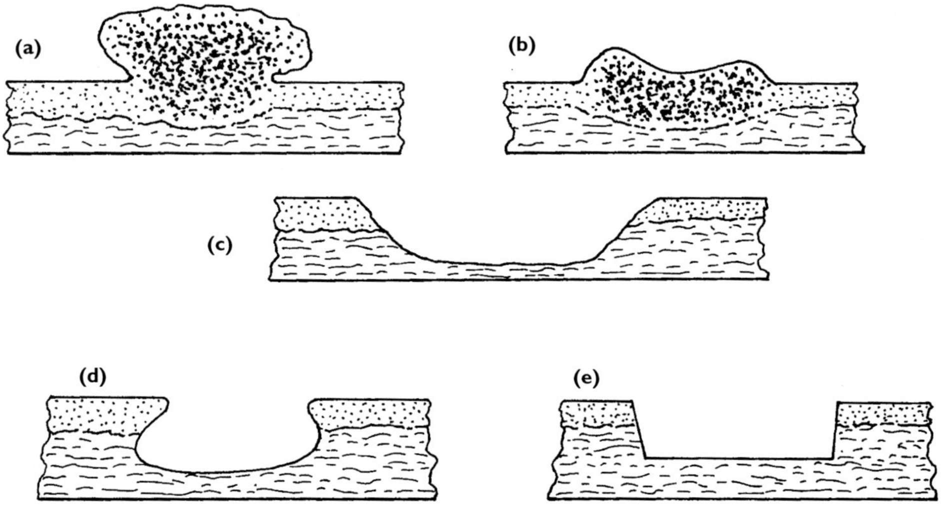

Figure 53 Varieties of ulcer.

(a) Fungating, exophytic carcinoma. The exposed surface is ulcerated.
(b) Rodent ulcer (basal cell carcinoma). The ulcer margins and rounded and raised.
(c) Septic ulcer. The ulcers have a shallow, open periphery.
(d) Amoebic or tuberculous ulcer. The transverse, colonic or ileal ulcers have overhanging edges.
(e) Syphilitic ulcer. Mucosal ulcers characterise secondary syphilis.

stenosis resulting from chronic duodenal ulceration is one example. Deep ulcers inevitably erode blood vessels. An active, chronic, posterior duodenal ulcer may cause haemorrhage by penetrating the retroduodenal artery; a chronic varicose ulcer may lead to bleeding from the long saphenous vein. Cancerous ulcers often have upturned margins composed of malignant tissue. Ulcers caused by chronic infection have sloping or shelved edges that contrast with the undermined periphery of tuberculous and amoebic ulcers. Penetration of the intestinal wall by a chronic ulcer may culminate in perforation of the gut. The consequences include peritonitis; the formation of an abscess; or the development of an internal fistula (p. 132).

Varieties of ulcer

- **Buruli ulcer.** In Buruli ulcer, *Mycobacterium ulcerans* is acquired from reeds at river margins in Australia, Africa and other countries. It causes a chronic, sclerotic, lesion with extensive undermining of nearby tissue.
- **Curling's ulcer.** Curling's stress ulcer, acute haemorrhagic gastritis, is a consequence of extensive burns or severe injury. The cause is defective tissue vascular perfusion.
- **Cushing's ulcer.** Cushing's ulcer of the first part of the duodenum is an analogous condition. It is a result of severe head injury.
- **Decubitus ulcer (bedsore).** Decubitus ulcers form at sites where there is persistent, sustained pressure on skin overlying bony prominences. Such ulcers are therefore frequent in areas of skin of the back and hips and occur particularly in elderly and debilitated patients confined to bed or to a chair. Ulceration is especially likely when there is circulatory and neurological impairment, for example in diabetes mellitus (p. 117).
- **Fissure.** A fissure is a linear ulcer.
- **Hunner's ulcer.** Hunner's ulcer is a large, intractable and painful ulcer affecting the whole thickness of the wall of the urinary bladder in either males or females. The development of Hunner's ulcer follows the persistence of cystitis. However, the precise reason for such ulceration remains uncertain.
- **Malignant ulcer.** Many carcinomas undergo ulceration. They progress from minute, epithelial lesions to become exophytic growths, to which the host arterial blood supply becomes critical when the tumour exceeds ~1 mm in diameter (p. 246). For this reason and because of the actions of cytokines such as TNFα, central necrosis of the tumour mass is followed by ulceration.
- **Marjolin's ulcer.** Marjolin's ulcer is a well-differentiated but aggressive squamous carcinoma arising at the epidermal margin of a long-standing varicose ulcer. Similar tumours may arise in burn scars and in a sinus draining the site of a chronic osteomyelitic abscess.
- **Oriental ulcer.** Oriental ulcer or sore is a name given to an ulcerating focus of cutaneous leishmaniasis (p. 282). It is one of many examples of tropical skin ulcers caused by protozoa, worms and fungi.
- **Peptic ulcer.** Peptic ulcers occur at the lower end of the oesophagus, in the stomach, in the duodenum and in relation to the stoma formed at gastrojejunostomy. They may arise in Meckel's diverticulum.
- **Rodent ulcer.** An ulcerated basal cell carcinoma of the skin (p. 296) is a 'rodent' ulcer.
- **Schistosomal ulcer.** Schistosomal ulcers are among the most frequent of those that occur in tropical and subtropical countries. Ulceration of the bladder is caused by *Schistosoma haematobium* (p. 338), that of the large intestine by *Schistosoma mansoni*.
- **Trophic ulcer.** Where the tissues are affected by a metabolic defect such as diabetes mellitus, they tend to beak down.
- **Varicose ulcer.** Varicose ulcers are very frequent. They develop on the skin of the lower leg where oxygen transport to the tissues is normal but cell metabolism is impeded. Those of long duration may be precancerous.

ULTRASOUND

Ultrasonic vibrations are sound waves of high frequency. They are inaudible to man. The lower limit of ultrasonic vibration is 20 KHz. The much higher range used in surgery is 1–15 MHz. Ultrasonic vibrations may be pulsed or continuous. They are measured in watts per square centimetre (W/cm^2). A watt is a unit of power that, in 1 second, produces 1 joule of energy.

Diagnostic ultrasound is described under Imaging (p. 169).

THERAPEUTIC ULTRASOUND

High-intensity vibrations affect the tissue through which the waves pass. Energy is given up in the form of heat. This property can be exploited to promote the resolution of soft-tissue injuries. At higher levels of intensity, cavitation can be produced. This destructive capability permits the ablation of the vestibular labyrinth in patients with Menière's disease. Urinary tract, biliary and pancreatic calculi can be shattered by ultrasonic vibrations. In the case of renal calculi, this technique, **lithotripsy**, has found wide application. The hazards of high-intensity ultrasound are mentioned on p. 169.

Now read Imaging (p. 169)

URETER

Biopsy diagnosis of ureteric disease

Specimens for microscopy are often obtained at ureterorenoscopy.

DEVELOPMENTAL AND CONGENITAL DISORDERS

The embryonic ureter is formed as the mesonephric (Wolffian) duct. It grows proximally towards the metanephros, the primitive kidney. A range of defects may develop during this complex process and some cause functional disorders, particularly obstruction. Varieties of duplication of the ureter are frequent. There may be:

- Simple, partial duplication.
- Simple, complete duplication.
- Duplication with an ectopic ureter.
- Duplication with an ectopic ureterocoele.

The abnormalities predispose to infection. **Ureterocoele** is a developmental anomaly in which the distal part of an ectopic ureter terminates in a ballooned segment in the wall of the urinary bladder. Other defects include the possibility that the ureter may lie behind the inferior vena cava and be partially obstructed. Folds of tissue, valves, may be present within the ureter. Diverticula may persist and the presence of congenital mega-ureter can lead to defective ureteric peristalsis.

INFLAMMATION AND INFECTION

The renal pelvis, the ureter and the urinary bladder are susceptible to epithelial changes that accompany persistent infection.

Acute

Ureteritis cystica

Inflammation of the ureter with cystic changes, ureteritis cystica, is associated with the deep, intramural sequestration of foci of epithelial cells. The epithelial islands enlarge. Fluid is retained so that many small, balloon-like, thin-walled structures project into the lumen of the affected duct, superficial (internal) to the surface of the surrounding urothelium.

Chronic

Fibrosis

There are many causes of ureteric fibrosis. A ureter may be injured or even ligated during surgery or become the site for tuberculous and other chronic infections. It may also be implicated in retroperitoneal fibrosis (p. 131).

MECHANICAL DISORDERS

Primary obstructive mega-ureter

In this condition, of unknown cause, there is obstruction and dilatation of the whole ureter except the terminal segment. The wall of the lower, narrowed segment, and the proximal, dilated part, contain excess, fibrous collagen. Vesico-ureteral reflux does not develop. Primary obstructive mega-ureter is analogous to idiopathic hydronephrosis.

Secondary obstruction

Secondary obstruction to a ureter may be caused by external agencies; by lesions within the wall; or by objects lodged in the lumen. Obstruction may be transient and physiological, as in the case of pressure caused by the enlarging pregnant uterus, or persistent and pathological, as in the case of mechanical obstruction provoked by the infiltrating tissue of a uterine cervical carcinoma.

Calculus

Calculi originating in the renal pelvis frequently lodge in a ureter. The calculi that form in the ureter closely resemble those originating in the urinary bladder and kidney (p. 196).

Ureterocoele

The effects of this malformation include urinary stasis and infection but vesico-ureteric reflux may be the predominant feature. In the absence of surgery, obstructive uropathy may develop. Hydro-ureter and hydronephrosis may precipitate infection. They culminate in pyonephrosis and unilateral renal failure.

TUMOURS

Metastatic ureteric tumours are rare. The most frequent of those infiltrating the wall of the ureter are carcinomas of the colon, uterine cervix and ovary. Lymphoma may behave in the same way.

Primary tumours of the ureter are very uncommon. Their structure and behaviour closely resemble those of transitional cell carcinoma of the urinary bladder. Hydro-ureter, hydronephrosis and ascending, bacterial infection are among the consequences of any form of ureteric cancer.

Now read Kidney (p. 195), Urinary bladder (below)

URETHRA

Biopsy diagnosis of urethral disease

Condylomata acuminata are diagnosed following excision. Tissue from suspected tumours of the urethra is obtained at urethroscopy.

DEVELOPMENTAL AND CONGENITAL DISORDERS

The male urethra is occasionally the site of epispadias or hypospadias (p. 268). Valves may exist in the posterior urethra.

INFECTION AND INFLAMMATION

Particularly in the female, the urethra forms the common route for ascending infections of the bladder (p. 338) and kidney (p. 197). The male urethra normally contains a small number of bacteria and, in spite of all aseptic precautions, urinary infection is frequent in patients undergoing catheterisation of the bladder. Urethritis may be due to acute infection with *Neisseria gonorrhoeae* but is frequently caused by *Escherichia coli*, *Chlamydia trachomatis*, *Mycoplasma hominis* or *Ureaplasma urealyticum*. In non-specific urethritis, no organisms may be identified and the condition may precede conjunctivitis and arthritis as part of the triad of Reiter's syndrome. Condyloma acuminata, the result of venereal infection with human papilloma viruses (HPV) 6 and 11, form papillary growths on the distal part of the penis and can obstruct the urethra.

MECHANICAL DISORDERS

Rupture

Severe trauma, particularly fracture of the pelvis, may disrupt the membranous part of the male urethra. The male urethra may also be damaged by injudicious attempts at catheterisation.

Obstruction

Obstruction of the anterior part of the male urethra is caused by chronic gonococcal infection; fibrosis; and stricture. Obstruction of the membranous part is a result of injuries that include pelvic fracture. Other causes of urethral obstruction are the presence of a calculus; a diverticulum; or the rare growth of squamous or transitional cell carcinoma.

Now read Penis (p. 267)

URINARY BLADDER

Biopsy diagnosis of urinary bladder disease

Many diseases of the urinary bladder have characteristic cystoscopic appearances. Infective and neoplastic conditions are diagnosed by cytological examination of the urine and by histological examination of endoscopic biopsies. Exophytic tumours are resected from the bladder wall, to determine the depth of invasion. The site of these lesions is recorded upon printed diagrams.

DEVELOPMENTAL AND CONGENITAL DISORDERS

Congenital diverticulum may be due to a persistent urachus or the obstruction of bladder outflow during intrauterine life by a posterior urethral valve. Such diverticula retain muscle in their walls and contract during micturition. There is therefore little risk of infection.

INFECTION AND INFLAMMATION

Cystitis

Inflammation of the urinary bladder, cystitis, may be acute or chronic. At all ages, cystitis is much more frequent in females than males, an observation attributable to the shorter female urethra. Inflammation is particularly likely to occur with the onset of sexual activity and during pregnancy. In men, obstruction due to benign prostatic hyperplasia (p. 277) is the commonest cause. In both sexes, other mechanisms of stagnation such as congenital mucosal valves; bladder calculi; tumours; diverticula; and neurological disorders, may be responsible. Infection often follows catheterisation (p. 34) and this procedure accounts for 60% of the urinary infections encountered in hospital practice. Such infections are largely unavoidable. The most common initiating organisms are faecal. They include *Escherichia coli*, Klebsiella, Proteus and Pseudomonas. Skin organisms may also be responsible. Among them are: *Staphylococcus epidermidis*, *Staph. saprophyticus* and *Staph. aureus*. In some countries, *Schistosoma haematobium* and *Mycobacterium tuberculosis* are the responsible agents.

Malakoplakia

In occasional cases of chronic cystitis, ovoid or round, yellow plaques form on the internal surface of the urinary bladder (Gk. *malakos:* soft, flat place). Within the plaque are many granular macrophages forming islands among vascular granulation tissue. The granules are degraded bacterial residues. Malakoplakia may be confused with carcinoma.

Calculus

Some vesical calculi arise in bladder diverticula or when there is outflow obstruction, particularly if there is co-existent infection. Urinary calculi may also form around foreign bodies such as hair grips; pieces of catheter; or sutures introduced from outside.

DIVERTICULUM

Acquired diverticula are much more common than congenital lesions and are a late consequence of benign prostatic hyperplasia (p. 277). The regions of the bladder near the ureteric orifices are especially vulnerable. Diverticula are composed of bladder mucosa that protrudes through the hypertrophic muscle coats. An initial exaggeration of the mucosal folds (trabeculation) is followed by sacculation from which the diverticula evolve. They do not contract during micturition. As they enlarge, there is urinary stasis with infection; calculus formation; and epithelial metaplasia. Malignant transformation occurs in 5% of affected patients.

TUMOURS

Transitional cell carcinoma

Urinary bladder cancer is a common disorder in both sexes. It is the fifth most frequent form of male cancer. The condition is encountered more often in urban than in rural areas and in lower than in higher social classes. Carcinogens promoting bladder tumours invoke a field change (p. 80) so that the entire bladder urothelium is at risk.

Causes

Bladder cancer is three to four times more likely in smokers than non-smokers. Transitional cell papilloma is a notifiable disease of workers in the aniline dye and rubber industries where there has been exposure to 2-naphthylamine and benzidine, respectively. Bladder cancer is 50 times more frequent in these workers than in the normal adult population. Naphthylamine and benzidine are conjugated in the liver and excreted as glucuronides. The urinary bladder wall contains the enzyme beta-glucuronidase. At the normal, slightly acid pH of the urine, this enzyme releases the carcinogens to act selectively on the bladder epithelium. The latent period before a tumour is detected may be as much as 20 years.

Now read Carcinogenesis (p. 76)

Structure

No true distinction between papilloma and well-differentiated transitional cell carcinoma is possible and, in the UK, virtually all transitional cell tumours are regarded as carcinomas, with only very occasional lesions diagnosed as true transitional cell papilloma. The tumours are divided into papillary and solid groups. By contrast with almost all other neoplasms, invasion is not a prerequisite for the diagnosis of malignancy.

Behaviour and prognosis

The assessment of the presence or absence of invasion can be very difficult since it is not possible to orientate biopsy specimens in terms of the structure of the urinary bladder. The most important group of tumours are those that extend into the muscularis propria, the detrusor muscle.

In terms of the TNM assessment of the anatomical extent of tumours, a T1 vesical carcinoma invades only the subepithelial connective tissue (Fig. 54). A T2 tumour invades bladder wall muscle while a T3 tumour invades the perivesical tissues. In the case of carcinoma that infiltrates further, to perivesical organs and tissues, the designation T4 is used.

Vesical tumours are graded in three categories. In general, the papillary tumours are mainly of low grade (G1 or G2) while the solid tumours are more likely to be of high grade (G3). Almost all grade 1 transitional cell carcinomas show evidence of invasion. Grade 2 tumours may infiltrate but not as far as the muscularis propria. The majority of grade 3 tumours are highly invasive.

Squamous metaplasia is occasionally recognised. Transitional cell carcinomas are characterised by their multifocal nature and the high frequency of local recurrence after treatment. Many so-called recurrent tumours lie at sites other than that of the primary lesion and are therefore a manifestation of multifocality, the urothelial field change typical of this condition.

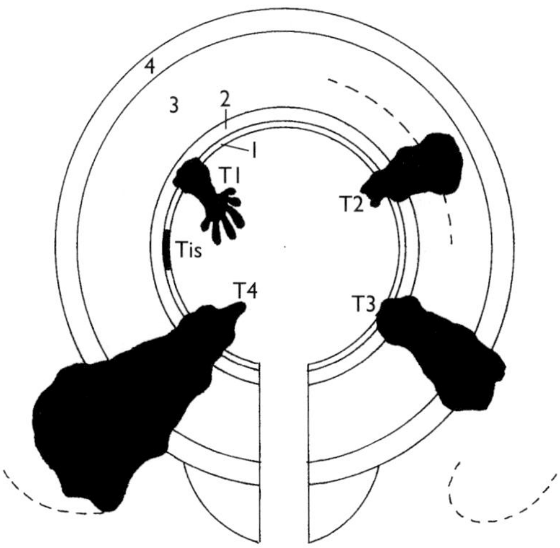

Figure 54 Carcinoma of urinary bladder.
TNM system facilitates staging of cancers. Here, simplified diagram shows carcinoma *in-situ* (Tis); tumour invading subepithelial connective tissue (T1); invading deep muscle (T2); extending macroscopically to extravesical tissue (T3); and invading pelvic wall and/or abdominal wall (T4). 1, Epithelium; 2, subepithelial connective tissue; 3, muscle; 4, perivesical fat. (Redrawn from International Union Against Cancer *TNM Atlas* 1997.)

Squamous carcinoma

Malignant change in the bladder urothelium is common in countries such as Egypt where bladder infestation by *Schistosoma haematobium* is frequent. In these cases, squamous metaplasia is an underlying change and squamous carcinoma may result.

Anaplastic carcinoma

When anaplastic carcinoma is recognised, there is early invasion of the muscular coats of the bladder, lymphatic permeation and venous spread. The response to treatment by cystectomy and/or radiotherapy is poor.

Adenocarcinoma

Adenocarcinoma may originate at the bladder apex from urachal remnants and is a common complication of ectopia vesicae.

UTERUS, CERVIX

Biopsy diagnosis of uterine disease

Cervical cancer may be suspected from cytological smears. Invasion is confirmed by subsequent cone biopsy. Endometrial cancer can be recognised by cytological examination of fluid obtained by a pipette inserted into the cervical canal. Confirmation of this diagnosis can be obtained from curetted tissue or from uteroscopic biopsies. Fallopian tube tumours can be diagnosed in the same way.

INFLAMMATION AND INFECTION

Cervicitis

The crypts within the cervical canal provide a site for the proliferation of micro-organisms that include *Neisseria gonorrhoeae*, the gonococcus; herpes viruses, particularly herpes simplex virus 2 (HSV 2); and *Chlamydia trachomatis*. Mycobacterial and trichomonal infections are less common and lesions caused by *Treponema pallidum* (p. 314) are now rare.

Cervical ectopy

Cervical ectopy is a physiological change, observed at puberty or in pregnancy, in which there is eversion of the thin, vascular, columnar epithelium of the endocervix onto the pale, squamous epithelium of the ectocervix. In essence, the central part of the squamous epithelium undergoes columnar epithelial metaplasia. The change is in part a response to exposure to the acid environment of the vagina. Formerly, the process was described incorrectly as 'erosion'. Histological examination reveals a transformation zone separating the two forms of epithelium. It is here that cervical cancer is most likely to arise.

TUMOURS

Malignant

Cervical carcinoma was previously the most common form of cancer in females. In recent years, it has declined to eighth position. The annual incidence of cervical cancer in England and Wales is now ~$70/10^6$ female adults. The frequency has fallen dramatically since the introduction of cytopathological screening, a cervical examination now offered to all adult women annually until the age of 64 years. The purpose of the examination is to detect signs of pre-malignant change.

Now read Cytodiagnosis (p. 114)

Squamous carcinoma

Squamous carcinoma (p. 303) constitutes more than 95% of malignant cervical tumours.

Causes

Squamous carcinoma is clearly related to the early onset and frequency of sexual activity. It is a sequel to squamous intra-epithelial lesions (SIL) that range from low grade, condyloma, to high grade, carcinoma-*in-situ*. Genetic factors have been implicated and a proportion of cervical cancers displays a loss of that part of somatic chromosome 11 that bears the *Ha-ras* gene.

To allow the detailed recording and comparative study of uterine cervical cytology, the entire spectrum of precancerous cervical epithelial disorders is described as **cervical intra-epithelial neoplasia (CIN)**. These dysplastic and neoplastic changes can be identified by exfoliative cytological examination of cervical mucus and are graded CIN 1, CIN 2 and CIN 3 according to precise definitions. The changes were formerly entitled mild dysplasia; moderate dysplasia; and severe dysplasia/carcinoma *in-situ*, respectively.

Human papilloma viruses (HPV) are demonstrable within the nuclei of the cells of the superficial parts of the cervical epithelium and are the candidate viruses for cervical squamous carcinoma. Forty per cent of otherwise normal females have a latent HPV infection; 5 to 10% of these individuals develop SIL but fewer than 1% progress to cancer. Low grade intra-epithelial lesions (CIN 1) are associated with the presence of human papilloma viruses (HPV) 6 or 11, high-grade lesions (CIN 2 and 3) with HPV 16 or 18. There is a relationship between the persistence of a high viral load and the risk of cancer.

Structure

The appearances of cervical squamous carcinoma closely resemble those of squamous carcinoma at other sites. The degree of differentiation varies but the formation of epithelial pearls and keratin is unusual.

Now read Squamous carcinoma (p. 303)

Behaviour

Squamous carcinoma develops over a period of several years with progression from dysplastic epithelium to carcinoma *in-situ*. Exophytic tumours grow outwards into the vaginal vault. Endophytic tumours invade deeply into the cervical canal. Early, local spread is characteristic and ulceration commonplace. The tumour readily extends through the paracervical connective tissues so that the ureters are frequently involved. Hydronephrosis is one result. Lymphatic spread occurs early but blood-borne metastasis is delayed.

It is possible to treat dysplastic and intra-epithelial neoplastic changes effectively by diathermy, cryotherapy or laser energy, preventing the development of invasive carcinoma. The 5-year survival rate in tumours confined to the cervix at the time of diagnosis is 85%.

Adenocarcinoma

Fewer than 5% of malignant cervical tumours are adenocarcinomas. These tumours are common in the nulliparous. They are usually well differentiated and arise in the endocervix.

UTERUS, ENDOMETRIUM

ENDOCRINE AND GROWTH DISORDERS

Endometriosis

Endometriosis describes the presence and growth of ectopic endometrial tissue at sites beyond the endometrium.

Causes

The genesis of endometriosis lies in the cycle of glandular, stromal and vascular changes that occur during the menstrual cycle and that are closely regulated by a complex series of hormonal interrelationships. The ectopic spread of endometriosis at distant locations cannot be explained simply by the dissemination of cells and fragments of endometrial glandular tissue through the Fallopian tubes and is highly suggestive of haematogenous spread.

Structure

The usual sites for endometriosis are within the Fallopian tubes, close to the uterus; on the ovarian surfaces; on the peritoneal surfaces of the pouch of Douglas; and on the pelvic peritoneum covering the rectum. However, endometriosis is not confined to abdominal locations and distant sites that are implicated include the umbilicus; abdominal scars; lymph nodes; lungs; pleura; and synovium. Foci of endometrial tissue comprise typical endometrial glands and stroma. The ovarian lesions are often cystic and contain altered blood, leading to the appearance termed **chocolate cyst** (p. 259). Elsewhere, the foci are seen as islands of fibrous tissue within which haemosiderin accumulates.

Behaviour and prognosis

The glands retain their sensitivity to hormones so that bleeding occurs into the lesions at the time of menstruation. The original glandular structure is often lost. One consequence of the fibrotic reaction is the fusion of adjacent tissues and organs. Fibrosis leads to the formation of adhesions and to complications such as intestinal obstruction. The hormonal-responsive changes of endometriosis subside at the menopause.

Endometrial polyp

Endometrial polyp describes a focus of hyperplastic endometrial tissue that protrudes into the cavity of the uterus.

TUMOURS

Malignant

Adenocarcinoma

Adenocarcinoma, a disorder of the elderly, is much the most common malignant endometrial tumour.

Causes

The effect of oestrogen excess in promoting endometrial adenocarcinoma is well established. There is an association with obesity. Obese individuals can readily convert adrenal androstenedione to oestrogen. There is an additional link with nulliparity.

Structure

Adenocarcinoma arises as a diffuse island of thickened endometrial tissue or as a more localised focus in the upper part of the uterine endometrium. Necrosis, ulceration and bleeding are characteristic. As the tumour grows, the uterus enlarges. The tumour is well differentiated with a uniform glandular structure. Loss of nuclear polarity, the presence of excess mitotic figures and hyperchromatism are among the changes recognised. There are variants, however, and a solid, cellular structure; a papillary formation; and a cribriform, sieve-like pattern, are those most often recognised. Individual glands may display foci of squamous metaplasia. When islands of malignant squamous cells form a distinct part of the tumour, the neoplasm is designated **adenosquamous carcinoma**.

Behaviour and prognosis
Although adenocarcinoma may extend locally, by lymphatic permeation and by metastasis, it is relatively non-aggressive. When tumour invasion takes place, the myometrium may be widely infiltrated and tumour cells reach the serosa where they establish carcinomatous deposits on the pelvic peritoneum and in the pouch of Douglas. Direct extension via the lumina of the Fallopian tubes is a feature of those tumours situated at the cornua. Metastatic deposits are frequently recognised in the vaginal wall. Lymphatic dissemination is, first, to the para-aortic nodes and, later, to those of the hypogastric and obturator regions. Blood-borne metastasis is to the liver and lungs but death is commonly the result of pelvic disease, with hydronephrosis and renal failure. Adverse prognostic features include poor tumour cell differentiation and evidence of extra-uterine tumour extension.

The majority of adenocarcinomas are confined to the uterus. They are treated effectively by hysterectomy. Surgical extirpation is followed by radiotherapy if the tumour has extended into the outer half of the myometrium. The mean 5-year survival rate is >60%.

Mixed mesodermal tumour

Mixed mesodermal tumours are very uncommon. They are highly malignant. In the majority, death occurs within 2 years of diagnosis. There are two groups: homologous and heterologous. In the former, the tumour is of stromal or smooth-muscular origin. In the latter, other cellular elements not normally present in the uterus are seen. They include cartilage and striated muscle cells, rhabdomyoblasts.

Endometrial sarcoma

Endometrial sarcoma is rare.

UTERUS, MYOMETRIUM

TUMOURS

Benign

Fibroleiomyoma

Fibroleiomyoma ('fibroid') is an exceedingly common tumour of smooth muscle origin. It grows during the active reproductive years. The tumour regresses but does not disappear after the menopause.

Causes
Fibroleiomyomas respond to female sex hormones. Cyclic hormonal changes are believed to play an important part in their genesis. The tumours become larger when oral contraceptives have been taken.

Structure
Fibroleiomyomas are firm or hard, circumscribed masses with pale grey–red cut surfaces on which a characteristic whorled pattern is evident. They arise within the substance of the myometrium where they occupy an intramural situation. They are often multiple. As growth slowly proceeds, fibroleiomyoma may protrude from a submucosal location into the uterine cavity and extend through the uterine cervix as a polypoidal mass. Other fibroleiomyomas are recognised beneath the serous surface of the uterus. They protrude into the pelvic cavity or invade a broad ligament. Rarely, a subserosal tumour may become pedunculated. When the supporting 'stalk' of vascular connective tissue is severed, such a mass can become attached to an alternative blood vascular source, such as the surface of the peritoneum or the omentum, where it assumes an independent existence as a 'parasitic' leiomyoma.

Fibroleiomyoma is formed of whorled islands of smooth-muscle cells, interspersed with extensive zones rich in fibroblasts and fibrous collagen. There are many thick-walled arteries. Dystrophic calcification; hyalinisation of collagen; necrosis; and lipid accumulation are secondary, 'degenerative' changes. They are consequences of diminishing vascularity. When ischaemia is brought about abruptly, by torsion of the pedicle of a pedunculated tumour or by haemorrhagic infarction ('red degeneration'), the tumour mass undergoes necrosis.

Behaviour and prognosis

The significance of uterine fibroleiomyoma extends beyond gynaecological practice in which they may cause every sign and symptom except amenorrhoea. Anaemia is frequent. Fibroleiomyoma is readily removed surgically but operation may be late and the enlargement of the uterus so great that urinary obstruction and infection occur. Occasionally, fibroleiomyoma provides a focus for metastasis from very common cancers such as carcinoma of the breast. However, transformation to leiomyosarcoma is rare.

Adenomatoid tumour

In this uncommon benign tumour, a resemblance to a form of benign mesothelioma (p. 274) is indicated. Endothelial cell-lined channels lie within a vascular connective tissue stroma and the tumour forms a nodule situated beneath the uterine serosa near the origin of the Fallopian tubes.

V

VACCINATION

The word vaccine derives from vaccinia, the virus of cowpox (Jenner – p. 372). Vaccination describes the administration of live or of dead micro-organisms, or of parts of them, in order to produce active immunity against viral, bacterial or protozoal infection.

Antigens given for prophylactic immunisation, such as the vaccine of yellow fever virus, are administered intramuscularly or subcutaneously. There is quick absorption and brisk antibody formation (p. 19). Antigen absorption can be slowed by the addition of adjuvant, an action that boosts the response. Alternatively, an intradermal injection may be chosen or the antigen given as a preformed antigen–antibody complex.

Vaccination has been employed with great success, not only in the reduction in frequency of infection (enteric fever, tetanus, hepatitis B, poliomyelitis, tuberculosis, schistosomiasis) but in its elimination (smallpox). Attempts are being made to manufacture an antiplasmodial, malaria vaccine.

Vaccines were at first manufactured empirically. Viruses, bacteria or protozoa were inactivated with formalin, for example, destroying the virulence of the organisms while retaining antigenicity. The disadvantages to this form of vaccine included:

- Difficulties of storage and transport.
- Accidental retention of live organisms.
- Reversion to a virulent strain.
- Inclusion of parts of the organisms not contributing to immunity but damaging to the recipient (**reactogenicity**).

The complete genomic sequences of many micro-organisms have now been established so that it is possible to isolate genes coding for virulence and to develop vaccines directed specifically at the gene product. The sequence of methods (p. 142) used to make safe, effective and cheap vaccines is:

- Identify the gene encoding a cell surface polypeptide that coats a virus such as hepatitis B.
- Clone the gene to a suitable vector.
- Induce replication of the nucleotide sequence.
- Manufacture unlimited amounts of the anti-viral protein.

Protection against common diseases such as tuberculosis and tetanus can be met by these strategies.

Structure

In the majority of patients with acute appendicitis, the lumen is not obstructed and the cause of the inflammatory reaction remains unknown. In some patients, however, the initiating event is obstruction of the appendix by a faecolith or by hypertrophic lymphoid tissue. Much less often, obstruction is attributable to a neoplasm such as a carcinoid tumour (p. 168) or to torsion.

The early phases of inflammation are recognised: vascular congestion, oedema, a polymorph exudate and fibrinous exudation. Whether or not there is obstruction, mucin continues to be secreted by mucosal cells. Compression of the appendiceal wall and dilatation of the lumen result. Vascular engorgement and tissue oedema threaten tissue viability. Deprived of normal venous drainage, infection supervenes. The accumulation of pus results in abscess formation. Appendicular artery thrombosis may then occur, leading to gangrene. The grey–green discoloration of vascular occlusion and gangrene, with a purulent exudate, is evident in any part of the viscus but may be confined to the distal part, beyond an obstruction.

Behaviour and prognosis

If inflammation is not localised, the spread of infection is diffuse. Untreated, the wall of the appendix perforates and peritonitis ensues. The likelihood of abscess formation is much greater in those infected with *Streptococcus intermedius* (*S. milleri*) and anaerobes than with other micro-organisms. Pus may track to the pelvis or to the right subphrenic space. Portal pyaemia may culminate in liver abscess (p. 210) and death (Treves, p. 376). Occasionally, when diagnosis and treatment are delayed, inflammation may subside spontaneously. Residual fibrous tissue and adhesions to adjacent omental tissue and bowel loops remain as signs of earlier disease.

MUCOCOELE

In the absence of continuing inflammation, fibrous tissue may obstruct the lumen of the appendix. Mucin secretion dilates the viscus and the appearances come to resemble those of cystadenoma or cystadenocarcinoma. Rupture of this mucocoele is one cause of pseudomyxoma peritonei (pp. 247, 260).

TUMOURS

Metastatic tumour cells occasionally lodge on the peritoneal surface. Blood-borne deposits within the organ are rare.

Benign

Carcinoid

Six of every seven neoplasms of the appendix are carcinoids; they comprise nearly half of all such tumours. A carcinoid is identified incidentally in ~1 in 300 cases where appendicectomy has been undertaken for inflammatory disease. The tumour is small, single and benign; it is usually located at the distal end of the appendix. The histological structure is closely similar to that of carcinoid of the small intestine (p. 168). The tumour extends within the mucosa and submucosa, infiltrates the muscularis and reaches the serous surface. When a tumour exceeds 15 mm in diameter, it is agreed that right hemicolectomy should be undertaken. By contrast with carcinoid of the ileum, metastasis and the development of the carcinoid syndrome (p. 82) occur in only 2% of cases.

Now read Carcinoid (p. 82)

Adenocarcinoid

Adenocarcinoid tumour, goblet cell carcinoid, is an uncommon variant that combines the histological features of carcinoid with those of carcinoma. The cells display the granules and markers characteristic of neuro-endocrine tumours (p. 127) with the mucin secretion common in intestinal adenocarcinoma. The dual character of the tumour may be explicable on the basis of an origin from the stem cells of the crypts of Lieberkühn. The prognosis is intermediate between that of carcinoid and carcinoma. Direct spread to the caecum, terminal ileum and peritoneum is probable, with metastasis to the liver and ovary.

Adenoma

The appearances and behaviour of adenoma of the appendix are similar to those of adenoma in other parts of the large intestine. With the exception of small tubular neoplasms, the tumour is associated with mucocele and resembles a mucinous cystadenoma in its pattern of secretion, obstruction and mural compression. The mass is often multiloculated. Papillary infolding of the mucosa is seen and dysplastic change in the lining epithelium is a reminder that adenoma and cystadenoma are premalignant conditions. They may coincide with other, similar tumours elsewhere in the intestinal tract.

Malignant

Adenocarcinoma and cystadenocarcinoma

These are rare appendiceal tumours. They closely resemble other carcinomas of the large intestine (p. 106). Their behaviour and prognosis depend upon the same criteria of extent of mucosal invasion and grade. Local recurrence is frequent, with involvement of the meso-appendix and ileocaecal lymph nodes. After right hemicolectomy, the 5-year survival rate is ~60%.

Now read Ileum (p. 168), Colon (p. 106)

PSEUDOMYXOMA PERITONEI

Pseudomyxoma peritonei is the massive accumulation within the peritoneal cavity of a gelatinous exudate of mucin-rich material. It is a potentially fatal complication of mucin-secreting tumours of the appendix, ovary, stomach and, rarely, other primary sites such as the testis. Secondary spread of such a tumour to the peritoneum allows the growth of relatively small clusters of neoplastic cells among a large, and sometimes enormous, volume of the secretion that cannot be removed easily by aspiration because of its high viscosity. Pseudomyxoma is an occasional complication of mucocoele. Whether it complicates benign appendicular tumours is uncertain.

Now read Peritoneum (p. 268)

VIRUS

Viruses are very small infective agents, incapable of independent life and multiplication outside living cells.

Structure

An infective virus particle is a **virion**. The particle comprises nucleic acid and a surrounding protein coat. The protein coat is the **capsid**. It is made up of **capsomeres**, the arrangement of which gives virus particles their characteristic shape; they are either compact, 20-sided icosahedrons or elongated cylinders in which the protein is arranged around the nucleic acid as a helix (Fig. 55).

Viruses are distinguished from other forms of life by the following characteristics:

- **Size**. Only the largest, the pox viruses, can be seen by light microscopy.
- **Organisation**. There is no cell wall and neither mitochondria nor ribosomes.
- **Structure**. By comparison with the structure of bacteria, the chemical form is simple. Each virus contains a single nucleic acid and a small number of protein molecules. Some viruses can be crystallised.
- **Shape**. Viruses display an orderly construction with an icosahedral or helical shape.
- **Interferons**. A response to interferons is usual.
- **Antibiotic sensitivity**. There is resistance to conventional antibiotics but sensitivity to a small number of antiviral agents.

Classification

Viruses are classified by the nature of their nucleic acid (Table 55) and by their size. The nucleic acid is DNA or RNA; it is arranged as single strands (ss) or double strands (ds). Size can be determined by passing viruses through filters of known pore size and by high-speed centrifugation. The classes of virus are divided into families and genera (Table 55).

Routes of infection

Many viruses, such as poliovirus and hepatitis A, are swallowed with food or water. Some, such as measles and influenza, are inhaled. Others, including HIV and hepatitis B and C viruses, can be inoculated directly from blood and blood products via contaminated instruments and needles, or spread by sexual contact. A further category, exemplified by the viruses of yellow fever, dengue and the arboviruses, is conveyed to the human host by intermediary vectors such as mosquitoes, sandflies and ticks, respectively.

Effects on the host

Infection

Infection begins when virus attaches to cell surfaces by adsorption. As virus penetrates the cell wall, the nucleocapsid is covered by plasma membrane

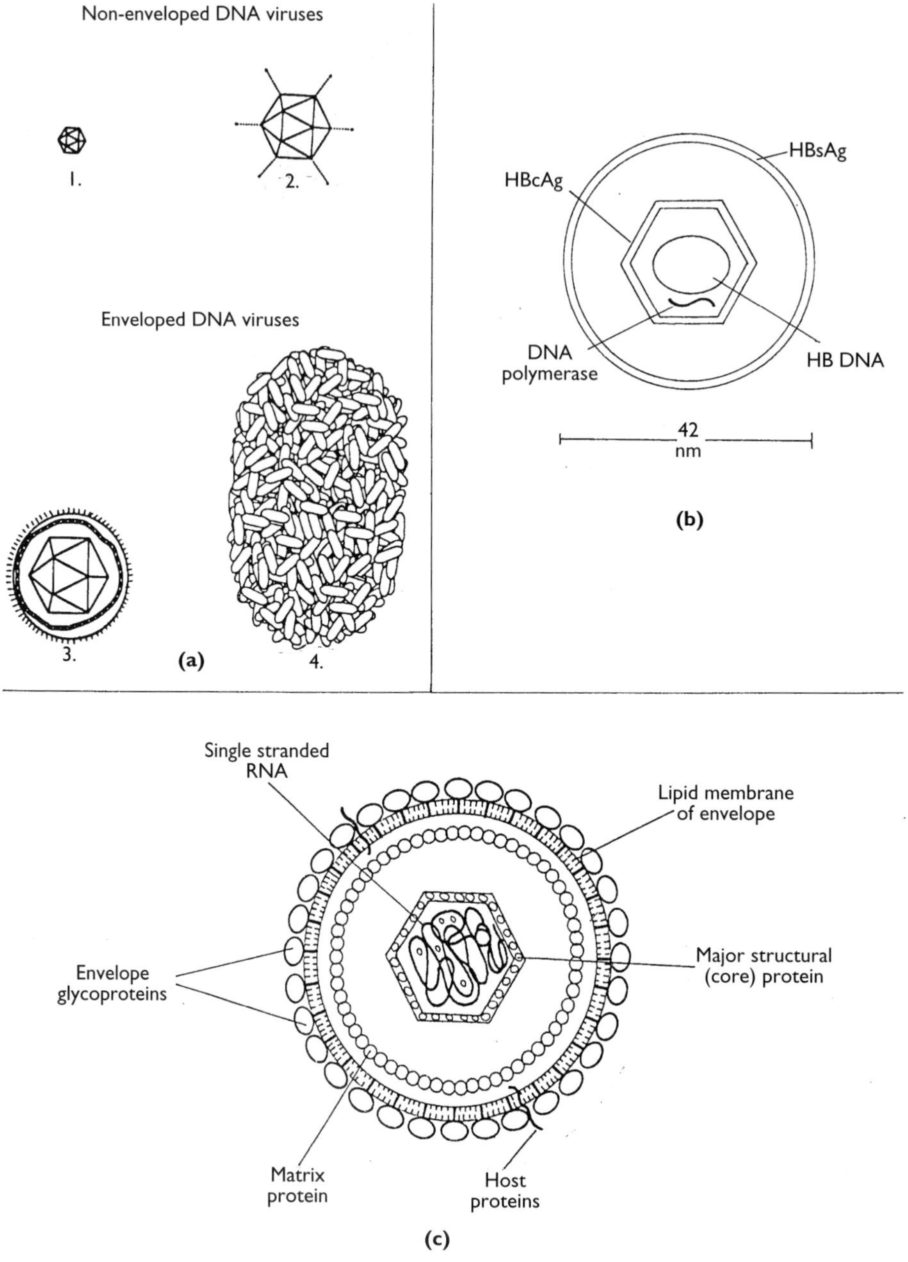

Figure 55 DNA and RNA virus sizes and structures.

(a) Comparative size and morphology of viruses. Viruses range in size from very small (poliovirus (1), parvovirus (2)) to large (herpes virus (3), pox virus (4)). Pox viruses approach size of bacteria. At top: non-enveloped DNA viruses. At bottom: enveloped DNA viruses.

(b) Hepatitis B virus particles. In the plasma of patients with severe, acute infection, and in the case of certain carriers, there may be as many as 10^6–10^7 infectious (Dane) particles and 10^{12} HBsAg particles per μL.

(c) Structure of human immunodeficiency virus (HIV). At height of infection, ~10^9 particles of HIV are produced daily. Variants of virus often appear. There are frequent changes in virus nucleic acid structure. They signify difficulty in predicting responses to treatment since new strains emerge that are resistant both to immune system and to antiviral drugs.

Table 55 Some viruses of importance in surgery in the UK and other countries

Virus family	Example of virus	Resultant diseases	Identification	Transmission	Treatment and Prevention
DNA Viruses					
Papovaviruses (45–55 nm; dsDNA)	Papillomaviruses	Skin, genital warts; HPV16, 18 associated with carcinoma of cervix	Cytology; EM; PCR	Direct skin or mucosal contact; indirect	No antiviral agents or vaccines
Herpesviruses (180–200 nm; dsDNA)	Cytomegalovirus	HSV 1: cold sores; HSV 2: genital herpes; HSV 3: varicella zoster; HHV 8: Kaposi sarcoma; EBV: Burkitt's lymphoma	Multinucleated cells or inclusions in smears (HSV); cell culture (HSV, CMV); Abs (all viruses); heterophil Abs (EBV)	Saliva; sexual contact; vesical fluid; seminal lymphocytes; saliva	Acyclovir (HSV); ganciclovir (CMV); immune globulin; no vaccines
Adenoviruses (70–90 nm; ds DNA)	42 types: 3,4,7,14,21 associated with pneumonia	Mesenteric adenitis, intussusception Pharyngoconjunctival fever Acute respiratory infections	Rise in CF antibody titre; cell culture – Ags (fluorescence) or virions (EM)	Faecal; eye-to-eye via towels; air droplets	No specific treatment
Hepadnaviruses (42 nm; ds DNA)	Hepatitis B virus	Hepatitis B	Antigens in blood: HBsAg = acute/persistent infection; HBeAg = high infectivity Antibodies in blood: anti-HBc early, then anti-HBs; anti-HBs, anti-HBc and anti-HBe together show immunity from recent or past infection	Blood; sexual; transplacental	No specific treatment; non-specific treatment with IFN effective; prevention by recombinant HBsAg vaccine
Picornaviruses (25–30 nm; ssDNA)	Hepatitis type A virus (enterovirus 72)	Hepatitis A	Identify in cell culture (enterovirus); rising Ab titre (Coxsackie B)	Faecal–oral (enteroviruses); respiratory	No specific treatment; vaccine or immunoglobulin
Togaviruses (60–70; ssDNA)	Rubivirus	Rubella; yellow fever 80 other arthropod-borne diseases	Specific Ab shows recent infection; rubella virus in cell culture	Respiratory (rubella); arthropod-borne (yellow fever)	No specific treatment; live rubella vaccine
Rhabdoviruses (180 nm; ss DNA)	Rabies virus	Rabies	Negri bodies in brain at autopsy; corneal scrapings, skin biopsy: anti-rabies Ab	Bite of infected dog, cat and other mammals including bat	No specific treatment; preventable by inactivated vaccine
RNA VIRUSES					
Retroviruses (80–100; ssRNA)	HIV–1, HIV–2	HIV (AIDS-related complex; AIDS) HTLV 1 (T-cell leukaemia)	HIV: Abs to CD4-binding gp 120	HIV: blood, semen, transplacental; HTLV 1: blood, milk	HIV: AZT and other antiviral agents on trial
Arenaviruses (50–300 nm; ss RNA)	Lassa fever virus	Lassa fever; Korean haemorrhagic fever	Specific Ab; virus isolation	Contact with rodent excreta	Ribavirin (Lassa fever); no vaccines
Filoviruses (filamentous; ssRNA	Ebola virus	Ebola disease	Cell culture; ELISA: anti-Ebola virus Abs; PCR	Blood and body fluids	No specific treatment; no vaccine
OTHER AGENTS					
Scrapie type agents (prion protein but no nucleic acid)		(In man): Spongiform encephalopathies: Creutzfeld–Jacob disease (CJD); new-type CJD (In cattle) Bovine spongiform encephalopathy (BSE)	Spongiform changes in brain sections. No Ab tests. Isolation of agent not routinely practicable	Consumption of untreated, infected foodstuffs	No specific treatment; no vaccine. Iatrogenic disease now preventable

Ab: antibody; Ag: antigen; AIDS: acquired immunodeficiency syndrome; AZT: azidothymidine (zidovudine); CF: complement fixation; CMV: cytomegalovirus; ELISA: enzyme-linked immunosorbent assay; EM: electron microscopy; HIV: human immunodeficiency virus; HSV: herpes simplex virus; PCR: polymerase chain reaction; RSV: respiratory syncytial virus.

lipoprotein. Entering the cell, virus loses this protein and becomes uncoated. The synthesis of viral protein and the replication of virus nucleic acid then begin. In this phase of multiplication, the formation of new infective particles is latent and there are no clinical signs of disease. Virus may kill cells by lysis. Infection may be manifest or abortive. Alternatively, infective virus may persist within the cell, in a steady state, without killing the cell. Virus can be integrated into cell nucleic acid, remaining latent, or can transform cells, causing them to behave as tumours (p. 242).

Primary viraemia

Virus particles localise in individual organs and tissues. The affected cells are injured or killed. Virus particles pass from the extracellular tissue fluid, enter the lymphatics and are taken up by macrophages. Relatively small numbers reach the bloodstream via the thoracic duct leading to a phase of primary viraemia.

Secondary viraemia and clinical disease

Settling in individual organs after clearance from the blood, virus multiplies in large numbers. The **secondary viraemia** that follows marks the acute onset of the clinical signs and symptoms.

Retroviruses

Retroviruses express the enzyme reverse transcriptase and are incorporated into the DNA of the host genome. Retroviruses include the agents of Rous sarcoma and AIDS. Characteristically, they bud from the cell surface, acquiring a surface layer composed of the phospholipids of the cell (Fig. 56).

Now read Carcinogenesis, Cancer (p. 76)

Individual viruses

The viruses of AIDS (human immunodeficiency viruses – HIV), cervical cancer (human papilloma

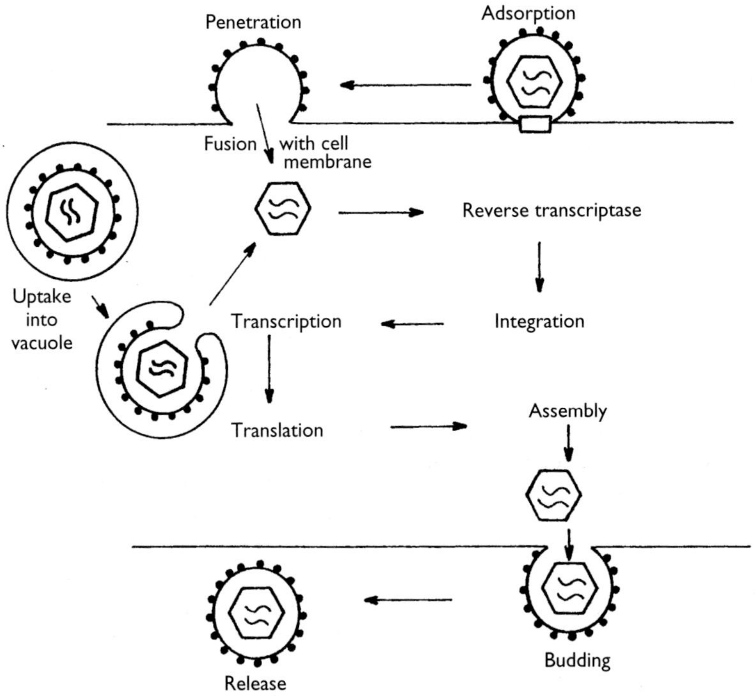

Figure 56 Human immunodeficiency virus (HIV) replication.
HIV is a retrovirus. It enters body and fuses with cell surface, penetrating directly or being taken into cell in vacuole. Virus reverse transcriptase leads to integration of viral-generated DNA into genome of host cell. Transcription and translation result in manufacture of more viral protein. New virus is assembled, acquires envelope, protrudes from cell surface and is released.

viruses – HPV) and hepatitis B (hepatitis B virus – HBV) are described on pp. 2, 340 and 152 respectively. Epstein–Barr virus (EBV) is mentioned on p. 224. Among other viruses of surgical significance are:

- **Cytomegalovirus**. Cytomegalovirus, a herpes virus, is a frequent cause of serious morbidity after solid organ transplantation. Infection may be acquired during **blood transfusion**.
- **Human herpes viruses**. HHV 6 is one herpes virus. It shows close homology with cytomegalovirus and with HHV 7 but does not infect B-cells efficiently, other than those carrying EB virus. The A variant is more common in those infected with HIV. Infection with HHV 6 usually occurs in infants aged 6 to 24 months. It causes an exanthem known as roseola. In adults, infection is recognised in immunocompromised patients with solid organ transplants or with HIV. There is a possible association with multiple sclerosis. HHV 8 may be a cause of **Kaposi's sarcoma** (p. 49).
- **Epstein–Barr virus (EBV)** is a further member of the herpes virus family. Latent infection persists in B-cells of the oropharynx for the lifetime of 90% of humans. Epstein–Barr virus is the cause of **infectious mononucleosis**, a relatively common disease of adolescents and young adults; it is also the agent of the rare chronic active EBV syndrome. The virus is closely associated with **Burkitt's B-cell lymphoma** (p. 224) in malaria-ridden parts of Africa, and with nasopharyngeal carcinoma (p. 240). EB virus infection results in humoral antibody formation. More virus is formed in immunosuppressed persons than in normal persons. Because patients with X-linked agammaglobulinaemia (p. 175) lack B-cells, however, they cannot be infected.
- **Transmissable spongiform encephalopathies (TSE-scrapie-type agents)**. Some very small, infective agents provoke diseases with incubation periods of 2 to 20 years. They were previously termed 'slow' viruses. The particles are extremely resistant to conventional methods of sterilisation (p. 304). However, they do not contain nucleic acids and are not true viruses; they are, in fact, derivatives of natural, body proteins. The term **prion**, protein infectious agent, has been introduced to describe them. They do not convey genetic information (p. 138).

In Western countries, the agents of TSE include those causing **Creutzfeld–Jacob disease** (CJD). In Papua New Guinea, **kuru**, a result of cannibalism of human offal by women and children, was an analogous condition. The corresponding agent in cattle results in **bovine spongiform encephalopathy** (BSE). In sheep, the analogue is **scrapie**.

In CJD, a rare form of progressive dementia, spongiform lesions of the central nervous system lead to death. The infective agent multiplies in lymphoid tissues and has been identified in the tonsils and vermiform appendix. When clinical manifestations eventually appear, progress is rapid. In many instances, the source of infection is unknown but the infection has been contracted from contaminated instruments, grafts and tissue preparations. A variant, **new-type CJD**, is transmitted by the consumption of beef derived from cattle infected with the agent of BSE.

Now read Sterilisation (p. 304)

VITAMINS

Vitamins are essential nutrients that cannot be synthesised in the body. They are required in very small quantities for specific purposes, for example to act as co-enzymes. Vitamins A, D, E and K are soluble in lipid; vitamins B and C in water.

LIPID SOLUBLE

Vitamin A

Vitamin A (retinol) is required for the normal survival and growth of epithelia of the gastro-intestinal, genito-urinary and respiratory systems, and of the retina. Retinol also modulates the integrity of cartilage. Vitamin A deficiency causes keratinisation and metaplasia of the epithelia. An excess may **impair development of the central nervous system**. The prophylactic administration of excess vitamin A should be avoided in pregnancy.

Vitamin D

Vitamin D is a steroid that is modified metabolically before it can exert its biological activities. Most vitamin D comes from the conversion of 7-

changes of VIN III. However, the neoplasm may originate in previously intact skin.

Structure
The appearances are those of an exophytic, wart-like mass on the labia, a hard or firm zone of induration, or an ulcer with firm, rolled edges. The tumour is a well-differentiated squamous carcinoma, the cellular features of which closely resemble those encountered in other sites (pp. 296, 303).

Behaviour and prognosis
Squamous carcinoma of the vulva spreads initially to the inguinal lymph nodes and thence to those of the femoral, iliac and para-aortic regional glands. Ultimately, dissemination via the bloodstream to the liver and lungs is recognised. Treatment is by early surgical excision. Adverse prognostic features are poor differentiation of the tumour cells and early involvement of local or regional lymph nodes. The mean 5-year survival rate ranges from 30% for those with lymph node disease to 90% when the tumour is small, localised and subject to complete excision.

Now read Squamous carcinoma (p. 303)

Other malignant tumours

Among the other malignant tumours encountered in vulval skin are malignant melanoma, adenocarcinoma of Bartholin's glands, and basal cell carcinoma (p. 296).

Malignant melanoma

Malignant melanoma of the vulva presents significant differences from malignant melanoma in other locations. Although the area of the vulval skin is ~ 1 to 2% of the total body surface, malignant melanoma of this region comprises 3 to 7% of all these tumours in females.

Vulval malignant melanoma is a disease of older women. One third of the tumours is polypoid, one quarter amelanotic. Whereas the 5-year survival of all skin melanomas in the female is ~80%, the 5-year survival rate for vulval tumours is only 47%. By contrast with other areas, superficial spreading melanoma of the vulva is the least frequent variety. Mucosal lentiginous melanoma, the equivalent of acral lentiginous melanoma, is the most common.

Now read Malignant melanoma (p. 227)

W

WART

VERRUCA VULGARIS

Verruca vulgaris, the common wart, is a frequent, virus-induced tumour of the skin of the hands and fingers of children and young persons. It is a squamous papilloma and affects a number of different anatomical sites. A wart is a raised, circumscribed, keratotic nodule varying in size from 1 to 15 mm in diameter.

Causes
Each form of wart is caused by a different human papilloma virus. The most frequent agents are HPV 1, 2 or 4. Some warts on the hands, and the majority of those on the face, are only slightly elevated. They are plane warts, **verruca plana**, a response to HPV 3 infection. Genital warts, condylomata acuminata (p. 294) are found on the penile, vulval and nearby skin surfaces.

Now read Human papilloma virus (pp. 80, 340), Virus (p. 347)

Structure
Warts are grey–brown in colour but there is no excess of melanin. The hyperplastic, thickened epidermis forms papillary folds and contours that display hyperkeratosis and parakeratosis alternately. The cytoplasm of the superficial keratinocytes is vacuolated. The majority contain eosinophilic inclusion bodies. A smaller proportion has kerato-hyaline bodies while basophilic nuclear inclusions may be detected. The dermal rete processes are long. The marginal processes are orientated centrally.

Behaviour and prognosis
Warts often disappear spontaneously but are effectively ablated by cryotherapy, laser or diathermy; excised by scissors or scalpel; or treated by applications of podophyllin, sodium salicylate or silver nitrate.

Now read Skin tumours (p. 295)

WATER

Water comprises ~60% of the body weight in adult males, 50% in females. The water content of the body is relatively less in the obese and elderly than in those of normal build and lower age. The distribution of water between the tissues is differential so that articular cartilage (p. 82) contains 71 to 76% water whereas compact bone (p. 50) contains no more than 15%. The major intracellular and extracellular compartments are separated by cell walls freely permeable to water, semi-permeable to electrolytes but impermeable to macromolecules, particularly proteins. This is a crucial factor in homeostasis and changes in membrane permeability induced by disease have profoundly deleterious effects. Many switches in membrane permeability to electrolytes are the result of the altered function of Ca^{2+} regulated ion channels. The regulation of water intake in response to thirst is by vasopressin (p. 273).

WATER DEPLETION

Water depletion may be a consequence of inadequate intake or excessive loss. In a temperate climate, the healthy adult has a daily requirement of ~1.4 L of drinking water. Approximately 1.0 L is taken in each day with food, and ~0.2 L 'metabolic' water is released by the oxidation of hydrogen contained in energy substrates, particularly carbohydrates.

In temperate climates, the daily water loss is ~600 mL through the skin, ~400 mL from healthy lungs, ~100 mL in the faeces and ~1500 mL via the kidneys, a total of ~2600 mL. The principal variations in water intake/output are attributable to the volume of water drunk, the volume of urine excreted. Patients with tracheostomies may lose ~2000 mL/day, particularly if the inspired air is not humidified. In patients with pyloric or intestinal obstruction, vomiting or nasogastric aspiration increase gastric loss significantly.

Each day, ~7.0 L water is secreted into and reabsorbed from the gastro-intestinal tract. This is the volume of which the body is effectively deprived in intestinal obstruction (p. 166). It is a so-called **'third-space' loss**. A similar change can affect the peritoneal cavity in peritonitis (p. 269) or ascites, and the pleural cavities, in hydrothorax. Large volumes of water, accompanied by varying amounts of electrolytes are excreted in severe diarrhoea and from fistulae.

In unacclimatised individuals, living and working in hot, humid environments, insensible loss through the skin and lungs can increase dramatically. A central failure of water regulation, with the excessive diurnal loss of very large amounts of fluid, is caused by the deficiency of pitressin in diabetes insipidus (p. 273).

Now read Peritonitis (p. 269), Shock (p. 290)

WATER EXCESS

The excessive accumulation of body water may be due to a high level of secretion of mineralocorticoids or ADH; to cardiac failure; or to renal failure. Water retention, with hyponatraemia and a reduction in plasma osmolality, may also result from the secretion of excess vasopressin by functioning small cell carcinoma of the bronchus. In surgical patients, the most frequent cause of water excess is injudicious intravenous infusion.

Now read Oedema (p. 251)

WORMS

Worms (helminths) are elongate, legless animals. They are classified as metazoa and fall into three groups:

Nematodes (roundworms)

This is the largest group and includes *Ascaris lumbricoides*; *Trichinella spiralis*; *Trichiuris trichiuria*; *Strongyloides stercolis*; *Enterobius vermicularis* (the pinworm or threadworm); *Toxocara canis;* and *Dracunculus medinensis* (the guinea worm). It also embraces the hookworm group, *Ancylostoma duodenale* and *Necator americanus*, and the tropical, filarial worms *Wuchereria bancrofti* and *Loa loa*.

Cestodes (tapeworms)

This group comprises *Taenia solium* (pig tapeworm); *Taenia saginata* (cattle tapeworm); *Echinococcus granulosus* (dog tapeworm); and *Diphylobothrium latum* (fish tapeworm).

Trematodes (flukes)

The most important members of this group are the Schistosoma species e.g. *Schistosoma mansoni*, *S. haematobium* and *S. japonicum*. There are also the liver flukes, *Fasciola hepatica* and *F. buskii*; the bile duct fluke, *Clonorchis sinensis*; and the lung fluke, *Paragonimus westermani*.

DISEASES CAUSED BY WORMS

Helminths cause widespread disease in countries where the opportunities for infestation are frequent. Worm infestation may also arise under poor conditions of food hygiene (echinococcosis – hydatid disease; ascariasis); by the larval penetration of the skin in infected water (schistosomiasis); and by arthropod bites (elephantiasis and onchocerciasis). Other helminthic diseases, such as ascariasis; toxocariasis; trichinosis; taeniasis; and echinococcosis, are ubiquitous. The complete genome of a multicellular nematode, *Caenorhabditis elegans*, has recently been described. Soon, the genetic structure of other worms will be unravelled yielding new opportunities for prophylaxis and treatment.

Although the most frequent diseases caused by worms are enterobiasis (*Enterobius vermicularis*); trichinosis (*Trichinella spiralis*); ascariasis (*Ascaris lumbricoides*); and taeniasis (*Taenia solium* or *T. saginata*), the infestations of greatest significance in surgical practice, listed by category, are:

Schistosomiasis

It is estimated that there may be 2×10^8 individuals with this worm infestation worldwide. The parasitic disease is widespread in South America and the Caribbean; in Africa and Arabia (*Schistosoma mansoni*); in the Middle East (*S. haematobium*); and in South-East Asia (*S. japonicum*). These three species cause intestinal ulceration and fistulas with papillomas; precancerous bladder irritation; and intestinal fibrosis and cirrhosis, respectively.

Ascariasis

Ascariasis is contracted by eating food contaminated with human faeces. The agent is *Ascaris lumbricoides*. Ileal obstruction; biliary obstruction; acute suppurative cholangitis; and acute pancreatitis are among the mechanical effects that may complicate the presence of these large helminths of which several hundreds may be found in one person.

Toxocariasis

This infestation is caused by *Toxocara canis* or *T. felicis* and is contracted by young children from soil contaminated by puppies or kittens. Retinal invasion can cause choroidoretinitis, or a localised mass resembling neuroblastoma or retinoblastoma.

Trichinosis

Trichinosis is conveyed by eating undercooked pork containing the larvae of *Trichinella spiralis*. The larvae encyst in skeletal muscle. Myalgia, orbital oedema and eosinophilia are three of the pathological effects. Deltoid muscle biopsy may reveal an encysted worm.

Taeniasis

Taeniasis, with the intestinal development of the pig tapeworm *Taenia solium* or of the cattle tapeworm *T. saginata*, causes no symptoms. However, **cysticercosis**, the consequence of swallowing the eggs of *T. solium*, may cause focal lesions in skeletal and cardiac muscle; subcutaneous tissue; and brain. Multiple sclerosis may be simulated. Hydrocephalus can result.

After a long latent period, epileptifom attacks predispose to accidental injuries such as burns.

Echinococcosis

Echinococcosis (hydatidosis) arises from ingestion of the dog tapeworm *Echinococcus granulosus* and may be contracted in the UK by consuming unwashed plants such as watercress. Eggs are ingested and hatch in the duodenum. Embryos are carried in the blood to the liver, lungs, spleen, bones and brain. The resultant **hydatid cysts** (p. 113), found in these organs, may be single or multiple.

Filariasis

Filariasis is a group of disorders. The causative agents are transmitted by biting insects. The female worms produce microfilarial embryos that parasitise blood, skin and eyes. One parasite is *Wuchereria bancrofti*. It leads to inflammation of enlarged lymph nodes, **elephantiasis** (p. 224) and tropical pulmonary eosinophilia. Another is *Brugia malayi*.

Onchocerciasis

Onchocerciasis ('river blindness') results from infestation by *Onchocerca volvulus*. Subcutaneous nodules develop resembling those of rheumatoid arthritis.

Loiasis

Loiasis is due to infestation by *Loa loa*. Migratory, subcutaneous Calabar swellings appear.

Fascioliasis

The liver fluke *Fasciola hepatica* parasitises human tissues in the Far East. Abdominal pain and malabsorption are among the consequences.

Other worm infestations include those due to *Diphylobothrium latum* and *Clonorchis sinensis*, contracted by eating undercooked fish; and *Dracunculus medinensis*, guinea worm infestation, contracted from contaminated water.

WOUND

A wound is an interruption or break in the continuity of the external surface of the body or the surface of an internal organ, caused by surgical or other forms of injury or trauma. The pathological results of wounding are **direct** or **indirect**. Tissue destruction exemplifies the former, blood loss (p. 42) the latter. Wounds may be **open** or **closed**. A surgical wound may be **incised** or **excised**.

Abrasion

An abrasion is an epidermal injury caused by friction. It is the mechanical rubbing or scraping away of part or the whole of the epidermis. Healing is usually rapid and complete.

Contusion

A contusion or bruise is a lesion caused by a crushing injury that does not break the epithelium. Capillaries and small vessels within and deep to the epithelium are damaged, with extravasation of small quantities of blood.

Laceration

A laceration is an interruption in the continuity of an epithelium, produced by a tearing injury.

Incision

An incision (Fig. 57) is an interruption to a body tissue produced by cutting.

Excision

During surgical operations, the skin and other tissues may be deliberately excised (Fig. 58).

Puncture and penetrating wounds

Sharp, pointed objects or instruments can pass long distances into the body tissues, easily, painlessly and at great speed. In classical times, puncture wounds were caused by rapiers and daggers. Now, knife wounds are very frequent. Cardiac tamponade, pneumo- and haemothorax are among the results. Irreparable damage to thoracic and abdominal organs is commonplace. Arrows, bolts and harpoons comprise a special category of injury: they cannot be pulled from the body directly. Pitchforks and long pieces of furniture thrown by explosion may impale arteries as well as causing extensive soft tissue and organ injury.

Now read Needle-stick injury (p. 362)

Bites

Apparently superficial bites may be accompanied by fractures; lacerated tendons, blood vessels or nerves; extension of injury into body cavities or joint spaces; or damage to critical structures such as the eye. There is a particular risk of tetanus (p. 94). The majority of teeth harbour potentially pathogenic micro-organisms. Human bites can transmit HIV, hepatitis B and syphilis. Animal bites convey a very large range of aerobic and anaerobic bacteria, including Pasteurella spp., but many others that are not identified routinely. The bite of any mammal can transmit rabies. In countries where rabies is endemic, rat bites offer low risks, bat bites high risks.

Blunt injuries

Blunt injuries caused by rubber bullets; by cricket balls or base-balls; or by impacts in car or aeroplane accidents, can cause hazardous, indirect effects including cardiac arrest and, in survivors, pericarditis.

Gunshot wounds

Gunshot and missile wounds are produced both by the combined effects of tissue penetration and the sudden dissipation of energy in the tissues. The kinetic energy of a missile is directly proportional to its mass but to the square of the velocity ($e = 0.5\ mv^2$). In earlier times, low-velocity, low-energy missiles, such as musket balls, caused relatively little tissue damage. Modern, high-velocity, high-energy rifle bullets cause great damage. Three main properties of the missile therefore determine the severity of a gunshot wound:

- Velocity.
- Mass.
- Composition.

High-energy rifle wounds are much more severe than those produced by small-calibre handguns. High-energy missiles produce widespread tissue cavitation due to the creation of pressure waves transmitted radial to the trajectory. There is therefore a small entry wound, a very much larger exit wound. Although the size of a wound is proportional to the calibre of a bullet, small, soft bullets often fragment upon impact and produce a correspondingly larger wound. Shrapnel fragments lead to multiple injuries.

Explosions

Explosions disrupt, tear and cause disintegration. In addition to the tissue injuries due to metal fragments, the explosions caused by grenades and small bombs in enclosed spaces provoke shock waves and produce lung injury. For the same reason, the underwater shock waves attributable to mines or torpedoes, injure the unprotected abdominal viscera.

WOUND HEALING

Wound healing may be by regeneration or by fibrous repair. Injuries to liver, skeletal muscle, nerve, renal tubules and adrenal cortex, heal wholly or partly by regeneration (p. 285). Injuries to hyaline – and to fibrocartilage – heal poorly or by fibrous repair. A fibrous, reparative response characterises the healing of wounds in which healing is delayed.

Good nutritional status; the absence of anaemia or debilitating disease; a competent immune system; and the avoidance of stress, are factors contributing to rapid wound healing. Gunshot, war wounds suffered under dry, sunny conditions heal more easily than those sustained in a wet, cold environment. In circumstances of neglect, maggots thrive on wounds and assist in the removal of necrotic tissue.

Incised wound healing

It is impossible to divide the whole thickness of healthy skin without causing cell injury, vascular damage and bleeding. Primary and secondary haemostasis occur. The early response is acute inflammation (p. 179) that soon subsides.

When the edges of a clean, sterile surgical wound are directly opposed, the rapid division of epidermal cells and the localised formation of a young, subepidermal fibrovascular scar (p. 290) lead to healing by **first intention** (Fig. 57). This process is encouraged by careful wound closure but is impeded around the tracks of sutures. A localised, limited, flurry of mitotic activity takes place in the cells at the margins of the avascular epidermis that adjoin the wound edge. Cell division is initiated by cytokines, and by products of cell damage such as nucleic acids. The role of chalones, wound hormones, is obscure. Epidermal cells extend cytoplasmic processes and begin to cover the wound surface. They meet, establishing a new surface. Cell division ceases.

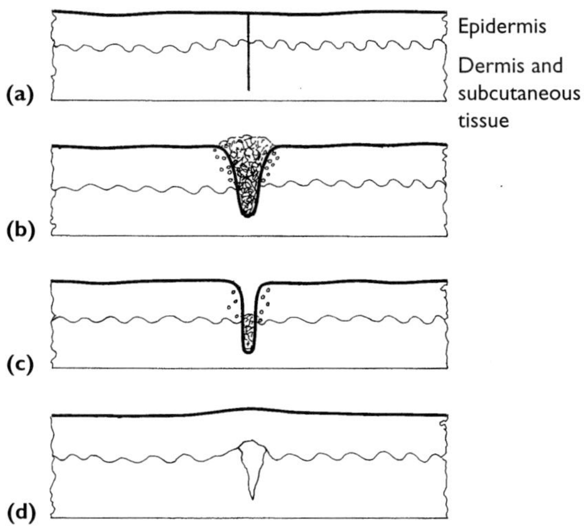

Figure 57 Healing of incised wound.
Surgical incisions of skin are normally made in the axis in which are supporting collagen fibre bundles.
(a) Incision of sterilised skin sufficiently deep to cut into vascular dermis, using a clean and sterile scalpel, causes immediate bleeding. Blood fills narrow space between separated surfaces. Coagulation occurs.
(b) Mitotic activity among epithelial cells at wound margins follows within 4 to 6 hours. Cells from opposing edges meet. Mitotic activity ceases as surface is reconstituted.
(c) Dividing epidermal cells migrate centrally. Nearby fibroblasts synthesise new type III collagen. Myofibroblasts initiate wound contraction.
(d) Continued collagen synthesis forms scar. Scar contracts, partly because of actions of contractile filaments within cells, later because of collagen cross-linking and maturation. Scar tissue remains visible but is soon covered by reformed epithelium.

In the underlying dermis, capillary buds advance into the wound accompanied by elongated and dividing fibroblasts. Fibrous, type III collagen is secreted and slowly matures. **Organisation** (pp. 131, 290) takes place. It is the conversion to, and replacement of, an inflammatory exudate or thrombus by granulation tissue. Organisation results in the formation of scar tissue, bands and adhesions. It is a feature of healing by fibrous repair.

Now read Fibrosis (p. 131), Healing (p. 147), Regeneration (p. 285), Scar (p. 290)

Excised wound healing

When tissue is excised, the initial cellular response at the wound margins is similar to that described for incision. However, the multiplying epidermal cells now extend downwards, deep to the fibrin coagulum and scab that covers the wound (Fig. 58). They grow across the base of the wound until they establish contiguity, constructing a covering for the wound base. Young, vascular granulation tissue forms beneath this neo-epidermis. As the quantity of extracellular matrix increases in amount, the floor of the excised wound is gradually raised until it reaches the level of the surrounding, intact skin. The resulting scar tissue is covered by epidermal cells. Healing is complete.

In pre-Listerian days (p. 373), surgical wounds were allowed to remain open, the edges separate. The purpose was to minimise sepsis. Granulation tissue formed the base of the healing wound and healing

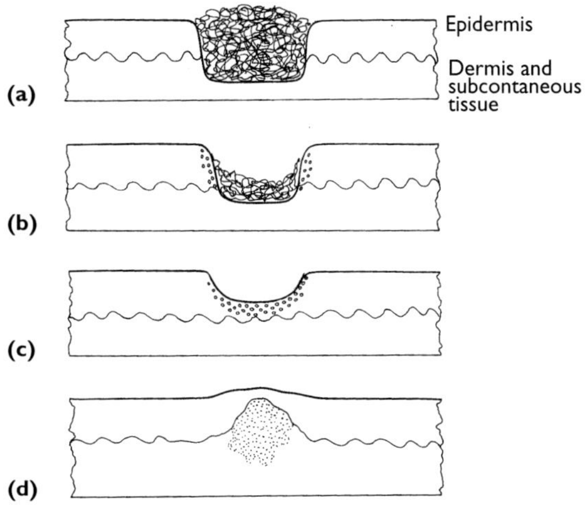

Figure 58 Healing of excised wound.
Removal of parts of epidermis, for example, during excision biopsy, leaves large, exposed area of vascular dermis and subcutaneous tissue. Healing that follows has many features in common with healing of incised wound.
(a) Bleeding is immediate. Exposed surface is quickly covered by fibrin clot.
(b) At edges of artificial 'ulcer', mitotic cell division of epithelial cells starts within 4 to 6 hours. Fibroblasts extend in from wound edges. These cells divide and form increasing quantities of fibrous type III collagen.
(c) Dividing cells cover whole base of exposed dermis/subcutis. As fibrin clot resolves, cells gradually form new surface.
(d) Buds of capillary endothelial cells migrate into wound and granulation tissue is formed. Fibroblasts synthesise increasing quantities of collagen. Myofibroblast filaments and maturing collagen cause wound to contract. Irregular-shaped scar remains.

was then said to be by **second intention**. This approach is still practiced today in dealing with heavily contaminated wounds.

Growth factors

The form and rate of wound healing are strongly influenced by many growth factors (Table 56). For example:

- Insulin-like growth factor 1 (IGF-1) increases the production of integrins.
- Integrins act as cell surface receptors for fibronectin (p. 88).
- Fibronectin provides a microskeleton for the migration of epithelial cells.

The expression of these growth factors is affected by cytokines such as tumour necrosis factor alpha (TNFα) derived from neutrophil polymorphs and other cells. They are part of the inflammatory response (p. 179) to wounding.

Now read Growth factors (p. 144)

Wound contraction

In a large wound, contraction causes centripetal movement of the skin edges and lessens the need for epithelial replacement. There is a lag period of 3–4 days before contraction begins; it is usually complete by the 14th day after a clean, sterile surgical incision. Contraction is an important component of wound healing. When healing is by second intention, a wound may be reduced by as much as 80% in size.

Contraction of wound tissue is determined by myofibroblasts. These cells have large bundles of actin filaments disposed along the cytoplasmic face of the plasma membrane. Contraction of these filaments leads to active cell movement. However, contraction is also effected by cell–cell and cell–matrix linkages. It is stimulated by TGFβ1, TGFβ2 and PDGF. Fibroblasts attach to the extracellular, collagen matrix through integrin receptors. The collagen matures and interfibrillar cross-linking accentuates contraction.

Contracture (excessive contraction) (p. 112) or **cicatrisation** occur after wound healing is complete and may, for example, produce immobilisation of joints in patients who have sustained severe burns.

Cicatrisation – scar formation

Between the 5th and 15th day of wound healing there is a rapid increase in the collagen content of the affected tissue and a great increase in the strength of the wound. The granulation tissue becomes less vascular and less cellular. There is remodelling of collagen with continually increasing cross-linkage between collagen fibrils. This relatively avascular tissue, composed largely of collagen, is a **scar** (p. 290). The process is **cicatrisation**. Replacement of collagen is a continual, slow process in old wounds; they may break down if the tissue is treated with large doses of corticosteroids (p. 6) or subjected to irradiation.

Wounds gain only 20% of their final strength in the first 3 weeks. They never attain a physiological, tensile

Table 56 Growth factors that influence wound healing

Cytokine	Principal source	Target cell – effects
Epidermal growth factor family e.g. EGF	Platelets	Epidermal and connective tissue regeneration; cell motility and proliferation
Fibroblast growth factor family e.g. FGFb	Macrophages, endothelial cells	Angiogenesis, fibroblast proliferation
Transforming growth factor beta family e.g. TGFβ1 and β2	Platelets, macrophages	Fibrosis, increased tensile strength; epidermal cell motility; macrophage chemotaxis; extracellular connective tissue synthesis, remodelling
Platelet derived growth factor (PDGF)	Platelets, macrophages, epidermal cells	Fibroblast proliferation and chemo-attraction; macrophage chemo-attraction

strength so that a cutaneous scar is only 70% as strong as normal skin.

WOUND COVERING

The protective covering of most surgical wounds is possible with synthetic or natural dressings. The healing of more extensive or recalcitrant wounds may be helped by employing skin substitutes. The use of these substances does not require painful or invasive procedures. They can therefore be positioned without admission to hospital. They offer an attractive alternative to autografting (p. 329). Although skin substitutes do not persist indefinitely, they stimulate cytokine (p. 114) production. In turn, these cytokines encourage the formation of basement membrane components, prevent dehydration and encourage granulation tissue formation.

Substitute grafts

There are three varieties:

- **Cultured allogeneic epidermal cells** that do not express HLA-DR antigens and are not 'contaminated' with Langerhans cells, the antigen-presenting cells (p. 173) of the epidermis.
- **Dermal tissue**. There are different forms. Allografted human cadaver skin, treated to remove antigenic cell elements, is one. A composite, collagen-based dermal lattice with an outer silicon covering, is another. A nylon mesh containing viable human fibroblasts with an outer Silastic (p. 280) layer has been used as a temporary covering.
- **A combination of epidermal and dermal tissue** comprising bovine type I collagen with live allogeneic human skin fibroblasts and epidermal cells.

IMPAIRED WOUND HEALING

The common causes of defective healing are infection; ischaemia; the presence of foreign materials such as road particles; the co-existence of malignant tumour cells; damage caused by chemicals or ionising radiation; and immunosuppression. Impaired wound healing may result from the inflammatory response at sites of sutures. The administration of corticosteroids may delay healing.

Wound infection

Small numbers of bacteria gain access to every surgical wound. Larger numbers invariably contaminate open wounds incurred by accident. Before the introduction of antiseptic surgery, the majority of incisions became infected and septicaemia and gangrene were common causes of death. Wounds may be infected by bacteria present within or on the patient (**endogenous infection**) or by bacteria introduced from the environment (**exogenous infection**). In **cross-infection**, there is bacterial spread from person to person, either from another patient, from hospital staff or from a visitor. The organisms that survive on the skin of the patient are likely to be staphylococci. The bacteria that gain access to wounds from endogenous, faecal sources include Bacteroides, Enterobacteria, Streptococcus, Enterococcus and Clostridia.

Now read Hospital acquired infection (p. 159)

Estimating infection

Whether overt clinical infection is likely to develop or not can be estimated clinically by the degree of bacterial contamination. It is relevant to relate the effects of this hazard to the rate of bacterial growth (p. 32). Four categories of contaminated wound are recognised:

- **Clean wounds**. These are incisions in patients in whom aseptic techniques have been observed; in whom a hollow, muscular organ has not been opened; and in whom no infection has been found.
- **Potentially contaminated wounds**. These are incisions for operations in which organs have been opened but in which contamination due to a failure of aseptic technique has not occurred.
- **Contaminated wounds**. In this category are traumatic wounds of less than 4 hours duration; surgical wounds following operations for acute inflammatory conditions without the formation of pus; and wounds in patients in whom there has been a failure of aseptic technique, for example inadvertent contamination during colectomy.
- **Dirty wounds**. These wounds include those that have been untreated for longer than 4 hours, and incisions in patients in whom a perforated viscus or pus is found at operation.

Clinical infection is likely in 2% of clean wounds, 10% of potentially contaminated wounds, 20% of contaminated wounds and 40% of dirty wounds. In surgical practice, the frequency of overt infection rises exponentially with the length of operation, probably because of increases in the extent both of tissue trauma and contamination. A haematoma is a fruitful site for bacterial multiplication. The frequency of infection also rises with the duration of pre-operative hospital stay since there is a growing opportunity for the skin to be colonised by pathogens. Many pathogens acquire resistance to the prophylactic antibiotics in common use in hospitals.

Systemic factors that predispose to wound infection include extreme youth or age; diabetes mellitus; malnutrition; and immunosuppression. Wound infection is unexpectedly frequent in the presence of jaundice.

Now read Hospital acquired infection (p. 159)

NEEDLE-STICK INJURY

The risk of transmission by needle-stick injury or other contaminated sharp instrument is much greater than exposure of broken epithelia to the same pathogens. To minimise this hazard, gloves are worn when staff are nursing patients considered to constitute a high risk. The hazard can also be reduced by employing blunt-tipped, suture needles.

The risk of becoming infected from a single exposure to blood from a patient carrying the HBe antigen of the hepatitis B virus (p. 152) may be as high as 30%. For hepatitis C (HVC), the risk is ~3%, for the human immunodeficiency virus (HIV) ~0.3%. Each hospital has its own protocol for such an injury. Injured staff are obliged to:

- Attend the Accident and Emergency Department immediately.
- Contact the Consultant Microbiologist or Occupational Health Officer.
- Complete an accident report form.

Prophylactic treatment should be started within 2 hours. Subsequent counselling enables the injured person and any known donor to be advised and tested for blood-borne virus.

Now read AIDS (p. 2), Hepatitis (p. 152)

X, Y & Z

XERODERMA PIGMENTOSUM

Xeroderma pigmentosum is a rare, heritable disorder in which an enzyme necessary for the repair of DNA is absent or deficient. The skin changes that result are exacerbated by sunlight. They are precancerous (p. 78).

YERSINIA

Yersinia pseudotuberculosis and *Y. enterocolitica* are environmental Gram-negative coccobacilli that may be transmitted by animals. In man, they can cause acute inflammation in the region of the terminal ileum, caecum (caecitis – typhlitis) and vermiform appendix. The acute inflammatory disease may mimic acute appendicitis (p. 345). A granulomatous lymphadenitis may develop that requires to be distinguished from Crohn's disease (pp. 104, 165) and tuberculosis (p. 332). The diagnosis of Yersinia infection can be made by detecting rising titres of anti-Yersinia serum antibodies, or by the isolation of the organisms from the lymph nodes or blood.

The inflammatory reaction usually resolves spontaneously but may be responsible for a characteristic form of postinfective arthropathy (p. 192) that is sometimes epidemic and that displays a predilection for the joints of the spine. It is a spondylo-arthropathy (p. 300).

ZOLLINGER–ELLISON SYNDROME

The Zollinger–Ellison syndrome is described on p. 121.

Copper	13–24	μmol/L
Creatinine	55–120	μmol/L
Fatty acids		
total	3.6–18	mmol/L
free, non-esterified	0.30–1.25	mmol/L
Gamma glutamyl transferase (GGT)	10–55 (male)	IU/L
	5–35 (female)	IU/L
Globulin	20–41	g/L
Glucose, fasting	3.6–5.8	mmol/L
Ketones	80–140	mmol/L
Immunoglobulin		
IgG	5–13	g/L
IgA	0.5–4.00	g/L
IgM	0.3–2.2 (male)	g/L
	0.4–2.5 (female)	g/L
Iron	14–32 (male)	μmol/L
	10–28 (female)	μmol/L
iron binding capacity	45–72	μmol/L
transferrin		
newborn	1.30–2.75	g/L
adult	2.20–4.00	g/L
transferrin saturation	20–50	per cent
Lactate	0.4–1.4	mmol/L
Lactate dehydrogenase (LDH)	230–460	IU/L
Magnesium	0.75–1.0	mmol/L
Phosphate (inorganic)	0.8–1.4	mmol/L
Phospholipid	1.25–3.2	g/L
Potassium[1] (serum)	3.6–5.1	mmol/L
Protein (total)	60–80	g/L
Pyruvate	34–103	μmol/L
Sodium	132–144	mmol/L
Triglycerides, fasting	0.6–1.7 (male)	mmol/L
	0.4–1.5 (female)	mmol/L
Urea	2.5–6.6	mmol/L
Zinc	11–22	μmol/L

[1] Levels often vary between plasma and serum.

CELLS AND OTHER CONSTITUENTS

Haemoglobin	130–180 (male)	g/L
	115–165 (female)	g/L
Red blood cells	4.5–6.5 (male)	$\times 10^{12}$/L
	3.8–5.8 (female)	$\times 10^{12}$/L
Mean corpuscular volume	76–100	fL
White blood cells (total)	4.0–11.0	$\times 10^{9}$/L
Neutrophils	2.0–7.5	$\times 10^{9}$/L
Lymphocytes	1.5–4.0	$\times 10^{9}$/L
Monocytes	0.2–0.8	$\times 10^{9}$/L
Eosinophils	0.04–0.4	$\times 10^{9}$/L
Basophils	0.01–0.1	$\times 10^{9}$/L
Platelets	150–350	$\times 10^{9}$/L
Fibrinogen	1.5–4.0	g/L
Fibrinogen degradation products (d-dimer)	<0.2	mg/L
Prothrombin time	8.0–10.5	sec
Erythrocyte sedimentation rate	0–10 (male)	mm/h
	3–15 (female)	mm/h

CEREBROSPINAL FLUID

Constituent	Value	Unit
Chloride	96–106	mmol/L
Glucose	2.5–4.0	mmol/L
Protein	100–400	mg/L
pH	7.31–7.34	
Cells	<6	$\times 10^{3}$/L

URINE

Constituent	Value	Unit
pH	4.6–8.0	
Sodium	100–200	mmol/24h
Potassium	25–100	mmol/24h
Phosphate	15–50	mmol/24h
Urea	170–600	mmol/24h
Creatinine	10–20 (male)	mmol/24h
	10–18 (female)	mmol/24h
Urate	1.2–3.0	mmol/24h
Oxalate	0.08–0.49 (male)	mmol/24h
	0.04–0.32 (female)	
Protein[1]	<0.3	g/L
Calcium[2]	<12	mmol/24 h
Amylase	1–17	IU/24h

[1] At rest. May be higher after severe exercise

[2] 1.2–3.7 mmol/24h on low calcium diet.

BRIEF BIOGRAPHIES OF SOME PIONEERS WHO LAID THE FOUNDATIONS OF SURGERY

Aschoff (Reticulo-endothelial system, p. 286)

Aschoff introduced the concept of a widely distributed system of phagocytic cells that were found in the bone marrow, spleen, liver and other vascular sites (*Münch. Med. Wschr.* 1922; 69;1352–6).

Karl Albert Ludwig Aschoff (1866–1942) was Professor of Pathology at Marburg and, later, at Freiburg im Breislau. He was the author of a well-known textbook, and contributed to understanding of appendicitis; jaundice and gall stones; renal sepsis; and thrombosis.

Banting and Best (Diabetes mellitus, p. 117)

The experimental removal of the pancreas provokes diabetes. The mechanism of this response became clear in 1922 when Banting and Best isolated insulin. They showed that, after ligation of the pancreatic duct, the acinar cells of the pancreas, but not those of the islets, soon atrophied. An extract of the degenerate gland contained a substance that caused glycosuria and hypoglycaemia (*Am. J. Physiol.* 1922; 59: 479). Eight months after the experiments began, clinical trials were started of the new anti-diabetogenic substance, insulin.

At the time of their discoveries, Frederick (later Sir Frederick) Grant Banting (1891–1941) was a demonstrator in physiology in the Department of Physiology of the University of Toronto. Charles Herbert Best (1899–1978) was a young graduate.

Barnard (Transplantation of the heart, p. 149)

Barnard completed the first successful transplantation of a human heart on December 3rd 1967 (*S. Afr. Med. J.* 1967; 41: 1271–4). Barnard's first patient, Louis Washkansky, survived only 18 days but his second patient, Dr Philip Blaiberg, lived long enough (583 days) to develop atheroma of the coronary arteries of the transplanted heart.

Christiaan Neethling Barnard (1922–2001) graduated from the University of Cape Town.

Barrett (Barrett's oesophagus, p. 254)

Barrett described the development of a metaplastic gastric epithelial lining of the oesophagus in response to persistent reflux (*Br. J. Surg.* 1950; 38: 175–82).

Norman Rupert Barrett (1903–1979) was a British thoracic surgeon and consultant to St Thomas's and the Brompton Hospitals.

Becquerel (Irradiation, p. 186)

Becquerel's name was given to the SI unit for the measurement of ionising radiation.

Antoine Henri Becquerel (1852–1908) discovered radioactivity (*Comptes Rend. Acad. Sci. (Paris)* 1896;122: 420–1). The discovery came in part from the accidental burn he received when he carried radium in his pocket.

Bennett (Leukaemia, p. 207)

In 1845, Bennett reported the case of a patient studied *post-mortem* in whom the gelatinous part of the coagulated blood resembled thick pus (*Edin. Med. Surg.* 1845; 64: 413–23). Microscopically, the coagulum contained many 'pus corpuscles' (neutrophil polymorphs). He called the disease 'leucocytaemia' but did not understand that the condition was a disorder of the blood itself. The essentially neoplastic nature of the disease, leukaemia, was recognised by Rudolph Virchow 6 weeks later.

John Hughes Bennett (1812–1875) was born in London. He graduated in Edinburgh and initiated an outstanding course of lectures on normal and pathological histology before becoming Professor of the

Institutes of Medicine of the University of Edinburgh in 1848.

Boerhaave (Spontaneous perforation of the oesophagus, p. 254)
Boerhaave established a hospital in Leiden and introduced the concept of bedside, clinical teaching.

Hermann Boerhaave (1668–1738) was educated for the Church but studied Medicine, Botany and Chemistry, holding Chairs in each subject. His reputation rests on *Institutiones Medicae* (1708), *Aphorismi de Cognoscendis et Curandis Morbis* (1709) and *Opera omnia medica* (1742).

Burkitt (Lymphoma, p. 224)
The African B-cell lymphoma recognised by Burkitt (*Br. J. Surg.* 1958–9, 59: 218–23) had apparently been described by the missionary Sir Albert Cook, in an unpublished report. The Epstein–Barr virus, with which the transmission of the tumour is associated, was identified soon afterwards (Epstein *et al.*, *Lancet* 1964;1:702–3).

Denis Burkitt (1911–1993) devoted his life to the study of geographical diseases. He became convinced that diet, rich in fibre, protected against both carcinoma of the colon and phlebothrombosis.

Calne (Liver transplantation, p. 214)
In 1968, Calne undertook the first successful liver transplant in Europe (*Br. Med. J.* 1968;630:262–5). He had previously begun an extensive programme of renal transplantation, benefiting from the introduction of azathioprine as an immunosuppressive drug. When cyclosporin became available through the work of Kostakis, immunosuppression was enhanced and the results of renal, hepatic and other forms of transplantation were greatly improved.

Sir Roy Calne (1930–) began research on organ transplantation in 1959, at the Royal College of Surgeons of England. He used 6-mercaptopurine for immunosuppression. He is Professor of Surgery at the University of Cambridge. He was Harkness Research Fellow at the Peter Bent Brigham Hospital, Harvard Medical School from 1960 to 1961 and it was there that his pioneering studies of organ transplantation first flourished.

Chagas (Chagas' disease, pp. 149, 254 and 282)
Chagas found flagellate trypanosomes, *T. cruzi*, in Reduvid bugs that bit inhabitants of the state of Minas Geraës of Brazil, transferring the organism to the human host (*Mem. Inst. Osw. Cruz.* 1909;1:159–218). Children were affected by anaemia and weakness, adults by mental defect, paralysis and disease of the oesophagus, colon and heart. Populations were particularly at risk when the natural, mammalian hosts had been dispersed by shrub and forest clearances.

Carlos Justiniano Ribiero Chagas (1879–1934) was awarded the Schaudinn prize in 1912 for his studies of protozoology and microbiology. He worked at the Oswaldo Cruz Institute, where he was Director from 1917 until 1934, and in 1925 became Professor of Tropical Medicine of the College of Medicine of Rio de Janeiro.

Chain (Antibiotics, p. 17)
Chain (1906–1979) shared the Nobel prize for Medicine with H.W. Florey and A. Fleming for their contributions to the discovery and exploitation of penicillin (Chain EB *et al. Lancet* 1940;2:226–8).

Ernst Boris Chain was born in Berlin. He graduated from the Friedrich-Wilhelm University in 1930. After 2 years in Cambridge, he was invited to Oxford in 1933. Following his pioneering studies in Oxford, he became Professor of Biochemistry at Imperial College, London in 1961.

Crohn (Crohn's disease, pp. 104, 165)
Crohn, with Ginzburg and Oppenheimer, described 'regional ileitis' (*J. Am. Med. Ass.* 1932; 99:1323–9). A similar condition had been reported by Combe and Sanders (1806), by Moynihan (1907) and by Dalziel (1913).

Burrill Bernard Crohn (1884–1984) was a minor contributor to the 1932 paper and was unhappy that his name should be given to the disease that is now eponymously associated with him.

Curie (Irradiation; radium, p. 185)
Working under conditions of great hardship in an outdoor shed in Paris, Marie and Pierre Curie isolated the radioactive substance polonium from Bavarian pitchblende (*Comptes Rend. Acad. Sci. (Paris)* 1898; 127: 175–8). Within a few months, they had extracted a second new radioactive element, radium (*Comptes Rend. Acad. Med. (Paris)* 1898; 127: 1215–17). Radium came to be used to treat cancer but was itself dangerously carcinogenic.

Marie Sklodowski (1867–1934) was Polish. She married Pierre Curie (1859–1906) in 1895. He was killed in a road accident in 1906 and Marie Curie succeeded to his position as Professor of Physics. She was awarded Nobel prizes for both physics and chemistry but died of aplastic anaemia in 1934.

Curling (Duodenal ulcer, p. 308)

Curling reported the association between burns and duodenal ulcer (*Medico Chir. Trans.* 1842; 25:260–81). In one typical case, a child, 11 years of age with no history of indigestion, sustained severe burns of the arms and chest and later died from profuse haematemesis. At autopsy, Curling found a half inch diameter ulcer 1 inch beyond the gastroduodenal junction.

Thomas Blizard Curling (1811–1888) was Consultant Surgeon to the London Hospital. He gave the first description of absence of the thyroid gland in cases of cretinism 20 years before Gull defined the features of myxoedema.

Cushing (Cushing's disease, p. 273; Cushing's syndrome, pp. 6, 126)

In his monograph *The Pituitary Body and its Disorders* (1912), Cushing described the first case of the syndrome that now bears his name. His concept that a tumour of the anterior pituitary gland was responsible for hyperadrenocorticalism could not be confirmed anatomically until 1932 (*Bull. Johns Hopk. Hosp.* 1932; 50: 137–95). By that time, Cushing was able to report the consecutive study of 2000 intracranial tumours (*Intracranial Tumours*, 1932).

Harvey Williams Cushing (1869–1939) was an internationally renowned neurosurgeon, Professor of Surgery at Harvard University, and the generous friend and colleague at the Johns Hopkins School of Medicine of the physician William Osler and, later, his biographer. Cushing's reports were often embellished with his sketches – like Charles Bell, he was an accomplished draughtsman and a masterly writer. He was also an eminent medical historian.

Dupuytren (Dupuytren's contracture, pp. 112, 131)

Dupuytren is now chiefly remembered for the description of an operation for the correction of the palmar fibrous contracture that is named after him (*J. Univ. Hebd. Méd. Chir. Pract.* 1832; 2 sér 15: 352–65) but he made many other important surgical advances. He classified burns, was the first surgeon to excise the mandible, amputate the uterine cervix for carcinoma, and ligate the subclavian and external iliac arteries.

Born a pauper, Baron Guillaume Dupuytren (1777–1835) became the leading French surgeon of his time. Self-opinionated, overbearing and mean, he was immensely hard-working and successful.

Fleming (Penicillin, p. 17)

Seven years after his discovery of lysozyme in tears and nasal secretions (*Proc. Roy. Soc. B* 1922;93:306–17), Fleming reported the antibacterial action of a mould, *Penicillium notatum*, on the growth of staphylococcal colonies (*Br. J. Exp. Path.* 1929;10:226–36). Fleming did not pursue his discovery to the point of isolating, characterising and testing the agent, penicillin, that was responsible for this phenomenon but he predicted its therapeutic value.

Alexander (later Sir Alexander) Fleming (1881–1955) was a Scot from Dumfriesshire with a liking for rifle shooting. He settled in London and worked at St. Mary's Hospital, Paddington.

Florey (Penicillin, p. 17)

Under conditions of war, Florey, Chain and their colleagues exploited Fleming's (1929) discovery of penicillin. They isolated the antibacterial substance, penicillin, and proved its efficacy as a chemotherapeutic agent (*Lancet* 1940; 2: 226–8). By 1942, a sufficient quantity of the antibiotic was available to allow war-wounded to be treated but it was not until bulk culture of the parent fungus was introduced in the USA that enough penicillin became available for the routine treatment of diseases such as cellulitis, septicaemia and meningitis.

Howard Walter (later Lord) Florey (1898–1968) was born and educated in Adelaide, Australia. His pioneering work on penicillin was undertaken in the Department of Pathology in Oxford. Florey, Chain and Fleming were awarded the Nobel prize, jointly, in 1945.

Gray (Irradiation (p. 186)

Gray demonstrated the increased sensitivity of tumour cells to X-rays when they are irradiated in a well-oxygenated environment (*Br. J. Radiol.* 1953;26:638–48). His name was given to the SI unit for the measurement of the dose of absorbed ionising radiation.

Louis Harold Gray, FRS, (1905–1965) worked in

the Cavendish Laboratory, Cambridge where he published his first paper in 1929 on *The absorption of penetrating radiation*. He became President of the British Institute of Radiology, and President of the 2nd International Congress of Radiation Research.

Halsted (Surgical gloves, p. 142)

Although it is possible that rubber gloves had been employed previously in surgery, Halsted certainly advocated their use (*Johns Hopkins Hospital Reports* 1891;2:308–10) and arranged for them to be made. However, the gloves were manufactured, not to prevent infection, but to protect the hands of an operating theatre nurse whose skin was sensitive to mercuric chloride.

William Stewart Halsted (1852–1922) was the first Professor of Surgery at the Johns Hopkins Medical School, Baltimore. Like Sigmund Freud and other famous physicians and surgeons of the time, Halsted was a cocaine addict – Osler was his doctor – but addiction did not prevent his success in the surgery of breast cancer and many other fields.

Hirschprung (Hirschprung's disease, p. 105)

Hirschprung's 1887 paper 'Constipation in the newborn due to dilatation and hypertrophy of the colon' provided the first full and clear account of this important paediatric disorder (*Jb Kinderheilk*. 1887–88; n.F, 27: 1–7). Treves later (1898) explained the obstruction on the basis of spasm of the hypertrophic, distal segment of the colon.

Harald Hirschprung (1830–1916) qualified in Copenhagen and became Senior Physician to the Children's Hospital of that city.

Hodgkin (Hodgkin's lymphoma, p. 223)

Hodgkin presented his historic paper entitled 'On some morbid appearances of the absorbent glands and spleen' to the Medical and Chirurgical Society, London (*Med-Chir. Trans.* 1832; 17: 68–114). Re-examination of the original tissues cast doubt on the correctness of the microscopic diagnosis in several of Hodgkin's own cases but the concept of Hodgkin's lymphoma became established when Samuel Wilks in 1866 added further cases and introduced the designation 'Hodgkin's disease'.

Thomas Hodgkin (1798–1866) was an Edinburgh graduate and a Quaker. He became Curator of the Pathological Museum of Guy's Hospital but failed to be appointed to the staff of the hospital, abandoned medical practice and died of dysentery in Jaffa.

Jenner (Vaccination, p. 343)

In an account of one of the most important discoveries in the history of medicine (*An enquiry into the causes and effects of the variolae vaccinae*. London: S. Low, 1798), Jenner described how he had been able to protect individuals against smallpox by inoculating them with lymph from the lesions of cowpox (vaccinia). His revolutionary method superceded the practice of inoculating fluid from smallpox lesions themselves.

Edward (later Sir Edward) Jenner (1749–1823) was a country practitioner in Gloucestershire. Before making his crucial experiment, he considered for many years the comment of a milkmaid who told him the she could not take smallpox because she had had cowpox.

Kaposi (AIDS, p. 2; Kaposi's sarcoma, p. 49)

Kaposi reported his multiple idiopathic haemorrhagic sarcoma in 1872 (*Arch. Derm. Syph. (Prag.)* 1872;4:265–73). In Virchow's *Handbuch der speziellen Pathologie und Therapie* 1876, 2:182, he described xeroderma pigmentosum.

Moritz Kaposi (1837–1902) was a Hungarian dermatologist who became Professor of Dermatology of the University of Vienna. Among his works were *Handbook of Diseases of the Skin* (1872) and *Pathology and Treatment of Syphilis* (1872).

Kelling (Laparoscopy, p. 269)

Minimally invasive surgery became possible with the advent of laparoscopic cholecystectomy. Gynaecologists had induced pneumoperitoneum with CO_2 gas as a means of effecting laparoscopy. The inspiration for this procedure was the work of Kelling (*Münch. Med. Wschr.* 1902; 49: 21–4) who proposed endoscopy as a means of understanding disease and used a cystoscope to produce pneumoperitoneum in an experimental animal.

Georg Kelling (1866–1945) was a German surgeon whose work centred on Dresden. He had studied medical science in Leipzig with the eminent Georg Ludwig. Attempting to control intra-abdominal bleeding, he invented *lufttamponade*, a procedure for high-pressure insufflation.

Koch (Koch's postulates, p. 202; tuberculosis, p. 332)
During 10 years of patient research conducted in his own home, Koch resolved the problem of how to grow bacteria in culture. He was able to show (*Beitr. Biol. Pflanzen* 1876; 2: 277–310) that a single disease, anthrax, was caused by a single bacterial genus, the organism now called *Bacillus anthracis*. Later, Koch reported his discovery of *Mycobacterium tuberculosis* (*Berl. Klin. Wschr.* 1882;19:221–30).

Robert Koch (1843–1910) was at first a general practitioner in Niemegk and Rakwitz, later an army surgeon and finally Director of the Institute for Infectious Diseases in Berlin. He investigated cholera in Egypt and discovered *Vibrio cholerae* in 1883.

Krukenberg (Krukenburg's tumour, pp. 247, 260)
Krukenberg described intra-abdominal secondary tumours of the ovaries in a thesis published when he was only 25 (*Arch. Gynäk.* 1896; 50: 287–321).

Friedrich Ernst Krukenberg (1870–1946) was Professor of Ophthalmology at Halle.

Langerhans (Diabetes mellitus, p. 117)
Langerhans described the pancreatic islets in 1869 in an inaugural dissertation (*Beiträge zur mikroskopischen Anatomie der Bauchspeicheldrüsen* (*Communication on the Microscopic Anatomy of the Pancreas*) Berlin: G. Lange, 1869). The work, conducted on fresh rabbit tissue, followed injection of the pancreatic duct with glycerine and the dye Berlin blue. In 1893, Laguesse proposed that the islets might be the source of an internal secretion and named them the 'islets of Langerhans'.

Paul Langerhans (1847–1888) was a pupil of Rudolph Virchow who was a friend of his family. Langerhans survived the Franco-Prussian war but died of pulmonary tuberculosis at the early age of 41.

Langhans (Tuberculosis, p. 333)
Langhans noted the presence of giant cells in lymphadenoma (Hodgkin's lymphoma) (*Virch. Arch. Path. Anat.* 1872; 54: 509–37) and described the multinucleated giant cells of tuberculosis. He also drew attention to the giant cells of the cytotrophoblast (*Arch. Gynäk.* 1870;1:317–34).

Born in 1839, Theodor Langhans died in 1915.

Lewis (Inflammation, p. 179)
In *Heart* (1924;11:209–65), and in *Studies of the Blood Vessels of the Human Skin and Their Responses* (1927), Lewis suggested that a histamine-like substance (H-substance) was responsible for the skin changes in anaphylaxis.

Thomas (later Sir Thomas) Lewis (1881–1945) was a distinguished London cardiologist. He was a pioneer of electrocardiography and a well-known advocate of the string galvanometer (*The Mechanism and Graphic Registration of the Heart Beat*, 1920). Lewis's book *Pain* appeared in 1942.

Lister (Antisepsis, p. 23, 159)
Lister revolutionised the entire practice of surgery when he reported his successful adoption of the methods of antisepsis (*Lancet* 1867; 1: 326–9; 357–9; 387–9; 507–9; 2: 95–6; 353–6; 668–9). Until that time, the average mortality from civilian surgical operations was at least 25% and from military surgery 80%. Lister's demonstration of the value of carbolic acid dressings and a carbolic acid spray showed that, with their use, operative mortality from sepsis could be reduced twenty-fold. The success of his work rested on meticulous experiments, many conducted in his own home, over a 40-year period.

Joseph (later Lord) Lister (1827–1912) came from a Yorkshire, Quaker family. Educated in London, he worked for 7 years in Edinburgh and married the daughter of Professor James Syme. Appointed Regius Professor of Clinical Surgery in Glasgow at the age of 33, Lister returned to Edinburgh in 1868 and to London, his birthplace, in 1877.

Mallory (Mallory–Weiss syndrome, p. 309)
Mallory and Weiss described the syndrome of gastric rupture with which their names are now eponymously associated (*Am. J. Med. Sci.* 1929; 178; 506–15).

G.K. Mallory (1900–) was Assistant in Pathology at the Boston City Hospital.

Soma Weiss (1899–1942) was appointed in 1939 as Hersey Professor of the Theory and Practice of Physic at Harvard, and Chief of Medicine at the Peter Bent Brigham Hospital. He was a noted clinical teacher.

Meckel (Meckel's diverticulum, p. 164)
The younger Meckel, one of the greatest comparative anatomists, is remembered not only for his accounts of intestinal diverticula (*Arch. Physiol. Halle* 1809; 9:

421–53) but also for his description of Meckel's cartilage, the first branchial cartilage.

Johann Friedrich Meckel (1781–1833), 'Meckel the Younger', graduated from Halle and succeeded his father as Professor of Anatomy in 1808.

Meigs (Meigs' syndrome, p. 261)

Meigs and Cass described ascites in association with ovarian fibroma (*Am. J. Obstet. Gynek.* 1937; 33: 249–67).

J.V. Meigs (1892–1963) was Professor of Gynecology at Harvard University Medical School.

Meleney (Necrotising fasciitis, p. 137)

Necrotising fasciitis represents a spectrum of fulminant disease, including Fournier's gangrene and Meleney's synergistic gangrene. Fournier developed the concept of a spreading gangrene of the scrotum (*Sem. Med.* 1883;56: 345). Meleney (*Arch. Surg.* 1924;9:317–64) described a 'Haemolytic streptococcus gangrene'. The term 'necrotising fasciitis' was introduced by B. Wilson (*Am. Surgeon* 1952; 18: 416–31).

J.A. Fournier (1832–1915) was an eminent French syphilologist and Director of the Saint Louis Hospital, Paris.

Frank L. Meleney (1889–1963) pioneered bacteriology in surgery. He was Professor of Surgery at the Presbyterian Hospital, New York, and Head of the Laboratory for bacteriological research.

Mendel (Genes, p. 138; Inheritance, p. 182)

Mendel's painstaking studies of the mathematical basis of the inherited characteristics of peas attracted no interest during his lifetime (*Verh. naturf. Vereines Brünn* 1866;4:3–47). Rediscovered in 1900, his work is now seen as a cornerstone of modern genetics.

Gregor Johann Mendel (1822–1884) was a highly educated monk who lived in the monastery in Brno. English translations of his work were published in 1909 and 1965.

Moynihan (Calculus, p. 75; Peptic ulcer, pp. 121, 308)

Moynihan made pioneering advances in gastrointestinal surgery (*Diseases of the Stomach and their Surgical Treatment*, 1901), introducing the concept of 'hunger pain' in peptic ulcer (*Duodenal Ulcer*, 1910). He suggested that 'a gallstone is a tombstone to the memory of the germ which lies within it'.

Berkeley George Andrew Moynihan (1865–1936), first Baron Moynihan of Leeds and President of the Royal College of Surgeons of England, was the son of a soldier awarded the VC in the Crimean War of 1854. Moynihan became Professor of Surgery at the University of Leeds, where he married the daughter of his predecessor, Professor Jessop. He founded the *British Journal of Surgery*.

Paget (Paget's disease of bone, p. 51; Paget's disease of the breast, p. 68)

Paget described the skin changes of intraduct carcinoma of the breast, Paget's disease of the nipple (*St. Barth. Hosp. Rep.* 1874;10:87–9) and osteitis deformans, Paget's disease of bone (*Med.–Chir. Trans.* 1877;60:37–44), adding further cases in 1882.

Sir James Paget, Bart (1814–1899) was a keen observer. He had identified the worm *Trichinella spiralis* in muscle that he was dissecting as a first-year student. He was also a fine surgical pathologist. Paget was a Curator of the Museum of St. Bartholomew's Hospital; he was elected President of the Royal College of Surgeons of England and became Surgeon to Queen Victoria.

Paré (Antisepsis, p. 23)

At least until the Napoleonic wars, it was the practice to apply boiling oil or hot tar to the ends of amputated limbs. In the course of his work as a military surgeon during the attack on Turin (1537), Paré's supply of oil was exhausted and he discovered that a mild dressing made with eggs, oil of roses and turpentine was better tolerated and much more effective. An alternative was a balm made by boiling together, in turpentine, oil of lilies, young whelps and earthworms.

Ambroise Paré (1510–1590) became the greatest surgeon of the Renaissance period. He was wise, humane, scholarly and skilful and is often portrayed as a model for all surgeons. His Turin experiences were described in his journal *Voyages faits en divers lieux*.

Pasteur (Disinfection, p. 119)

Pasteur founded the science of microbiology. A brilliant publicist, he demonstrated the staphylococcal cause of boils and the streptococcal origin of puerperal sepsis (*Bull. Acad. Med. (Paris)* 2 sér 1879;8:505–8. Later, he successfully protected sheep against virulent anthrax and devised a vaccine for the prophylactic treatment of patients bitten by rabid wolves or dogs (*Comptes Rendu Acad. Sci. (Paris)* 1885;101:765–74).

Born in Dole in the Jura, Louis Pasteur (1822–1895) was educated in Besançon and Paris. He was appointed Professor of Physics in Dijon in 1848, making fundamental studies of crystals before becoming Professor of Chemistry at Lille in 1854. His investigations of fermentation led to proof that micro-organisms do not multiply by spontaneous generation (*Ann. Sci. Nat. Zool. (Paris)* 1861;16:5–98). They also enabled him to make recommendations that saved the wine industry and rescued silk worms from a destructive parasitic disease. Some of Pasteur's greatest work was completed during the years after he had suffered a stroke and partial left hemiplegia.

Plummer (Plummer–Vinson syndrome (p. 257)

Plummer described cardiospasm (*J. Am. Med. Ass.* 1912;58:2013–5). Independently, Vinson described case of cardiospasm with dilatation and angulation of the oesophagus (*Medical Clinics of North America* 1919;3:623–7). In the same year, A. Brown Kelly (*J. Otolaryngol* 1919;34:285–9) and D.R. Paterson (*J. Layrnyngol.* 1919;34:289–91) drew attention to the same syndrome.

Porter Paisley Vinson (1890–1959) was an American surgeon, Henry Stanley Plummer (1874–1937) an American physician. In 1924, Plummer advocated the pre-operative administration of iodine in cases of toxic goitre. Adam Brown Kelly (1865–1941) was an eminent otolaryngologist appointed to the Victoria Infirmary of Glasgow in 1892.

Pott (Tuberculosis of the spine, p. 54; Occupational cancer, p. 80)

Pott described occupational cancer in 1775 in *'Chirurgical observations relative to the cataract, the polypus of the nose, the cancer of the scrotum, etc.'*.

Percival Pott (1714–1788) survived a compound fracture of the tibia without amputation in 1758. The injury was not a 'Pott's fracture'. During his convalescence, he wrote his book on Hernia. In 1769, he published his book on fractures and dislocations. Later, he described spinal curvature due to tuberculosis osteitis in *Remarks on that kind of palsy of the lower limbs, which is frequently found to accompany a curvature of the spine* (1779).

Raynaud (Raynaud's phenomenon, p. 284)

Raynaud achieved lasting fame through his 1862 doctoral thesis *De l'asphyxie locale et de la gangrène symetrique des extemitiés* (Local asphyxia and symmetrical gangrene of the extremities). Characteristic of his 25 case reports was the description of a young woman who, under the influence of very moderate cold and even at the height of summer, saw her fingers become ex-sanguine, completely insensible, and of a whitish-yellow colour, a phenomenon lasting a variable time and terminating by a period of very painful reaction.

Maurice Raynaud (1834–1881), a Paris graduate and French physician, was greatly revered but never attained a high academic appointment, even in the field he liked most, medical history. He died suddenly after suffering for some years from cardiac disease.

Röntgen (Irradiation – X rays, Table 36, p. 185)

Röntgen began his experiments with cathode-ray tubes in June 1894 and discovered that a high-voltage current passed through such a tube caused emissions which penetrated the bones of Frau Röntgen's hand, a large book, and wood blocks. The emissions, which he called 'rays', were visualised on a screen painted with barium platinocyanide. A translation of his 1895 report in *S. B. phys.-med. Ges. Würtzburg* was quickly published in English (*Nature* 1896;53:274–27). It was not long before the damaging effects of the X-rays were recognised, and, within a few years, radiation-induced cancers were reported. The name Roentgen as a unit of radiation was adopted in 1928 in his honour.

After a controversial youth during which he was refused entry by the University of Utrecht, Wilhelm Konrad Röntgen (1845–1923) graduated in Zurich. He held a series of senior academic appointments before returning to Würtzburg in 1888 to become Professor of Physics.

Rous (Viral causes of cancer, p. 80)

In 1908, Henry Wade investigated a transmissible sarcoma of the dog but was unable to isolate the agent (*J. Path. Bacteriol.* 1908;12:384–425). Shortly afterwards, Rous successfully isolated a transmissible agent from a fowl sarcoma (*J. Exp. Med.* 1910;12:696–705; 13:397–411).

Francis Peyton Rous (1879–1970) had joined the staff of the Rockefeller Institute, New York only a short time before starting his epoch-making experiments. At the age of 87, he was awarded the Nobel prize jointly with Charles Huggins. Huggins had successfully pioneered the use of the synthetic oestrogen, stilboestrol, for the treatment of cancer of the prostate gland.

Schaumann (Sarcoidosis, p. 289)

Schaumann described the systemic nature of sarcoidosis (Boeck's sarcoid – Besnier–Boeck–Schaumann disease). He recognised cytoplasmic inclusion bodies in the giant cells of granulomatous conditions such as sarcoidosis and berylliosis (*Ann. Derm. Syph. (Paris)* 1917;5 sér., 6:357–73).

Jörgen Nilsen Schaumann (1879–1953) was a Swedish dermatologist.

Schwann (Schwannoma, p. 250)

Schwann's name is associated with neurilemmoma because it was given to the perineuronal, so-called Schwann cell from which this tumour is thought to arise.

Theodor Schwann (1810–1882) identified the nucleus as part of a 'cell' but mistook its origin (*Mikroskopischen Untersuchungen über die Uebereinstimmung in der Struktur und dem Wachstum der Thiere und Pflanzen.* Berlin: Sander, 1839). He was a friend of the botanist, Matthias Jacob Schleiden with whom he discussed tissue structure. He concluded that even complex animal tissues developed only from cells. Although he referred to Schleiden's work on plants, neither understood that new cells form only by division. Schwann subsequently became Professor of Anatomy at Louvain and at Liège. He proved that putrefaction is caused by living bodies (1837); that gastric juice contains pepsin (1836); and that bile is indispensable for digestion (1850).

Semmelweiss (Antisepsis, p. 23)

Semmelweiss made unique epidemiological studies on puerperal sepsis in the years 1841–1846. He showed that, depending on whether pregnant women were attended by students and doctors, on the one hand, or by midwives, on the other, the maternal mortality varied five-fold. Students were encouraged to take part in autopsy studies and did not wash their hands before entering the wards; midwives were forbidden to attend the autopsy room. These observations, made 20 years before Lister's observations on surgical sepsis, were controversial but the statistical analyses recorded in detail in his epoch-making (1861) book *Die Aetiologie, der Begriff und der Prophylaxis des Kindbettfiebers* (The Aetiology, Concept and Prophylaxis of Childbed Fever) were incontrovertible.

Ignaz Phillipp Semmelweiss (1818–1865), born in Buda and Magyar by birth, graduated in Vienna. Sadly, he developed a mental illness and died from cellulitis and septicaemia contracted during an autopsy.

Sievert (Irradiation, p. 185)

Sievert developed important techniques for measuring the dose of ionising radiation absorbed by tumours and invented the Sievert chamber. He studied the effects of unavoidable, background radiation, anticipating the harmful effects of radioactive fallout. The Sv, the sievert, was accepted in 1979 as the international unit for expressing the dose equivalent for ionising radiation. and the influences of radiation on radiologists.

Rolf Maximilian Sievert (1898–1966) was the first Professor of Medical Radiation Physics at the Karolinska Hospital, Stockholm. He held the chair from 1941 until 1965.

Sipple (MEN 2A – Sipple syndrome, p. 127)

Sipple described the concurrence of medullary carcinoma of the thyroid and phaeochromocytoma, occasionally with parathyroid adenoma, neurofibromas, diabetes and diarrhoea (*Am. J. Med.* 1961;31:163–6). It is the multiple endocrine neoplasia syndrome 2A and is inherited as a Mendelian dominant characteristic.

J. H. Sipple (1930–) is an American respiratory physician. He was born in Cleveland, Ohio and became Professor of Medicine at the State University of New York Medical Centre in 1977.

Treves (Appendicectomy, p. 346)

Treves advocated the surgical treatment of acute appendicitis in a subacute or chronic phase, after the immediate period of acute inflammation had subsided. He published his book on *Intestinal Obstruction* on 1884 and achieved notoriety with the successful appendicectomy he performed upon King Edward VII shortly before the 1902 London Coronation.

Frederick (later Sir Frederick) Treves (1853–1923) was Surgeon to the London Hospital where he became known for his interest in and description of the Elephant Man, John Merrick, who suffered from generalised neurofibromatosis.

Virchow (Amyloid, p. 9; leukaemia, p. 207; thrombosis, p. 320)

Virchow defined amyloid, thrombus and leukaemia. Following the work of Schleiden, Schwann, and many others, he argued that, just as the cell is the unit of normal structure and function, so it is the unit of disease.

Rudolf Ludwig Karl Virchow (1821–1902), author of *Cellular Pathology* (1858) and the 'father' of modern pathology, was Professor of Pathology in Würtzburg and Berlin. In a life of unending and brilliantly rapid work, Virchow published more than 2000 papers or cases, edited 169 volumes of the Archives he had founded at the age of 26 with Reinhardt, undertook much palaeopathological research, including studies with Schliemann at Troy, and became Leader of the Opposition in the German Parliament when Bismarck was Chancellor.

von Recklinghausen (Osteitis fibrosa cystica, p. 51; hyperparathyroidism, p. 267; neurofibromatosis, p. 250)

Von Recklinghausen is remembered for his beautifully illustrated accounts of generalised osteitis fibrosa cystica (1891) in which, however, he failed to distinguish the bone changes from those of polyostotic fibrous dysplasia (*Die fibröse oder deformirende ostitis, die Osteomalacie und die osteoplastische Carcinose in ihren gegenseitigen Beziehungen.* In: Festschrift R. Virchow Berlin; G. Reimer, 1891). He is also known for his description of neurofibromatosis (*Ueber der multiplen Fibrome der Haut und ihre Beziehung zu den multiplen Neuromen* Berlin: Hirschwald, 1882). Both conditions are still often designated 'von Recklinghausen's disease'. Von Recklinghausen gave haemochromatosis its present name.

Friedrich Daniel von Recklinghausen (1833–1910) was born in Gütersloh, Westphalia. He studied under Virchow and became Professor of Pathology, first at Königsberg, then at Wurtzbürg and finally at Strasbourg.

Wermer (MEN 1–Wermer syndrome, p. 126)

Wermer described the coexistence of multiple adenomas of the endocrine glands, in particular of the parathyroid, pancreas, anterior pituitary and adrenals (*Am. J. Med.* 1954;16:363–71). The condition constitutes the multiple endocrine adenomatosis syndrome (MEN 1).

P. Wermer was an American physician in the Department of Medicine of Columbia University, Presbyterian Hospital, New York.

Wilms (Wilms' tumour, p. 200)

Wilms greatly clarified understanding of mixed tumours in his 1899 book *Mischgeschwülste, I. Die Mischgeschwülste der Niere.*

Max Wilms, born in Aachen, was a graduate of Bonn, becoming Professor of Surgery at Basel in 1907 and at Heidelberg in 1910. He was the editor of a famous Textbook of Surgery.

Zollinger (Zollinger–Ellison syndrome (p. 266)

The names of Zollinger and Ellison are given eponymously to a syndrome in which primary peptic ulcerations of the duodenum were found to be associated with islet cell tumors of the pancreas (*Ann. Surg.* 1955;142:709–28).

Robert Milton Zollinger (1903–) was Chairman of the Department of Surgery of Ohio State University, USA. He became President of the American College of Surgeons. Edwin Homer Ellison (1918–1970) became Professor of Surgery at Ohio State University, USA, in 1957.

FURTHER READING

Biochemistry

Williams DL, Marks, V. *Scientific Foundations of Biochemistry in Clinical Practice,* 2nd edition. Oxford: Butterworth-Heinemann, 1994.

Mayne, PD. *Clinical Chemistry in Diagnosis and Treatment,* 6th edition. London: Arnold, 1994.

Cancer

Franks LM, Teich NM. *Introduction to the Cellular and Molecular Biology of Cancer*, 3rd edition. Oxford: Oxford University Press, 1998.

Hermanek P, Hutter RVP, Sobin LH, Wagner G, Wittekind CH. *TNM Atlas: Illustrated Guide to the TNM/pTNM Classification of Malignant Tumours*, 4th edition, corrected second printing. Berlin, Heidelberg, New York: Springer-Verlag, 1999.

Basic surgical training

Forsling ML, Briggs T, Dickinson A, Turner Gareth. *FRCS MCQ Practice Exams in Applied Basic Sciences.* Knutsford: Pasttest, 1995.

Self-assessment MCQs for the AFRCSED in Surgery in General Edinburgh: the Royal College of Surgeons of Edinburgh, 1998.

SELECT. The Royal College of Surgeons of Edinburgh Educational Programme for the MRCS Examination. Edinburgh: The Royal College of Surgeons of Edinburgh, 2000.

STEP – MRCS Distance Learning Course. Surgeons in Training Education Programme for Membership of the Royal College of Surgeons of England, 2000.

Genetics

Bonthron DT, FitzPatrick DR, Porteous Mary EM, Trainer Alison H. *Clinical Genetics: A Case-Based Approach.* London, Philadelphia: WB Saunders, 1998.

Immunology

Lydyard, PM, Whelan, A, Fanger MW. *Instant Notes in Immunology.* Oxford: BIOS Scientific Publishers Limited, 2000.

Playfair JHL *Immunology at a Glance.* Oxford, London, Edinburgh: Blackwell Science Ltd, 1996.

Internet

Bride, M. *Teach Yourself the Internet.* London: Hodder & Stoughton, 2001.

Kiley R. *The Doctor's Internet Handbook.* London: Royal Society of Medicine Press Ltd, 2000.

Microbiology

Mims C, Playfair J, Roitt, I, Wakelin D, Williams R. *Medical Microbiology*, 2nd edition. London Philadelphia: Mosby, 1998.

Pathology

Cotran RS, Kumar V, Collins T. *Robins Pathologic Basis of Disease*, 6th edition. Philadelphia, London, Toronto: WB Saunders Company, 1999.

Kumar V, Cotran RS, Robbins SL. *Basic Pathology*, 6th edition. Philadelphia, London: WB Saunders Company, 1997.

Underwood JCE. *General and Systemic Pathology.* 3rd edition. Edinburgh, London: Churchill Livingstone 2000

Walter JB, Talbot, IC. *Walter and Israel General Pathology*, 7th edition. New York, Edinburgh, London: Churchill Livingstone, 1996.

Statistics

Brown RA, Swanson Beck J. *Medical Statistics on Personal Computers. A Guide to the Use of Statistical Packages*, 2nd edition. London: BMJ Publishing group, 1994.

Campbell MJ, Machin D. *Medical Statistics. A Commonsense Approach*, 3rd edition. Chichester: John Wiley & Sons Ltd, 1999.

Surgery

Deitch, EA. *Tools of the Trade and Rules of the Road. A Surgical Guide.* Philadelphia, New York: Lippincott-Raven, 1997.

Burnand KG, Young AE, editors. *The New Aird's Companion to Surgical Studies*, 2nd edition. Edinburgh, London, New York: Churchill Livingstone, 1998.

INDEX